THE NEUROBIOLOGY OF DRUG
AND ALCOHOL ADDICTION

ANNALS OF THE NEW YORK ACADEMY OF SCIENCES
Volume 654

THE NEUROBIOLOGY OF DRUG AND ALCOHOL ADDICTION

Edited by Peter W. Kalivas and Herman H. Samson

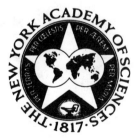

The New York Academy of Sciences
New York, New York
1992

Library of Congress Cataloging-in-Publication Data

The Neurobiology of drug and alcohol addiction / edited by Peter W. Kalivas and Herman H. Samson.
    p.   cm. – (Annals of the New York Academy of Sciences, ISSN 0077-8923 ; v. 654)
    Includes bibliographical references and index.
    ISBN 0-89766-711-5 (cloth : alk. paper). – ISBN 0-89766-712-3 (paper : alk. paper)
    1. Drug abuse–Physiological aspects–Congresses. 2. Alcoholism–Physiological aspects–Congresses. 3. Neuropsychopharmacology–Congresses. I. Kalivas, Peter W., 1952– . II. Samson, Herman H. III. Series.
    [DNLM: 1. Neurobiology–congresses. 2. Substance Abuse–genetics–congresses. 3. Substance Abuse–therapy–congresses. W1 AN626YL v. 654]
    Q11.N5 vol. 654
    [RC563.2]
    500 s–dc20
    [616.86′07]
    DNLM/DLC
for Library of Congress   92-18792
                                      CIP

CCP
Printed in the United States of America
ISBN 0-89766-711-5 (cloth)
ISBN 0-89766-712-3 (paper)
ISSN 0077-8923

ANNALS OF THE NEW YORK ACADEMY OF SCIENCES

Volume 654
June 28, 1992

THE NEUROBIOLOGY OF DRUG AND ALCOHOL ADDICTION[a]

Editors and Conference Organizers
PETER W. KALIVAS and HERMAN H. SAMSON

CONTENTS

[a] This volume is the result of a conference entitled **The Neurobiology of Drug and Alcohol Addiction** held by The New York Academy of Sciences on July 23–26, 1991 in Spokane, Washington.

Financial assistance was received from:

Major Funders

• University of Washington
• Washington State University

Supporter

• National Institute on Alcohol Abuse and Alcoholism/NIH

Contributors

• DuPont/Medical Products Department
• Johnson & Johnson Consumer Products, Inc.
• R.W. Johnson Pharmaceutical Research Institute
• Merck Sharp & Dohme Research Laboratories
• Pfizer Central Research
• Syntex Research
• The Upjohn Company

Foreword

The understanding of the neurobiology of drug and alcohol abuse has progressed rapidly over the last decade. Much of this advancement has been parallel to the development of the neurosciences in general. But in some cases, the study of the mechanisms of substance abuse has led the way towards the development of general principles of brain function. As demonstrated by the diversity of papers in this volume, the levels of analysis of the neurobiology of alcohol and substance abuse spans the range from molecular biology to clinical treatment. A major goal of the meeting which generated the papers of this volume was to foster a cross-level interaction between substance abuse researchers which would further our understanding of substance abuse and provide direction for future studies.

The meeting was organized to begin at the molecular level and progress through each level of analysis, ending with the current clinical perspectives of treatment—which is the basic organization of this book. The section on molecular mechanisms examines the current knowledge of various receptor and transduction mechanisms related to alcohol and other drugs of abuse. The concepts of sensitization following repeated exposure to drugs covered in the next section span the molecular, anatomical, and behavioral levels of analysis. The section on reinforcement of drugs links the molecular with the anatomical, with more emphasis on the neural circuitry involved with drug self-administration. The genetics and clinical neurobiology section provides a bridge between the molecular and behavioral levels, with emphasis on the role of genetics in drug action. The final sessions examined the behavioral levels of conditioning and their potential implication for treatment. While immediate application of the information presented at this meeting to drug and alcohol abuse treatment was not a primary goal, it was hoped that the interaction among the various disciplines would stimulate the translation of this basic knowledge into new and more effective treatment protocols.

PETER W. KALIVAS
HERMAN H. SAMSON

Acknowledgments

We wish to thank Jenny Baylon for her help in organizing the meeting and keeping the correspondence moving. We also wish to thank the New York Academy of Sciences and Renée Wilkerson in particular for an outstanding job of overcoming various organizational difficulties and natural disasters. Also, Joyce Hitchcock did an excellent job in efficiently organizing the production of the *Annal*, and we are grateful to David Soifer for helpful comments on the composition of the program and on white water rafting. Finally, we want to thank the session chairs who sparked lively conversation and maintained a smooth and stimulating exchange of ideas.

PETER W. KALIVAS
HERMAN H. SAMSON

Cellular Actions of Opiates and Cocaine

R. ALAN NORTH

Vollum Institute for Advanced Biomedical Research
Oregon Health Sciences University
3181 S.W. Sam Jackson Park Road
Portland, Oregon 97201

INTRODUCTION

The mesolimbic dopamine system has been increasingly implicated in the reinforcing actions of opiates and cocaine, implying that neurons within this system should be directly affected by these drugs.[1-5] Such direct actions have been studied by removing tissue slices containing parts of the ventral tegmental area and nucleus accumbens, and measuring the actions of the drugs by electrophysiological methods. The neurons from which the recordings are made can be identified, either histologically or by their unique membrane electrical properties. Two kinds of information have been sought. First, intracellular recording of membrane potential or current allows any direct actions of the drugs on the ion channels of the neuron to be assessed. Second, intracellular recording of synaptic potentials gives a sensitive measure of drug action on the neurons that provide synaptic inputs to the region.

VENTRAL TEGMENTAL AREA

The ventral tegmental area and medial part of the zona compacta contain the cell bodies of the mesolimbic system. Intracellular recording from these cells *in vitro* distinguishes two types of neuron; about 85% of cells (termed principal neurons) correspond to the dopamine-containing cells and about 15% of cells (secondary neurons) are believed to correspond to cells that do not contain dopamine.[6-10]

Opiates

Several drugs of abuse have the common action of increasing the extracellular dopamine levels in the nucleus accumbens,[5] implying that they increase the frequency of firing of midbrain dopamine neurons. Extracellular recordings *in vivo* show such an excitation.[11,12] However, μ-opioid receptors in the ventral tegmental area are not located on the dopamine cells themselves, because their number is unaltered by destruction of most of the dopamine-containing neurons.[13] This suggests the hypothesis that opiates excite the dopamine-containing neurons indirectly, by inhibiting another class of cell that provided an ongoing synaptic input to the dopamine cell.

1

Recent experiments with intracellular recording have sought to identify this other class of cell. The dopamine-containing cells are unaffected by opioids, but secondary neurons within the VTA are hyperpolarized.[8,9,14] Conversely, principal cells but not secondary cells are hyperpolarized by dopamine, acting through D_2 receptors. The hyperpolarization by opioids results from an increase in membrane conductance to potassium ions, as has been observed for opioids in many other mammalian neurons.[14-16] Opioids hyperpolarize the secondary cells by acting at μ receptors.[8,9]

Further studies indicate that the secondary cells which are hyperpolarized are local γ-aminobutyric acid (GABA)-containing interneurons that provide inhibitory synaptic input to the principal cells.[17] In the intact animal, this inhibition is thought to be continually active, perhaps because of excitatory afferents to the interneurons originating in the cortex. In the tissue slice, the GABA-mediated synaptic potentials are recorded in the principal (dopamine) cells only when the secondary neurons are depolarized to fire action potentials (e.g., by a small increase in the extracellular potassium concentration). The synaptic potentials are prevented by μ-selective opioids, suggesting that the hyperpolarization of the secondary cells prevents action potential discharge.[17] As a consequence, the principal (dopamine-containing) cells are excited.[17]

Thus, intracellular recording in vitro indicates that dopamine cells are excited by μ-selective opioids because they inhibit local circuit interneurons. A similar explanation was previously proposed to account for the excitation of hippocampal pyramidal cells by opioids; they inhibit a set of local inhibitory interneurons.[18-20] Further experiments will be necessary to clarify the strength and number of the synaptic connections between secondary neurons and principal cells; this can be approached in the brain slice by recording from pairs of synaptically connected neurons.

Cocaine

One characteristic of the amine-containing cell groups of the mammalian brain is that they fire spontaneously. This occurs both in vivo, where it is modified by synaptic inputs arising from other brain regions, and in vitro.[21] The spontaneous firing occurs principally because calcium ions enter the cell, depolarizing it to a potential at which a sodium-dependent action potential occurs; the entering calcium also activates a potassium conductance, and the outward movement of potassium ions repolarizes the neuron and terminates the action potential. A second characteristic, mentioned briefly above, is that the cells express on their surface one type of receptor for their own transmitter (α_2 receptors on noradrenaline cells,[22] 5-HT_{1A} receptors for 5-hydroxytryptamine cells,[23] and D_2 receptors for dopamine cells[14]). In each case, receptor activation leads to potassium conductance increase, hyperpolarization, and inhibition of cell firing. Under resting circumstances, the spontaneously firing cells release small amounts of their cognate transmitter, which acts back on the same or neighboring cells to inhibit their firing.

Cocaine inhibits the spontaneous action potentials of principal (dopamine-containing) VTA neurons, in vivo[24] and in vitro.[25] This is not a direct action of cocaine, but results from blockade of reuptake of dopamine released by the spontaneously firing cells within the nucleus.[25] The extracellular dopamine concentration then rises to a level at which it hyperpolarizes the cells. The evidence for this is that the inhibitory action of cocaine is prevented by antagonists at dopamine D_2 receptors, which have little or no effect on the cells in the absence of cocaine. The inhibition produced by cocaine is therefore self-limiting; as more VTA neurons are silenced, less dopamine will be released and there will be less potentiating action of cocaine. The effective concentrations of cocaine (1–10 μM) are similar to but slightly higher than the plasma levels associated with subjective effects.[26]

NUCLEUS ACCUMBENS NEURONS

Opiates

Behavioral studies indicate that opiates are reinforcing when administered into the nucleus accumbens itself[24,27]; conversely, local administration of a naloxone homolog into the accumbens will prevent intravenous self-administration of morphine.[28,29] Opiate-binding sites are found in the nucleus accumbens, with μ receptors most heavily concentrated in the ventromedial "shell" of the nucleus.[30] In vivo experiments indicate that opiates applied locally will inhibit the firing of a subset of the neurons in the accumbens, but it remains unclear whether this is mostly a direct action on the accumbens neurons or a presynaptic inhibition of excitatory inputs from elsewhere.[31]

There have been no systematic studies of opiate actions on accumbens neurons using in vitro methods. The abundant medium spiny output neurons of the dorsal striatum, with which the nucleus accumbens has considerable homology, are unaffected by opioids; however, a small subpopulation of cells (<4%) having distinct electrical properties are hyperpolarized.[32] The main effect of opioids in the striatum is indirect: namely, presynaptic inhibition of the release of both excitatory amino acids from corticostriate fibers, and of GABA from intrinsic striatal neurons.[32] The presynaptic inhibition is consistent with the results of in vivo studies mentioned above.[31] There is a need for similar experiments to be performed in the nucleus accumbens itself, particularly on neurons that can be identified with respect to their functional role and connections.

Cocaine

The principal direct action of dopamine released onto accumbens neurons is inhibition of firing[33–35]: activation of D_1 receptors leads to increase intracellular levels of cyclic adenosine 3', 5'-monophosphate, and this results in potassium channel opening and hyperpolarization.[34,35] Extracellular recording in vivo suggests that cocaine potentiates the action of dopamine because it inhibits reuptake, and cocaine therefore inhibits the firing of accumbens neurons.[36,37]

When studies are carried out with intracellular recordings in vitro, only the terminal axons of the dopamine-containing cells remain, and there is little spontaneous release of dopamine occurring in the tissue slice. This contrasts with the situation in the VTA (see above), and probably explains why cocaine has no effect on the membrane properties of the accumbens neurons recorded in vitro.[35] However, the effect of cocaine can be detected readily when exogenous dopamine is added. Dopamine (acting at D_1 receptors) hyperpolarizes the neurons, and cocaine causes a leftward shift in the concentration-response curve, indicating that it prevents uptake into the slice of the added dopamine.[35] At 1 μM, cocaine doubles the sensitivity to applied dopamine and at 30 μM the sensitivity to dopamine is increased 50-fold.

Cocaine causes an even greater increase in the sensitivity of the cells to added 5-HT, presumably because it also blocks the reuptake of 5-HT.[35] At 1 μM, cocaine potentiates the effect of 5-HT by 13-fold, and at 30 μM by 120 times. The finding that the uptake of 5-HT is more affected by cocaine than the uptake of dopamine is in general agreement with results of biochemical studies of the inhibition by cocaine of the uptake of tritiated analogs of 5-HT and dopamine.[38]

These studies indicate that dopamine (or 5-HT) added to the tissue slice undergoes very considerable uptake; the ambient concentration at the surface of the recorded neuron can be increased 50–100 times by complete block of uptake. If these findings pertain to synaptically released dopamine, then cocaine would be expected to increase greatly the time for which dopamine acts on the accumbens neurons, and probably the number of accumbens neurons that fell the influence of dopamine released from a set of dopamine-containing fibers.

CONCLUSIONS

The results can be interpreted with respect to the overall actions of opiates and cocaine when applied systemically. First, bear in mind that actions of these substances outside the mesolimbic pathway may critically affect the inputs to the VTA and/or the accumbens. Second, drugs taken systemically will act at the same time both in the VTA and accumbens. For example, if the firing of dopamine cells is stopped by an action at the cell bodies there can be no potentiation of dopamine action in target regions such as the accumbens.

Excitation of dopamine cells by opiates has been clearly shown and is now known to result from inhibition of local inhibitory interneurons. At the level of target cells of the nucleus accumbens the principal action of released dopamine seems to be inhibitory. Opiates may also add to this inhibition by reducing corticostriate synaptic input, but the detailed actions of opiates on single accumbens neurons remain to be studied in vitro.

Cocaine inhibits rather than excites dopamine cells: it does so by blocking the reuptake of dopamine tonically released from cell bodies and/or dendrites and, therefore, the inhibition is self-limiting. The predominant action of systemically administered cocaine seems to be in the accumbens, where uptake blockade means that any released dopamine can diffuse over greater distances and a longer time, presumably to inhibit more target cells.

Further research at the cellular level will be required to determine the cellular basis of opiate action within the nucleus accumbens proper, and to develop a more detailed understanding of the local synaptic interactions between neurons in both the accumbens and the VTA.

REFERENCES

1. KOOB, G. F. & F. E. BLOOM. 1988. Cellular and molecular mechanisms of drug dependence. Science **242:** 715–723.
2. WISE, R. A. 1984. Neural mechanisms of the reinforcing action of cocaine. Res. Mon. Natl. Inst. Drug Abuse **50:** 15–33.
3. WISE, R. A. 1987. The role of reward pathways in the development of drug dependence. Pharmacol. Ther. **35:** 227–263.

4. KOOB, G. F. & N. E. GOEDERS. 1989. Neuroanatomical substrates of drug self-administration. In The Neuropharmacological Basis of Reward. J. M. Liebman & S. J. Cooper, Eds.: 214–263. Oxford University Press. New York.
5. DICHIARA, G. & A. IMPERATO. 1988. Drugs abused by humans preferentially increase synaptic dopamine concentrations in the mesolimbic system of freely moving rats. Proc. Natl. Acad. Sci. USA 85: 5274–5278.
6. JOHNSON, S. W. & R. A. NORTH. 1991. Two types of neurone in the rat ventral tegmental area and their synaptic inputs. J. Physiol. In press.
7. GRACE, A. A. & S.-P. ONN. 1989. Morphology and electrophysiological properties of immunocytochemically identified rat dopamine neurons recorded in vitro. J. Neurosci. 9: 3463–3481.
8. LACEY, M. G., N. B. MERCURI & R. A. NORTH. 1989. Two cell types in rat substantia nigra zona compacta distinguished by membrane properties and the actions of dopamine and opioids. J. Neurosci. 9: 1233–1241.
9. YUNG, W. H., M. A. HAEUSSER & J. J. B. JACK. 1991. Electrophysiology of dopaminergic and non-dopaminergic neurones of the guinea-pig substantia nigra pars compacta in vitro. J. Physiol. 436: 643–667.
10. MATSUDA, Y., K. FUJIMURA & S. YOSHIDA. 1987. Two types of neurons in the substantia nigra pars compacta studied in a slice preparation. Neurosci. Res. 5: 172–179.
11. GYSLING, K. & R. WANG. 1983. Morphine-induced activation of A10 dopamine neurons in the rat. Brain Res. 277: 119–127.
12. MATHEWS, R. T. & D. C. GERMAN. 1984. Electrophysiological evidence for excitation of rat ventral tegmental area by dopamine. Neuroscience 11: 617–625.
13. DILTS, R. P. & P. W. KALIVAS. 1989. Autoradiographic localization of μ-opioid and neurotensin receptors within the mesolimbic dopamine system. Brain Res. 488: 311–327.
14. LACEY, M. G., N. B. MERCURI & R. A. NORTH. 1987. Dopamine acts on D_2 receptors to increase potassium conductance in neurones of the rat substantia nigra zona compacta. J. Physiol. 392: 397–416.
15. NORTH, R. A. 1989. Drug receptors and the inhibition of nerve cells. The XII Gaddum Lecture. Br. J. Pharmacol. 98: 13–28.
16. NORTH, R. A. 1991. Opioid actions on membrane ion channels. In Handbook of Experimental Pharmacology. A. Herz, H. Akil & E. J. Simon, Eds. Springer-Verlag. Berlin. In press.
17. JOHNSON, S. W. & R. A. NORTH. 1992. Opioids excite dopamine neurons by hyperpolarization of local interneurons. J. Neurosci. 12: 483–488.
18. LEE, H. K., T. DUNWIDDLE & B. HOFFER. 1980. Electrophysiological interactions of enkephalins with neuronal circuitry in the rat hippocampus. II. Effects on interneuron excitability. Brain Res. 184: 331–342.
19. ZIEGLGANSBERGER, W., E. D. FRENCH, G. R. SIGGINS & F. E. BLOOM. 1979. Opioid peptides may excite hippocampal pyramidal neurons by inhibiting adjacent inhibitory interneurons. Science 205: 415–417.
20. MADISON, D. V. & R. A. NICOLL. 1988. Enkephalin hyperpolarizes interneurons in the rat hippocampus. J. Physiol. 398: 123–130.
21. GRACE, A. A. 1988. In vivo and in vitro intracellular recordings from rat midbrain dopamine neurons. Ann. N.Y. Acad. Sci. 537: 51–76.
22. YOSHIMURA, M. & H. HIGASHI. 1985. 5-hydroxytryptamine mediates inhibitory postsynaptic potentials in rat dorsal raphe neurons. Neurosci. Lett. 53: 69–74.
23. PAN, Z. Z., W. F. COLMERS & J. T. WILLIAMS. 1989. 5-HT mediated synaptic potentials in the dorsal raphe nucleus: Interaction with excitatory amino acid and GABA neurotransmission. J. Neurophysiol. 62: 481–486.
24. EINHORN, L. C., P. A. JOHANSEN & F. J. WHITE. 1988. Electrophysiological effects of cocaine in the mesoaccumbens dopamine system: Studies in the ventral tegmental area. J. Neurosci. 8: 100–112.
25. LACEY, M. G., N. B. MERCURI & R. A. NORTH. 1990. Actions of cocaine on rat dopaminergic neurones in vitro. Br. J. Pharmacol. 99: 731–735.
26. JAVAID, J. I., M. W. FISCHMAN, C. R. SCHUSTER, H. DEKIRMENJIAN & J. M. DAVIS. 1978. Cocaine plasma concentration: Relation to physiological and subjective effects in humans. Science 202: 227–228.

27. GOEDERS, N. E., J. D. LANE & J. E. SMITH. 1984. Intracranial self-administration of methionine enkephalin into the nucleus accumbens. Pharmacol. Biochem. Behav. **20**: 451–455.
28. CORRIGAL, W. A. & F. J. VACCARINO. 1988. Antagonist treatment in nucleus accumbens or periaqueductal grey affects heroin self-administration. Pharmacol. Biochem. Behav. **30**: 442–450.
29. VACCARINO, F. J., F. E. BLOOM & G. F. KOOB. 1985. Blockade of nucleus accumbens opiate receptors attenuates the intravenous heroin reward in the rat. Psychopharmacology **86**: 37–42.
30. MANSOUR, A., H. KHACHATURIAN, M. E. LEWIS, H. AKIL & S. J. WATSON. 1987. Autoradiographic differentiation of mu, delta, and kappa opioid receptors in the rat forebrain and midbrain. J. Neurosci. **7**: 2445–2464.
31. HAKAN, R. L. & S. J. HENRIKSEN. 1989. Opiate influences on nucleus accumbens neuronal electrophysiology: Dopamine and non-dopamine mechanisms. J. Neurosci. **9**: 3538–3546.
32. JIANG, Z.-G. & R. A. NORTH. 1991. Membrane properties and synaptic responses of rat striatal neurones in vitro. J. Physiol. **443**: 533–553.
33. WOODRUFF, G. N., P. S. McCARTHY & R. J. WALKER. 1976. Studies on the pharmacology of neurons in the nucleus accumbens of the rat. Brain Res. **115**: 233–242.
34. UCHIMURA, N., H. HIGASHI & S. NISHI. 1986. Hyperpolarizing and depolarizing actions of dopamine via D-1 and D-2 receptors on nucleus accumbens neurons. Brain Res. **375**: 368–372.
35. UCHIMURA, N. & R. A. NORTH. 1990. Actions of cocaine on rat nucleus accumbens neurones *in vitro*. Br. J. Pharmacol. **99**: 736–740.
36. WHITE, F. J., S. R. WACHTEL, P. A. JOHANSEN & L. C. EINHORN. 1987. Electrophysiological studies in the rat mesoaccumbens dopamine system: Focus on dopamine receptor subtypes, interactions, and the effects of cocaine. *In* Neurophysiology of Dopaminergic Systems: Current Status and Clinical Perspectives. L. A. Chiodo & A. S. Freeman, Eds.: 317–365. Lakeshore. Detroit.
37. HENRY, D. J., M. A. GREENE & F. J. WHITE. 1989. Electrophysiological effects of cocaine in the mesoaccumbens dopamine system: Repeated administration. J. Pharmacol. Exp. Ther. **251**: 833–839.
38. RITZ, M. C., R. J. LAMB, S. R. GOLDBERG & M. J. KUHAR. 1987. Cocaine receptors on dopamine transporters are related to self-administration of cocaine. Science **237**: 1219–1223.

Purification, Reconstitution, and Cloning of an NMDA Receptor-Ion Channel Complex from Rat Brain Synaptic Membranes: Implications for Neurobiological Changes in Alcoholism[a]

ELIAS K. MICHAELIS,[b,c,e] MARY L. MICHAELIS,[b,c]
KESHAVA N. KUMAR,[b,c] NANDA TILAKARATNE,[b,f]
DAVID B. JOSEPH,[b] PETER S. JOHNSON,[b]
KENT K. BABCOCK,[b] GARY L. AISTRUP,[d]
AND RICHARD L. SCHOWEN[c,d]

[b] Department of Pharmacology and Toxicology
[c] Center for Biomedical Research
[d] Department of Biochemistry
University of Kansas
Lawrence, Kansas 66045

HIROTSUGU MINAMI, MASAO SUGAWARA,
KAZUNORI ODASHIMA, AND YOSHIO UMEZAWA

Department of Chemistry
University of Hokkaido
Sapporo 060, Japan

INTRODUCTION

L-Glutamate forms the most widespread excitatory transmitter network in the mammalian central nervous system.[1-3] The excitation produced by L-glutamic acid is important not only in transmission of information between neurons, but also in early

[a] This work was supported by Grants AA04732 from NIAAA and DAAL03-88-K-0017 and DAAL03-91-G-0167 from the ARO to E.K.M. P. S. J. is supported by an institutional Training Grant #GM07775-12 from NIGMS to the University of Kansas.
[e] Author to whom correspondence should be addressed: Dr. Elias K. Michaelis, Center for Biomedical Research, 2099 Constant Ave., West Campus, University of Kansas, Lawrence, KS 66047.
[f] Present address: Department of Psychiatry, Medical College of Pennsylvania, EPPI, 3200 Henry Ave., Philadelphia, PA 19129.

7

developmental events in the nervous system,[4–6] abnormal excitability,[7,8] and neuronal degeneration.[9,10] There is also evidence that changes in glutamate transmission may be involved in the adaptive changes that occur in brain during chronic alcoholism. Several years ago we suggested that one way in which the brain might adapt to the presence of ethanol is to increase the number of receptors for the major excitatory neurotransmitter in the CNS, namely, L-glutamic acid.[11–13]

We demonstrated that a period of chronic ethanol administration to experimental animals resulted in a significant increase in sensitivity of the treated animals to the convulsant effects of kainic acid, a potent glutamate analog that activates a select population of receptors.[11] Furthermore, we observed an increase in the brain synaptic membrane binding sites for L-[^{3}H]-glutamate in the alcohol-treated animals[12,13] and an increase in immunoreactivity of an antibody raised against a brain glutamate-binding protein.[14] These observations were replicated more recently in studies with brain membranes from human alcoholics[15] and led us to suggest that the adaptive responses of brain neurons to chronic ethanol administration either in experimental animals or humans include an apparent increase in glutamate receptors associated with neuronal plasma membranes.

PHYSIOLOGICAL AND PHARMACOLOGICAL PROPERTIES OF THE NMDA RECEPTOR AND SITES OF ACTION OF ETHANOL

On the basis of many pharmacological, physiological and biochemical studies, a classification scheme for glutamate receptors has been developed. The receptors fall into two major classes, those that are coupled to the enzyme phospholipase C and lead to the formation of 1,4,5-inositol triphosphate, a metabolic response, and those that form ligand-gated ion channels.[16,17] The receptors that form ion channels are further subclassified according to their sensitivity to specific agonists. One major class of receptors are those activated by glutamate and its analog N-methyl-D-aspartate (NMDA), and the other major class are those that are activated by glutamate and its analogs kainate, quisqualate, and α-3-hydroxy-5-methyl-4-isoxazolepropionic acid (AMPA),[16] the "non-NMDA" receptors. The NMDA subtype of glutamate receptors has been the focus of many recent investigations because of its role in important physiological and neuropathological processes such as long term potentiation, a physiological analog of learning and memory,[18] the initiation of neuronal damage induced by ischemia and hypoglycemia,[19] and the generation of seizure activity.[7,8]

Potent inhibitory effects of low concentrations of ethanol on the NMDA receptor-ion channel have been demonstrated in a number of different types of assays[20–23] and results of very recent studies suggest a similar inhibitory effect of ethanol on kainate receptors expressed in frog oocytes.[24] The observation that the NMDA receptor-ion channel is remarkably sensitive to physiologically relevant concentrations of ethanol (5–50 mM)[20,21] has served to focus much attention on the glutamatergic system and, in particular, on NMDA receptor-mediated synaptic transmission as a target for many of the CNS actions of ethanol. Therefore, a more detailed examination of the mechanisms underlying this inhibition is warranted as are studies to elucidate the molecular structure of the NMDA receptors.

The NMDA receptors contain a number of distinct ligand binding domains through which their function is regulated. There are ligand binding sites for the agonists L-glutamate and NMDA, the competitive antagonists ($\pm$)3-carboxypiperazin-

4-yl-propylphosphonic acid (CPP), 2-amino-5-phosphonopentanoic acid (2-AP5) and 2-amino-7-phosphonoheptanoic acid (2AP7), the co-activator glycine, and the ion channel blockers phencyclidine (PCP), 1-[1-(2-thienyl)cyclohexylpiperidine (TCP), and dizocilpine (MK-801).[16] One major component of our studies has been focused on exploring the site or sites through which ethanol acts to disrupt the activity of these receptors.

We have made use of an *in vitro* biochemical assay for NMDA receptor activation which, in some respects, parallels the receptor-controlled opening of the cation channel. This involves monitoring the activation of [³H]TCP binding to brain membranes by glutamate, NMDA, and glycine or various combinations of these agents. Use of this assay system has made it possible to begin identifying which of the multiple sites on the NMDA receptor complex are targets through which ethanol inhibits receptor activation. The results of our recent studies indicated that the site with which glycine interacts to enhance ion channel activation is most sensitive to inhibition by very low concentrations of ethanol ($IC_{50} \sim 0.6$ mM) (D. B. Joseph, M. Michaelis, and E. Michaelis, manuscript submitted). The activation of [³H]TCP binding produced by glutamate, on the other hand, was nearly insensitive to this drug, since ethanol at 100 mM concentration produced only a marginal inhibition of the activation by glutamate and had no effect on the affinity of the site for glutamate. Since most of the investigators reporting ethanol-induced inhibition of physiological responses used NMDA rather than glutamate to activate the receptor, we also examined the effects of ethanol on [³H]TCP binding activated by NMDA. In these studies we observed that in the presence of 100 mM ethanol, the K_{act} of the receptor for NMDA was shifted an order of magnitude to the right, suggesting the receptor was much less sensitive to NMDA in the presence of ethanol. In addition, the maximal NMDA-induced TCP binding (B_{max}) was reduced by 25% from 106 fmol/mg protein to 73 fmol/mg protein. These observations of differential sensitivity of the glutamate versus NMDA-activation of [³H]TCP binding suggest that the molecular events involved in the opening of the ion channel by NMDA differ somewhat from those involved in the channel activation brought about by glutamate. Clearly a full understanding of these observations is likely to require a complete molecular characterization of the NMDA receptor complex. The second major component of our work is directed toward this goal and involves efforts to clone the proteins and to elucidate their biochemical and molecular properties.

MOLECULAR CHARACTERISTICS OF TWO TYPES OF NMDA RECEPTORS

Two alternative structures have been presented in the literature for glutamate/NMDA receptor-ion channel complexes. One structure, identified by functional expression cloning of brain cDNA, is a large protein which has all expected characteristics of an NMDA receptor-ion channel when it is expressed in frog oocytes.[25] The inferred structure of this protein based on the cDNA sequence is that of a 105 kDa protein that has substantial homology to some of the previously cloned kainate/AMPA receptor proteins, especially the GluR1 to GluR4 proteins.[26-28] Functional activity of the NMDA receptor-ion channel complexes in frog oocytes following expression of the 105 kDa protein presumably involves the formation of homomeric multi-subunit structures of this protein.

The second type of NMDA receptor-ion channel structure that we and others have identified is a hetero-oligomeric structure isolated from brain neuronal membranes.[29-31] It was suggested previously[29-31] that this protein complex consists of four subunits that have molecular sizes of 67–70, 57–60, 42–46, and 31–36 kDa as determined by SDS-PAGE. This complex exhibited [3H]TCP binding sites with properties that fit those of an NMDA receptor-ion channel, *i.e.*, glutamate- and glycine-activated

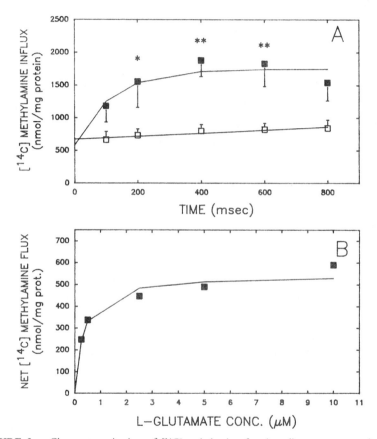

FIGURE 1. L-Glutamate activation of [14C]methylamine flux into liposomes reconstituted with partially purified glutamate-binding proteins. (**A**) Rapid kinetics of [14C] methylamine influx were measured in the absence (□) or presence (■) of 5 μM L-glutamic acid. The purification of glutamate-binding proteins and their reconstitution into liposomes were performed as described in Ly and Michaelis.[30] All values shown are the mean ($\pm$SEM) from five separate protein purification and reconstitution experiments. The constants estimated by fitting the data for glutamate-induced methylamine flux to a pseudo-first order equation are: k = 8.6 sec^{-1} and I_{∞} = 1,173 nmol/mg protein. Values of glutamate-induced flux that are significantly different from background flux are indicated (* $p \leqslant 0.05$, ** $p \leqslant 0.01$, 8 d.f.). (**B**) Concentration-dependent stimulation by L-glutamate of [14C] methylamine influx. The values shown are the mean net influx at 100 msec from 3 or 4 protein isolation and reconstitution experiments. The constants estimated from the optimal fit to the Michaelis-Menten type of equation are: K_{act} = 0.32 μM and I_{max} = 547 nmol/mg protein. (This figure is reproduced from *Biochemistry* with the permission of the American Chemical Society.[30])

TCP binding to this protein complex in a concentration-dependent manner.[29] A partially purified complex that contained proteins similar in molecular size to those described above was isolated in our laboratory from brain synaptic membranes by affinity chromatography through an L-glutamate-derivatized matrix and reconstituted into liposomes.[30] These proteins, upon reconstitution, formed L-glutamate and NMDA-sensitive ion channels that were detected by rapid-kinetic measurements of cation fluxes into liposomes[30] (FIGS. 1 and 2). Activation of these channels by L-glutamate was inhibited by the selective antagonist of NMDA receptors, 2-AP5, and by antibodies raised against a 71 kDa protein that was previously isolated in our laboratories[31]

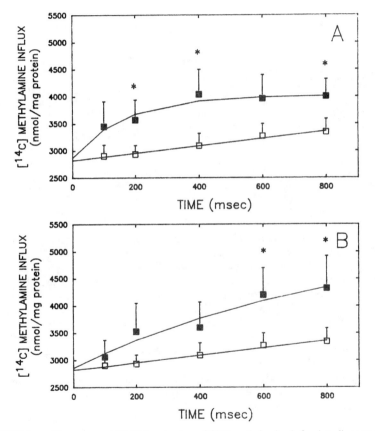

FIGURE 2. L-Glutamate and NMDA activation of [¹⁴C] methylamine influx into liposomes reconstituted with partially purified glutamate-binding proteins. Rapid kinetics of methylamine flux were measured in the presence (■) or absence (□) of 10 μM L-glutamate (A) or in the presence (■) or absence (□) of 10 μM NMDA (B). Each value represents the mean (± SEM) from six protein isolation and reconstitution experiments. Values of glutamate and NMDA-induced flux that are significantly different from background flux are indicated (* $p \leqslant 0.05$, 10 d.f.). Data analysis and curve-fitting were performed as described in FIGURE 1A. Estimated constants for glutamate-activated ion flux are: k = 6.1 sec⁻¹ and I_∞ = 1,152 nmol/mg protein; those for NMDA-stimulated methylamine flux are: k = 1.2 sec⁻¹ and I_∞ = 2,412 nmol/mg protein. (Figure is reproduced from *Biochemistry* with the permission of the American Chemical Society.[30])

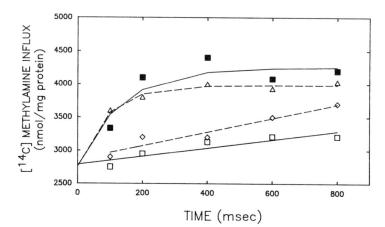

TIME (msec)

FIGURE 3. Effects of preincubation with immune and pre-immune IgG's on L-glutamate-induced [14C] methylamine flux in liposomes reconstituted with partially purified glutamate-binding proteins. Proteoliposomes were pre-incubated for 1 h at 4°C with either buffer (■) or 5 μg/ml pre-immune IgG (△) or 5 μg/ml immune IgG (◊). These proteoliposomes were subsequently employed in determinations of [14C] methylamine flux in the presence or absence of 10 μM L-glutamic acid. Each value shown is the mean from 4 protein isolation and reconstitution experiments. The constants for glutamate-activated flux are: k = 7.4 sec^{-1} and I_∞ = 1,502 nmol/mg protein; those for glutamate-activated flux in the presence of pre-immune IgG are: k = 10.9 sec^{-1} and I_∞ = 1,232 nmol/mg protein. Methylamine flux in samples incubated with L-glutamate following preincubation with immune IgG was a linear process. (Figure is reprinted from *Biochemistry* with the permission of the American Chemical Society.[30])

(FIG. 3). One of the proteins of the multisubunit complex isolated from synaptic membranes was identified on Western blots as identical or related to the 71 kDa glutamate-binding protein previously purified from synaptic membranes.[30]

We recently reported on several modifications of the techniques used by Ly and Michaelis[30] that have produced more highly purified proteins which may form functional glutamate/NMDA receptors.[32] These modifications included the use of the detergents CHAPS (1.5% w/v) and *n*-octylglucoside (10% v/v) together with glycerol in the solubilization buffer, a glutamate-derivatized ReactiGel support as the affinity chromatography matrix,[33] and NMDA as the displacing ligand to elute proteins specifically bound to the ReactiGel. The protein fraction eluted from the glutamate-ReactiGel matrix by introducing 5 mM NMDA into the elution buffer contained proteins with estimated molecular sizes based on migration in SDS-PAGE that are equal to 70, 62, 43 and 41 (doublet), and 36 and 31 (doublet) kDa.[32] The proteins at 41–43 and 31–36 kDa frequently migrated on SDS-PAGE either as diffuse bands or as doublets[32] (FIG. 4).

LIGAND BINDING CHARACTERISTICS OF THE HETERO-OLIGOMERIC COMPLEX OF NMDA RECEPTOR PROTEINS

The complex of proteins eluted from the affinity matrix by NMDA displacement represented a four to five-thousand-fold enrichment of L-glutamate-sensitive L-

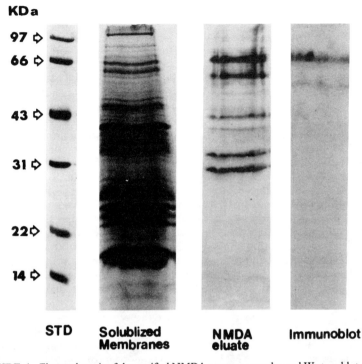

FIGURE 4. Electrophoresis of the purified NMDA receptor complex and Western blot analysis of the isolated proteins. The fraction eluted from the affinity chromatography column by 5 mM NMDA was probed on a Western blot with polyclonal antibodies against the 71 kDa glutamate-binding protein. (Figure is reprinted from *Nature* by permission.[32])

[3H]glutamate, strychnine-insensitive [3H]glycine, and MK-801-sensitive [3H]TCP binding entities when compared with brain homogenates (K. Kumar, P. Johnson, K. Babcock, G. Aistrup, R. Schowen, and E. Michaelis, manuscript submitted). Nearly all L-[3H]glutamate-binding sites in the isolated protein complex were sensitive to NMDA. The fraction eluted by NMDA also had ligand-binding sites for the competitive inhibitor of NMDA receptors, [3H]CPP. These data indicate that there is a co-purification of these important recognition sites of the NMDA receptor complex. This protein complex did not contain either kainate- or quisqualate-sensitive AMPA binding sites.

The estimated equilibrium dissociation constant (K_D) for L-glutamate binding to the agonist recognition site was 99 nM. This K_D is similar to that reported for glutamate binding to synaptic membranes and to the K_{act} for L-glutamate enhancement of [3H]TCP binding[34,35] or activation of cation fluxes in liposomes reconstituted with a partially purified preparation of this complex.[30] The K_i for NMDA displacement of L-[3H]glutamate bound to this protein complex was 490 nM. However, the Hill coefficient for NMDA displacement of L-[3H]glutamate bound to the complex was 0.52, which is suggestive of a complex interaction of NMDA with the agonist recognition sites of the protein. The estimated K_D for [3H]TCP binding to the complex was 56 nM, a value that is comparable to that determined for binding of this ligand to synaptic membranes.[35] The K_D for strychnine-insensitive [^{3}H]glycine binding to the isolated protein complex was 3.6 μM, a value that is ten-fold higher than the K_D for the binding of this ligand to synaptic membrane receptors.[36]

If the isolated proteins associate to form a macromolecular NMDA receptor complex, then occupation of the agonist sites by L-glutamate and the allosteric co-activator sites by glycine should produce an increase in the rate of [^{3}H]TCP binding to the ion channel. This presumably would be caused by a conformational change that leads to the opening of an ion channel.[35] L-Glutamate and glycine added at micromolar concentrations to the NMDA-eluted fraction produced an increase in the binding of [^{3}H]TCP to the purified protein complex and this increase was apparently due to altered kinetics of binding. If the incubation was carried out for only 10 min, then the increase in TCP binding produced by the same concentrations of glutamate and glycine over that measured in their absence is 113%. The NMDA receptor complex is also known to have recognition sites for various polyamines such as spermine and spermidine, and occupation of these sites by the polyamines is known to enhance the rate of [^{3}H]TCP binding.[37] When 1 mM concentrations of the polyamines spermine and spermidine were tested using non-equilibrium conditions, i.e., a 10 min incubation period with [^{3}H]TCP, binding increased 200 to 400%. These observations are indicative of the presence of an intact NMDA receptor-ion channel complex in which the agonists, co-activator, and polyamine binding sites interact with and open the ion channel component of this complex.

We have obtained additional evidence that the proteins isolated by glutamate-affinity chromatography form a complex in experiments utilizing molecular size-exclusion chromatography in order to determine the size and structure of the isolated ligand-binding entities. The NMDA-eluted fraction obtained from glutamate-affinity chromatography was subjected to chromatography on a Sephacryl S-400 HR column, and the highest activities of both NMDA-sensitive glutamate-binding and MK-801-sensitive TCP-binding proteins eluted in the same fractions. The NMDA-sensitive L-[^{3}H]glutamate-binding activity associated with the proteins in these fractions represented a 6,100-fold purification of these entities as compared with their levels in brain homogenates, and the average Stokes radius of the proteins in this fraction had an estimated average value of 5.1 nm. The Stokes radius was very close to that of catalase (5.2 nm), a protein with molecular size equal to 232 kDa. The protein fractions with the highest ligand-binding activity contained the four major subunits described above, though some of the proteins formed doublets or diffuse bands upon analysis by SDS-PAGE, also as described previously.[32] An important question is whether the protein subunits of the complex isolated from synaptic membranes and identified by gel chromatography and SDS-PAGE are indeed part of a complex of proteins in synaptic membranes or whether they are the result of protein degradation occurring during the purification process. We have recently shown that organophosphorous compounds such as diisopropyl fluorophosphate (DFP) selectively inhibit the binding of [^{3}H]CPP to NMDA receptor sites in synaptic membranes without having any effect on either strychnine-insensitive [^{3}H]glycine or MK-801-sensitive [^{3}H]TCP binding to the NMDA receptor or on quisqualate- and kainate-sensitive [^{3}H]AMPA binding to the kainate/AMPA receptors.[38] DFP inhibited CPP binding to synaptic membranes covalently, and thus it was used to label the proteins related to the CPP binding sites of the NMDA receptors in synaptic membranes. As shown in FIGURE 5, two major peaks of proteins were labeled by [^{3}H]DFP in a 2-AP5-sensitive manner, a protein of 47–50 kDa and

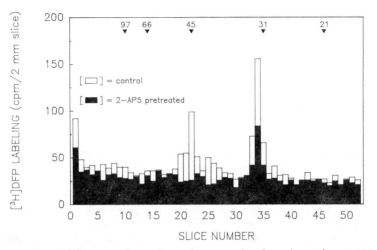

FIGURE 5. [³H]DFP labeling of synaptic membrane proteins. Synaptic membranes were pre-treated with either Tris/SO₄ buffer (□) or 10 mM 2-AP5 in the same buffer for 15 min (■) prior to being exposed to 25 μM [³H]DFP. Following a 45-min incubation in the presence of [³H]DFP, the membranes were precipitated by centrifugation, washed, solubilized, and the labeled proteins were analyzed by SDS-PAGE. The histogram represents a composite of the mean cpm/slice from four separate experiments. (The figure is reproduced from *Molecular Pharmacology* with permission of the American Society for Pharmacology and Experimental Therapy.[38])

a 32-kDa protein. The proteins labeled by DFP have molecular sizes very similar to those observed in the isolated complex of proteins described above and are an indication that the smaller molecular size proteins are present as part of an NMDA receptor complex in synaptic membranes.

RECONSTITUTION OF THE PURIFIED NMDA RECEPTOR PROTEINS INTO PLANAR LIPID BILAYER MEMBRANES

We have recently reported that the protein complex that we have purified by affinity chromatography can be reconstituted in planar lipid bilayer membranes and that, following such reconstitution, L-glutamic acid can activate ion channels that have some of the characteristics of an NMDA receptor.[39,40] The isolated proteins were first reconstituted into phosphatidylethanolamine/cholesterol liposomes according to the procedures described in Minami *et al.*[39] The liposomes were allowed to fuse with the leaflet of a planar lipid bilayer that faces the "*cis*" chamber of a Montal-Mueller cell and all agonists and antagonists were introduced into the "*trans*" chamber. All measurements were performed in the presence of 5 μM glycine and in the absence of Mg²⁺. If liposomes that did not contain any proteins were allowed to fuse with the membrane bilayer, then the introduction of L-glutamate into the "*trans*" chamber did not produce any increase in ion current or in background noise across the bilayer. However, the introduction of the same concentrations of L-glutamate to the "*trans*" chamber following fusion of protein-containing liposomes produced currents that had the characteristics of single ion channel conductances. These currents exhibited a linear voltage-current relationship and apparently represented opening of single channels to three different conductance states. The reversal potential for all three states of glutamate-induced openings of the ion channels was approximately 0 mV. The estimated slope conductances for the three types of channel open states were 23, 47, and 67 pS.[40] The integral of the current through these ion channels over a 10-sec period was dependent on the glutamate concentration used to activate the ion channels. The estimated K_{act} for glutamate was 0.8 μM.

Further evidence that the reconstituted proteins of the complex function as NMDA-sensitive ion channels was obtained from experiments in which NMDA only was used as the agonist to activate these ion channel responses. The NMDA responses were consistently observed only after the glycine concentration in the "*trans*" chamber was raised from 5 μM, the concentration present in both chambers during all experiments, to 10 μM. Concentrations of NMDA ranging between 100 and 200 μM were required to produce consistent activation of these channels in the reconstitution studies. Additional experiments were performed employing preparations of proteins obtained following affinity chromatographic isolation through glutamate-derivatized ReactiGel and molecular size-exclusion chromatography on Sephacryl S-400 HR. The fractions representing the complex of proteins eluted from the Sephacryl S-400 HR columns exhibited characteristics of glutamate-activated ion-conducting channels, and the glutamate-activated conductance of these channels was partially blocked by the introduction of Mg^{2+} into the buffer medium of the cell chambers. We have also observed an apparent voltage sensitivity of the Mg^{2+} blockade as the imposition of high positive potentials (+130 to +180 mV) rescued these channels from Mg^{2+} inhibition. On the other hand, at all negative potentials the Mg^{2+} inhibition of the ion channels was nearly complete.

CLONING OF THE GLUTAMATE BINDING SUBUNIT OF THE HETERO-OLIGOMERIC COMPLEX OF THE NMDA RECEPTOR

We have recently reported on the cloning of the cDNA for the glutamate-binding protein subunit of the NMDA receptor complex that we had previously isolated.[32] The cloning of the cDNA for this subunit was achieved through screening of expression cDNA libraries from rat brain hippocampus with polyclonal and monoclonal antibodies raised against the purified rat brain glutamate-binding protein. The structure of the protein inferred from the sequence of this cDNA is that of a 57 kDa membrane protein with four transmembrane domains. This protein has no significant homology to the structure of either the 105 kDa NMDA receptor protein[25] or the ~100 kDa kainate/AMPA receptor proteins.[26-28] This protein has a structural motif for the second transmembrane domain similar to that in some other ligand-gated ion channel proteins such as the α-subunits of the nicotinic acetylcholine and γ-aminobutyric acid receptors[32] but lacks homology to any of these receptor proteins. Although the single isolated protein retains its glutamate-binding activity and immunoreactivity with antibodies raised against the purified brain glutamate-binding protein, this protein did not produce ion channel activity when expressed in frog oocytes following injection of cRNA derived from the cloned cDNA (unpublished observations). We are assuming that the glutamate-binding subunit is not sufficient by itself to produce a glutamate and NMDA-sensitive ion channel. We had reached the same conclusion previously on the basis of reconstitution studies with this protein subunit in liposomes. The results of our cloning studies thus far point out the need to clone the remaining subunits and to determine the stoichiometries and cooperative interactions of the subunits in order to understand the minimum structure of an active NMDA receptor-ion channel.

CONCLUSIONS

The molecular and functional characteristics of the protein complex described in this paper are consistent with the idea that this complex of four proteins is a type of NMDA receptor that is present in neuronal membranes. Additional information about the location and function of this receptor complex in neurons has been accumulated through the use of specific antibodies raised against one of the protein subunits of this complex, the glutamate-binding protein. Light microscopic examination of the location of antigenic sites that react with antibodies raised against this protein revealed that it is localized in dendritic processes of neurons in the hippocampus.[41,42] At the electron microscopic level these immunoreactive proteins are most heavily represented in the post-synaptic membranes of neurons.[42] Expression of this protein in hippocampal neurons and granule cells of the cerebellum in primary cultures correlates most closely with the appearance of functional NMDA receptors and not with the presence of kainate or AMPA receptors.[42,43] Furthermore, the antibodies raised against the glutamate-binding subunit of the complex protected hippocampal neurons against NMDA-induced, but not against kainate or quisqualate-induced cell degeneration.[42] Based on these findings at the cellular level, it appears that the isolated protein complex or the cloned and expressed subunits of this complex will be useful molecular models in the study of drug interactions with the NMDA receptor such as those described above for ethanol.

ACKNOWLEDGMENTS

We acknowledge the support of the Center for Biomedical Research and we thank Kim Bland for her assistance in the preparation of this paper.

REFERENCES

1. FONNUM, F. 1984. J. Neurochem. **42:** 1–11.
2. COTMAN, C. W., D. T. MONAGHAN, O. P. OTTERSEN & J. STORM-MATHISEN. 1980. Trends Neurosci. **10:** 273–280.
3. COTMAN, C. W. & D. T. MONAGHAN. 1988. Annu. Rev. Neurosci. **11:** 61–80.
4. BALAZS, R., N. HACK & O. S. JORGENSEN. 1988. Neurosci. Lett. **87:** 80–86.
5. BREWER, G. J. & C. W. COTMAN. 1989. Neurosci. Lett. **99:** 268–273.
6. MATTSON, M. P., P. DOUG & S. P. KATER. 1988. J. Neurosci. **8:** 2087–2100.
7. CHAPMAN, A. G., B. S. MELDRUM, N. WANG & J. C. WATKINS. 1987. Eur. J. Pharmacol. **149:** 91–96.
8. GEAN, D. W. & A. SHINNICK-GALLAHER. 1988. Neuropharmacology **27:** 557–562.
9. WEILOCH, T. 1987. Science **230:** 681–683.
10. CHOI, D. W. 1987. J. Neurosci. **7:** 369–379.
11. FREED, W. J. & E. K. MICHAELIS. 1978. Biochem. Behav. **8:** 509–514.
12. MICHAELIS, E. K., M. J. MULVANEY & W. J. FREED. 1978. Biochem. Pharmacol. **27:** 1685–1691.

13. MICHAELIS, E. K., M. L. MICHAELIS & W. J. FREED. 1980. *In* Biological Effects of Alcohol. H. Begleiter, Ed.: 43–56. Plenum Publishing Corp. New York.
14. MICHAELIS, E. K., S. ROY, N. GALTON, M. CUNNINGHAM, E. LeCLUYSE & M. L. MICHAELIS. 1987. Neurochem. Int. 11: 209–218.
15. MICHAELIS, E. K., W. J. FREED, N. GALTON, J. FOYE, M. L. MICHAELIS, I. PHILLIPS & J. E. KLEINMAN. 1990. Neurochem. Res. 15: 1055–1063.
16. WATKINS, J. C., P. KROGSGAARD-LARSEN & T. HONORE. 1990. Trends Pharmacol. Sci. 11: 25–33.
17. RECASENS, M., J. GUIRAMAND, A. NOURIGAT, I. SASSETTI & G. DEVILLIERS. 1988. Neurochem. Int. 13: 463–467.
18. COTMAN, C. W., D. T. MONAGHAN & A. H. GANONG. 1988. Ann. Rev. Neurosci. 11: 61–80.
19. SIMON, R. P., J. H. SWAN, T. GRIFFITHS & B. S. MELDRUM. 1984. Science 226: 850–852.
20. LOVINGER, D. M., G. WHITE & F. F. WEIGHT. 1989. Science 243: 1721–1724.
21. HOFFMAN, P. L., C. S. RABE, F. MOSES & B. TABAKOFF. 1989. J. Neurochem. 52: 1937–1940.
22. DILDY-MAYFIELD, J. E. & S. W. LESLIE. 1991. Neurochemistry 56: 1536–1543.
23. SIMSON, P. E., H. E. CRISWELL, K. B. JOHNSON, R. E. HICKS & G. R. BREESE. 1991. J. Pharmacol. Exp. Ther. 257: 225–231.
24. DIDLY-MAYFIELD, J. E., J. M. SIKELA & R. A. HARRIS. 1991. Soc. Neurosci. Abstr. 17: 1167.
25. MORIYOSHI, K., M. MASU, T. ISHII, R. SHIGEMOTO, N. MIZUNO & S. NAKANISHI. 1991. Nature 354: 31–37.
26. HOLLMAN, M., A. O'SHEA-GREENFIELD, S. W. ROGERS & S. HEINEMANN. 1989. Nature 342: 643–648.
27. KEINANEN, K., W. WISDEN, B. SOMMER, P. WERNER, A. HERB, T. A. VERDOOM, B. SAKMAN & P. H. SEEBURG. 1990. Science 249: 556–560.
28. BOULTER, J., M. HOLLMANN, A. O'SHEA-GREENFIELD, M. HARTLEY, E. DENERIS, C. MARON & S. HEINEMANN. 1990. Science 249: 1033–1037.
29. IKIN, A. F., Y. KLOOG & M. SOKOLOVSKY. 1990. Biochemistry 29: 2290–2295.
30. LY, A. M. & E. K. MICHAELIS. 1991. Biochemistry 30: 4307–4316.
31. CHEN, J. W., M. D. CUNNINGHAM, N. GALTON & E. K. MICHAELIS. 1988. J. Biol. Chem. 263: 417–426.
32. KUMAR, K. N., N. TILAKARATNE, P. S. JOHNSON, A. E. ALLEN & E. K. MICHAELIS. 1991. Nature 354: 70–73.
33. WANG, H., K. N. KUMAR & E. K. MICHAELIS. 1992. Neuroscience 46: 793–806.
34. MONAGHAN, D. T. & C. W. COTMAN. 1986. Proc. Natl. Acad. Sci. USA 83: 7532–7536.
35. KLOOG, Y., R. HARING & M. SOKOLOVSKY. 1988. Biochemistry 27: 843–848.
36. KESSLER, M., T. TERRAMANI, G. LYNCH & M. BAUDRY. 1989. J. Neurochem. 52: 1319–1328.
37. RANSOM, R. W. & N. L. STEC. 1988. J. Neurochem. 51: 830–836.
38. JOHNSON, P. S. & E. K. MICHAELIS. 1992. Mol. Pharmacol. 41. In press.
39. MINAMI, H., M. SUGAWARA, K. ODASHIMA, Y. UMEZAWA, M. UTO, E. K. MICHAELIS & T. KUWANA. 1991. Anal. Chem. 63: 2787–2795.
40. EGGEMAN, K. T., G. AISTRUP, K. N. KUMAR, E. K. MICHAELIS & R. L. SCHOWEN. 1991. Neurosci. Abs. 17: 74.
41. EATON, M. J., J.-W. CHEN, K. N. KUMAR, Y. CONG & E. K. MICHAELIS. 1990. J. Biol. Chem. 265: 16196–16204.
42. MATTSON, M., H. WANG & E. K. MICHAELIS. 1991. Brain Res. 565: 94–108.
43. BALAZS, R., A. RESINK, N. HACK, J. B. F. VAN DER VALK, K. N. KUMAR & E. K. MICHAELIS. 1992. Neurosci. Lett. In press.

Cannabinoid Receptor Localization in Brain: Relationship to Motor and Reward Systems

MILES HERKENHAM

Section on Functional Neuroanatomy
National Institute of Mental Health
Building 36, Room 2D-15
Bethesda, Maryland 20892

INTRODUCTION

Marijuana (*Cannabis sativa*) is one of the oldest and most widely used drugs in the world, with a history of use dating back over 4,000 years.[1,2] It was not until about twenty years ago that the principal psychoactive ingredient of the marijuana plant was isolated and found to be Δ^9-tetrahydrocannabinol (Δ^9-THC).[3-5] Δ^9-THC and other natural and synthetic cannabinoids produce characteristic behavioral and cognitive effects,[6,7] most of which can be attributed to actions on the central nervous system.[8] Marijuana use in this country is widespread, with approximately 40 million Americans having at least tried the drug.[9] Compulsive use is associated with social and psychological problems in individuals.[10] There is little evidence of adverse health side effects or toxicity.[7,11-13]

Until recently, very little was known about the cellular mechanisms through which cannabinoids act. The unique spectrum of cannabinoid effects and the stereoselectivity (enantioselectivity) of action of cannabinoid isomers in behavioral studies (see below) strongly suggested the existence of a specific cannabinoid receptor in brain, but early attempts to identify and characterize such a recognition site were not successful (discussed in refs. 14–16).

Without evidence that cannabinoids act through a specific receptor coupled to a functional effector system, researchers were prone to study the effects of cannabinoids on membrane properties, membrane-bound enzymes, eicosanoid production, metabolism, and other neurotransmitter systems *in vitro*.[8,17-19] As pointed out before,[20] most of the biochemical studies employed concentrations of Δ^9-THC that were in excess of physiologically meaningful concentrations that might be found in brain (for review, see refs. 8, 18). In addition, the criterion of structure-activity relationship was not met—that is, the potencies of various cannabinoids in the *in vitro* assays did not correlate with their relative potencies in eliciting characteristic behavioral effects.[8,20] Particularly damaging to the relevance of these *in vitro* studies was the absence of enantioselectivity.[20]

However, several groups have reported enantioselectivity of THC isomers in various behavioral tests *in vivo*. Martin's group found that the potencies of (−) and (+) forms of each of the *cis* and *trans* isomers of Δ^9-THC differ by 10- to 100-fold in producing static ataxia in dogs, depressing schedule-controlled responding in monkeys, and in producing hypothermia and inhibiting spontaneous activity in mice.[21] Hollister *et al.*[22] showed cannabinoid enantioselectivity in human studies using indices of the subjective experience, or "high." May's group found enantioselectivity of a series of synthetic cannabinoids in tests of motor depression and analgesia.[23-25]

One of May's compounds, (−)-9-nor-9β-hydroxyhexahydrocannabinol (β-HHC), was used as a lead compound by Johnson and Melvin[26] for the synthesis of a rather large series of structurally novel, classical and nonclassical, cannabinoids for studies of their potential use as analgesics (FIG. 1). The synthetic cannabinoids share physicochemical properties with the natural cannabinoids and produce many behavioral and physiological effects characteristic of Δ9-THC, but are 5–1000 times more potent and show high enantioselectivity.

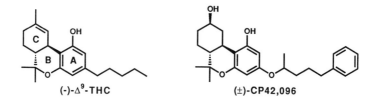

(-)-Δ9-THC   (±)-CP42,096

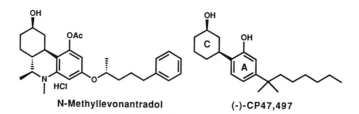

N-Methyllevonantradol   (-)-CP47,497

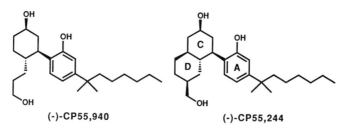

(-)-CP55,940   (-)-CP55,244

FIGURE 1. Chemical structures of Δ9-tetrahydrocannabinol (Δ9-THC) and three synthetic cannabinoids. According to the nomenclature of Johnson and Melvin,[26] Δ9-THC and 9-Nor-9β-hydroxyhexahydrocannabinol (β-HHC) are defined as members of the ABC-tricyclic cannabinoid class. CP 55,940 is a hydroxypropyl analog of a 2-(3-hydroxycyclohexyl)phenol, defined as an AC-bicyclic cannabinoid. CP 55,244 is an ACD-tricyclic cannabinoid with a rigidly positioned hydroxypropyl moiety. (Reproduced from Herkenham *et al.*[16])

The availability of the nonclassical compounds revolutionized the study of the biochemical basis of cannabinoid activity. Howlett's group used them in neuroblastoma cell lines to show inhibition of adenylate cyclase activity.[27] Such inhibition is enantioselective, and the pharmacological profile correlates well with that observed by Martin's group in tests of mouse spontaneous activity, catalepsy, body temperature, and analgesia.[28]

One of the nonclassical compounds, CP 55,940, was tritiated and used by Howlett's group to identify and fully characterize a unique cannabinoid receptor in membranes from rat brain.[14] The results from the centrifugation assay showed that [³H]CP 55,940 receptor binding is saturable, has high affinity and enantioselectivity, and exhibits characteristics expected for a neuromodulator receptor associated with a guanine nucleotide regulatory (G) protein.

Recently, we characterized and validated the binding of [³H]CP 55,940 in slide-mounted brain sections and described assay conditions to autoradiographically visualize the CNS distribution of cannabinoid receptors in a number of mammals, including humans.[29] Autoradiography revealed a unique distribution that is similar in all mammalian species examined; binding is most dense in outflow nuclei of the basal ganglia—the substantia nigra pars reticulata and globus pallidus—and in the hippocampus and cerebellum.

The localization of dense receptors in the outflow nuclei of the basal ganglia may account for some of the actions of cannabinoids. Dense binding localized in the globus pallidus, entopeduncular nucleus, and substantia nigra pars reticulata suggests an association of cannabinoid receptors with striatal efferent projections to these nuclei and, therefore, a role for cannabinoids in motor control. In addition, binding may be localized on mesostriatal dopaminergic neurons, which would implicate a role for cannabinoids in direct control of dopamine release and, therefore, brain reward mechanisms.

This report summarizes several key features of our cannabinoid receptor localization studies: 1) validation that the in vitro binding in brain sections is the same binding that mediates the effects of cannabinoids in vivo; 2) general features of brain distribution in several species, including human; and 3) neuronal localization of cannabinoid receptors to motor and/or limbic components of the basal ganglia, assessed by making selective chemical lesions of either the striatal GABAergic efferent or dopaminergic afferent pathways interconnecting the caudate-putamen (CPu) and the substantia nigra.

MATERIALS AND METHODS

Binding Assays

Cannabinoid Receptor Binding

The procedures for obtaining cryostat-cut sections of fresh, frozen brain mounted on "subbed" microscope slides were described previously.[15,29] Assay conditions yielding 80–90% specific binding are: incubation of slide-mounted sections at 37°C for 2 h in 50 mM Tris-HCl buffer, pH 7.4, with 5% bovine serum albumin (BSA) and 1–10 nM [³H]CP 55,940 (sp. act. 76 Ci/mmole). Slides are washed at 0°C for 4 h in the same buffer with 1% BSA and then dried. For use in competition studies to characterize and validate binding, natural and synthetic cannabinoid ligands were obtained from the

National Institute of Drug Abuse and Pfizer, Inc. Names and stereochemical configurations of some of the cannabinoids are shown in FIGURE 1.

Autoradiography was performed on 15–25 μm-thick brain sections of rat (Sprague-Dawley), guinea pig (Hartley), dog (beagle), rhesus monkey and human (dying of non-neurological disorders). Sections were incubated in 10 nM [³H]CP 55,940 using optimized conditions, then washed, dried, and exposed to tritium-sensitive film (LKB or Amersham) for 3 to 4 weeks before developing. Developed films were digitized with a solid-state video camera and Macintosh II computer-based system for densitometry. Receptor densities were quantified using IMAGE® software (Wayne Rasband, Research Services Branch, NIMH).

Dopamine D_1 and D_2 Receptor Binding

Both the D_1 and D_2 receptor assays were carried out as previously described.[30–32] For D_1 receptor binding, slides were warmed to room temperature and incubated at 25°C for 2.5 h in 25 mM Tris-HCl buffer, pH 7.5, with 100 mM NaCl, 1 mM $MgCl_2$, 0.001% ascorbate, and 0.55 nM [³H]SCH 23390 (sp. act. 74.8 Ci/mmole). Slides were washed for 10 min in the same buffer at 4°C, dipped in deionized water, and dried. Nonspecific binding was determined by addition of 2 μM cis-flupenthixol and was typically <5% of total binding. Sections were exposed to film for 2 weeks.

For D_2 receptor binding, sections were incubated at 25°C for 1.5 h in 25 mM Tris-HCl buffer, pH 7.5, with 200 mM NaCl, 1 mM $MgCl_2$, 0.001% ascorbate, and 1.5 nM [³H]raclopride (sp. act. 64 Ci/mmole). They were washed for 3 min in the same buffer at 4°C with 100 mM NaCl. Nonspecific binding, determined by addition of 5 μM sulpiride, was typically <5% of total binding. Sections were exposed to film for 3 weeks.

Dopamine Uptake Site

Assay conditions were described previously.[33,34] Slides were incubated at 2°C for 30 h in 50 mM sodium phosphate buffer, pH 7.5, with 120 mM NaCl, 0.01% BSA, 0.001% ascorbate, 500 nM trans-flupenthixol, and 0.25 nM [³H]GBR 12935 (sp. act. 53.1 Ci/mmole). They were washed for 2 h in same buffer at 2°C. Nonspecific binding, determined by addition of 20 μM mazindol, was typically <15% of total binding. Sections were exposed to film for 8 weeks.

Lesions

Striatal Ibotenate Lesions

Male rats (Sprague Dawley) were anesthetized and placed in a stereotaxic frame. A cannula was lowered into the caudate-putamen. Via an infusion pump and tubing, 1.5 μl (7.5 μg) of ibotenate dissolved in normal saline was infused over 8 min. Animals survived for 2 or 4 weeks before sacrifice by decapitation.

6-OHDA Lesions

Rats were prepared as above but were injected i.p. with desmethylimipramine (15 mg/kg) 30 min before infusion. The cannula was lowered into the medial forebrain bundle (mfb). Four μl (8 μg) of 6-OHDA dissolved in normal saline with 0.1% ascorbate added was infused over 8 min. Animals survived for 4 weeks before sacrifice; at 2 weeks post-lesion they were tested for rotational behavior 40 min after administration of 5 mg/kg of *d*-amphetamine sulfate (Sigma). Only those rats showing greater than 10 rotations per min during a 5-min test were used in the binding experiment.

RESULTS

A large series of cannabinoid and non-cannabinoid drugs was assayed to test for competitive displacement of [³H]CP 55,940 (TABLE 1). The competition curves and derived inhibition constants (K_i's) for the natural and synthetic cannabinoids provided a test for validation of binding. We found that highly significant ($p < 0.0001$) correlations exist between the K_i's and potencies of the drugs in tests of dog ataxia and human subjective experience, the two most reliable markers of cannabinoid activity.[6,7] The K_i's also correlate very closely with relative potencies in tests of motor function (ataxia, hypokinesia, catalepsy), analgesia, and inhibition of contractions of guinea pig ileum and adenylate cyclase in neuroblastoma cell lines *in vitro*.[29] Enantioselectivity is striking; the (−) and (+) forms of CP 55,244 differ by more than 10,000-fold *in vitro*, a separation predicted by the rigid structure of the molecule (FIG. 1)[26] and by potencies *in vivo*. Natural cannabinoids lacking psychoactive properties, such as cannabidiol, show extremely low potency at the receptor, and all tested non-cannabinoid drugs have no potency (TABLE 1).

Autoradiography showed that in all species very dense binding is found in the globus pallidus, substantia nigra pars reticulata (SNR), and the molecular layers of the cerebellum and hippocampal dentate gyrus (FIGS. 2 and 3). Dense binding is also found in the cerebral cortex, other parts of the hippocampal formation, and striatum. In rat, rhesus monkey and human, the SNR contains the highest level of binding (FIG. 3). In dog, the cerebellar molecular layer is most dense (FIG. 2H). In guinea pig and dog, the hippocampal formation has selectively dense binding (FIG. 2E, F). Neocortex in all species has moderate binding across fields, with peaks in superficial and deep layers. Very low and homogeneous binding characterizes the thalamus and most of the brainstem, including all of the monoamine-containing cell groups, reticular formation, primary sensory, visceromotor and cranial motor nuclei, and the area postrema. The exceptions—hypothalamus, basal amygdala, central gray, nucleus of the solitary tract, and laminae I–III and X of the spinal cord—show slightly higher but still sparse binding (FIGS. 2 and 3).

Quantitative autoradiography reveals very high numbers of receptors, exceeding 1 pmole/mg protein in densely labeled areas. Thus, cannabinoid receptor density is far in excess of densities of neuropeptide receptors and is similar to levels of cortical benzodiazepine,[35] striatal dopamine,[30,36] and whole-brain glutamate receptors.[37]

TABLE 1. Potencies of Some Cannabinoids in the Section Binding and Other Assays

Compound	Ki (nM)	Catalepsy/ Ataxia (mg/kg)	Mouse Analgesia (mg/kg)	Cyclase Inhibition (nM)	Human "High" (mg)
CP 55,940 (−AC)	15 (Kd)	0.35	0.7	25	
CP 56,667 (+AC)	470	>10	>15	>5,000	
CP 55,244 (−ACD)	1.4	0.09	0.09	5	
CP 55,243 (+ACD)	18000	>10	>10	>10,000	
CP 50,556	14	1.5	0.4	100	0.5
CP 53,870	26000	>10	6.5	>5,000	
CP 54,939	14	0.05	0.7	7	
Nabilone	120	0.03		100	1
β-HHC	124	0.1	1.6		
α-HHC	2590	0.5	>50		
(−)Δ⁹-THC	420	0.5	10	100	1
(+)Δ⁹-THC	7700	>2.0	>100		
Δ⁸-THC	498	0.5	8.8		2
11-OH-Δ⁹-THC	210	0.05	1.9		1
TMA-Δ⁸-THC	2300				
8β-OH-Δ⁹-THC	4200				10
8α-OH-Δ⁹-THC	8700				10
11-OH-Cannabinol	800				
Cannabinol	3200				>15
Cannabidiol	53000	inactive	>100		>30
Cannabigerol	275000	>7			
9-COOH-11-nor-Δ⁹-THC	75000	>40	10		
9-COOH-11-nor-Δ⁸-THC	Inactive				

CP analogs were synthesized at Pfizer Central Research; their structures are given in Johnson and Melvin.[26] The first 6 analogs are enantiomeric pairs, as are α- and β-HHC and (−) and (+)Δ⁹-THC. CP 50,556 is levonantradol; CP 53,870 is dextronantradol; CP 54,939 is desacetyl levonantradol; TMA-Δ⁸-THC is trimethylammonium-Δ⁸-THC. The last two compounds are Δ⁹-THC metabolites. Ki's ± standard deviations are derived from binding surface analysis. Drugs which at 10 μM concentration show no inhibition of [³H]CP 55,940 binding are: amphetamine, β-estradiol, cis-flupenthixol (dopamine receptor ligand), cocaine, corticosterone, cyclohexyl-adenosine, dexamethasone, etorphine (opiate receptor ligand), γ-amino butyric acid (GABA), glutamate, leukotriene B₄ and D₄ (both at 1 μM), lysergic acid diethylamide (LSD), phencyclidine (PCP), prostaglandin E₂, Ro15-1788 (benzodiazepine receptor ligand), and thujone (the active ingredient of absinthe). (Modified from Herkenham et al.[29])

Striatal Ibotenate Lesions

The single injection of ibotenate into the caudate-putamen resulted in a small central site of nonspecific destruction marked by gliosis and a much larger (approximately 3 × 4 mm) surrounding area of selective neuronal degeneration, in accordance with previous descriptions of toxicity in the dose range and location used.[38] In the affected striatal territory, the losses on the lesion relative to corresponding territory on the control side were the most profound for the dopamine D_1 receptors, showing a 96% reduction in binding at 4 weeks (TABLE 2). Cannabinoid and D_2 receptors were reduced

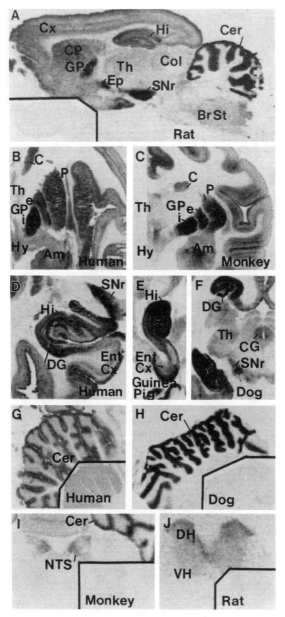

FIGURE 2. Autoradiography of 10 nM [³H]CP 55,940 binding in brain. Tritium-sensitive film exposed for 4 weeks, developed and computer digitized. Images were photographed directly from the computer monitor. Gray levels represent relative levels of receptor densities. Sagittal section of rat brain in **A**. Coronal brain sections of human in **B**, **D**, and **G**; rhesus monkey in **C** and **I**; dog in **F** and **H**; and rat in **J**. Horizontal section of guinea pig brain in **E**. *Insets* show non-specific binding in adjacent sections (miniaturized images are shown). *Abbreviations:* Am, amygdala; Br St, brain stem; Cer, cerebellum; CG, central gray; C, caudate; Col, colliculi; CP, caudate-putamen; Cx, cerebral cortex; DG, dentate gyrus; DH, dorsal horn of spinal cord; Ent Cx, entorhinal cortex; Ep, entopeduncular nucleus (homolog of GPi); GP, globus pallidus (e, external; i, internal); Hi, hippocampus; Hy, hypothalamus; NTS, nucleus of solitary tract; P, putamen; SNr, substantia nigra pars reticulata; Th, thalamus; VH, ventral horn of spinal cord. (Reproduced from Herkenham *et al.*[29])

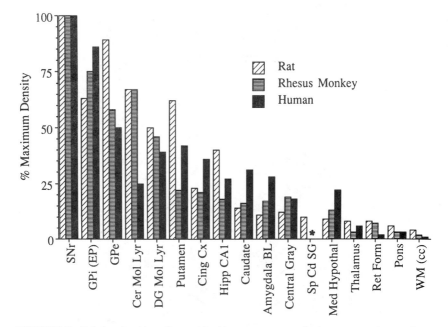

FIGURE 3. Relative densities of cannabinoid receptors across brain structures in rat, rhesus monkey, and human. Autoradiographic images were digitized by a solid-state camera and Macintosh II computer-based system for quantitative densitometry using Image® software (Wayne Rasband, Research Services Branch, NIMH). Transmittance levels were converted to fmoles/mg tissue using tritium standards, then normalized to the densest structure in each animal (SNr for all three). For every section incubated for total binding, an adjacent section was incubated in the presence of CP 55,244 to permit subtraction of nonspecific binding on a regional basis. Structure abbreviations not given in FIGURE 2 legend are: Cing Cx, cingulate cortex; Hipp CA1, hippocampal field CA1; Med Hypothal, medial hypothalamus; Sp Cd SG, substantia gelatinosa of spinal cord (* only rat measured); Ret Form, reticular formation; WM (cc), white matter of corpus callosum. (Reproduced from Herkenham et al.[29])

by 78–80% in the affected territory, and the dopamine uptake site, which resides on afferent dopaminergic axons, was slightly reduced at 4 weeks (not shown).

Both cannabinoid and D_1 dopamine receptors are lost in similar patterns (FIG. 4) and amounts (TABLE 2) in projection zones of lesioned striatal efferent neurons. In agreement with known medial-lateral topography of striatal projections,[39] receptor losses in both GP and SNR were greatest medially, with sparing of binding in lateral parts receiving projections from unlesioned parts of the lateral and posterior caudate-putamen (FIG. 4). For cannabinoid receptor binding, losses in the labeled striatonigral pathway were also evident (not shown).

Mfb 6-OHDA Lesions

Nissl-stained sections of the substantia nigra showed unilateral loss of neurons in the SNC (FIG. 4e). Autoradiography showed no change in cannabinoid receptor

TABLE 2. Effects of Unilateral Striatal Ibotenate Lesions at 4 Week Survival ($n = 5$)

Structure	Cannabinoid Receptor	L % R	D-1 Receptor	L % R	D-2 Receptor	L % R
CPu (L)	536 ± 37	20	69 ± 18	4	54 ± 25	18
(R)	2843 ± 849		1558 ± 111		299 ± 22	
GP (L)	719 ± 182	15	13 ± 6	12		
(R)	4763 ± 969		106 ± 28			
EP (L)	905 ± 340	22	57 ± 23	24		
(R)	4159 ± 834		240 ± 39			
SNR (L)	1023 ± 174	16	164 ± 16	13		
(R)	6421 ± 635		1254 ± 97			

Values are in fmoles/mg protein and are the means and standard deviations of specific binding to approximately 50% of the total number (B_{max}) of receptors and 10% of uptake sites in each region, since ligand concentrations were near the K_d or below, in the case of [^{3}H]GBR-12935, for each drug. Corresponding locations on the control (R) side were outlined and measured. All left–right differences are significant at the $p < 0.005$ level of confidence except for the dopamine uptake site, which is significant at the $p < 0.05$ level (Student's paired t-test). Abbreviations: CPu, caudate putamen; EP, entopeduncular nucleus; GP, globus pallidus; SNR, substantia nigra pars compacta. (Data are from Herkenham et al.[32])

binding in either the striatum (FIG. 4d) or the nigra (FIG. 4e), whereas dopamine uptake sites were lost throughout the striatum and nigra on the lesioned side (FIG. 4f). Quantitative densitometry showed major losses of dopamine uptake sites in the caudate-putamen, accumbens nucleus (ACb), and substantia nigra pars compacta (SNC), but no loss of cannabinoid receptors (TABLE 3).

DISCUSSION

The section binding assay is easy to perform, is reliable, and shows high sensitivity to manipulations of binding conditions, such as the addition of guanine nucleo-

TABLE 3. Effect of Unilateral 6-OHDA Lesions at 4 Week Survival ($n = 4$)

Structure	Cannabinoid Receptor	L % R	Dopamine Uptake Site	L % R
CPu (L)	4395 ± 266	99	62 ± 57	20
(R)	4422 ± 282		311 ± 60	
ACb (L)	2533 ± 384	102	38 ± 30	39
(R)	2491 ± 463		98 ± 13	
SNC (L)	1709 ± 320	95	1 ± 1	7
(R)	1807 ± 264		17 ± 7	

Values are in fmoles/mg protein and are the means and standard deviations of specific binding to approximately 50% and 10% of the total number (B_{max}) of receptors and uptake sites in each region, respectively. Densitometric measures of caudate-putamen (CPu), nucleus accumbens (ACb), and substantia nigra pars compacta (SNC) were each taken from the entire structure at the levels shown in FIGURE 3. Left–right cannabinoid receptor differences were not significant (Student's paired t-test); dopamine uptake site left–right differences were significant in the CPu ($p < 0.01$), ACb ($p = 0.05$), and SNC ($p < 0.03$). (Data are from Herkenham et al.[32])

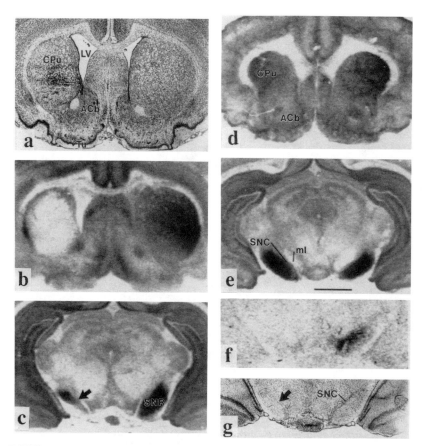

FIGURE 4. Lesion data showing localization of cannabinoid receptors to striatonigral neurons
(a–c) and not to dopaminergic nigrostriatal neurons (d–g). As shown in a–c, a unilateral deposit
of ibotenate was placed into the caudate-putamen. Nissl-stained section in a shows the area of
selective neuronal loss and the enlarged lateral ventricle (LV). At 4 weeks survival, the losses of
cannabinoid receptors in the caudate-putamen (b) and substantia nigra pars reticulata (SNR)
(*arrow* in c) are shown autoradiographically. The losses are topographic; note sparing of laterally
situated striatal neurons and their nigral projections. As shown in d–g, a unilateral lesion of the
mesencephalic ascending dopamine system was made by depositing 6-OHDA into the medial
forebrain bundle. At 4 weeks survival, degeneration of dopamine neurons in the substantia nigra
pars compacta (SNC) is evident in the Nissl stain (*arrow* in g) and by the losses of dopamine uptake
sites in the SNC (f), whereas cannabinoid receptor binding is unaffected in the striatum (d) and
nigra (e). *Abbreviations*: ACb, nucleus accumbens; ml, medial lemniscus; Tu, olfactory tubercle.
Magnification bar measures 2 mm. (Modified from Herkenham *et al.*[32])

tides.[29] BSA appears to act as a carrier to keep cannabinoids in solution without appreciably affecting binding kinetics. The low nonspecific binding and absence of
binding in white matter indicates that the autoradiographic patterns are not affected
by ligand lipophilia. The inclusion of BSA in the incubation medium may actually
mimic the disposition of cannabinoids administered *in vivo*, as they would quickly complex with serum albumin or other carriers in the blood.

The structure-activity profile suggests that the receptor defined by the binding of [³H]CP 55,940 is the same receptor that mediates many of the behavioral and pharmacological effects of cannabinoids (TABLE 1), including the subjective experience termed the human "high." All other tested psychoactive drugs, neurotransmitters, steroids, and eicosanoids at 10 μM concentrations failed to bind to this receptor. There was no compelling evidence for receptor subtypes from that analysis.

Autoradiography of cannabinoid receptors reveals a heterogeneous distribution pattern that conforms to cytoarchitectural and functional subdivisions in the brain. The distribution is unique–no other pattern of receptors is similar–and it is similar across several mammalian species, including human, suggesting that cannabinoid receptors are phylogenetically stable and conserved in evolution. The distribution appears to be similar to the distribution of the mRNA probe hybridized to a rat brain cannabinoid receptor gene.[40]

The locations of cannabinoid receptors help to understand cannabinoid pharmacology. High densities in the hippocampus and cerebral neocortex implicate roles for cannabinoids in cognitive functions. High densities in axons and terminals of the GABAergic striatal neurons of the basal ganglia and of glutamatergic granule cells of the cerebellum suggest a modulatory role in movement systems. Sparse densities in lower brainstem areas controlling cardiovascular and respiratory functions may explain why high doses of Δ^9-THC are not lethal.

The results of the 6-OHDA lesions indicate that cannabinoid receptors do not reside on mesencephalic dopamine neurons projecting to either the caudate-putamen or the ACb. Systemically administered Δ^9-THC has been shown to elevate extracellular levels of dopamine in the caudate-putamen[41] and ACb.[42] The mechanism of action appears to be indirect, as the effects are attenuated by naloxone.[42] Nevertheless, it has been proposed that drugs which elevate dopamine levels in the striatum are those that are known to have abuse liability in humans.[43,44] In humans, cannabinoids can produce a feeling of euphoria as part of the subjective experience known as the marijuana "high," but dysphoria, dizziness, thought disturbances, and sleepiness are also reported.[6,7,26] Animals generally will not self-administer Δ^9-THC.[45,46] Cannabinoids did not lower the threshold for electrical self-stimulation in one study.[47] In another study they did,[48] but apparently both this phenomenon and the enhancement of basal dopamine efflux from the ACb by Δ^9-THC are strain-specific, occurring only in Lewis rats.[49] Thus, the effects of cannabinoids on dopamine circuits thought to be common mediators of reward are indirect and different from those of drugs such as cocaine and morphine which directly affect extracellular dopamine levels and produce craving and powerful drug-seeking behavior.

Accounts of cannabis use in humans stress the loosening of associations, fragmentation of thought, and confusion on attempting to remember recent occurrences.[7,50] These cognitive effects may be mediated by receptors in the cerebral cortex, especially the receptor-dense hippocampal cortex. The hippocampus "gates" information during memory consolidation and codes spatial and temporal relations among stimuli and responses.[51,52] Δ^9-THC causes memory "intrusions,"[53] impairs temporal aspects of performance,[54] and suppresses hippocampal electrical activity.[55]

The localization of cannabinoid receptors in motor areas suggests therapeutic applications. Cannabinoids exacerbate hypokinesia in Parkinson's disease but are beneficial for some forms of dystonia, tremor, and spasticity.[6,7,56-58] The association of cannabinoid receptors with GABAergic striatal projection neurons suggests roles for cannabinoids in control of movement, perhaps therapeutic roles in hyperkinesis and dystonia. Cannabinoids have been shown to be beneficial for some forms of dystonia, tremor, and spasticity.[6,7,56-59] Lack of association of cannabinoid receptors with dopamine neurons indicates that cannabinoids do not directly affect dopamine release associated with reward and drug-seeking behavior. Further work may show the basis for the reported usefulness in controlling nausea and stimulating appetite in patients receiving chemotherapy for cancer or AIDS. Finally, the development of an antagonist could lead to additional therapeutic applications. The section binding assay can be used to screen the potencies of novel drugs and serve to identify cannabinoid receptor subtypes, which could lead to renewed interest in developing cannabinoid drugs without unwanted side effects.

REFERENCES

1. HARRIS, L. S., W. L. DEWEY & R. K. RAZDAN. 1977. Cannabis. Its chemistry, pharmacology, and toxicology. In Handbook of Experimental Pharmacology. W. R. Martin, Ed. 45/II: 371–429. Springer-Verlag. New York.
2. MECHOULAM, R. 1986. The pharmacohistory of Cannabis sativa. In Cannabinoids as Therapeutic Agents. R. Mechoulam, Ed.: 1–19. CRC Press. Boca Raton, FL.
3. GAONI, Y. & R. MECHOULAM. 1964. Isolation, structure, and partial synthesis of an active constituent of hashish. J. Am. Chem. Soc. 86: 1646.
4. MECHOULAM, R., A. SHANI, H. EDERY & Y. GRUNFELD. 1970. Chemical basis of hashish activity. Science 169: 611–612.
5. MECHOULAM, R. 1973. Cannabinoid chemistry. In Marihuana. Chemistry, Pharmacology, Metabolism, and Clinical Effects. R. Mechoulam, Ed.: 1–99. Academic Press. New York.
6. DEWEY, W. L. 1986. Cannabinoid pharmacology. Pharmacol. Rev. 38: 151–178.
7. HOLLISTER, L. E. 1986. Health aspects of cannabis. Pharmacol. Rev. 38: 1–20.
8. MARTIN, B. R. 1986. Cellular effects of cannabinoids. Pharmacol. Rev. 38: 45–74.
9. KOZEL, N. J. & E. H. ADAMS. 1986. Epidemiology of drug abuse: An overview. Science 234: 970–974.
10. AMERICAN PSYCHOLOGICAL ASSOCIATION. 1987. Position statement on psychoactive substance use and dependence: Update on marijuana and cocaine. Am. J. Psychiatry 144: 698–702.
11. BERKOW, R. 1987. The Merck Manual of Diagnosis and Therapy. 15. Merck Co. Rahway, NJ.
12. HAYES, J. S., M. C. DREHER & J. K. NUGENT. 1988. Newborn outcomes with maternal marihuana use in Jamaican women. Pediatr. Nurs. 14: 107–110.
13. DILL, J. A. & A. C. HOWLETT. 1988. Regulation of adenylate cyclase by chronic exposure to cannabimimetic drugs. J. Pharmacol. Exp. Ther. 244: 1157–1163.
14. DEVANE, W. A., F. A. I. DYSARZ, M. R. JOHNSON, L. S. MELVIN & A. C. HOWLETT. 1988. Determination and characterization of a cannabinoid receptor in rat brain. Mol. Pharmacol. 34: 605–613.
15. HERKENHAM, M. 1991. Characterization and localization of cannabinoid receptors in brain: An in vitro technique using slide-mounted tissue sections. NIDA Res. Monogr. 112: 129–145.
16. HERKENHAM, M., A. B. LYNN, M. R. JOHNSON, L. S. MELVIN, B. R. DE COSTA & K. C. RICE. 1991. Characterization and localization of cannabinoid receptors in rat brain: A quantitative in vitro autoradiographic study. J. Neurosci. 11: 563–583.
17. HILLIARD, C. J., R. A. HARRIS & A. S. BLOOM. 1985. Effects of the cannabinoids on physical properties of brain membranes and phospholipid vesicles: Fluorescent studies. J. Pharmacol. Exp. Ther. 232: 579–588.
18. PERTWEE, R. G. 1988. The central neuropharmacology of psychotropic cannabinoids. Pharmacol. Ther. 36: 189–261.
19. REICHMAN, M., W. NEN & L. E. HOKIN. 1988. Δ^9-Tetrahydrocannabinol increases arachadonic acid levels in guinea pig cerebral cortex slices. Mol. Pharmacol. 34: 823–828.
20. HOWLETT, A. C., M. BIDAUT-RUSSELL, W. A. DEVANE, L. S. MELVIN, M. R. JOHNSON & M. HERKENHAM. 1990. The cannabinoid receptor: Biochemical, anatomical and behavioral characterization. Trends Neurosci. 13: 420–423.

21. MARTIN, B. R., R. L. BALSTER, R. K. RAZDAN, L. S. HARRIS & W. L. DEWEY. 1981. Behavioral comparisons of the stereoisomers of tetrahydrocannabinols. Life Sci. **29:** 565–574.
22. HOLLISTER, L. E., H. K. GILLESPIE, R. MECHOULAM & M. SREBNIK. 1987. Human pharmacology of 1S and 1R enantiomers of delta-3-tetrahydrocannabinol. Psychopharmacology **92:** 505–507.
23. WILSON, R. S. & E. L. MAY. 1975. Analgesic properties of the tetrahydrocannabinols, their metabolites, and analogs. J. Med. Chem. **18:** 700–703.
24. WILSON, R. S., E. L. MAY, B. R. MARTIN & W. L. DEWEY. 1976. 9-Nor-9-hydroxyhexahydrocannabinols. Synthesis, some behavioral and analgesic properties, and comparison with the tetrahydrocannabinols. J. Med. Chem. **19:** 1165–1167.
25. WILSON, R. S., E. L. MAY & W. L. DEWEY. 1979. Some 9-hydroxycannabinoid-like compounds. Synthesis and evaluation of analgesic and behavioral properties. J. Med. Chem. **22:** 886–888.
26. JOHNSON, M. R. & L. S. MELVIN. 1986. The discovery of nonclassical cannabinoid analgetics. *In* Cannabinoids as Therapeutic Agents. R. Mechoulam, Ed.: 121–145. CRC Press. Boca Raton, FL.
27. HOWLETT, A. C., M. R. JOHNSON, L. S. MELVIN & G. M. MILNE. 1988. Nonclassical cannabinoid analgesics inhibit adenylate cyclase: Development of a cannabinoid receptor model. Mol. Pharmacol. **33:** 297–302.
28. LITTLE, P. J., D. R. COMPTON, M. R. JOHNSON & B. R. MARTIN. 1988. Pharmacology and stereoselectivity of structurally novel cannabinoids in mice. J. Pharmacol. Exp. Ther. **247:** 1046–1051.
29. HERKENHAM, M., A. B. LYNN, M. D. LITTLE, M. R. JOHNSON, L. S. MELVIN, B. R. DE COSTA & K. C. RICE. 1990. Cannabinoid receptor localization in brain. Proc. Natl. Acad. Sci. USA **87:** 1932–1936.
30. RICHFIELD, E. K., A. B. YOUNG & J. B. PENNEY. 1986. Properties of D2 dopamine receptor autoradiography: High percentage of high-affinity agonist sites and increased nucleotide sensitivity in tissue sections. Brain Res. **383:** 121–128.
31. RICHFIELD, E. K., A. B. YOUNG & J. B. PENNEY. 1987. Comparative distribution of dopamine D-1 and D-2 receptors in the basal ganglia of turtle, pigeon, rat, cat, and monkey. J. Comp. Neurol. **262:** 446–463.
32. HERKENHAM, M., A. B. LYNN, B. DE COSTA & E. K. RICHFIELD. 1991. Neuronal localization of cannabinoid receptors in the basal ganglia of the rat. Brain Res. **547:** 267–274.
33. RICHFIELD, E. K. & M. HERKENHAM. 1989. Quantitative autoradiography of the dopamine uptake complex in the central nervous system. Soc. Neurosci. Abstr. **15:** 1230.
34. RICHFIELD, E. K. 1990. Quantitative autoradiography of the dopamine uptake complex in rat brain using [³H]GBR 12935: Binding characteristics. Brain Res. **540:** 1–13.
35. ZEZULA, J., R. CORTÉS, A. PROBST & J. M. PALACIOS. 1988. Benzodiazepine receptor sites in the human brain: Autoradiographic mapping. Neuroscience **25:** 771–795.
36. BOYSON, S. J., P. McGONIGLE & P. B. MOLINOFF. 1986. Quantitative autoradiographic localization of the D1 and D2 subtypes of dopamine receptors in rat brain. J. Neurosci. **6:** 3177–3188.
37. GREENAMYRE, J. T., A. B. YOUNG & J. B. PENNEY. 1984. Quantitative autoradiographic distribution of L-[³H]glutamate binding sites in rat central nervous system. J. Neurosci. **4:** 2133–2144.
38. KÖHLER, C. & R. SCHWARCZ. 1983. Comparison of ibotenate and kainate neurotoxicity in rat brain: A histological study. Neuroscience **8:** 819–835.
39. ALTAR, C. A. & K. HAUSER. 1987. Topography of substantia nigra innervation by D1 receptor containing striatal neurons. Brain Res. **410:** 1–11.
40. MATSUDA, L. A., S. J. LOLAIT, M. J. BROWNSTEIN, A. C. YOUNG & T. I. BONNER. 1990. Structure of a cannabinoid receptor: Functional expression of the cloned cDNA. Nature **346:** 561–563.
41. NG CHEONG TON, J. M., G. A. GERHARDT, M. FRIEDEMANN, A. M. ETGEN, G. M. ROSE, N. S. SHARPLESS & E. L. GARDNER. 1988. The effects of Δ⁹-tetrahydrocannabinol on potassium-evoked release of dopamine in the rat caudate nucleus: An in vivo electrochemical and in vivo microdialysis study. Brain Res. **451:** 59–68.
42. CHEN, J., W. PAREDES, J. LI, D. SMITH, J. LOWINSON & E. L. GARDNER. 1990. Δ⁹-

Tetrahydrocannabinol produces naloxone-blockable enhancement of presynaptic basal dopamine efflux in nucleus accumbens of conscious, freely-moving rats as measured by intracerebral microdialysis. Psychopharmacology 102: 156–162.

43. KORNETSKY, C. 1985. Brain-stimulation reward: A model for the neuronal bases for drug-induced euphoria. NIDA Res. Monogr. 62: 30–50.

44. DI CHIARA, G. & A. IMPERATO. 1988. Drugs abused by humans preferentially increase synaptic dopamine concentrations in the mesolimbic system of freely moving rats. Proc. Natl. Acad. Sci. USA 85: 5274–5278.

45. HARRIS, R. T., W. WATERS & D. McLENDON. 1974. Evaluation of reinforcing capability of Δ⁹-tetrahydrocannabinol in rhesus monkeys. Psychopharmacologia 37: 23–29.

46. LEITE, J. R. & E. A. CARLINI. 1974. Failure to obtain "cannabis-directed behavior" and abstinence syndrome in rats chronically treated with cannabis sativa extracts. Psychopharmacologia 36: 133–145.

47. STARK, P. & P. B. DEWS. 1980. Cannabinoids. I. Behavioral Effects. J. Pharmacol. Exp. Ther. 214: 124–130.

48. GARDNER, E. L., W. PAREDES, D. SMITH, A. DONNER, C. MILLING, D. COHEN & D. MORRISON. 1988. Facilitation of brain stimulation reward by Δ⁹-tetrahydrocannabinol. Psychopharmacology 96: 142–144.

49. GARDNER, E. L., J. CHEN, W. PAREDES, J. LI & D. SMITH. 1989. Strain-specific facilitation of brain stimulation reward by Δ⁹-tetrahydrocannabinol in laboratory rats is mirrored by strain-specific facilitation of presynaptic dopamine efflux in nucleus accumbens. Soc. Neurosci. Abstr. 15: 638.

50. MILLER, L. L. 1984. Marijuana: Acute effects on human memory. In The Cannabinoids: Chemical, Pharmacologic, and Therapeutic Aspects. S. Agurell, W. L. Dewey & R. E. Willette, Eds.: 21–46. Academic Press. New York.

51. DOUGLAS, R. J. 1967. The hippocampus and behavior. Psychol. Bull. 67: 416–442.

52. EICHENBAUM, H. & N. J. COHEN. 1988. Representation in the hippocampus: What do hippocampal neurons encode? Trends Neurosci. 11: 244–248.

53. HOOKER, W. D. & R. T. JONES. 1987. Increased susceptibility to memory intrusions and the Stroop interference effect during acute marijuana intoxication. Psychopharmacology 91: 20–24.

54. SCHULZE, G. E., D. E. McMILLAN, J. R. BAILEY, A. SCALLET, S. F. ALI, W. J. SLIKKER & M. G. PAULE. 1988. Acute effects of Δ-9-tetrahydrocannabinol in rhesus monkeys as measured by performance in a battery of complex operant tests. J. Pharmacol. Exp. Ther. 245: 178–186.

55. CAMPBELL, K. A., T. C. FOSTER, R. E. HAMPSON & S. A. DEADWYLER. 1986. Effects of Δ⁹-tetrahydrocannabinol on sensory-evoked discharges of granule cells in the dentate gyrus of behaving rats. J. Pharmacol. Exp. Ther. 239: 941–945.

56. MARSDEN, C. D. 1981. Treatment of torsion dystonia. In Disorders of Movement, Current Status of Modern Therapy, Vol. 8. A. Barbeau, Ed.: 81–104. Lippincott. Philadelphia.

57. PETRO, D. J. & C. E. ELLENBERGER. 1981. Treatment of human spasticity with delta-9-tetrahydrocannabinol. J. Clin. Pharmacol. 21: 413s–416s.

58. CLIFFORD, D. B. 1983. Tetrahydrocannabinol for tremor in multiple sclerosis. Ann. Neurol. 13: 669–671.

59. MEINCK, H.-M., P. W. SCHONLE & B. CONRAD. 1989. Effect of cannabinoids on spasticity and ataxia in multiple sclerosis. J. Neurol. 236: 120–122.

Opioid and Cannabinoid Receptor Inhibition of Adenylyl Cyclase in Brain[a]

STEVEN R. CHILDERS,[b] LYNNE FLEMING,[c]
CHRIS KONKOY,[c] DON MARCKEL,[c] MARY PACHECO,[c]
TAMMY SEXTON,[b] AND SUSAN WARD[d]

[b] Department of Physiology and Pharmacology
Bowman Gray School of Medicine
Wake Forest University
300 S. Hawthorne Road
Winston-Salem, North Carolina 27103

[c] Departments of Pharmacology and Neuroscience
University of Florida College of Medicine
Gainesville, Florida 32610

[d] Sterling Research Group
Sterling Drug Inc.
Rensselaer, New York 12144

INTRODUCTION

One of the major superfamilies of neurotransmitter receptors is G-protein-coupled receptors (reviewed in refs. 1 and 2). These receptors are pharmacologically distinct, but share many properties, including the fact that agonist binding to these receptors is regulated by guanine nucleotides, and that coupling of these receptors to their respective effectors require GTP. Among the most common effectors for these receptors are regulation of adenylyl cyclase (both stimulation and inhibition), stimulation of phosphoinositol turnover, and direct coupling through G-proteins to ion channels.

At least two major classes of drugs of abuse bind directly to G-protein-linked receptors: opioids and cannabinoids. For opioid receptors, this classification has

[a] This work was supported in part by Public Health Service Grant DA-02904 and DA-06784 from the National Institute on Drug Abuse.

Abbreviations: AAI: aminoalkylindole; App(NH)p: 5'-adenylyl-imidodiphosphate; D-Ala enk: D-ala$_2$-met$_5$-enkephalinamide; DAMGO: tyr-D-ala-gly-NMe-phe-gly-ol; DSLET: D-ser$_2$-thr$_6$-leu-enkephalin; DMEM: Dulbecco's modified Eagles Medium; EGTA: ethylene glycol bis-(β-aminoethyl ether) N,N,N',N'-tetraacetic acid; G$_i$: inhibitory GTP coupling protein; GTP-γS: guanosine-5'-O-(3-thiotriphosphate); IBMX: iso-butylmethylxanthine; nor-BNI: nor-binaltorphimine; NTI: naltrindole; U-50,488H: (trans-(dl)-3,4-dichloro-N-methyl-N-[2-(1-pyrrolidinyl)cyclohexyl]-benzeneacetamide) methane sulfonate.

been known for some years, dating from the initial discoveries that opioid agonists inhibited adenylyl cyclase in brain membranes[3] and neuroblastoma cells,[4-6] to the finding that agonist binding sites were regulated by guanine nucleotides.[7,8] Since then, two major effector systems have been associated with opioid receptors: inhibition of adenylyl cyclase and direct coupling of receptors to Ca^{2+} and K^+ channels through G-proteins.[9-11]

In contrast, the binding of cannabinoids to G-protein-coupled receptors is a recent discovery. The discovery of putative cannabinoid receptor sites was long hampered by lack of suitable ligands, and a clear discovery of cannabinoid receptors did not occur until Howlett's group reported that cannabinoids inhibited adenylyl cyclase in neuroblastoma cells.[12,13] The suggestion that putative cannabinoid receptors were coupled to G-protein-linked receptors was confirmed when a receptor binding assay using the potent radioligand [³H]CP 55,940 demonstrated that cannabinoid agonist binding was sensitive to guanine nucleotides.[14] Later, this receptor was cloned and its deduced amino acid sequence was consistent with other members of this receptor super-family.[15] At this time, the only effector confirmed for the cannabinoid receptor is inhibition of adenylyl cyclase, although preliminary data have suggested that G-protein-linked K^+ channels may be coupled to these receptors (S. Deadwyler, personal communication).

One of the major questions unanswered by previous work on both opioid and cannabinoid receptors involves the biological roles for these second messenger systems. This is particularly true in the case of receptor-mediated inhibition of adenylyl cyclase, whose precise role in the brain has not been clear. In several systems, opioid receptor actions on ion channels do not involve diffusible second messengers like cyclic AMP,[10,11] although one group has reported that opioid effects on Ca^{2+} channels in spinal cord require cyclic AMP.[16] The purpose of the present study was to explore several possible alternatives for the role of receptor-mediated inhibition of adenylyl cyclase for both opioids and cannabinoids. Since the primary role of cyclic AMP is to affect protein phosphorylation,[17] one set of experiments examined the ability of opioid-inhibited adenylyl cyclase to inhibit membrane protein phosphorylation. Another set of studies examined the effect of receptor-inhibited adenylyl cyclase on regulation of pro-enkephalin mRNA levels, since the proenkephalin gene contains a cyclic AMP-responsive element which increases gene expression in the presence of cyclic AMP.[18] A final set of experiments examined the relationship between opioid and cannabinoid actions in cerebellar granule cells, a cell type in which both classes of receptor exist on the same cell and produce the same effect on cyclic AMP levels.

METHODS

Adenylyl Cyclase Assay

Various brain regions were dissected from male Sprague-Dawley rats (150–200 g), and homogenized in Tris-Mg^{2+} buffer (50 mM Tris-HCl, 3 mM $MgCl_2$, pH 7.4) with a Polytron. After centrifugation at $48,000 \times g$ for 10 min, the pellet was resuspended in 1 ml of pH 4.5 buffer (50 mM sodium acetate, 5 mM $MgCl_2$, 1 mM dithiothreitol, 1 mM EGTA, pH 4.5) and incubated with occasional mixing at 0°C for 10 min. The membranes were then diluted with a fivefold excess of Tris-Mg^{2+} buffer, centrifuged, then resuspended in fresh Tris-Mg^{2+} buffer.[19] Adenylyl cyclase activity was assayed as previously described using [^{3}H]ATP as a substrate with an HPLC procedure.[20] Conditions for opioid- and cannabinoid-inhibited adenylyl cyclase have been described previously.[21-23]

Phosphorylation Assay

Rat brain regions were dissected on ice and homogenized by Polytron in Tris-Mg^{2+} buffer containing a cocktail of protease inhibitors (20 μl/ml of a solution containing 0.2 mg/ml each of aprotinin, bestatin, pepstatin, and leupeptin in 50% ethanol-water), and centrifuged at 48,000 $\times$ *g* for 10 min. Brain membranes were pretreated at pH 4.5 (19, 21) and resuspended in assay buffer (50 mM Tris-HCl, 3 mM MgSO$_4$, 2 mM IBMX, pH 7.4) at a concentration of 10 mg protein/ml. Membranes (100 μg protein) were preincubated with 500 μM App(NH)p, 50 μM GTP, 50 mM NaCl, 1 mM EGTA, and various drugs (total volume 40 μl) in assay buffer for 5 min at 30°C. The phosphorylation reaction was initiated by addition of 10 μl [^{32}P]ATP (10 μCi/tube) together with unlabeled ATP (final concentration: 1 μM) and incubated for 20 sec at 30°C. The reaction was terminated by addition of 50 μl electrophoresis buffer (125 mM Tris-HCl, pH 6.8, 4% SDS, 2% glycerol, 10% β-mercaptoethanol, 0.0025% bromphenol blue). The samples were then boiled for 2 min. Aliquots were separated by electrophoresis on a 7%–20% linear gradient acrylamide slab gel.[24] The gels were dried and subjected to autoradiography on Kodak XAR film. Radioactive bands on the autoradiograms were quantitated either by scanning on a Betagen Betascope or by densitometry on a Zeineh densitometer.

Cell Culture Methods

Primary rat forebrain neuronal cultures were prepared by the method of Sumners *et al.*[25] Briefly, brains from one day old Sprague-Dawley rats were removed and placed in an isotonic salt solution containing an antibiotic mixture (100 units/ml penicillin, 0.1 mg/ml streptomycin and 2.5 mg/ml amphotericin B), pH 7.4. The forebrains were minced and suspended in 0.25% trypsin for 10 min at 37°C. DNAse I (160 μg) was added to the suspension for the final 5 min of incubation. The enzymatic dissociation was stopped by addition of 3 vol Dulbecco's modified Eagles Medium (DMEM) with 10% horse serum. Cells were centrifuged at 200 $\times$ *g* for 4 min and resuspended in fresh media supplemented with 10% horse serum and antibiotics, and strained through sterile cheesecloth. Cells were seeded at 3 $\times$ 10^6 cells/ml on tissue culture plates coated with poly-L-lysine and incubated in a humidified atmosphere of 5% CO$_2$/95% air at 37°C. After 3 days, 10 μM cytosine arabinoside (ara-c) was added and cultures were incubated for 2 days. The cultures were then incubated without ara-c for 10–15 days.

Rat cerebellar granule cells were cultured as described previously.[26] Cerebella were removed from 8-day-old rats, minced and incubated with trypsin and DNase as described above for rat forebrain cultures. The cells were resuspended in 10 ml of fresh DMEM with fetal bovine serum (FBS) and 25 mM KCl, triturated 30–40 times and filtered through two layers of sterile gauze. Cells (2 $\times$ 10^6 cells/ml) were plated on 6-well tissue culture plates coated with poly-L-lysine and placed in a humidified (5% CO$_2$/95% air) incubator at 37°C. After 24 h, the medium was replaced with fresh medium containing 25 mM KCl, 10% FBS, antibiotics and 10 μM ara-c. Medium was replaced every 2–3 days and experiments were performed after 8–12 days. For experiments with opioids and cannabinoids, cultures were switched to serum-free DMEM at least 1 h before drug additions, and all cultures were serum-deprived for the same length of time.

Northern Blot Analysis of Pro-Enkephalin mRNA

Primary cultures of rat neonatal forebrain were lysed with 4 M guanidinium isothiocyanate, 25 mM sodium citrate, pH 7.0, 0.5% sarkosysl, 0.1 mM β-mercaptoethanol after two washes in ice-cold phosphate-buffered saline. Total RNA was extracted by the method of Chomczynski and Sacchi.[27] Individual RNA samples were denatured by heating to 65°C in 1.9 M formaldehyde and 50% formamide with 0.5 μg/μl ethidium bromide. Samples were electrophoresed in 1.5% agarose gels containing 1 M formaldehyde, transferred to Zeta-probe nylon membranes (Bio Rad) by capillary action and immobilized by drying at 80°C *in vacuo* for 30 min. For analysis of α-tubulin mRNA, blots were then prehybridized in 5x SSC (1x = 0.15 M NaCl, 15 mM NaH$_2$PO$_4$, 1 mM EDTA), 20 mM Na$_2$HPO$_4$ (pH 7), 7% SDS, 10x Denhardt's solution (1x = 0.02% each of polyvinylpyrrolidone, bovine serum albumin and Ficoll 400), and 100 μg/ml denatured salmon sperm DNA at 50°C for 1–2 h. Blots were hybridized in the same solution with a 5'-phosphorylated 30-base oligonucleotide probe (New England Nuclear) to α-tubulin at 50°C for 4 h. Blots were washed twice in 3x SSC, 25 mM Na$_2$HPO$_4$, 5% SDS and once in 1x SSC, 1% SDS at 50°C for 20 min each. Autoradiography was performed by exposing blots to Kodak X-Omat film with intensifying screens for 4–7 days at −70°C. For analysis of proenkephalin mRNA, blots were stripped by washing in 0.1x SSC and 1% SDS at 95°C for 1 h. Blots were then prehybridized in 4x SSPE, 1% SDS, 5x Denhardt's solution, 50% formamide and 500 μg/ml denatured salmon sperm DNA at 65°C for 1–4 h. Blots were hybridized in the same solution with a 950-base riboprobe (synthesized from pYSEA1 [28], kindly provided by Dr. Steven Sabol) for 20 h at 65°C. Blots were then washed once in 2x SSC and 0.1% SDS and four times in 0.1x SSC and 0.1% SDS at 70°C for 20 min each. Blots were exposed to X-ray film with intensifying screens at −70°C for 1–3 days. All autoradiograms were analyzed on an LKB densitometer. Levels of proenkephalin mRNA were reported as PE (pro-enkephalin mRNA) units, obtained by scanning bands and expressing proenkephalin mRNA levels relative to α-tubulin mRNA. In each blot, 1 PE unit was the ratio between pro-enkephalin and α-tubulin mRNA levels in the control (basal) lane. Each blot represents a typical experiment which was repeated at least twice with similar results.

RESULTS

Properties of Opioid-inhibited Adenylyl Cyclase

Although all opioid receptor types (μ, δ and $\varkappa$) are coupled to G-proteins,[9] the nature of the effector systems coupled to all of these receptor types has not been clear until recently. Both δ[4-6] and μ[29] receptors inhibit adenylyl cyclase in transformed neuroblastoma cells. The present studies explored whether they produce the same effect in non-transformed brain tissue. These experiments were aided by the use of low pH pretreatment of brain membranes, a technique which increases opioid-inhibited adenylyl cyclase.[19,21,22] Under these conditions, in rat brain membranes, both μ and δ receptors produced similar levels of inhibitory activity (FIG. 1). The highest level of μ-inhibited activity was observed in thalamus, using the μ-selective compound DAMGO as an agonist. The highest level of δ-inhibited activity was seen in striatum or frontal cortex (data not shown), using DSLET as an agonist. The selectivity of these responses was confirmed using antagonist blockade experiments (FIG. 2). Addition of 50 nM naloxone, which is relatively μ-selective, completely blocked DAMGO-inhibited adenylyl cyclase while 500 nM naloxone blocked only 50% of the DSLET-inhibited activity. On the other hand, 1 μM naltrindole (NTI), a δ-selective antagonist, had no effect on DAMGO inhibition in thalamus, although 100 nM NTI completely blocked DSLET inhibition in striatum.

The question of whether $\varkappa$ receptors are also coupled to adenylyl cyclase is not straightforward, because currently there is no simple cell culture system which expresses $\varkappa$ receptors. Although one study[30] reported that $\varkappa$ receptors did not inhibit adenylyl cyclase, another study in rat spinal cord demonstrated inhibition of adenylyl cyclase by $\varkappa$ agonists.[31] We[22] showed that the guinea pig cerebellum was an excellent model for $\varkappa$-inhibited adenylyl cyclase. In these membranes, $\varkappa$ agonists, including dynorphin, inhibited basal adenylyl cyclase activity by 40% (FIG. 3). The $\varkappa$ specificity of this response was demonstrated by the finding that the $\varkappa$-selective antagonist nor-binaltorphimine (nor-BNI) was 25 times more potent in blocking dynorphin inhibition than naloxone (FIG. 3). Unlike rat brain, where there is no region which contains only one type of opioid receptor response, the guinea pig cerebellum is totally selective for $\varkappa$-inhibited adenylyl cyclase. In these membranes, neither μ nor δ agonists had any effect on adenylyl cyclase activity up to 10 μM concentrations.[22]

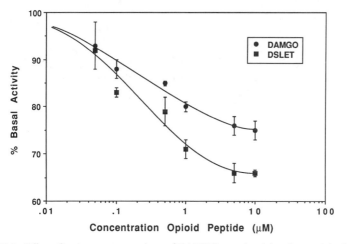

FIGURE 1. Effect of various concentrations of DAMGO on adenylyl cyclase activity in membranes from thalamus, and effect of DSLET in membranes from striatum. In all experiments, opioid-inhibited adenylyl cyclase was enhanced by pretreatment of membranes at pH 4.5 before assay of adenylyl cyclase at pH 7.4. Results are expressed as % of basal activity, assayed in the absence of agonist.

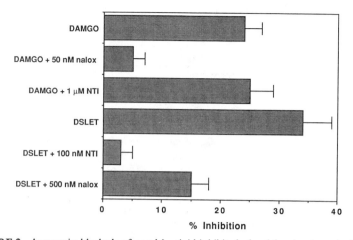

FIGURE 2. Antagonist blockade of μ and δ opioid-inhibited adenylyl cyclase in rat brain membranes. Adenylyl cyclase activity was assayed in striatal membranes in the presence and absence of 10 μM DSLET, and in thalamus membranes in the presence and absence of 10 μM DAMGO. Antagonists (naloxone for μ receptors and naltrindole [NTI] for δ receptors) were added at 0.1 μM. Results are expressed as % inhibition of basal adenylyl cyclase by each agonist.

Properties of Cannabinoid-inhibited Adenylyl Cyclase

Receptor-mediated inhibition of adenylyl cyclase by cannabinoids was previously established in neuroblastoma cells[12] and in brain.[32] In both cases, the agonists were either traditional cannabinoids like THC, or potent cannabinoid analogs like CP-

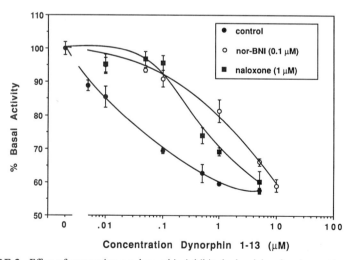

FIGURE 3. Effect of antagonists on dynorphin-inhibited adenylyl cyclase in membranes from guinea pig cerebellum. Adenylyl cyclase was assayed in low pH pretreated cerebellar membranes with various concentrations of dynorphin A_{1-13}, in the presence and absence of 0.1 μM nor-BNI or 1 μM naloxone. Data are expressed as % of basal activity assayed in the absence of agonist.

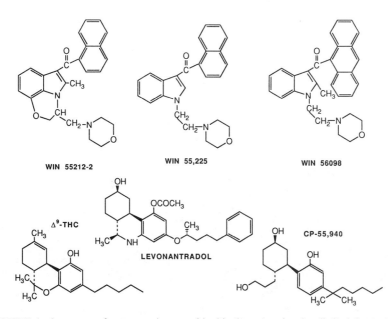

FIGURE 4. Structures of representative cannabinoids (*bottom*) and aminoalkylindoles (*top*). In the aminoalkylindole series, WIN 55212-2 and WIN 55225 are agonists, while WIN 56098 is a putative antagonist.

55,940. A major breakthrough in the pharmacology of the cannabinoids occurred with the development of aminoalkylindoles (AAI's). These compounds were not originally synthesized as THC analogs, but nevertheless bound with high affinity to cannabinoid receptors and produced THC-like biological effects.[23,33] The AAI series consists of both agonists and antagonists (FIG. 4). The AAI agonists are exemplified by WIN 55,212-2, the most potent AAI agonist, and WIN 55,225, an agonist of moderate potency. The AAI antagonists include WIN 56,098 which, although relatively weak (with pA_2 values in the μM range), represent the first authentic cannabinoid receptor antagonist to be developed.

In brain membranes (particularly in cerebellum), AAI agonists inhibited adenylyl cyclase in a GTP-dependent manner (FIG. 5). In this experiment, WIN 55212-2 inhibited adenylyl cyclase activity by 40% in the presence of 50 μM GTP, but had no effect on activity in the absence of GTP. These results suggested that AAI agonists acted through G-protein–linked receptors.[23]

The cannabinoid nature of this response in cerebellar membranes was demonstrated with AAI antagonists (FIG. 6). In FIGURE 6A, addition of 2 μM of the AAI antagonist WIN 56098 produced a fivefold rightward shift in the dose-response curve of the agonist WIN 55212-2. The cannabinoid analog levonantradol (FIG. 6B) inhibited adenylyl cyclase to the same extent as AAI agonists; furthermore, WIN 56098 (2 μM) produced a fourfold shift in the levonantradol dose-response curve. In contrast, the AAI antagonist had no effect on actions of other receptor agonists in several systems, including inhibition of adenylyl cyclase and contractions of mouse vas deferens.[23]

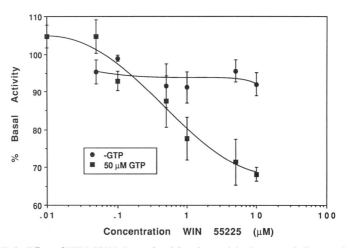

FIGURE 5. Effect of WIN 55212-2 on adenylyl cyclase activity in rat cerebellar membranes in the presence and absence of 50 μM GTP.

These data suggested that AAI's and cannabinoids may bind to the same receptors, and established the use of AAI antagonists as specific cannabinoid-blocking agents *in vitro*.

Receptor binding studies, using both the traditional cannabinoid radioligand [^{3}H]CP 55,940 as well as [^{3}H]WIN 55212-2, have established the cannabinoid nature of these putative AAI receptors.[33] These experiments have shown that unlabeled cannabinoids and AAI's inhibit the binding of [^{3}H]CP 55,940 and [^{3}H]WIN 55,212-2 with similar IC$_{50}$ values. Moreover, cannabinoids and AAI's inhibit adenylyl cyclase in brain membranes in a similar fashion. For example, the regional distributions of AAI-inhibited adenylyl cyclase (using WIN 55212-2 as an agonist) and cannabinoid-inhibited adenylyl cyclase (using levonantradol as an agonist) are identical (FIG. 7). In both cases, the highest level of inhibition occurred in cerebellum and striatum, with lower inhibition observed in the frontal cortex and no significant inhibition in other regions. Interestingly, this distribution parallels the localization of cannabinoid receptor binding as determined by autoradiography,[34] with the major exception of hippocampus, where relatively high levels of binding are not paralleled by significant cannabinoid inhibition of adenylyl cyclase.

Receptor-mediated Inhibition of Protein Phosphorylation: Immediate Targets of the Adenylyl Cyclase System

The long-established role for cyclic AMP is stimulation of protein kinase,[17] and receptor inhibition of adenylyl cyclase should inhibit phosphorylation of a variety of phosphoprotein substrates. In order to identify which membrane proteins would be most affected by receptor inhibition of adenylyl cyclase, we analyzed the effect of opioid agonists on protein phosphorylation under conditions where opioids inhibit adenylyl cyclase. These experiments utilized App(NH)p, an ATP analog which is a sub-

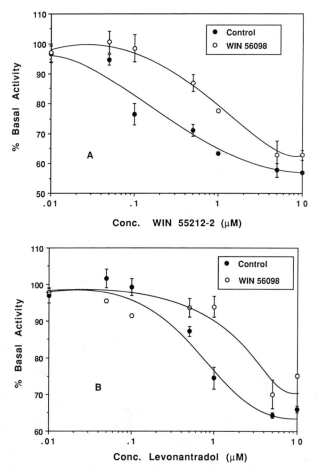

Conc.   WIN 55212-2 (μM)

Conc. Levonantradol (μM)

FIGURE 6. Effect of the AAI antagonist WIN 56098 (2 μM) on AAI and cannabinoid inhibition of adenylyl cyclase in rat cerebellar membranes. The agonists used were: **A**, WIN 55212-2; **B**, levonantradol.

strate for adenylyl cyclase but is not recognized by most protein kinases.[35] The reaction used in these studies was the following:

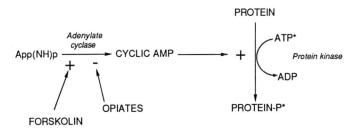

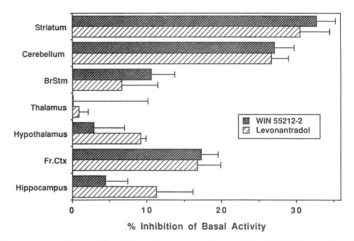

FIGURE 7. Comparison of the effects of levonantradol and WIN 55212-2 on adenylyl cyclase in various rat brain regions. Data are the mean values ±SD of experiments using maximally effective concentrations of each agonist (2 μM in each case).

In this reaction, brain membranes were preincubated with GTP, sodium, and unlabeled App(NH)p in the presence and absence of opioid agonists and forskolin. Then protein phosphorylation was initiated with $[\gamma\text{-}^{32}P]ATP$. Cyclic AMP formed by adenylyl cyclase acting on App(NH)p would be increased by forskolin and decreased by opioid-inhibited adenylyl cyclase. The effect of this reaction on protein phosphorylation in striatal membranes is shown in FIGURE 8. In the absence of App(NH)p (first three lanes), forskolin had no effect on protein phosphorylation because no substrate for adenylyl cyclase was present; similarly, the opioid agonist D-ala enk (which inhibited adenylyl cyclase by 30–35% in the same membranes) had no effect on protein phosphorylation. The last three lanes show the results when 500 μM App(NH)p was added during the preincubation step. App(NH)p alone had minimal effects on labeling, consistent with the idea that App(NH)p is not recognized by most protein kinases.[35] Forskolin (0.1 μM) stimulated the labeling of several bands in the presence of App(NH)p; two bands in particular, MW 65 and 83 kDa, were also stimulated by addition of cyclic AMP in the absence of App(NH)p (not shown). Finally, D-ala enk added together with forskolin and App(NH)p decreased labeling of these same two bands to levels similar to basal labeling without forskolin.

The inhibition of protein phosphorylation by opioid agonists is produced through opioid-inhibited adenylyl cyclase. This conclusion is supported by the data in TABLE 1, which shows the quantitative analysis of opioid effects under a variety of conditions, including: 1) the average opioid inhibition of labeling of both 63 kDa and 85 kDa bands was 25%, similar to the 30% inhibition of adenylyl cyclase activity in striatal membranes; 2) opioid-inhibited phosphorylation was blocked by naloxone; 3) opioid-inhibited phosphorylation required GTP, and was not detected either in the absence of GTP or in the presence of non-hydrolyzable GTP analogs such as GTP-γS; 4) opioid-inhibited phosphorylation was observed in rat striatum but not in rat cerebellum, an area devoid of opioid receptors; 5) opioid-inhibited phosphorylation required sodium. All of these data fit the criteria for receptor-mediated inhibition of adenylyl cyclase.

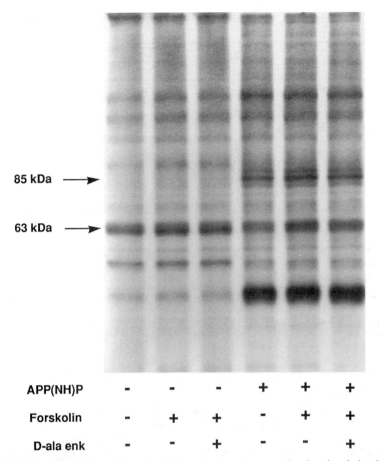

FIGURE 8. Effects of App(NH)p, forskolin and D-ala enk on protein phosphorylation in rat striatal membranes. Experiments in the first three lanes were conducted in the absence of App(NH)p, while those in the last three lanes were conducted in the presence of 500 μM App(NH)p. In each lane, the various additions refer to compounds added to the membranes during a 10 min preincubation step before addition of 1 μM [^{32}P]ATP to all experiments. *Lane 1*, basal (no additions); *lane 2*, 0.1 μM forskolin; *lane 3*, forskolin + 10 μM D-ala enk; *lane 4*, 500 μM App(NH)p; *lane 5*, App(NH)p + forskolin; *lane 6*, App(NH)p + forskolin + D-ala enk.

The identities of the 63 and 85 kDa bands are currently being determined. Interestingly, in two-dimensional electrophoresis (not shown), the 85 kDa band is extremely basic (pI > 9), while the 63 kDa band is neutral (pI ~ 7). These properties, together with their molecular weights and their ability to be phosphorylated by cyclic AMP, make it likely that these two bands are synapsins, with the 85 kDa band being synapsin I and the 63 kDa band being synapsin II.[17] These preliminary identifications are currently being confirmed with specific antibodies.

TABLE 1. Analysis of Opioid-Inhibited Phosphorylation of 63 kDa and 85 kDa Bands

Condition	D-Ala Enk (20 µM)	% Forskolin-stimulated Phosphorylation	
		85 kDa ± SEM	63 kDa ± SEM
Guanine nucleotides			
None	+	93 ± 4 (5)	95 ± 2 (5)
50 µM GTP	+	75 ± 9 (5)*	78 ± 7 (5)*
50 µM GTP-γ-S	+	95 ± 7 (5)	98 ± 12 (5)
NaCl			
None	+	108 ± 5 (3)	103 ± 5 (3)
50 mM	+	76 ± 11 (3)*	80 ± 10 (3)*
Naloxone			
None	+	76 ± 0.6 (4)*	78 ± 10 (4)*
1 µM Naloxone	+	106 ± 6 (4)	105 ± 7 (4)
1 µM Naloxone	−	104 ± 16 (4)	98 ± 12 (4)
Regions			
Striatum	+	75 ± 6 (13)*	75 ± 7 (13)*
Cerebellum	+	104 ± 9 (3)	102 ± 11 (3)

Data were calculated from scanning of bands as described in METHODS. All data are expressed as percent [32P] labeling in the presence of 0.1 µM forskolin and 500 µM App(NH)p. Forskolin stimulated labeling by approximately 200% (for both bands) compared to basal labeling. Data are mean values ± SE; ( ), number of separate experiments. * $p \leq 0.05$ vs. control (forskolin + App(NH)p), by Student's unpaired t-test.

Long-term Roles for Receptor-inhibited Adenylyl Cyclase: Regulation of Neuropeptide mRNA

One of the functions of cyclic AMP in the cell is to produce long-term changes through genomic regulation. For example, a number of neuropeptide genes contain cyclic AMP responsive elements (CRE's) which stimulate mRNA synthesis when activated by cyclic AMP.[18] To test the hypothesis that receptor-mediated inhibition of adenylyl cyclase might play a regulatory role in this process, we examined whether opioid-inhibited adenylyl cyclase could attenuate the expression of pro-enkephalin mRNA in cell culture. The system chosen for these studies was primary neuronal culture of neonatal rat forebrain.[25] These cultures were effective models since they could be enriched with neurons, and they contained both opioid-inhibited adenylyl cyclase as well as relatively high levels of pro-enkephalin mRNA. When these cells were cultured for 10–14 days from neonatal rat brain, assays of intracellular cyclic AMP levels were performed to determine whether opioid-inhibited adenylyl cyclase could be detected. Results (FIG. 9) showed that although δ- and µ-selective agonists had no effect, dynorphin A_{1-13} (1 µM) decreased intracellular cyclic AMP by more than 50%, with dynorphin A producing a smaller but still significant reduction. Moreover, the inhibition by dynorphin was blocked by naloxone.

These cells were then assayed for pro-enkephalin mRNA content by Northern

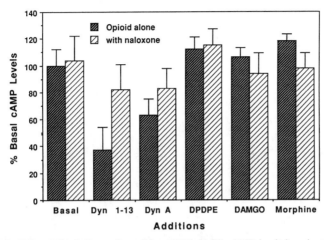

FIGURE 9. Effects of opioid agonists on intracellular cyclic AMP levels in primary neuronal cultures of neonatal rat forebrain. After leaving the cells in serum-free media overnight, cultures were incubated with the indicated agonists at 1 μM concentrations for 10 min in Hanks buffered saline solution before adding 1 μM forskolin and incubating for an additional 10 min. Cyclic AMP levels were determined in extracts from cultures as described in METHODS.

analysis (TABLE 2). In all cases, cells were incubated with forskolin in the presence and absence of 1 μM dynorphin A_{1-13} for 4 h before extraction of RNA. In this time period, forskolin (1 μM) increased pro-enkephalin mRNA levels by approximately two-fold. Moreover, dibutyryl cyclic AMP (600 μM) produced approximately the same increase. These results demonstrated that these cells contain active CREs which stimulated mRNA levels by cyclic AMP. To determine the effect of opioid agonists on the forskolin-stimulated pro-enkephalin mRNA levels, cells were treated for 4 h with forskolin and dynorphin A_{1-13} (1 μM). Results from 12 different experiments showed that dynorphin A_{1-13} decreased forskolin-stimulated pro-enkephalin mRNA levels by 38%, similar to the degree of inhibition of intracellular cyclic AMP levels by dynorphin A_{1-13}. As shown in TABLE 2, the dynorphin effect on forskolin-stimulated mRNA levels was blocked by naloxone, and was not detected in cells treated overnight with pertussis toxin (100 ng/ml). These data suggested that the dynorphin response was mediated through genuine opioid receptors coupled through G-proteins. To confirm that opioid-inhibited adenylyl cyclase was responsible for the dynorphin response, the effect of dynorphin A_{1-13} was compared in cells treated with forskolin or with dibutyryl cyclic AMP. If opioid-inhibited adenylyl cyclase were responsible for the dynorphin effect on pro-enkephalin mRNA, then the opioid agonist should have no effect on mRNA levels stimulated with dibutyryl cyclic AMP. Results (TABLE 2) showed that although dynorphin A_{1-13} decreased pro-enkephalin mRNA by 38% in forskolin-treated cells, it had no significant effect on cells treated with dibutyryl cyclic AMP. These data confirm that opioid-inhibited adenylyl cyclase plays a long-term role in regulating pro-enkephalin synthesis, and provides a mechanism for a negative feedback loop for opioid synthesis.

TABLE 2. Northern Analysis of Pro-enkephalin mRNA Levels in Primary Cultures of Neonatal Rat Forebrain Neurons

Treatment	PE Units	% Stimulated Levels
A. Untreated cells		
Basal	1.00	–
Forskolin (1 μM)	1.86	100
Forskolin + dynorphin A_{1-13} (1 μM)	1.15	62
Forskolin + dynorphin + naloxone (1 μM)	1.92	103
Dibutyryl cAMP (600 μM)	1.73	100
db-cAMP + dynorphin	1.75	104
B. Pertussis toxin-treated cells		
Basal	1.00	–
Forskolin	2.23	100
Forskolin + dynorphin	2.01	90

Primary cultures of neonatal rat forebrain neurons were cultured for 10–14 days. Before drug treatments, cells were deprived of serum for 24 h, then incubated with forskolin, dibutyryl cyclic AMP and appropriate concentrations of dynorphin A_{1-13} for 4 h before lysis of cells and extraction of RNA. Other cells were treated with pertussis toxin (100 ng/ml) for 18 h before addition of drugs. Following RNA extraction, pro-enkephalin mRNA levels were determined by Northern analysis as described in METHODS. Results are expressed as pro-enkephalin mRNA (PE) units determined by normalizing pro-enkephalin mRNA vs. α-tubulin mRNA as described.

Relationship between Cannabinoid and Opioid Adenylyl Cyclase Systems

Although cannabinoids and opioids bind to different receptors, they both inhibit adenylyl cyclase. This commonality of effector system suggests that if the two types of receptors exist on the same cells, they may produce the same biological response. This situation may exist in the cerebellum, where both receptors appear to be present on cerebellar granule cells. FIGURE 10 shows the results of an agonist additivity experiment, in which agonists for different receptors were added at maximally effective concentrations to an adenylyl cyclase assay containing guinea pig cerebellar membranes. In addition to an opioid agonist (U-50488H) and a cannabinoid agonist (WIN 55212-2), the experiment also contained a $GABA_B$ agonist (baclofen) and an adenosine A_1 agonist (phenylisopropyladenosine, PIA). Previous studies have shown that all of these receptors inhibit adenylyl cyclase in cerebellum, and in the rat, the $GABA_B$ and A_1 receptors exist together on cerebellar granule cells.[36] Results (FIG. 10) revealed that the 25–30% inhibition of activity by each agonist alone was increased to only 30–35% inhibition when two different agonist were added together. In other words, there was only a partial additivity of response, thus suggesting that at least some of these receptors may be co-localized in cerebellar granule cells. To confirm this hypothesis, granule cells were cultured from both rat and guinea pig cerebellum, and effects of both cannabinoids and opioids on intracellular cyclic AMP levels were determined (data not shown). In rat cerebellar granule cells, cannabinoid analogs inhibited forskolin-stimulated cyclic AMP levels by 50–70%; these actions were blocked by

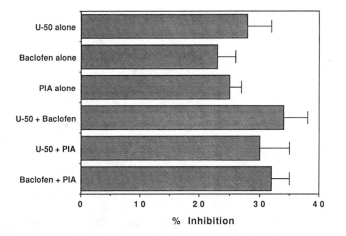

FIGURE 10. Additivity of various receptor agonists in inhibiting adenylyl cyclase in guinea pig cerebellar membranes. Each agonist was added either alone or in combination with a second agonist, and results were expressed as per cent of basal activity assayed in the absence of any agonist. All agonists were added at maximally effective concentrations, determined from dose response curves for each agonist alone (not shown).

AAI antagonists and by pertussis toxin. In guinea pig cerebellar granule cells, the same effect was observed with dynorphin A_{1-13} and U-50488H. These data suggest that these different receptor types exist on the same cells.

DISCUSSION

The coupling of opioid and cannabinoid receptors to adenylyl cyclase is typical of the G-protein-linked receptor superfamily. These reactions require GTP, they are not supported by non-hydrolyzable guanine nucleotide analogs, and they are abolished by pertussis toxin treatment. All three of the opioid receptor types (μ, $\varkappa$, and δ) inhibit adenylyl cyclase in brain membranes. Although the pharmacology of these receptor responses generally agree with the pharmacology of receptor binding assays, the potencies of agonists in inhibiting adenylyl cyclase are several orders of magnitude weaker than the potencies of the same agonists in displacing receptor binding in brain membranes. However, this discrepancy is explained by the requirement of sodium and GTP for receptor coupling to adenylyl cyclase.[6] Under these conditions, the nanomolar potencies of agonists are shifted to low affinity states in which micromolar potencies become common.[7,8] A similar discrepancy exists for cannabinoid inhibition of adenylyl cyclase compared to receptor binding,[14,23] and the explanation is the same.

Despite a considerable number of studies characterizing the inhibition of adenylyl cyclase in brain by both opioids and cannabinoids, the biological functions of these second messenger systems, and the roles that these systems play in the chronic actions of these drugs of abuse, are still not understood. In the opioid system, most (but not all) studies have agreed that the acute actions of opioid agonists in regulating ion channels are mediated through direct receptor-G-protein coupling to channels.[10] Although cyclic AMP may regulate some aspects of channel function,[11] the direct electrophysiological actions of opioids in these systems may not involve a diffusible second messenger. To examine the role of receptor-mediated inhibition of adenylyl cyclase in the actions of these drugs, the present study explored two possible actions of this second messenger system: inhibition of cyclic AMP-dependent phosphorylation of specific membrane proteins, and the regulation of pro-enkephalin mRNA by opioid-inhibited adenylyl cyclase.

Although a number of previous studies reported effects of opioid agonists on protein phosphorylation in brain membranes,[37,38] the present study represents the first effort to identify specific phosphoprotein substrates of the receptor-G_i-adenylyl cyclase cascade. These experiments required the development of a unique assay which utilized App(NH)p as an adenylyl cyclase substrate to characterize opiate-inhibited protein phosphorylation. It is important to note that this reaction should not be specific to opioid receptors. Indeed, the reaction is designed so that any receptor which inhibits adenylyl cyclase should produce similar results as long as the proper components are present in the membranes. These results suggest that the biological endpoints of cannabinoid- and opioid-inhibited adenylyl cyclase may be similar.

Two of the primary candidates for this reaction may be synapsins I and II. Such an identification provides a potential functional significance for opioid-inhibited adenylyl cyclase. It is well known that one of the primary actions of opioids is inhibition of neurotransmitter release.[39] In addition, studies using purified synapsin showed that phosphorylation of synapsin increases neurotransmitter release in the squid giant axon.[40] It is interesting to speculate that opiate-inhibited synapsin phosphorylation may contribute to opioid-inhibited neurotransmitter release. Preliminary results from our laboratory (L. Fleming and S. Childers, unpublished observations) have shown that the phosphorylation of these bands were increased during chronic morphine treatment. Again, it is tempting to speculate that cellular compensation for the acute inhibitory actions of opioids on synapsin phosphorylation may lead to increased phosphorylation, and thus blunt the actions of opioids in this system.

Other roles of opioid-inhibited adenylyl cyclase may include long-term regulatory functions in the cell. The finding that cyclic AMP increases pro-enkephalin mRNA expression[18] suggested that inhibition of intracellular cyclic AMP may produce the opposite effect. The well-known finding that chronic morphine treatment decreased pro-enkephalin mRNA levels in rat striatum[41] suggested that opioids could act through inhibition of adenylyl cyclase to regulate their own synthesis. Our studies located an ideal model to test this hypothesis: primary neuronal cultures from neonatal rat forebrain. These cells contained both opioid-inhibited adenylyl cyclase and pro-enkephalin mRNA, and they could be manipulated in various ways to test the hypothesis. The results showed that an opioid agonist, dynorphin A_{1-13}, reduced forskolin-stimulated pro-enkephalin mRNA levels by acting on a G-protein-linked opioid receptor. Moreover, since dynorphin had no effect on dibutyryl cyclic AMP-stimulated pro-enkephalin mRNA, these actions appeared to be mediated by opioid-inhibited adenylyl cyclase. These data suggest that one of the roles of opioid-inhibited adenylyl cyclase in brain is to act as a feedback regulator of endogenous opioid synthesis. In this model, high concentrations of enkephalin released from presynaptic stores would act at presynaptic opioid receptors to inhibit adenylyl cyclase and decrease pro-enkephalin gene expression. Such a mechanism would not only be important in the actions of opioid receptors, but also might be mediated by other receptors which inhibit adenylyl cyclase as well. Future studies will focus on these potential relationships.

Finally, the study of second messenger systems coupled to these receptors has also revealed an interesting potential relationship between cannabinoid and opioid receptors. The present studies have suggested that both cannabinoid and opioid receptors (together with adenosine A_1 and $GABA_B$ receptors) are present on cerebellar granule cells. The finding that maximally effective concentrations of these agonists do not provide an additive response further suggests that at least some of these receptors are present on the same cells and share common effectors.[36] Although cannabinoids and opioids bind to different receptor types with different pharmacological specificities, the fact that they share effectors suggests that they also share a common biological response. Because of common effectors, the phenomenon of receptor convergence may be important in certain cells in the central nervous system. In these cells, we predict that different receptor agonists would produce identical biological responses. Whether such receptor convergence is important in the relationship of effects of opioids and cannabinoids has yet to be determined.

SUMMARY

Both opioids and cannabinoids bind to G-protein-coupled receptors to inhibit adenylyl cyclase in neurons. These reactions were assayed in brain membranes, where maximal inhibitory activity occurred in the following regions: μ-opioid inhibition in rat thalamus, δ-opioid inhibition in rat striatum, $\varkappa$-opioid inhibition in guinea pig cerebellum, and cannabinoid inhibition in cerebellum. The inhibition of adenylyl cyclase by both cannabinoid and opioid agonists was typical of G-protein-linked receptors: they required GTP, they were not supported by non-hydrolyzable GTP analogs, and they were abolished (in primary neuronal cell culture) by pertussis toxin treatment. The immediate targets of this system were determined by assaying protein phosphorylation in the presence of receptor agonists and App(NH)p, a substrate for adenylyl cyclase. In striatal membranes, opioid agonists inhibited the phosphorylation of at least two bands of MW 85 and 63 kDa, which may be synapsins I and II, respectively. Other experiments determined the long-term effects of this second messenger system. In primary neuronal cultures, opioid-inhibited adenylyl cyclase attenuated forskolin-stimulated pro-enkephalin mRNA levels, thus providing a feedback regulation of opioid synthesis. Finally, in cerebellar granule cells, both cannabinoid and opioid receptors may exist on the same cells. In these cells, agonists which bind to different receptor types may produce similar biological responses.

REFERENCES

1. GILMAN, A. G. 1984. G proteins and dual control of adenylate cyclase. Cell 36: 577–579.
2. NEER, E. J. & D. E. CLAPHAM. 1988. Roles of G-protein subunits in transmembrane signalling. Nature 133: 129–133.
3. COLLIER, H. O. J. & A. C. ROY. 1974. Morphine-like drugs inhibit the stimulation by E prostaglandins of cyclic AMP formation by rat brain homogenates. Nature 248: 24–27.
4. SHARMA, S. K., M. NIREMBERG & W. KLEE. 1975. Morphine receptors as regulators of adenylate cyclase activity. Proc. Natl. Acad. Sci. USA 72: 590–594.

5. TRABER, F., R. GULLIS & B. HAMPRECHT. 1975. Influence of opiates on levels of adenosine 3',5'-monophosphate in neuroblastoma × glioma hybrid cells. Life Sci. **16:** 1863–1868.

6. BLUME, A. J., L. LICHTSHTEIN & G. BOONE. 1979. Coupling of opiate receptors to adenylate cyclase: Requirement for sodium and GTP. Proc. Natl. Acad. Sci. USA **76:** 5626–5630.

7. BLUME, A. J. 1978. Interactions of ligands with opiate receptors of brain membranes: Regulation by ions and nucleotides. Proc. Natl. Acad. Sci. USA **75:** 1713–1717.

8. CHILDERS, S. R. & S. H. SNYDER. 1980. Differential regulation by guanine nucleotide of opiate agonist and antagonist receptor interactions. J. Neurochem. **34:** 583–593.

9. CHILDERS, S. R. 1991. Opioid receptor-coupled second messenger systems. Life Sci. **48:** 1991–2003.

10. NORTH, R. A., J. T. WILLIAMS, A. SURPRENANT & M. J. CHRISTIE. 1987. μ and δ receptors belong to a family of receptors that are coupled to potassium channels. Proc. Natl. Acad. Sci. USA **84:** 5487–5491.

11. GROSS, R. A., H. C. MOISES, M. D. UHLER & R. L. MACDONALD. 1990. Dynorphin A and cAMP-dependent protein kinase independently regulate neuronal calcium currents. Proc. Natl. Acad. Sci. USA **87:** 7025–7029.

12. HOWLETT, A. C. 1985. Cannabinoid inhibition of adenylate cyclase. Biochemistry of the response in neuroblastoma cell membranes. Mol. Pharmacol. **27:** 429–436.

13. HOWLETT, A. C., J. M. QUALY & L. L. KHACHATRIAN. 1986. Involvement of G_i in the inhibition of adenylate cyclase by cannabimimetic drugs. Mol. Pharmacol. **29:** 307–313.

14. DEVANE, W. A., F. A. DYSARZ, M. R. JOHNSON, L. S. MELVIN & A. C. HOWLETT. 1988. Determination and characterization of a cannabinoid receptor in rat brain. Mol. Pharmacol. **34:** 605–613.

15. MATSUDA, L. A., S. J. LOLAIT, M. J. BROWNSTEIN, A. C. YOUNG & T. I. BONNER. 1990. Structure of a cannabinoid receptor and functional expression of the cloned cDNA. Nature **346:** 561–564.

16. CHEN, G. G., A. CHALAZONITIS, K. F. SHEN & S. M. CRAIN. 1988. Inhibitor of cyclic AMP-dependent protein kinase blocks opioid-induced prolongation of the action potential of mouse sensory ganglion neurons in dissociated cell cultures. Brain Res. **462:** 372–377.

17. NESTLER, E. J., S. I. WALAAS & P. GREENGARD. 1984. Neuronal phosphoproteins: Physiological and clinical implications. Science **225:** 1357–1364.

18. COMB, M., N. C. BIRNBERG, A. SEASHOLTZ, E. HERBERT & H. M. GOODMAN. 1986. A cyclic AMP- and phorbol ester-inducible DNA element. Nature **323:** 353–356.

19. CHILDERS, S. R. & G. LARIVIERE. 1984. Modification of guanine nucleotide regulatory components in brain membranes: II. Relationship of guanosine-5'triphosphate effects on opiate receptor binding and coupling receptors with adenylate cyclase. J. Neurosci. **4:** 2764–2771.

20. CHILDERS, S. R. 1986. A high performance liquid chromatography assay of brain adenylyl cyclase using [³H]-ATP as substrate. Neurochem. Res. **11:** 161–171.

21. CHILDERS, S. R. 1988. Opiate-inhibited adenylate cyclase in rat brain membranes depleted of Gs-stimulated adenylate cyclase. J. Neurochem. **50:** 543–553.

22. KONKOY, C. S. & S. R. CHILDERS. 1989. Dynorphin-selective inhibition of adenylyl cyclase in guinea pig cerebellum membranes. Mol. Pharmacol. **36:** 627–633.

23. PACHECO, M., S. R. CHILDERS, R. ARNOLD, F. CASIANO & S. J. WARD. 1991. Aminoalkylindoles: Actions on specific G-protein-linked receptors. J. Pharmacol. Exp. Ther. **257:** 170–183.

24. LAEMMLI, U. K. 1970. Cleavage of structural proteins during the assembly of the head of bacteriophage T4. Nature **227:** 680–685.

25. SUMNERS, C., M. I. PHILLIPS & M. K. RAIZADA. 1983. Rat brain cells in primary culture: Visualization and measurement of catecholamines. Brain Res. **264:** 265–275.

26. WOJCIK, W. J. & N. H. NEFF. 1983. Adenosine A₁ receptors are associated with cerebellar granule cells. J. Neurochem. **41:** 759–763.

27. CHOMCZYNSKI, P. & N. SACCHI. 1987. Single-step method of RNA isolation by acid guanidinium thiocyanate-phenol-chloroform extraction. Anal. Biochem. **162:** 156–159.

28. YOSHIKAWA, K., J. S. HONG & S. L. SABOL. 1985. Electroconvulsive shock increases pre-

proenkephalin messenger RNA abundance in rat hypothalamus. Proc. Natl. Acad. Sci. USA **82:** 589–593.

29. YU, V. C., S. EIGER, D. S. DUAN, J. LAMEH & W. SADEE. 1990. Regulation of cyclic AMP by the mu-opioid receptor in human neuroblastoma SH-SY5Y cells. J. Neurochem. **55:** 1390–1396.

30. POLASTRON, J., M. J. BOYER, Y. QUERTERMONT, J. P. THOUVENOT, J. C. MEUNIER & P. JAUZAC. 1990. Mu-opioid receptors and not kappa-opioid receptors are coupled to the adenylate cyclase in the cerebellum. J. Neurochem. **54:** 562–570.

31. ATTALI, B., D. SAYA & Z. VOGEL. 1989. Kappa-opiate agonists inhibit adenylate cyclase and produce heterologous desensitization in rat spinal cord. J. Neurochem. **52:** 360–369.

32. BIDAUT-RUSSELL, M., W. A. DEVANE & A. C. HOWLETT. 1990. Cannabinoid receptors and modulation of cyclic AMP in the rat brain. J. Neurochem. **55:** 21–26.

33. HAYCOCK, D. A., J. E. KUSTLER, J. I. STEPHENSON, S. J. WARD & T. D'AMBRA. 1990. Characterization of aminoalkylindole binding: Selective displacement by cannabinoids. NIDA Res. Monogr. **105:** 304–305.

34. HERKENHAM, M., A. B. LYNN, M. D. LITTLE, M. R. JOHNSON, L. S. MELVIN, B. R. DeCOSTA & K. C. RICE. 1990. Cannabinoid receptor localization in brain. Proc. Natl. Acad. Sci. USA **87:** 1932–1936.

35. YOUNT, R. G., D. BABCOCK, W. BALLANTYNE & D. OJALA. 1971. Adenylyl imidodiphosphate, an adenosine triphosphate analog containing a P-N-P linkage. Biochemistry **10:** 2484–2489.

36. Wojcik, W. J., D. Cavalla & N. H. NEFF. 1985. Co-localized adenosine A_1 and $GABA_B$ receptors of cerebellum may share a common adenylyl cyclase catalytic unit. J. Pharmacol. Exp. Ther. **232:** 62–66.

37. EHRLICH, Y. H., K. A. BONNET, L. G. DAVIS & E. G. BRUNNGRABER. 1978. Decreased phosphorylation of specific proteins in neostriatal membranes from rats after long-term narcotics exposure. Life Sci. **23:** 137–146.

38. NESTLER, E. J. & J. F. TALLMAN. 1988. Chronic morphine treatment increases cyclic AMP-dependent protein kinase activity in the rat locus coeruleus. Mol. Pharmacol. **33:** 127–132.

39. COX, B. M. & M. WEINSTOCK. 1966. The effects of analgesic drugs on the release of acetylcholine from electrically stimulated guinea-pig ileum. Br. J. Pharmacol. **27:** 81–92.

40. LLINAS, R., T. L. MCGUINNESS, C. S. LEONARD, M. SUGIMORI & P. GREENGARD. 1985. Intraterminal injection of synapsin I or calcium/calmodulin-dependent protein kinase II alters neurotransmitter release at the squid giant synapse. Proc. Natl. Acad. Sci. USA **82:** 3035–3039.

NMDA Receptors: Role in Ethanol Withdrawal Seizures

PAULA L. HOFFMAN,[a] KATHLEEN A. GRANT,
LAWRENCE D. SNELL,[a] LESLIE REINLIB,
AND KAREN IORIO[a]

Laboratory of Physiologic and Pharmacologic Studies
National Institute on Alcohol Abuse and Alcoholism
Rockville, Maryland 20852

BORIS TABAKOFF

Department of Pharmacology
University of Colorado Health Sciences Center
4200 East Ninth Avenue
Denver, Colorado 80262

MECHANISMS OF ETHANOL WITHDRAWAL

Physical dependence on ethanol is defined by the presence of an ethanol withdrawal syndrome that becomes apparent following cessation of ethanol intake and elimination of ethanol from the individual. This withdrawal syndrome has been well-characterized in humans as well as in animal models,[1] and consists of several symptoms that have been classified as early (tremor, diaphoresis, hallucinations, convulsions) and later (delirium tremens, increased autonomic activity and profuse sweating, profound disorientation).[2] Many neurochemical alterations have been described during ethanol withdrawal,[3,4] and it is likely that changes in the activity of certain neuronal systems contribute to specific withdrawal symptoms. In particular, recent studies have begun to elucidate the neurochemistry of ethanol withdrawal seizures. These seizures have certain characteristics of grand mal seizures, and are more likely to occur in individuals with a history of ethanol withdrawal or epileptic seizures.[1] In fact, it has been postulated that ethanol withdrawal may be likened to kindling,[5] in that repeated episodes of ethanol withdrawal result in more rapid development of physical dependence and a more severe withdrawal syndrome.[5,6] Therefore, the mechanisms that have been proposed to underlie the development of kindling may serve as a framework for studying the neurochemical basis for ethanol withdrawal seizures. Two neuronal systems that have been found to be very sensitive to modulation by ethanol (see below) have also been implicated in long-term synaptic potentiation (LTP), a model for neuroadaptation, as well as in kindling processes. These are the γ-amino-

---

[a] *Present address:* Department of Pharmacology, C236, University of Colorado Health Sciences Center, 4200 East Ninth Avenue, Denver, CO 80262.

butyric acid (GABA) and glutamate systems, which are the major inhibitory and excitatory neurotransmitter systems, respectively, of brain. In particular, the characteristics of the N-methyl-D-aspartate (NMDA) subtype of glutamate receptor have been postulated to contribute to the generation of seizure activity. These characteristics include the fact that the NMDA receptor is coupled to an ion channel that, when open, is permeable to calcium ions, as well as to monovalent cations. Furthermore, the response to glutamate at the NMDA receptor depends on the level of depolarization of the cell, since magnesium ion, which blocks the channel, is cleared from the channel upon cellular depolarization.[7] Thus, when glutamate interacts with other subtypes of receptor (*e.g.*, kainate, quisqualate),[7] the resulting rapid EPSP and cellular depolarization promote the activation of the NMDA receptor.

During high-frequency electrical stimulation that is used to produce LTP or kindling, both glutamate and GABA are released, and the interaction of GABA with the GABA$_A$ receptor results in hyperpolarization, which counteracts the depolarizing effect of glutamate, and thus tends to attenuate the activation of the NMDA receptor.[7] However, an important characteristic of the GABA$_A$ receptor is its desensitization following prolonged stimulation.[8] Therefore, it has been postulated that, during the stimulation that produces kindling or LTP, desensitization of the GABA$_A$ receptor leads to enhanced depolarization of the cell (*i.e.*, hippocampal cells), and a consequent increased activation of the NMDA receptor.[7] Since the response to glutamate at the NMDA receptor is of relatively long duration, these responses can summate, allowing for entry of large amounts of calcium into the cell, and leading to repetitive firing which contributes to seizure activity and possibly to synaptic potentiation.[7]

ETHANOL AND THE GABA$_A$ RECEPTOR

Both the GABA$_A$ receptor and the NMDA receptor are affected acutely by ethanol, and chronic ethanol exposure induces changes in these systems that, based on the scheme described above, would be expected to result in enhanced NMDA receptor activity and seizure activity. It had been postulated for some time that the depressant effects of ethanol in the CNS might be mediated by enhancement of the actions of GABA, but such enhancement has been difficult to demonstrate consistently in electrophysiological studies.[9] For example, under voltage clamp conditions with whole cell patch recording, ethanol was reported to enhance the initial response to GABA in dorsal root ganglion cells in one recent study,[10] but not in another.[11] Ethanol has also been reported to increase the response to GABA in cultured chick spinal cord neurons[12]; however, there was no enhancement of the GABA current by ethanol in adult rat locus coeruleus neurons in a brain slice preparation.[13] In addition, both in several earlier studies, and in a more recent examination of responses to GABA in cultured hippocampal neurons from embryonic rats, no effect of ethanol was observed.[9,14] One possible explanation for the variability of the response lies in the recent realization of the structural heterogeneity of the GABA$_A$ receptor-channel complex. Cloning of the GABA$_A$ receptor has demonstrated a large number of receptor subunits: at least 6 α subunits, 3 β subunits, 2 γ subunits, 1 δ subunit, 1 ϵ subunit and 1 ζ subunit.[15] Various combinations of these subunits can be expressed in reconstitution systems, and the resulting receptors show different pharmacological responses. For example, the γ-2 subunit seems to be required for the actions of benzodiazepines,[16] while the presence of the α-6 subunit allows the binding of the benzodiazepine partial inverse agonist Ro15-4513 (which is an antagonist of certain actions of ethanol) but not other benzodiazepines.[17] These findings suggest that ethanol may enhance the actions of GABA only at some isoforms of the GABA$_A$ receptor, and these isoforms may be distributed differentially among the brain regions and cells that have been studied. For example, it was reported that microinjection of the GABA$_A$ receptor agonist muscimol into the medial septal area, but not the lateral septum, enhanced the sedative/hypnotic response to ethanol. Similarly, the systemic administration of ethanol increased GABA-induced inhibition of rhythmically firing cells in the medial septal area, but not in the lateral septum.[18] Furthermore, in mouse hippocampal neurons, recent work using the patch clamp technique indicated that ethanol enhanced the action of GABA only in some cells, although all cells responded to GABA and benzodiazepines, as well as barbiturates.[19]

In contrast to the findings in electrophysiological studies, a consistent result in several laboratories has been that ethanol *in vitro* enhances GABA or GABA$_A$ agonist-stimulated $^{36}Cl^-$ flux in membrane preparations from certain regions of mouse and rat brain and spinal cord.[20-22] The consistency of this finding may reflect the cellular heterogeneity of the synaptoneurosome or microsac brain preparations used; these preparations should include various isoforms of the GABA$_A$ receptor, some of which are sensitive to ethanol. The biochemical effects of GABA are significantly enhanced by low concentrations of ethanol (25 mM; approximately 115 mg%) that can be achieved *in vivo*, and this effect of ethanol would therefore be expected to occur in the intact animal during ethanol ingestion.

Prolonged enhancement of the effects of GABA by ethanol could lead to a desensitization of the GABA$_A$ receptor following chronic ethanol exposure. Although the response to GABA$_A$ agonists in chronically ethanol-treated animals has not been systematically evaluated in electrophysiological studies, biochemical and behavioral measurements have, in some cases, suggested the occurrence of GABA$_A$ receptor desensitization. Both Harris and his colleagues[23,24] and Morrow et al.[25] examined muscimol-stimulated $^{36}Cl^-$ uptake in brain preparations of animals treated chronically with ethanol. Allan and Harris, using cerebellar tissue from mice fed ethanol in a liquid diet, found no change in the response to muscimol, but did report an attenuation of the muscimol-enhancing effect of ethanol.[23] In a later study, Buck and Harris reported that, in cerebral cortical tissue from chronically ethanol-fed mice, the response to pentobarbital was unchanged, while the effect of benzodiazepines was reduced.[24] Morrow et al., in contrast, found that the response to pentobarbital or muscimol was reduced in cortical tissue from rats exposed to ethanol by inhalation for 14 days. This desensitization was a function of the blood ethanol concentration at the end of the treatment period, and was not found when ethanol concentrations were lower than 150 mg%. Reduced behavioral effects of GABA (motor incoordination, locomotor activity) have also been reported in animals exposed chronically to ethanol.[26-28] Thus, while there are some conflicting results, the data suggest that desensitization of GABA responses can occur in animals treated chronically with ethanol. As for the acute studies, some discrepancies may arise from differential sensitivity to ethanol of the various isoforms of the GABA receptor, as well as the apparent necessity for a threshold blood ethanol concentration to be reached during chronic treatment.[25] Nonetheless, a decreased response to GABA may figure prominently in the expression of ethanol withdrawal seizures, as is suggested by the ability of administered GABA$_A$ agonists to attenuate these seizures.[29-32] The regional localization of GABA receptor desensitization is well illustrated in the studies of Breese and his colleagues who found that administration of bicuculline (a GABA$_A$ receptor antagonist) into the inferior colliculus, but not the medial geniculate nucleus or the substantia nigra, produced symptoms similar to audiogenic seizures in ethanol-withdrawn rats.[33] These authors also found that muscimol, injected into the inferior colliculus, suppressed audiogenic ethanol withdrawal seizures.[33] They suggested that reduced GABA sensitivity specifically in the inferior colliculus contributes to (audiogenic) ethanol withdrawal seizures.

ETHANOL AND THE NMDA RECEPTOR

As discussed above, desensitization of the GABA$_A$ receptor can also contribute to activation of the NMDA receptor. In animals treated chronically with ethanol, changes in the function of the NMDA receptor occur which would further enhance this activation. The effects of ethanol on NMDA receptor function have been relatively recently discovered, and, in contrast to the results with ethanol and the GABA$_A$ receptor, are very consistent among laboratories. Studies in primary cultures of cerebellar granule cells and in dissociated fetal brain cells showed that ethanol, acutely, is a potent and selective inhibitor of NMDA-induced increases in Ca^{++} flux.[34,35] Electrophysiological studies in cultured neonatal hippocampal neurons confirmed the inhibitory effect of ethanol on NMDA-induced currents.[36,37] Ethanol is also a potent inhibitor of NMDA-stimulated neurotransmitter release from slice preparations of several brain areas.[38-40] Recent work suggests that the site of action of ethanol at this receptor involves the interaction of NMDA or glutamate with glycine,[38,41] which binds to a strychnine-insensitive site and enhances the response to NMDA; glycine has been postulated to be required for NMDA actions (*i.e.*, glutamate and glycine are co-agonists at the NMDA receptor).[42] Inhibition of NMDA responses (or responses to glutamate at the NMDA receptor), like enhancement of GABA responses, occurs at very low *in vitro* concentrations of ethanol (10–50 mM),[34-40] and would therefore be expected to be expressed *in vivo* during ethanol ingestion. Chronic inhibition of NMDA responses could lead to a compensatory "up-regulation" of the receptor, and enhanced function.

The development of NMDA receptor up-regulation was evaluated in brains of mice fed ethanol in a liquid diet for seven days, which produced tolerance to and physical dependence on ethanol. In membrane binding studies, an increased number of hippocampal binding sites for [³H]MK-801 was found at the time of ethanol withdrawal.[43] MK-801 is a non-competitive antagonist at the NMDA receptor and is believed to bind within the ion channel; therefore, these results suggested that chronic ethanol ingestion resulted in an increased number of NMDA receptor-channel complexes in the hippocampus. Autoradiographic analysis showed that MK-801 binding was also increased in several other brain areas of ethanol-fed mice.[44] Recent studies, using membrane binding techniques, have also indicated an increased number of NMDA-specific glutamate binding sites in hippocampus of ethanol-fed mice, but no increase in the number of glycine binding sites or binding sites for a competitive NMDA antagonist.[45] These findings are of interest in view of current work that suggests that the various components of the NMDA receptor develop at different rates,[46] and that binding sites for different ligands may in fact be localized on different subunits of the receptor.[47] It will be of interest to determine whether the increases in MK-801 and glutamate binding sites reflect increased synthesis of receptor subunits, or may be indicative of altered sensitivity to factors such as glycine, which can increase glutamate binding to the NMDA receptor.[48] It has also been reported that treatment of brain tissue with reducing agents such as dithiothreitol produces an increase in MK-801 binding,[49] raising the possibility that chronic ethanol exposure may induce post-translational modifications of the receptor.

Assessment of receptor up-regulation by ligand binding studies does not address the question of alterations in the functional properties of the receptor. This issue has been approached by using primary cultures of cerebellar granule cells and exposing them chronically to ethanol *in vitro*. The response to NMDA was evaluated by measuring levels of intracellular calcium with the fluorescent dye Fura-2. After exposure of cells to 100 mM ethanol for 48 h, there was a significant increase in the maximum response to NMDA (in the presence of glycine), with no change in the EC_{50} for NMDA. The maximal response to glycine, in the presence of NMDA, was also significantly increased.[50] However, the EC_{50} for glycine was unaltered, and these data are consistent with an increase in the number of NMDA receptor-channel complexes in cells exposed chronically to ethanol, similar to the results found in binding studies in mouse brain, rather than increased sensitivity to glycine. Preliminary results indicate that a comparable change occurs in cells exposed to 20 mM ethanol for 3 days *in vitro*. Further evidence that the characteristics of the receptor-channel complexes were not altered after chronic ethanol exposure were the findings that there was no difference between control and ethanol-treated cells with respect to (percent) inhibition of the NMDA response by Mg^{++}, MK-801 or ethanol.[50] In addition, the increase in NMDA receptor-channel complexes in the cerebellar granule cells appeared to be selective, since, in preliminary studies, no change was found in the response to 25 mM KCl, which is expected to activate voltage-sensitive calcium channels. These results suggest that the NMDA receptor up-regulation resulting from chronic ethanol exposure consists of an increased number of functional receptor-channel complexes with properties comparable to those of the receptors in control cells or animals.

A priori, based on the known involvement of NMDA receptors in epileptiform seizure activity, and extrapolating from cells in culture to the intact animal, one might postulate that the enhanced function of NMDA receptors in brains of ethanol-treated animals would contribute to ethanol withdrawal seizures, once ethanol is eliminated from the animals. Several studies have been carried out to assess the relationship between the increased NMDA receptor-channel complexes and the symptoms of ethanol withdrawal. A time course of the alterations in hippocampal MK-801 binding showed that the increase was present at the time of ethanol withdrawal and at 8 h after withdrawal, when withdrawal seizures peak, and had dissipated by 24 h after withdrawal, when overt seizures no longer occur.[44] Thus, the time course of the biochemical change correlated well with the time course for ethanol withdrawal seizure activity; although MK-801 binding is increased at the time of withdrawal, seizures do not occur at this time because of the high blood and brain ethanol levels present in the animals. Perhaps a more direct demonstration of the role of the NMDA receptor in ethanol withdrawal seizures is the finding that these seizures can be attenuated by MK-801 and other antagonists at the NMDA receptor (although not by an antagonist at the glycine site),[43,51] and that seizures can be exacerbated by administration of NMDA at doses that are not convulsant in control animals.[43]

Finally, mice that have been selectively bred to be prone or resistant to ethanol withdrawal seizures have been used to assess the role of the NMDA receptor in these seizures. Selective breeding results in lines of animals that are genetically invariant for the trait which is selected, while genes associated with unrelated traits are randomly

distributed between lines.[52] Therefore, any biochemical characteristic that differs between the selected lines may be postulated to be related to the selected trait. Analysis
of MK-801 binding showed a significantly greater number of binding sites in hippocampus of ethanol withdrawal seizure-prone (WSP) mice than ethanol withdrawal
seizure-resistant (WSR) mice.[53] After chronic ethanol treatment, the number of hippocampal binding sites was increased in both lines of mice, but remained significantly
higher in brains of WSP mice (in ethanol-treated WSR mice, the number of sites was
similar to that in *control* WSP mice). These data strongly support a key role for the
NMDA receptor in ethanol withdrawal seizures. It should be noted that no difference
in flunitrazepam binding or GABA-stimulated flunitrazepam binding was seen between the WSP and WSR lines of mice[54]; however, GABA$_A$ receptors were not
studied in the hippocampus, nor was the effect of chronic ethanol treatment examined. On the other hand, differences in the chronic effects of ethanol on voltage-
sensitive calcium channels (L channels) have been reported between WSP and WSR
mice,[55] and the relative contributions of these channels and NMDA receptor-gated
channels to ethanol withdrawal seizures is still under investigation.[56]

ETHANOL WITHDRAWAL SEIZURES: NMDA AND GABA$_A$ RECEPTOR INTERACTIONS

The data obtained to date are compatible with the postulate that changes in NMDA
receptor function produced by chronic ethanol treatment are crucial to ethanol withdrawal seizures. However, reduced function of the GABA system may also be an essential factor in this withdrawal symptom. The changes in NMDA receptor function
in cerebellar granule cells, if they also occur in brains of intact animals, indicate that
the number, but not the characteristics, of NMDA receptors are altered by chronic ethanol treatment. Therefore, desensitization of the GABA$_A$ receptor, produced after
chronic ethanol treatment, may be a necessary alteration that allows activation of the
NMDA receptors *in vivo*. Once these receptors are activated, the increased number of
receptors leads to an enhanced response, which contributes to the seizure activity. Ca-
veats that must be kept in mind include the fact that various studies of NMDA and
GABA$_A$ receptors have been performed in different brain regions, as well as in cultured cells; in particular, ethanol did not enhance the response to GABA in hippocampal preparations.[20] It will be of special interest, therefore, to determine whether
hippocampal GABA receptor sensitivity is altered, with a time course similar to the
changes in NMDA receptor function, after chronic ethanol treatment. The concerted
effect of alterations in these systems may be important for the generation of ethanol
withdrawal seizures, and an understanding of the role of the two systems could facilitate the development of specific therapeutic methods to counteract certain symptoms
of ethanol withdrawal, without the drawback of using drugs, such as benzodiazepines,
at doses that may have significant addictive liability.

REFERENCES

1. TABAKOFF, B. & J. D. ROTHSTEIN. 1983. Biology of tolerance and dependence. *In* Medical
and Social Aspects of Alcohol Abuse. B. Tabakoff, P. B. Sutker & C. L. Randall, Eds.:
187–220. Plenum Press. New York.

2. VICTOR, M. & R. D. ADAMS. 1953. The effect of alcohol in the nervous system. Research Publication, Association for Research on Nervous and Mental Disorders **32:** 526–573.
3. TABAKOFF, B. & P. L. HOFFMAN. 1987. Biochemical pharmacology of alcohol. *In* Psychopharmacology: The Third Generation of Progress. H. Y. Meltzer, Ed.: 1521–1526. Raven Press. New York.
4. HOFFMAN, P. L. & B. TABAKOFF. 1985. Ethanol's action on brain biochemistry. *In* Alcohol and the Brain: Chronic Effects. R. E. Tarter, D. H. van Thiel & K. L. Edwards, Eds.: 19–68. Plenum Press. New York.
5. BALLENGER, J. C. & R. M. POST. 1978. Kindling as a model for alcohol withdrawal syndromes. Br. J. Psychiatry **133:** 1–14.
6. BROWN, M. E., R. F. ANTON, R. MALCOLM & J. C. BALLENGER. 1988. Alcohol detoxification and withdrawal seizures: Clinical support for a kindling hypothesis. Biol. Psychiatry **23:** 507–514.
7. COLLINGRIDGE, G. L. & R. A. J. LESTER. 1989. Excitatory amino acid receptors in the vertebrate central nervous system. Pharmacol. Rev. **40:** 143–210.
8. MCCARREN, M. & B. E. ALGER. 1988. Use-dependent depression of IPSPs in rat hippocampal pyramidal cells *in vitro.* J. Neurophysiol. **60:** 645–663.
9. SHEFNER, S. A. 1990. Electrophysiological effects of ethanol on brain neurons. *In* Biochemistry and Physiology of Substance Abuse. R. R. Watson, Ed. **2:** 25–53. CRC Press. Boca Raton, FL.
10. NISHIO, M. & T. NARAHASHI. 1990. Ethanol enhancement of GABA-activated chloride current in rat dorsal root ganglion neurons. Brain Res. **518:** 283–286.
11. WHITE, G., D. M. LOVINGER & F. F. WEIGHT. 1990. Ethanol inhibits NMDA-activated current but does not alter GABA-activated current in an isolated adult mammalian neuron. Brain Res. **507:** 332–336.
12. CELENTANO, J. J., T. T. GIBBS & D. H. FARB. 1988. Ethanol potentiates GABA- and glycine-induced chloride currents in chick spinal cord neurons. Brain Res. **455:** 377–380.
13. OSMANOVIC, S. S. & S. A. SHEFNER. 1990. Enhancement of current induced by superfusion of GABA in locus coeruleus neurons by pentobarbital but not ethanol. Brain Res. **517:** 324–329.
14. HARRISON, N. L., M. D. MAJEWSKA, J. W. HARRINGTON & J. L. BARKER. 1987. Structure-activity relationships for steroid interaction with the γ-aminobutyric acid$_A$ receptor complex. J. Pharmacol. Exp. Ther. **241:** 346–353.
15. VICINI, S. 1991. Pharmacologic significance of the structural heterogeneity of the GABA$_A$ receptor-chloride ion channel complex. Neuropsychopharmacology **4:** 9–15.
16. PRITCHETT, D. B., H. SONTHEIMER, B. SHIVERS, S. YMER, H. KETTENMANN, P. R. SCHOFIELD & P. H. SEEBURG. 1989. Importance of a novel GABA$_A$ receptor subunit for benzodiazepine pharmacology. Nature **338:** 582–585.
17. LÜDDENS, H., D. B. PRITCHETT, M. KÖHLER, I. KILLISCH, K. KEINÄNEN, H. MONYER, R. SPRENGEL & P. H. SEEBURG. 1990. Cerebellar GABA$_A$ receptor selective for a behavioral alcohol antagonist. Nature **346:** 648–651.
18. GIVENS, B. S. & G. R. BREESE. 1990. Site-specific enhancement of γ-aminobutyric acid-mediated inhibition of neural activity by ethanol in the rat medial septal area. J. Pharmacol. Exp. Ther. **254:** 528–538.
19. AGUAYO, L. G. 1990. Ethanol potentiates the GABA$_A$-activated Cl$^-$ current in mouse hippocampal and cortical neurons. Eur. J. Pharmacol. **187:** 127–130.
20. ALLAN, A. M. & R. A. HARRIS. 1986. Gamma-aminobutyric acid and alcohol actions: Neurochemical studies of long sleep and short sleep mice. Life Sci. **39:** 2005–2015.
21. MEHTA, A. K. & M. K. TICKU. 1988. Ethanol potentiation of GABAergic transmission in cultured spinal cord neurons involves γ-aminobutyric acid$_A$-gated chloride channels. J. Pharmacol. Exp. Ther. **246:** 558–564.
22. SUZDAK, P. D., R. D. SCHWARTZ, P. SKOLNICK & S. M. PAUL. 1986. Ethanol stimulates γ-aminobutyric acid receptor mediated chloride transport in rat brain synaptoneurosomes. Proc. Natl. Acad. Sci. USA **83:** 4071–4075.
23. ALLAN, A. M. & R. A. HARRIS. 1987. Acute and chronic ethanol treatments alter GABA receptor-operated chloride channels. Pharmacol. Biochem. Behav. **27:** 665–670.

24. BUCK, K. J. & R. A. HARRIS. 1990. Benzodiazepine agonist and inverse agonist actions on GABA$_A$ receptor-operated chloride channels. II. Chronic effects of ethanol. J. Pharmacol. Exp. Ther. **253:** 713–719.

25. MORROW, A. L., P. D. SUZDAK, J. W. KARANIAN & S. M. PAUL. 1988. Chronic ethanol administration alters γ-aminobutyric acid, pentobarbital and ethanol-mediated ^{36}Cl$^-$ uptake in cerebral cortical synaptoneurosomes. J. Pharmacol. Exp. Ther. **246:** 158–164.

26. DAR, M. S. & W. R. WOOLES. 1985. GABA mediation of the central effects of acute and chronic ethanol in mice. Pharmacol. Biochem. Behav. **22:** 77–84.

27. MARTZ, A., R. A. DEITRICH & R. A. HARRIS. 1983. Behavioral evidence for the involvement of γ-aminobutyric acid in the actions of ethanol. Eur. J. Pharmacol. **89:** 53–62.

28. TABERNER, P. V. & J. W. UNWIN. 1981. Behavioral effects of muscimol, amphetamine, and chlorpromazine on ethanol tolerant mice. Br. J. Pharmacol. **74:** 2761–2762.

29. FRYE, G. D., T. J. McCOWN & G. R. BREESE. 1983. Differential sensitivity of ethanol withdrawal signs in the rat to γ-aminobutyric acid (GABA)-mimetics: Blockade of audiogenic seizures but not forelimb tremors. J. Pharmacol. Exp. Ther. **226:** 720–725.

30. GOLDSTEIN, D. B. 1979. Sodium bromide and sodium valproate: Effective suppressants of ethanol withdrawal reactions in mice. J. Pharmacol. Exp. Ther. **208:** 223–227.

31. GOLDSTEIN, D. B. 1973. Alcohol withdrawal reactions in mice: Effects of drugs that modify neurotransmission. J. Pharmacol. Exp. Ther. **186:** 1–9.

32. GONZALEZ, L. P. & M. K. HETTINGER. 1984. Intranigral muscimol suppresses ethanol withdrawal seizures. Brain Res. **298:** 163–166.

33. FRYE, G. D., T. J. McCOWN & G. R. BREESE. 1983. Characterization of susceptibility to audiogenic seizures in ethanol-dependent rats after microinjection of γ-aminobutyric acid (GABA) agonists into the inferior colliculus, substantia nigra or medial septum. J. Pharmacol. Exp. Ther. **227:** 663–670.

34. HOFFMAN, P. L., C. S. RABE, F. MOSES & B. TABAKOFF. 1989. N-methyl-D-aspartate receptors and ethanol: Inhibition of calcium flux and cyclic GMP production. J. Neurochem. **52:** 1937–1940.

35. DILDY, J. E. & S. W. LESLIE. 1989. Ethanol inhibits NMDA-induced increases in free intracellular Ca^{++} in dissociated brain cells. Brain Res. **499:** 383–387.

36. LOVINGER, D. M., G. WHITE & F. F. WEIGHT. 1989. Ethanol inhibits NMDA-activated ion current in hippocampal neurons. Science **243:** 1721–1724.

37. LIMA-LANDMAN, M. T. R. & E. X. ALBUQUERQUE. 1989. Ethanol potentiates and blocks NMDA-activated single channel currents in rat hippocampal pyramidal cells. FEBS Lett. **247:** 61–67.

38. WOODWARD, J. J. & R. A. GONZALES. 1990. Ethanol inhibition of N-methyl-D-aspartate-stimulated endogenous dopamine release from rat striatal slices: Reversal by glycine. J. Neurochem. **54:** 712–715.

39. GONZALES, R. A. & J. J. WOODWARD. 1990. Ethanol inhibits N-methyl-D-aspartate-stimulated [^{3}H]norepinephrine release from rat cortical slices. J. Pharmacol. Exp. Ther. **253:** 1138–1144.

40. GÖTHERT, M. & M. FINK. 1989. Inhibition of N-methyl-D-aspartate (NMDA)- and L-glutamate-induced noradrenaline and acetylcholine release in the rat brain by ethanol. Arch. Pharmacol. **340:** 516–521.

41. RABE, C. S. & B. TABAKOFF. 1990. Glycine site directed agonists reverse ethanol's actions at the NMDA receptor. Mol. Pharmacol. **38:** 753–757.

42. KLECKNER, N. W. & R. DINGLEDINE. 1988. Requirement for glycine in activation of NMDA receptors expressed in *Xenopus* oocytes. Science **241:** 835–837.

43. GRANT, K. A., P. VALVERIUS, M. HUDSPITH & B. TABAKOFF. 1990. Ethanol withdrawal seizures and the NMDA receptor complex. Eur. J. Pharmacol. **176:** 289–296.

44. GULYA, K., K. A. GRANT, P. VALVERIUS, P. L. HOFFMAN & B. TABAKOFF. 1991. Brain regional specificity and time course of changes in the NMDA receptor-ionophore complex during ethanol withdrawal. Brain Res. **547:** 129–134.

45. SNELL, L. D., B. TABAKOFF & P. L. HOFFMAN. 1991. The density of NMDA but not glycine binding sites is increased in ethanol-dependent mice. Alcoholism: Clin. Exp. Res. **15:** 333.

46. McDONALD, J. W., M. V. JOHNSTON & A. B. YOUNG. 1990. Differential ontogenic development of three receptors comprising the NMDA receptor/channel complex in the rat hippocampus. Exp. Neurol. 110: 237–247.
47. MICHAELIS, E. K., K. N. KUMAR, N. TILAKARATRIE & A. M. LY. 1991. Purification and cloning of NMDA receptor proteins. Alcoholism: Clin. Exp. Res. 15: 323.
48. MONAGHAN, D. T., H. J. OLVERMAN, L. NGUYEN, J. C. WATKINS & C. W. COTMAN. 1988. Two classes of N-methyl-D-aspartate recognition sites: Differential distribution and differential regulation by glycine. Proc. Natl. Acad. Sci. USA 85: 9836–9840.
49. REYNOLDS, I. J., E. A. RUSH & E. AIZENMAN. 1990. Reduction of NMDA receptors with dithiothreitol increases [³H]-MK-801 binding and NMDA-induced Ca^{2+} fluxes. Br. J. Pharmacol. 101: 178–182.
50. IORIO, K. R., L. REINLIB, B. TABAKOFF & P. L. HOFFMAN. 1991. NMDA-induced $\Delta[Ca^{2+}]_i$ enhanced by chronic ethanol treatment in cultured cerebellar granule cells. Alcoholism: Clin. Exp. Res. 15: 333.
51. GRANT, K. A., L. SNELL & B. TABAKOFF. 1991. NMDA receptor complex antagonists and the suppression of ethanol withdrawal seizures. Alcoholism: Clin. Exp. Res. 15: 332.
52. PHILLIPS, T. J., D. J. FELLER & J. C. CRABBE. 1989. Selected mouse lines, alcohol and behavior. Experientia 45: 805.
53. VALVERIUS, P., J. C. CRABBE, P. L. HOFFMAN & B. TABAKOFF. 1990. NMDA receptors in mice bred to be prone or resistant to ethanol withdrawal seizures. Eur. J. Pharmacol. 184: 185–189.
54. FELLER, D. J., R. A. HARRIS & J. C. CRABBE. 1988. Differences in GABA activity between ethanol withdrawal seizure prone and resistant mice. Eur. J. Pharmacol. 157: 147–154.
55. BRENNAN, C. H., J. CRABBE & J. M. LITTLETON. 1990. Genetic regulation of dihydropyridine-sensitive calcium channels in brain may determine susceptibility to physical dependence on alcohol. Neuropharmacology 29: 429–432.
56. HOFFMAN, P. L. & B. TABAKOFF. 1991. The contribution of voltage-gated and NMDA receptor-gated calcium channels to ethanol withdrawal seizures. Alcohol and Alcoholism Suppl. 1: 171–175.

Possible Substrates of Ethanol Reinforcement: GABA and Dopamine

R. ADRON HARRIS,[a,c] MARK S. BRODIE,[b]
AND THOMAS V. DUNWIDDIE[a]

[a] Denver Veterans Administration Medical Center and
Department of Pharmacology (C236)
University of Colorado Health Sciences Center
4200 E. Ninth Avenue
Denver, Colorado 80262

[b] Department of Physiology and Biophysics
University of Illinois College of Medicine
Chicago, Illinois 60612

In this chapter we review two actions of ethanol that may be related to its reinforcing effects: activation of ventral tegmental neurons and augmentation of GABA action.

ETHANOL AND VENTRAL TEGMENTAL FUNCTION

In general terms, many drugs of abuse seem to have little in common, since a wide diversity of agents that act upon different neurotransmitter receptors and/or transmitter uptake systems all share abuse potential in humans, and are self-administered by laboratory animals. However, considerable evidence has developed to suggest that the *sine qua non* for abuse potential is the ability of a drug to interact with dopaminergic neurotransmitter systems, particularly the dopaminergic projection from the ventral tegmental area (VTA) to the nucleus accumbens, and to some extent other limbic regions such as frontal cortex.[1] With drugs such as cocaine and amphetamine, the link to dopamine (DA) systems is readily apparent; both of these drugs inhibit DA uptake and, in the case of amphetamine, release DA as well, and would be expected to potentiate DA's actions upon postsynaptic receptors.

With other classes of drugs, such as the opiates, the link to DA systems is not as apparent, and there remains some debate as to whether opiate "reward" and dopaminergic "reward" rely upon distinct and separate substrates. Wise and colleagues have suggested that opiate reward is dependent upon a dopaminergic substrate[2]; Kornetsky and Bain[3] suggest that the two systems may be complementary, whereas Ettenberg et al.[4] suggest that independent substrates mediate the two types of reward.

[c] Address correspondence to Dr. R. A. Harris at the Department of Pharmacology.

Regardless of the specific mechanisms involved, the evidence implicating the VTA-nucleus accumbens system in both types of pharmacological reward is extensive. For example, activation of opiate receptors in the VTA is not only a necessary but also a sufficient condition for opiate reinforcement; the reinforcing effects of systemic opiates can be blocked by local applications of opiate antagonists to the VTA,[5] and direct administration of opioids into the VTA in rats is by itself reinforcing.[6,7] While it would be overly simplistic to conclude that the DA-containing projections of the VTA constitute *the* substrate of reward, these findings identify some aspect of the VTA-NAC axis as an important link in pharmacological reward.

Given the critical importance of the VTA in at least some types of pharmacological reinforcement, it then becomes important to ask whether the VTA-nucleus accumbens axis is central to *all* types of pharmacological reinforcement. With other drugs of abuse support for this hypothesis is not as complete as for the opiates, but in general the evidence seems consistent with this conclusion.[1] However, in addition to behavioral studies that provide direct support for this hypothesis, there have been numerous electrophysiological studies involving the effects of drugs of abuse on the activity of the VTA that suggest commonalities among abused drugs at the cellular level. More specifically, VTA neurons are usually *activated* by parenteral administration of drugs with abuse potential, such as nicotine,[8-10] phencyclidine,[11] opiates,[12,13] and ethanol.[14] Although exceptions to this exist (*e.g.*, cocaine *inhibits* VTA activity[15]), these exceptions are usually drugs that potentiate the effects of synaptically released DA, and thus might be expected to have a net facilitatory effect upon dopaminergic systems despite the inhibition of firing of dopaminergic neurons.

The cellular mechanisms that underlie the excitatory effects of these drugs upon VTA neurons are in some cases not completely understood. Of particular interest are those drugs that generally inhibit neuronal activity, such as ethanol, benzodiazepines, and opiate drugs, but which *increase* the firing of DA-containing VTA neurons. In the case of the opiate drugs, the primary mechanism appears to be a disinhibitory one. The DA-containing neurons of the VTA are opiate-insensitive, whereas putative GABAergic interneurons are inhibited by activation of mu opiate receptors. The opiate inhibition of these interneurons is hypothesized to result in a decrease in tonic inhibition of the dopaminergic neurons, which leads to increased firing.[13]

In the case of ethanol, the mechanism underlying increases in DA neuron firing is less well-established. Given the ability of ethanol to potentiate GABAergic inhibition in some systems (see below), one might predict that ethanol would inhibit VTA neurons, yet this is clearly not the case[14,16] (see also FIG. 1). Behavioral and biochemical studies have also suggested that GABA$_A$ agonists *increase* rather than decrease dopaminergic output from the VTA.[17] This has led to the suggestion that the excitatory effects of ethanol on DA neurons in the VTA might come about as a result of an inhibition of inhibitory interneurons mediated via GABA$_A$ receptors. This might initially seem inconsistent with the mechanism proposed for opiate actions (where the DA cells are under tonic inhibitory GABAergic control mediated via GABA$_A$ receptors), but this is not necessarily the case. One possibility proposed by Kalivas *et al.*,[17] is that the inhibition of DA neurons by interneurons is mediated via GABA$_B$ receptors on the DA cells. If this were the case, then the ethanol-induced excitation could be mediated by an increased activation of GABA$_A$ receptors on interneurons. However, this suggestion is not consistent with electrophysiological studies, which have suggested that the DA neurons are primarily inhibited by GABA$_A$, not GABA$_B$ receptors (S. W. Johnson and R. A. North, unpublished). Another possibility is outlined in

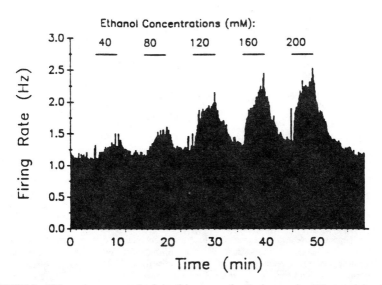

FIGURE 1. This ratemeter record of the firing rate of a single putative DA-containing VTA neuron in a brain slice preparation (taken from ref. 16) illustrates the effect of ethanol on spontaneous neuronal activity. Horizontal bars indicate duration of ethanol superfusion. The firing rate was averaged over 12 second intervals, and the height of each vertical bar indicates the mean firing rate in that 12 sec interval. Concentrations of from 40 to 200 mM ethanol produced a concentration-dependent increase in firing rate.

FIGURE 2; we have shown that not all $GABA_A$ responses are potentiated by ethanol.[18-20] If the $GABA_A$ receptors on interneurons are ethanol sensitive, and the receptors on DA neurons are ethanol insensitive, then the net of ethanol would be to disinhibit the DA neurons and increase their firing. As a final point in this regard, it should be kept in mind that all reinforcing effects need not originate in the VTA; drugs that mimic the effects of DA in the nucleus accumbens (usually an inhibition of cell firing[21]) could be reinforcing as well (see below).

Although some studies have suggested that ethanol-induced excitation of mesencephalic dopamine neurons is mediated indirectly, via ethanol-induced inhibition of GABA interneurons,[22] not all studies support this hypothesis. For example, studies using a brain slice preparation of the VTA indicate that ethanol can increase the rate of neuronal firing even under conditions where synaptic release of transmitter is blocked.[16] This suggests that ethanol acts directly on the DA neurons to increase their firing, not indirectly via the interneurons. It should be noted, however, that in many systems there is a Ca^{++}-independent component of GABA release,[23] so it is possible that under these conditions ethanol might be inhibiting the Ca^{++}-independent release of GABA. Further evidence suggesting that ethanol-induced excitation of DA neurons of the VTA is direct comes from intracellular studies of VTA neurons,[24] which have shown that ethanol decreases the amplitude of the afterhyperpolarizations (AHPs), which are likely to be a major regulator of firing rate in DA neurons of the VTA; it is unlikely that this effect is mediated indirectly by GABA. Furthermore, preliminary observations indicate that the excitatory effects of ethanol are *not* blocked by

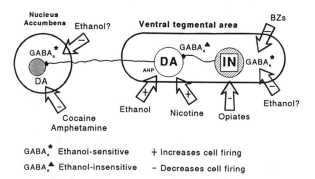

FIGURE 2. Putative substrates of pharmacological reinforcement. This illustrates schematically some of the ways in which drugs of abuse might interact with the ventral tegmental area/nucleus accumbens system. Cocaine and amphetamine are likely to act by potentiating DA effects in nucleus accumbens, which would have a primarily depressant effect on cell firing,[21] whereas nicotine appears to have a direct excitatory effect upon DA neurons (DA) in the VTA. Opiates, benzodiazepines (BZs), and ethanol may all act to inhibit the firing of inhibitory interneurons (IN) via effects on opiate receptors or an ethanol-sensitive GABA$_A$ receptor respectively, and these interneurons could then inhibit the DA cells via ethanol-insensitive GABA$_A$ receptors. Alternatively, ethanol might have a direct excitatory effect upon the DA cells via a mechanism that does not involve a GABAergic receptor.

the benzodiazepine inverse agonist Ro 15-4513, which reverses many GABA-related ethanol responses (M.S. Brodie, unpublished). Finally, bicuculline *increases* the rate of firing of putative DA-containing neurons in these brain slices[25] and antagonizes synaptically evoked IPSPs,[13] whereas if the GABA$_A$ receptors were only on interneurons, one would expect that bicuculline would inhibit rather that excite DA neurons of the VTA. The final resolution of this issue may depend upon determining whether the excitatory effects of ethanol persist when GABA$_A$ receptors are blocked.

ETHANOL AND GABAERGIC TRANSMISSION

Background

In the 1970s evidence emerged that the barbiturates and benzodiazepines produce many of their CNS actions by enhancement of GABAergic inhibition. This was shown to be due to allosteric modulation of the GABA$_A$ receptor subtype that activates chloride channels. Because of similarities in behavioral actions of ethanol and other sedative/antianxiety/anticonvulsant drugs such as barbiturates and benzodiazepines, it was hypothesized that ethanol might also enhance GABA action. Initial behavioral studies showed that GABA agonists increase actions of ethanol and GABA antagonists reduce these actions.[26] These studies provided evidence, albeit indirect, that ethanol might exert some of its actions through the GABA/benzodiazepine receptor. However, attempts to define actions of ethanol on these receptors using ligand binding were less successful. Pharmacologically relevant concentrations of ethanol (5–100 mM) generally produce little or no change in binding of ligands to GABA or benzodiazepine receptors, although higher concentrations (100–400 mM) inhibit the binding of [^{35}S]TBPS to the convulsant site on the receptor complex.[27] Despite the minimal effects on receptor binding, studies of receptor function have been more successful in detecting interactions between ethanol and GABA. Using the uptake of ^{36}Cl$^-$ by brain membrane vesicles or cultured neurons, several groups found that ethanol enhanced the action of GABA agonists and this interaction was seen with 5–50 mM ethanol (*e.g.*, see ref. 27). Electrophysiological results have been less consistent than chloride flux data, with reports of ethanol enhancing, inhibiting, and not affecting GABA actions.[27] Many of the electrophysiological studies showing no effect of ethanol on GABA action have been carried out in hippocampus, a brain region that also shows no action of ethanol on GABA-activated chloride flux.[28] Recent studies using the "patch-slice" technique for whole-cell voltage clamping of neurons of brain slices show that ethanol enhances the action of GABA on cortical neurons, but not on hippocampal neurons.[20] These results are important because they provide some of the first direct evidence that actions of synaptically released GABA are potentiated by ethanol, and that this action displays the regional specificity previously shown with the chloride flux technique. (Possible molecular explanations for ethanol-sensitive and -insensitive GABA receptors are discussed in the next section.) Another recent electrophysiological study noted that ethanol enhancement of GABA action on cerebellar Purkinje cells requires norepinephrine, suggesting neuromodulation is also involved in the ethanol-GABA interaction.[29]

The importance of GABA-activated chloride channels in the behavioral actions of ethanol has been evaluated by genetic techniques. In brief, lines of animals selected for differences in sensitivity to behavioral actions of ethanol provide an excellent approach to test hypotheses regarding alcohol actions.[30] The basic premise is that if common genes (alleles) are responsible for both the behavioral and neurochemical actions of ethanol, then they must co-segregate during the selection process. Indeed, the ability of ethanol to augment GABA-activated chloride flux of brain membranes differs with behavioral sensitivity to ethanol for many genetic models, such as Long-sleep/Short-sleep (LS/SS) mice, Diazepam Sensitive/Resistant (DS/DR) mice, individual HS mice, and High and Low Alcohol Sensitive (HAS/LAS) rats.[31,32] However, Alcohol Tolerant/Nontolerant (AT/ANT) rats do not differ in ability of ethanol to enhance GABA action.[33] Differences between LS and SS GABA-activated chloride channels have also been detected after expression of brain mRNA in Xenopus oocytes.[18] These genetic approaches provide considerable evidence that the augmentation of GABA-activated chloride flux observed *in vitro* is important for at least some of the behavioral actions of ethanol and provide justification for more a molecular analysis of this action of ethanol.

Molecular Basis of Ethanol–GABA Interactions

Each GABA-activated chloride channel appears to be formed from five protein subunits, and the drug sensitivity of the channel complex depends upon the subunit composition (see ref. 34). To date, four groups of subunits, α, β, δ, and γ, have been cloned and sequenced and each group has multiple members (*e.g.*, α_1 through α_6). These subunits have a distinct distribution at both the brain regional and cellular level. GABA agonists bind primarily to the β subunits whereas benzodiazepines bind to α subunits, although a γ subunit is required for augmentation of GABA action by benzodiazepines. In contrast, action of barbiturates is seen with all combinations of subunits and does not require any particular subunit. Ethanol, however, is remarkably specific in regard to subunit requirement for enhancement of GABA action. Expression of RNA in Xenopus oocytes and use of a hybrid arrest (antisense oligonucleotide) strategy indicates that a specific subunit, γ_{2L}, is required for ethanol action.[19] This is of particular interest because the γ_{2L} subunit differs from the γ_{2S} subunit by only eight amino acids, yet the γ_{2S} subunit does not confer ethanol sensitivity to the channel. These eight amino acids contain a consensus sequence for phosphorylation by protein kinase C (PKC) and site-directed mutagenesis of this sequence suggests that the γ_{2L} subunit must be phosphorylated in this region to confer ethanol sensitivity (K. Wafford, personal communication). These results suggest that a GABA receptor will be sensitive to ethanol only if it contains a phosphorylated γ_{2L} subunit. This may well account for the lack of ethanol–GABA interactions found in some studies. For example, numerous studies failed to find augmentation of GABA action by ethanol in the hippocampus and this may be due to low levels of the γ_{2L} subunit in this brain region.[35] (Although these investigators did not detect mRNA for γ_{2L} in rat hippocampus, we have detected this mRNA in mouse and rat hippocampus using a sensitive PCR technique [K. J. Buck and R. A. Harris, in preparation].) In addition, the phosphorylation state of γ_{2L} will depend on the activities of PKC and protein phosphatases, both of which are regulated by intracellular messengers (*e.g.*, calcium). This may explain why the action of ethanol is more sensitive to assay temperature and techniques of membrane preparation than are other drugs affecting chloride channel function.[36] In fact, the action of ethanol would be expected to be more sensitive to differences in brain region and assay parameters than actions of GABA, barbiturates or benzodiazepines, because these compounds have less rigorous subunit requirements.

The requirement of phosphorylation of the γ_{2L} subunit means that neuromodulators which affect PKC or phosphatase activity may play a role in ethanol action. This may explain why activation of $GABA_B$ receptors promotes the action of ethanol at $GABA_A$ receptors and, conversely, blockade of $GABA_B$ receptors antagonizes some behavioral and biochemical actions of ethanol.[32,37] Our recent studies suggest that $GABA_B$ receptors influence the function of $GABA_A$ receptors, perhaps due to activation of PKC.[38] Furthermore, the observation that norepinephrine promotes the action of ethanol on $GABA_A$ receptors of cerebellar Purkinje cells could possibly reflect changes in phosphorylation state of $GABA_A$ receptor subunits.[29] Thus, some of the complexity and controversy of the interactions between ethanol and GABA responses may be clarified by more detailed study of the role of specific receptor subunits, such as the γ_{2L} subunit, in GABAergic neurotransmission.

GABA and Ethanol Reinforcement

Several lines of evidence support a role for GABAergic systems in ethanol self-administration. Enhancement of GABA action by ethanol can be antagonized by Ro 15-4513, a benzodiazepine partial inverse agonist, which itself has little or no effect on GABA-activated chloride channels (or behavior).[39] This compound reduces ethanol intake of Long-Evans, Sprague-Dawley and Alcohol-Preferring (P) rats without altering food or water consumption.[40–43] In addition, another benzodiazepine inverse agonist, Ro 19-4603, reduced voluntary ethanol consumption by the Sardinian

Ethanol Preferring (sP) rats.[44] Conversely, the benzodiazepine agonist, diazepam, maintained alcohol preference during alcohol withdrawal.[45] Taken together, these behavioral results suggest that enhancement of GABAergic function by ethanol (or diazepam) is one mechanism responsible for ethanol reinforcement. This idea is supported by immunocytochemical data showing that the alcohol-preferring P and HAD rats have a higher density of GABAergic terminals in the nucleus accumbens than the alcohol non-preferring NP and LAD rats.[46] Again, an increase in GABAergic function is linked with ethanol preference. Finally, the electrophysiological evidence summarized above suggests that ethanol increases dopaminergic activity in the VTA, possibly by enhancing GABAergic inhibition of interneurons,[14] or by a direct effect upon the DA neurons themselves.

CONCLUSIONS

There is considerable evidence that ethanol enhances actions of GABA at a subpopulation of $GABA_A$ receptors, that GABAergic pathways are important in ethanol reinforcement and that ethanol activates mesolimbic dopaminergic pathways critical for reinforcement. However, the relationship between these three phenomena remains to be rigorously defined. Our understanding of the mechanism of action of other drugs activating dopaminergic pathways is due in part to microinjection of drugs into discrete mesolimbic regions.[5-7] Although the low potency and rapid movement of ethanol probably precludes detecting a localized pharmacological action of this drug, agents acting on other receptors (*e.g.*, $GABA_A$, $GABA_B$, benzodiazepine) have been underutilized to define the reinforcing actions of ethanol. Local injection of receptor-specific ligands combined with *in vivo* microdialysis or electrochemistry should provide considerable new information regarding the mechanism of activation of dopaminergic pathways by ethanol.

REFERENCES

1. WISE, R. A. & M. A. BOZARTH. 1987. A psychomotor stimulant theory of addiction. Psychol. Rev. **94:** 469–492.
2. BOZARTH, M. A. & R. A. WISE. 1981. Heroin reward is dependent upon a dopaminergic substrate. Life Sci. **28:** 551–555.
3. KORNETSKY, C. & G. T. BAIN. 1982. Biobehavioral bases of the reinforcing properties of opiate drugs. Ann. N.Y. Acad. Sci. **398:** 241–259.
4. ETTENBERG, A., H. O. PETTIT, F. E. BLOOM & G. F. KOOB. 1982. Heroin and cocaine self-administration in rats: Mediation by separate neuronal systems. Psychopharmacol. **78:** 204–209.
5. BRITT, M. D. & R. A. WISE. 1983. Ventral tegmental site of opiate reward: Antagonism by a hydrophilic opiate receptor blocker. Brain Res. **258:** 105–108.
6. BOZARTH, M. A. & R. A. WISE. 1981. Intracranial self-administration of morphine into the ventral tegmental area of rats. Life Sci. **28:** 551–555.
7. PHILLIPS, A. G., F. G. LEPIANE & H. C. FIBIGER. 1983. Dopaminergic mediation of reward produced by direct injection of enkephalin into the ventral tegmental area of the rat. Life Sci. **33:** 2505–2511.
8. MEREU, G., K. W. YOON, V. BOI, G. L. GESSA, L. NAES & T. C. WESTFALL. 1987. Preferential stimulation of ventral tegmental area dopaminergic neurons by nicotine. Eur. J. Pharmacol. **141:** 395–399.

9. BRODIE, M. S. 1991. Low concentrations of nicotine increase the firing rate of neurons of the rat ventral tegmental area in vitro. *In* Advances in Pharmacological Sciences. F. Adlkofer & K. Thurau, Eds.: 373–377. Birkhauser Verlag. Basel/Boston.

10. CALABRESI, P., M. G. LACEY & R. A. NORTH. 1989. Nicotinic excitation of rat ventral tegmental neurones in vitro studied by intracellular recording. Br. J. Pharmacol. **98:** 135–140.

11. CECI, A. & E. D. FRENCH. 1989. Phencyclidine-induced activation of ventral tegmental A10 dopamine neurons is differentially affected by lesions of the nucleus accumbens and medial prefrontal cortex. Life Sci. **45:** 637–646.

12. MATTHEWS, R. T. & D. C. GERMAN. 1984. Electrophysiological evidence for excitation of rat ventral tegmental area dopamine neurons by morphine. Neuroscience **11:** 617–625.

13. JOHNSON, S. W. & R. A. NORTH. 1990. Electrophysiological effects of opioids on neurons in the ventral tegmental area. Soc. Neurosci. Abstr. **16:** 1027.

14. GESSA, G. L., F. MUNTONI, M. COLLU, L. VARGIU & G. MEREU. 1985. Low doses of ethanol activate dopaminergic neurons in the ventral tegmental area. Brain Res. **348:** 201–203.

15. BRODIE, M. S. & T. V. DUNWIDDIE. 1990. Cocaine effects in the ventral tegmental area: Evidence for an indirect dopaminergic mechanism of action. Naunyn Schmiedebergs Arch. Pharmacol. **342:** 660–665.

16. BRODIE, M. S., S. A. SHEFNER & T. V. DUNWIDDIE. 1990. Ethanol increases the firing rate of dopamine neurons of the rat ventral tegmental area in vitro. Brain Res. **508:** 65–69.

17. KALIVAS, P. W., P. DUFFY & H. EBERHARDT. 1990. Modulation of A10 dopamine neurons by gamma-aminobutyric acid agonists. J. Pharmacol. Exp. Ther. **253:** 858–866.

18. WAFFORD, K. A., D. M. BURNETT, T. V. DUNWIDDIE & R. A. HARRIS. 1990. Genetic differences in the ethanol sensitivity of $GABA_A$ receptors expressed in Xenopus oocytes. Science **249:** 291–293.

19. WAFFORD, K. A., D. BURNETT, N. J. LEIDENHEIMER, D. BURT, J. B. WANG, P. KOFUJI, T. V. DUNWIDDIE, R. A. HARRIS & J. M. SIKELA. 1991. Ethanol sensitivity of the $GABA_A$ receptor expressed in *Xenopus* oocytes requires eight amino acids contained in the gamma2L subunit of the receptor complex. Neuron **7:** 27–33.

20. PROCTOR, W. R. & T. V. DUNWIDDIE. 1991. Differential effects of ethanol on hippocampal, cerebellar, and cortical neurons from rat brain slices. Alcoholism: Clin. Exp. Res. **15:** 325.

21. UCHIMURA, N., H. HIGASHI & S. NISHI. 1986. Hyperpolarizing and depolarizing actions of dopamine via D-1 and D-2 receptors on nucleus accumbens neurons. Brain Res. **375:** 368–372.

22. MEREU, G. & G. L. GESSA. 1985. Low doses of ethanol inhibit the firing of neurons in the substantia nigra, pars reticulata: A GABAergic effect? Brain Res. **360:** 325–330.

23. SCHWARTZ, E. A. 1989. Depolarization without calcium can release gamma-aminobutyric acid from a retinal neuron. Science **238:** 350–355.

24. BRODIE, M. S. & S. A. SHEFNER. 1989. The effect of ethanol on membrane properties of neurons of the ventral tegmental area in vitro. Soc. Neurosci. Abstr. **15:** 524.

25. STITTSWORTH, J. D., A. L. MUELLER & M. S. BRODIE. 1987. Cholecystokinin octapeptide (CCK8) potentiates GABA-induced inhibition of dopamine neurons in the ventral tegmental area in vitro. Soc. Neurosci. Abstr. **13:** 934.

26. ALLAN, A. M. & R. A. HARRIS. 1987. Involvement of neuronal chloride channels in ethanol intoxication, tolerance and dependence. *In* Recent Developments in Alcoholism, M. Galanter, Ed. **5:** 313–325. Plenum Publishing. New York.

27. DEITRICH, R. A., T. V. DUNWIDDIE, R. A. HARRIS & V. G. ERWIN. 1989. Mechanism of action of ethanol: Initial central nervous system actions. Pharm. Rev. **41:** 491–537.

28. ALLAN, A. M. & R. A. HARRIS. 1986. Gamma-aminobutyric acid and alcohol actions: Neurochemical studies of long sleep and short sleep mice. Life Sci. **39:** 2005–2015.

29. FREUND, R. K., M. Y. LIN, C. G. VAN HORNE, T. J. HARLAN & M. R. PALMER. 1990. Are ethanol-mediated depressions of neuronal activity mediated by a GABAa mechanism of action? Soc. Neurosci. Abstr. **16:** 260.

30. CRABBE, J. C. & R. A. HARRIS. 1991. The Genetic Basis of Alcohol and Drug Actions. Plenum Press. In press.

31. HARRIS, R. A. & A. M. ALLAN. 1989. Alcohol intoxication: Ion channels and genetics. FASEB J. **3**: 1689–1695.
32. ALLAN, A. M., D. BURNETT & R. A. HARRIS. 1991. Ethanol-induced changes in chloride flux are mediated by both GABAA and GABAB receptors. Alcoholism: Clin. Exp. Res. **15**: 233–237.
33. UUSI-OUKARI, M. & E. R. KORPI. 1989. Cerebellar GABA$_A$ receptor binding and function in vitro in two rat lines developed for high and low alcohol sensitivity. Neurochem. Res. **14**: 733–739.
34. OLSEN, R. W. & A. J. TOBIN. 1990. Molecular biology of GABAA receptors. FASEB J. **4**: 1469–1480.
35. WHITING, P., R. M. McKERNAN & L. L. IVERSEN. 1990. Another mechanism for creating diversity in the gamma-aminobutyrate type A receptors: RNA splicing directs expression of two forms of gamma-2 subunit, one of which contains a protein kinase C phosphorylation site. Proc. Natl. Acad. Sci. USA **87**: 9966–9970.
36. McQUILKIN, S. J. & R. A. HARRIS. 1990. Factors affecting actions of ethanol on GABA-activated chloride channels. Life Sci. **46**: 527–541.
37. ALLAN, A. M. & R. A. HARRIS. 1989. A new alcohol antagonist: Phaclofen. Life Sci. **45**: 1771–1779.
38. HAHNER, L., S. McQUIKLIN & R. A. HARRIS. 1991. Cerebellar GABAB receptors modulate function of GABAA receptors. FASEB J. **5**: 2466–2472.
39. TICKU, M. K. & S. K. KULKARNI. 1988. Molecular interactions of ethanol with GABAergic system and potential of RO15-4513 as an ethanol antagonist. Pharmacol. Biochem. Behav. **30**: 501–510.
40. JUNE, H. L., G. H. LUMMIS, R. E. COLKER, T. O. MOORE & M. J. LEWIS. 1991. Ro15-4513 attenuates the consumption of ethanol in deprived rats. Alcoholism: Clin. Exp. Res. **15(3)**: 406–411.
41. SAMSON, H. H., M. HARAGUCHI, G. A. TOLLIVER & K. G. SADEGHI. 1989. Antagonism of ethanol-reinforced behavior by the benzodiazepine inverse agonists Ro15-4513 and FG 7142: Relation to sucrose reinforcement. Pharmacol. Biochem. Behav. **33**: 601–608.
42. McBRIDE, W. J., J. M. MURPHY, L. LUMENG & T. K. LI. 1988. Effects of Ro 15-4513, fluoxetine and desipramine on the intake of ethanol, water and food by the alcohol-preferring (P) and -nonpreferring (NP) lines of rats. Pharmacol. Biochem. Behav. **30**: 1045–1050.
43. SAMSON, H. H., G. A. TOLLIVER, A. O. PFEFFER, K. G. SADEGHI & F. G. MILLS. 1987. Oral ethanol reinforcement in the rat: Effect of the partial inverse benzodiazepine agonist RO15-4513. Pharmacol. Biochem. Behav. **27**: 517–519.
44. BALAKLEEVSKY, A., G. COLOMBO, F. FADDA & G. L. GESSA. 1990. Ro 19-4603, a benzodiazepine receptor inverse agonist, attenuates voluntary ethanol consumption in rats selectively bred for high ethanol preference. Alcohol Alcoholism **25**: 449–452.
45. DEUTSCH, J. A. & N. Y. WALTON. 1977. Diazepam maintenance of alcohol preference during alcohol withdrawal. Science **198**: 307–309.
46. HWANG, B. H., L. LUMENG, J.-Y. WU & T.-K. LI. 1990. Increased number of GABAergic terminals in the nucleus accumbens is associated with alcohol preference in rats. Alcoholism (N.Y.) **14**: 503–507.

Common Intracellular Actions of Chronic Morphine and Cocaine in Dopaminergic Brain Reward Regions[a]

DANA BEITNER-JOHNSON,[b] XAVIER GUITART,
AND ERIC J. NESTLER

Laboratory of Molecular Psychiatry
Departments of Pharmacology and Psychiatry
Yale University School of Medicine
Connecticut Mental Health Center
34 Park Street
New Haven, Connecticut 06508

INTRODUCTION

Although the exact biological processes by which drug addiction develops are not fully understood, much progress has been made in recent years toward delineating the specific brain regions involved. Several lines of evidence have focused attention on the mesolimbic dopamine system [dopaminergic neurons originating in the ventral tegmental area (VTA) and certain of their projection regions, most notably the nucleus accumbens (NAc)] as being critical in mediating the rewarding properties of drugs of abuse, which may be at the core of their addiction liability (for reviews see refs. 1–5). Neurochemical lesions of the VTA and/or NAc have been shown to disrupt opiate, cocaine, and amphetamine self-administration,[6-11] and it is also reported that rats will self-administer opiates and/or stimulants directly into these brain regions (for review see ref. 2) or other mesolimbic dopaminergic projection areas.[12] In addition, virtually all drugs abused by humans, including opiates, cocaine, amphetamine, ethanol, nicotine, and tetrahydrocannabinol, when administered systemically to rats, lead to increased extracellular levels of dopamine in the NAc.[13,14] This characteristic acute action of drugs of abuse on the mesolimbic dopamine system is thought to contribute to their rewarding properties and suggests that the VTA and NAc are brain regions involved in a common mechanism of drug reward.

Drugs of abuse also have profound chronic effects on brain function. There is a growing body of evidence in animals and in humans that chronic use of opiates and psychostimulants increases drug craving.[15-17] Moreover, chronic exposure to these drugs leads to similar types of sensitization to their acute locomotor-activating

[a] This work was supported by US PHS Grants DA07359 and 2 P50 04060, by the VA–Yale Alcoholism Research Center, Department of Veterans Affairs, and by the Abraham Ribicoff Research Facilities, Connecticut Mental Health Center, State of Connecticut Department of Mental Health.

[b] Author to whom correspondence should be addressed; Tel.: (203) 789-7153; Fax: (203) 562-7079.

effects.[18-20] These chronic actions also appear to be mediated, at least in part, via the VTA/NAc pathway,[4,19-23] although the precise biochemical mechanisms involved remain unknown.

The various classes of abused drugs, including opiates, stimulants, alcohol, nicotine and cannabinoids, have distinct primary sites of action (that is, direct interactions with different receptors or other cell-surface proteins). Thus, if the addictive effects of these drugs of abuse are mediated via common chronic actions, it is likely that post-receptor (intracellular) targets are involved.[24,25] To address this possibility, we studied the biochemical effects of chronic morphine and chronic cocaine treatments on the cyclic AMP (cAMP) system and its intracellular targets within the mesolimbic dopamine system. These studies have identified a number of common intracellular actions of chronic opiates and cocaine in these dopaminergic brain reward regions. Furthermore, drug-naïve Fischer 344 and Lewis rats (two genetically inbred strains that show different levels of drug preference) exhibit similar inherent differences in the cAMP system and intracellular target proteins specific to the mesolimbic dopamine system. We propose that these drug-induced biochemical adaptations represent part of a general mechanism underlying drug craving and addiction, and that similar mechanisms may contribute to individual genetic vulnerability to drug addiction.

BACKGROUND: BIOCHEMICAL MECHANISMS OF OPIATE ACTION IN THE RAT LOCUS COERULEUS

Studies of the intracellular actions of acute and chronic opiates have begun to reveal information about the processes by which opiate addiction occurs. Early studies on cultured neuroblastoma x glioma cells indicated that in contrast to acute opiate inhibition of adenylate cyclase, chronic opiates increase adenylate cyclase activity.[26] It was hypothesized that this increase in adenylate cyclase represents a biochemical equivalent of opiate tolerance and dependence. Subsequent studies in the rat locus coeruleus (LC) have supported and expanded the cAMP hypothesis of opiate addiction.[24,27]

The LC, the major noradrenergic nucleus in brain, is thought to play a prominent role in mediating physical opiate addiction (*i.e.*, physical dependence and physical abstinence syndromes). Experiments in our laboratory have shown that chronic morphine up-regulates the intracellular cAMP system at multiple levels in the LC. Chronic morphine treatment increases levels of $G_{i\alpha}$ and $G_{o\alpha}$ (but not other G-protein subunits), adenylate cyclase, cAMP-dependent protein kinase, and a number of phosphoprotein substrates for the protein kinase in this brain region.[28-31] As these increases occur at the protein and messenger RNA level, it is likely that opiate regulation of gene expression is involved.[27,32] There is now substantial direct evidence to suggest that the up-regulation of the cAMP system plays a critical role in the development of opiate tolerance, dependence, and withdrawal in LC neurons.[33,34]

A GENERAL ROLE FOR G-PROTEINS AND THE CYCLIC AMP SYSTEM IN DRUG ADDICTION IN THE MESOLIMBIC DOPAMINE SYSTEM

The LC is generally not thought to be involved in drug reward mechanisms.[1] Thus, we examined the possibility that similar adaptations in the intracellular cAMP system may be involved in the chronic actions of opiates in dopaminergic brain reward regions. We found that chronic morphine *decreases* levels of the inhibitory G-protein $G_{i\alpha}$ and *increases* levels of adenylate cyclase and cAMP-dependent protein kinase activities in the NAc, but not in several other brain regions.[24] These results raised the interesting possibility that adaptations in the cAMP pathway may contribute to mechanisms of drug reward and craving mediated via the NAc.

This hypothesis was tested further by determining whether similar intracellular adaptations occur in the NAc in response to chronic cocaine. Indeed, chronic cocaine produced very similar alterations as chronic morphine, with decreased levels of $G_{i\alpha}$ and $G_{o\alpha}$ and increased levels of adenylate cyclase and cAMP-dependent protein kinase observed[24,35] (FIG. 1). Similar effects were not seen in a number of other brain regions studied, including the caudate/putamen (a projection area of substantia nigra dopamine neurons) generally considered not to be involved in brain reward processes. The effects of cocaine in the NAc were not seen after acute drug administration, indicating that these changes are a result of chronic exposure to the drug. In contrast to morphine and cocaine, chronic administration of several other psychotropic drugs without prominent reinforcing properties [haloperidol (an antipsychotic drug which acts as a dopamine antagonist), and imipramine and fluoxetine (antidepressant drugs which act as monoamine re-uptake blockers)] did not produce changes in these intracellular messengers in the NAc.[24]

In the case of chronic cocaine, these biochemical alterations can be understood within a functional context of known electrophysiological effects of cocaine on NAc neurons. Chronic cocaine has been shown to produce supersensitivity of NAc neurons to the effects of D_1-dopaminergic agonists on these cells.[36] This cocaine-induced functional supersensitivity occurs in the absence of detectable changes in levels of the receptor *per se*,[37,38] suggesting the involvement of post-receptor mechanisms. As D_1 receptors are generally thought to exert their effects via activation of the cAMP pathway, the observed increase in adenylate cyclase and cAMP-dependent protein kinase, to-

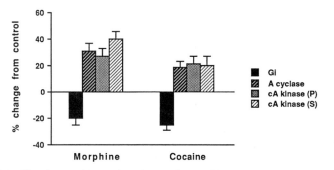

FIGURE 1. Chronic morphine and cocaine produce similar adaptations in G-proteins and the cAMP system in the NAc. Rats were treated chronically with either morphine: 1 subcutaneous pellet of morphine daily for 5 days (75 mg, NIDA), or cocaine: 15 mg/kg intraperitoneal injections twice daily for 14 days. Rats were then sacrificed on day 6 for morphine, or day 15 for cocaine. The NAc was dissected from control and treated rats and duplicate aliquots of tissue extracts were analyzed for levels of $G_{i\alpha}$, adenylate cyclase activity, or cAMP-dependent protein kinase activity in particulate (P) and soluble (S) fractions. The data are expressed as percent change from control ± SEM ($n = 8$–14). All changes shown are statistically significant ($p < 0.05$ by χ^2 test). (Data are from refs. 24 and 35.)

gether with the observed decrease in $G_{i\alpha}$, without a change in $G_{s\alpha}$ or G_β, could account for D_1 receptor supersensitivity observed electrophysiologically. Although it is not known how NAc neurons respond to chronic morphine treatment, we would predict similar effects (at least under our treatment conditions) compared to chronic cocaine based on our biochemical findings. These results indicate that adaptations in the intracellular cAMP system may represent common responses of NAc neurons to drugs of abuse.

G-PROTEINS AND THE CYCLIC AMP SYSTEM IN FISCHER AND LEWIS RATS: MODELS FOR GENETIC DETERMINANTS OF DRUG ADDICTION

Genetic factors are generally thought to contribute to individual differences in susceptibility to drug addiction in both animals and people, although the specific factors involved remain unknown. One model system for such differences are Fischer F344 and Lewis rats, inbred strains that show, respectively, lower and higher levels of self-administration of opiates, cocaine, and alcohol.[40-42] Lewis rats also develop greater degrees of conditioned place preference to systemic morphine and cocaine compared to Fischer rats[42] (FIG. 2). As a way to understand the biological basis of these strain differences in drug preference, we studied G-proteins, adenylate cyclase, and cAMP-dependent protein kinase activities in the NAc of drug-naïve Fischer and Lewis rats. Interestingly, levels of these proteins in drug-naïve Lewis rats, compared to drug-naïve Fischer rats, resembled the effects of chronic morphine and chronic cocaine on these proteins in outbred Sprague-Dawley rats.[42] That is, levels of adenylate cyclase and

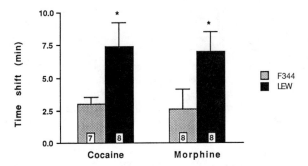

FIGURE 2. Lewis rats develop greater degrees of conditioned place preference to systemic morphine and cocaine compared to Fischer rats. Conditioned place preference was carried out according to published procedures.[66] Briefly, Lewis or Fischer 344 rats (200 g) were placed in opened conditioned place preference chambers for 30 min to obtain baseline scores. On each of the subsequent 4 days, rats received single injections of cocaine hydrochloride (15 mg/kg i.p.) or morphine sulfate (4 mg/kg s.c.) and were placed in a designated side of the chambers for 60 min. On the following day, rats were returned to opened chambers for 30 min to obtain test scores. Differences between test and baseline scores for each rat reflect conditioned place preference. Both strains developed significant place preference to morphine and to cocaine, although the magnitude was significantly greater for the Lewis rats (* $p < 0.05$ by student's *t*-test). In contrast, neither strain developed significant place preference for vehicle injections. (From refs. 42 and 58.)

cAMP-dependent protein kinase activities in the NAc are higher in Lewis rats compared to Fischer rats, whereas levels of $G_{i\alpha}$ are lower. These strain differences were not observed in a number of other brain regions. These findings suggest that different levels of expression of components of the cAMP pathway in the NAc may contribute to individual genetic vulnerability to drug addiction (see ref. 43).

MORPHINE AND COCAINE EXERT COMMON CHRONIC ACTIONS ON TYROSINE HYDROXYLASE

To further investigate possible intracellular targets of chronic opiate and cocaine action in the VTA and NAc, we focused on the effects of these drugs on the next step in the cAMP signal transduction pathway, namely, individual phosphoprotein substrates of cAMP-dependent protein kinase. Cyclic AMP-dependent protein phosphorylation was studied in these brain regions by use of a back phosphorylation procedure, whereby proteins present in acid extracts of brain tissue are phosphorylated by purified cAMP-dependent protein kinase and $[\gamma\text{-}^{32}P]ATP$. Phosphorylated proteins are then analyzed by 2-dimensional gel electrophoresis and autoradiography. This procedure offers a sensitive way to identify individual proteins involved in a wide array of neural phenomena.[31,44] Using these techniques we found that chronic morphine and chronic cocaine regulated many of the same phosphoproteins in these brain regions. FIGURES 3 and 4 show autoradiograms of 2-dimensional gels that illustrate the effect of chronic morphine (FIG. 3) and chronic cocaine (FIG. 4) on back phosphorylation in the VTA. While the overall phosphoprotein pattern in control and drug-treated rats was very similar, a number of individual phosphoproteins were consistently altered by the drug treatments. Prominent among these morphine- and cocaine-regulated phosphoproteins (or MCRPPs) is a 58 kD protein known to be tyrosine hydroxylase (the rate-limiting enzyme in dopamine biosynthesis), whose level of back phosphorylation was increased in the VTA in response to chronic morphine and cocaine.[45]

Differences observed in levels of back phosphorylation (*i.e.*, $^{32}PO_4$ incorporation) can reflect differences in the state of phosphorylation of individual phosphoproteins or differences in their total amounts. Increased levels of tyrosine hydroxylase as measured by back phosphorylation techniques under different conditions implied that chronic morphine and cocaine treatments increased the total amount of tyrosine hydroxylase in the VTA without altering its phosphorylation state. We confirmed these interpretations directly by measuring levels of enzyme immunoreactivity with immunoblotting procedures. As shown in FIGURE 5, chronic morphine and chronic cocaine increased levels of tyrosine hydroxylase immunoreactivity by ~30–40% in the VTA. In contrast, these drug treatments had no effect on enzyme levels in the NAc, substantia nigra, or caudate/putamen.[45]

The up-regulation of tyrosine hydroxylase immunoreactivity in the VTA by both chronic morphine and chronic cocaine treatments may reflect common functional changes induced in VTA neurons by these drugs of abuse. The expression of tyrosine hydroxylase in adrenal medulla, peripheral sympathetic neurons, and central catecholaminergic neurons appears to be induced by conditions that increase synaptic activation of the cells (for references see ref. 32). An increase in tyrosine hydroxylase expression in the VTA in response to morphine or cocaine may, therefore, result from an elevated level of VTA neuronal activity. Indeed, such an increase has been reported to occur in response to chronic cocaine treatment. Henry *et al.*[21] showed that there

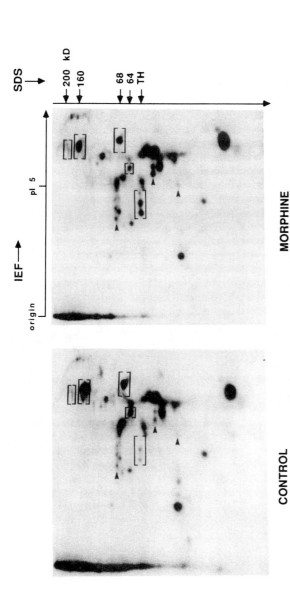

FIGURE 3. Autoradiograms of 2-dimensional gels illustrating the effect of chronic morphine on back phosphorylation in the VTA. Rats were treated chronically with morphine as described in the legend to FIGURE 1. Isolated VTA nuclei from control and drug-treated rats were then subjected to direct back phosphorylation with cAMP-dependent protein kinase and [γ-^{32}P]ATP and to 2-dimensional gel electrophoresis (see ref. 31). Resulting gels were dried and autoradiographed. *Brackets* indicate the positions of phosphoproteins of M$_r$ 200, 160, 68, and 64 kD (known to be neurofilament proteins) whose direct back phosphorylation is decreased by both chronic morphine and chronic cocaine. *Brackets* also indicate the position of a 58 kD phosphoprotein (known to be tyrosine hydroxylase, TH) whose direct back phosphorylation is increased by chronic morphine and chronic cocaine. Several other unknown phosphoproteins, which are not discussed here, also appeared to be drug-regulated (indicated by *arrowheads*). (From ref. 48.)

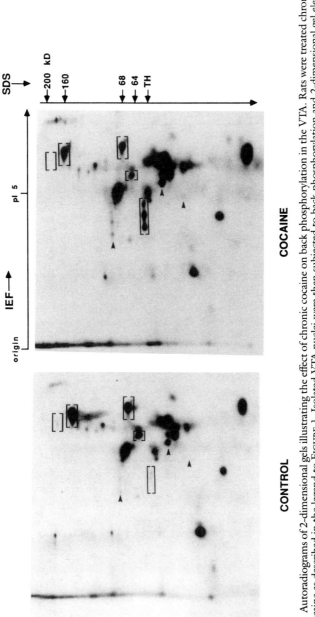

FIGURE 4. Autoradiograms of 2-dimensional gels illustrating the effect of chronic cocaine on back phosphorylation in the VTA. Rats were treated chronically with cocaine as described in the legend to FIGURE 1. Isolated VTA nuclei were then subjected to back phosphorylation and 2-dimensional gel electrophoresis, as in FIGURE 3. *Brackets* indicate the positions of phosphoproteins of M_r 200, 160, 68, and 64 kD (known to be neurofilament proteins) whose direct back phosphorylation is decreased by both chronic morphine and chronic cocaine. *Brackets* also indicate the position of a 58 kD phosphoprotein (known to be tyrosine hydroxylase, TH) whose direct back phosphorylation is increased by chronic morphine and chronic cocaine. Several other unknown phosphoproteins, which are not discussed here, also appeared to be drug-regulated (indicated by *arrowheads*). (From ref. 48.)

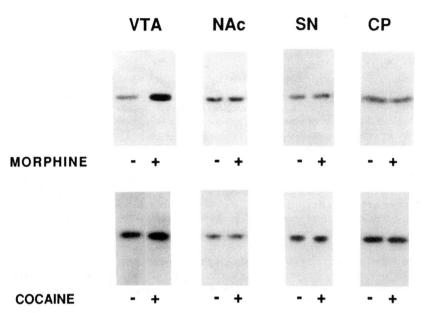

FIGURE 5. Autoradiograms illustrating the effect of chronic morphine and chronic cocaine on tyrosine hydroxylase immunoreactivity. Rats were treated chronically with morphine or cocaine, as described in the legend to FIGURE 1. The VTA, NAc, SN (substantia nigra), and CP (caudate/putamen) were isolated from control (−) or drug-treated (+) rats and then analyzed by SDS-polyacrylamide gel electrophoresis and tyrosine hydroxylase (TH) immunolabeling. Levels of TH immunoreactivity in the VTA relative to control were 143% ± 12 (n = 8) for morphine and 131% ± 12 (n = 12) for cocaine (p < 0.05 by χ^2 test). TH levels were not different from control in the NAc, SN, or CP in response to either drug treatment. (From ref. 45.)

are more spontaneously active VTA neurons and that their firing rates are significantly higher in cocaine-treated rats compared to controls. Again, it is not known how VTA neurons respond electrophysiologically to chronic morphine treatment, but it is reasonable to hypothesize that chronic morphine may also increase the firing rate or intrinsic excitability of VTA neurons.

In contrast to drug actions in the VTA, chronic morphine and chronic cocaine decreased the phosphorylation state of tyrosine hydroxylase in the NAc, with no change in the total amount of the enzyme.[45] In contrast, no effect on enzyme phosphorylation was observed in the caudate/putamen. As cyclic AMP-dependent protein kinase and other protein kinases are known to phosphorylate and activate tyrosine hydroxylase, dephosphorylation of the enzyme would suggest reduced catalytic activity in response to chronic morphine and cocaine. This dephosphorylation of tyrosine hydroxylase could account for reduced levels of *in vivo* dopamine synthesis observed in response to chronic cocaine in the NAc,[46] and for reduced levels of *in vivo* basal and morphine-stimulated dopamine release in this brain region in response to chronic morphine.[47] Because tyrosine hydroxylase present in the NAc is located in dopaminergic nerve terminals derived from the VTA, it appears that chronic morphine and chronic cocaine regulate the enzyme differently within VTA cell bodies and their nerve terminals (see below).

TYROSINE HYDROXYLASE LEVELS DIFFER IN DRUG-NAÏVE
FISCHER AND LEWIS RATS

Tyrosine hydroxylase levels were also markedly different in the mesolimbic dopamine system between Fischer and Lewis rat strains. The VTA of drug-naïve Lewis (drug-preferring) rats had ~45% higher levels of tyrosine hydroxylase immunoreactivity than drug-naïve Fischer rats, whereas the NAc contained ~45% lower levels.[43] In contrast, no differences in tyrosine hydroxylase immunoreactivity levels were seen in the substantia nigra or caudate/putamen (FIG. 6).

The pattern of tyrosine hydroxylase levels in the VTA and NAc of drug-naïve Lewis versus Fischer rats resembles the influence of chronic morphine and chronic cocaine on the enzyme in these brain reward regions of Sprague-Dawley rats. That is, higher levels of enzyme are seen in the VTA both in drug-treated versus control Sprague-Dawley rats and in drug-naïve Lewis versus Fischer rats. Moreover, lower levels of enzyme activity would appear to occur in the NAc under each of these conditions, with lower levels of enzyme catalytic activity achieved in the drug-treated state through decreases in enzyme phosphorylation and with lower total levels of the enzyme in Lewis versus Fischer rats. The observation of higher enzyme levels in the VTA, but lower levels in the NAc, supports the view that dopaminergic neurotransmission within these two brain regions subserves different functional roles (as will be discussed further below).

MORPHINE AND COCAINE EXERT COMMON
CHRONIC ACTIONS ON NEUROFILAMENT PROTEINS

It can be seen in FIGURES 3 and 4 that in addition to increasing levels of tyrosine hydroxylase back phosphorylation in the VTA, chronic morphine and chronic cocaine also alter a number of other phosphoproteins in similar ways. In particular, phosphoproteins of 200, 160, 68, and 64 kD are all decreased by back phosphorylation in response to both drug treatments. Using specific antibodies with 2-dimensional immunoblotting methods, these drug-regulated phosphoproteins have now been identified

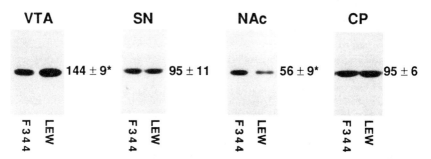

FIGURE 6. Autoradiograms of immunoblots comparing levels of tyrosine hydroxylase immunoreactivity in brain regions of Lewis and Fischer 344 rats. Brain regions isolated from drug-naïve Lewis and Fischer rats were isolated and analyzed for tyrosine hydroxylase as described in the legend to FIGURE 4. Data are expressed as mean levels in Lewis rats as a percent of levels in Fischer rats ± SEM and represent the results from 7–14 rats of each strain. * $p < 0.025$ by χ^2 test. (From ref. 43.)

as neurofilament (NF) proteins.[48] The 200 kD phosphoprotein corresponds to NF-200 or NF-H (high), 160 kD corresponds to NF-160 or NF-M (middle), 68 kD corresponds to NF-68 or NF-L (low),[49] and 64 kD corresponds to the novel NF protein known alternatively as NF-66[50] or α-internexin.[51]

By use of immunoblotting and Coomassie-blue staining, we found that chronic morphine- and cocaine-induced decreases in NF-200, NF-160 and NF-68 back phosphorylation are associated with equivalent decreases in the total amounts of these proteins.[48] The NF-66 protein, however, was regulated differently by chronic morphine and chronic cocaine. Chronic cocaine induced a decrease in NF-66 immunoreactivity as well as decreasing its back phosphorylation. Chronic morphine did not alter NF-66 immunoreactivity,[48] but did decrease its back phosphorylation. This result can be interpreted to indicate that chronic morphine increases the phosphorylation state of NF-66, without changing its total amount (for a detailed discussion of back phosphorylation see refs. 31 and 44). Such differential drug regulation of NF-66 presumably underlies some of the distinct functional changes induced in VTA neurons by chronic morphine and by chronic cocaine.

Morphine and cocaine regulation of NFs exhibited temporal, regional, and pharmacological specificity.[48] Regulation of the proteins was not observed in response to acute drug administration, and chronic drug treatment failed to alter levels of the proteins in several other brain regions studied. Moreover, chronic treatment of rats with imipramine and haloperidol did not alter levels of NFs in the VTA. As NFs are major components of the neuronal cytoskeleton, the finding that they are decreased by chronic morphine and chronic cocaine raised the possibility that these drug treatments may be disrupting the general cytoskeletal architecture in the VTA. Therefore, we examined a variety of other cytoskeletal proteins in the VTA, including α- and β-tubulin, actin, vimentin, synaptophysin, tau, and synapsin I. None of these other major structural proteins were altered by chronic morphine treatment, suggesting that NFs 68, 160, and 200 were selectively down-regulated.[48]

It is uncertain what impact such alterations in NFs exert on the functional integrity of VTA neurons. NFs are known to be associated with axonal transport, as a variety of *in vivo* manipulations which alter NF proteins, including axotomy, aluminum, or β,β'-iminodiproprionitrile intoxication, are all associated with decreased rates of axonal transport.[53-55] Given this evidence, our findings that NFs are decreased in response to chronic morphine and cocaine raise the possibility that these drug treatments decrease the rate of axonal transport in VTA neurons (see below). NFs are also thought to function as determinants of neuronal structure[56-58]: decreases in NF proteins could, therefore, also induce major alterations in the structural features of VTA cell bodies, dendrites, and/or axons.

DIFFERENT LEVELS OF NEUROFILAMENT PROTEINS IN FISCHER AND LEWIS RATS

Fischer and Lewis rat strains exhibited different levels of NFs specifically in the VTA: drug-naïve Lewis rats had markedly lower levels of NFs in this but not other brain regions compared to drug-naïve Fischer rats.[42,58] Such strain differences in the VTA were observed for NF-200, NF-160, and NF-68. These strain differences in NFs resemble the effects of chronic morphine and cocaine treatment on NFs in the VTA of Sprague-Dawley rats, where the drugs decrease NF levels.

A MODEL FOR THE BIOCHEMICAL BASIS OF DRUG ADDICTION

The findings presented here document a number of common chronic actions of morphine and cocaine on intracellular messenger proteins in the mesolimbic dopamine system. These common actions are particularly striking given that systemic morphine and cocaine have markedly different acute behavioral effects (sedative versus stimulant), as well as opposite acute electrophysiological actions on VTA neurons.[59,60] Yet after chronic systemic administration, these drugs elicit some important common behavioral effects that are thought to be mediated, at least in part, via the mesolimbic dopamine system: e.g., drug craving and locomotor sensitization (see INTRODUCTION). The common intracellular adaptations in the cAMP system elicited by chronic morphine and chronic cocaine could be part of the biochemical basis of these behavioral phenomena. The mechanism by which these common chronic actions are achieved is unknown, but probably involves a concert of factors that integrate to produce common functional effects on these neurons, reflected in the biochemical changes described here.

Such an association between the biochemical adaptations and drug craving is suggested by several lines of evidence. First, it appears that these changes in G-proteins, adenylate cyclase, cAMP-dependent protein kinase, tyrosine hydroxylase, and NF proteins are long-term adaptations that occur in the VTA and/or NAc in response to repeated exposure to morphine and cocaine, as these changes were not seen in response to acute treatment with the drugs. Second, chronic morphine and chronic cocaine regulate tyrosine hydroxylase in the VTA and NAc, where dopamine is thought to play a central role in drug reward mechanisms. Third, the various biochemical alterations show regional specificity, in that they were not seen in a number of other brain regions, including the nigrostriatal dopamine system, which is generally not correlated with drug reward. Fourth, none of these biochemical changes were produced by chronic treatment of rats with haloperidol or imipramine, two psychotropic drugs that are not reinforcing. Finally, these various effects of chronic morphine and chronic cocaine on intracellular messengers in the mesolimbic dopamine system of Sprague-Dawley rats are similar to differences seen in the same dopaminergic brain regions of drug-naïve Fischer and Lewis rats, two genetically inbred strains that show, respectively, lower and higher levels of drug preference for morphine, cocaine, and alcohol. Such similarities between phosphoprotein regulation in the VTA by chronic morphine and cocaine, and basal levels of the proteins in the VTA of Lewis versus Fischer rats, are summarized in FIGURE 7. Based on the remarkably similar biochemical profiles of the mesolimbic dopamine system in morphine-treated rats, cocaine-treated rats, and drug-naïve Lewis rats (compared to Fischer rats), we would propose that a drug-addicted (or drug-preferring) state is associated with higher levels of tyrosine hydroxylase and lower levels of NFs in dopaminergic cell bodies of the VTA, and with decreased levels of tyrosine hydroxylase activity and an up-regulated cAMP pathway in the NAc. These results and interpretations are summarized schematically in FIGURE 8.

These findings have a number of potentially important implications for understanding the neurobiology of morphine and cocaine addiction. One major conclusion of these studies is that the activity of the mesolimbic dopamine system is regulated differentially in dopaminergic cell bodies in the VTA versus dopaminergic nerve terminals in the NAc. This is consistent with the view, alluded to above, that dopaminergic neurotransmission subserves different functional roles in these two brain regions. In the VTA, where dopamine is known to act upon inhibitory D_2 autorecep-

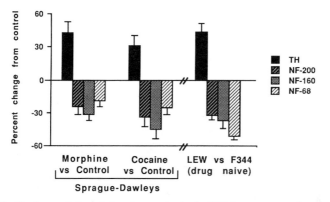

FIGURE 7. Similar regulation of phosphoproteins in the VTA in response to chronic morphine or chronic cocaine or in drug-naïve Lewis versus Fischer 344 rats. Sprague-Dawley rats received chronic morphine or chronic cocaine as described in the legend to FIGURE 1. Drug-naïve Lewis rats were compared to drug-naïve Fischer 344 rats. Tyrosine hydroxylase (TH) and neurofilaments (NFs) were analyzed by immunoblotting techniques. Data are expressed as percent difference from control (for morphine- and cocaine-treated rats), or percent change from Fischer 344 (for Lewis rats). Shown are levels of TH, NF-200, NF-160, and NF-68. Data are expressed as mean ± SEM and represent the results from 8–16 rats in each group. (Based on data in refs. 45, 48, and 58.)

tors and possibly on non-dopaminergic terminals as well, increased levels of tyrosine hydroxylase could reflect increased local dopaminergic tone, consistent with increased VTA firing rates that occur with chronic cocaine treatment.[21] In the NAc, where dopamine has distinct physiological and biochemical actions on multiple subtypes of receptors localized both pre- and postsynaptically, decreased tyrosine hydroxylase phosphorylation probably reflects lower enzyme activity and decreased dopamine synthesis. As described above, recent *in vivo* microdialysis studies have provided corroborating evidence that dopamine synthesis is decreased after chronic morphine or cocaine.[46,47] Moreover, sensitization of D_1 dopamine receptor function observed in the NAc[36] could reflect a compensatory response to decreased dopamine synthesis (and presumably decreased dopamine release[c]) in rats after repeated cocaine administration.

---

[c] In the case of morphine, it has been reported that chronic morphine decreases basal levels of dopamine release in the NAc.[47] The state of basal extracellular dopamine levels in the NAc after chronic cocaine remains controversial. It has been reported that 7 days after chronic cocaine treatment, basal levels of dopamine release in the NAc are reduced.[61] However, Justice and colleagues did not find a difference in basal levels of dopamine release 1 day after chronic cocaine treatment,[22] and report in another study that electrically stimulated dopamine release is increased in the NAc after chronic cocaine.[62] There is also considerable evidence that chronic cocaine treatment increases the ability of a subsequent dose of cocaine to stimulate extracellular dopamine levels,[22] although this effect may be due at least in part to pharmacokinetic considerations.[63,64] Taken together with a cocaine-induced decrease in dopamine synthesis,[46] these various findings are difficult to interpret, but may indicate that chronic cocaine induces a redistribution of dopamine stores into readily releasable pools, such that in response to specific types of stimuli, dopamine overflow is temporarily increased in the NAc.[62]

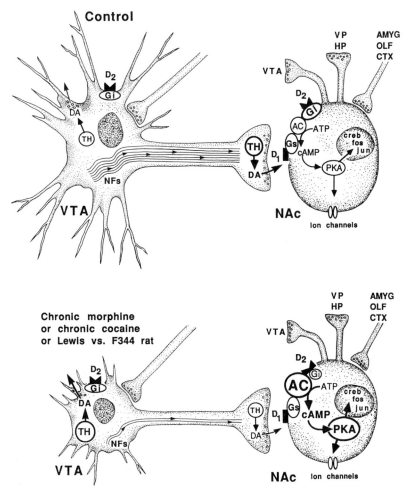

FIGURE 8. Schematic summary of similar biochemical manifestations of the "drug-addicted" and "drug-preferring" state. The top figure depicts a control VTA neuron projecting to the NAc. Shown in the VTA cell are tyrosine hydroxylase (TH), dopamine (DA), presynaptic dopamine receptors (D_2) coupled to G-proteins (G_i), and neurofilaments (NFs). Shown in the NAc are, in addition to TH and DA, dopamine receptors (D_1 and D_2), G-proteins (G_i and G_s), components of the intracellular cyclic AMP system (AC, adenylate cyclase activity; PKA, cAMP-dependent protein kinase activity; and possible substrates for the kinase–ion channels and the nuclear transcription factors, CREB, fos, and jun), as well as major inputs and outputs of this region (VP, ventral pallidum; HP, hippocampus; AMYG, amygdala; OLF, olfactory cortex; CTX, other cortical regions).

The bottom figure depicts a VTA neuron projecting to the NAc after chronic morphine or cocaine treatment, or from a Lewis (drug-preferring) rat, as compared to a Fischer (F344) rat. In the drug-addicted or drug-preferring animal, TH levels are *increased* in the VTA, and *decreased* in the NAc (due to either decreased phosphorylation as for morphine and cocaine, or decreased enzyme levels as in Lewis versus Fischer rats). In addition, NF levels are decreased in the VTA in the drug-addicted and drug-preferring state. This decrease in NFs may be associated with alterations in neuronal structure, decreases in axonal caliber and/or decreases in axonal transport

Another important implication of our findings is the possibility that the differential regulation of dopaminergic transmission in the VTA and NAc may be achieved via decreased levels of NFs in the VTA. Thus, decreased levels of NFs could lead to decreases in axonal diameter and axonal transport in these neurons, as implied in FIGURE 8. Indeed, we have recently found that chronic morphine does impair axonal transport in the mesolimbic dopamine system.[65] This may explain the finding that while chronic morphine and cocaine treatments increase tyrosine hydroxylase levels in the VTA, this increase is not reflected in the nerve terminals, indicating that less tyrosine hydroxylase may be reaching the NAc. This differential distribution of tyrosine hydroxylase is also reflected in Lewis versus Fischer rats: Lewis rats have more tyrosine hydroxylase in the VTA, but less in the NAc, which could be explained by the correspondingly lower levels of NF proteins in their VTA.

Although tentative, our findings suggest the possibility that chronic use of morphine or cocaine may alter the structural features of mesolimbic dopamine neurons, in such a way as to reduce the ability of these cells to transmit dopaminergic signals to postsynaptic cells in the NAc. Thus, long-term opiate or stimulant use may impair the brain's endogenous reward system, which could have a major impact, in humans, on motivation and affect. Our similar findings with Lewis and Fischer rats suggest that populations that are genetically predisposed to drug addiction may have a similar type of mesolimbic dopamine impairment inherently.

A third important implication of our studies is that up-regulation of the cAMP system may be part of the biochemical basis of the D_1 receptor supersensitivity observed under chronic cocaine conditions[36] and predicted on the basis of our biochemical studies under chronic morphine conditions. Altered levels of $G_{i\alpha}$, adenylate cyclase, and cAMP-dependent protein kinase would be expected to change the synaptic responsiveness of the NAc neurons not only to dopamine, but also to a host of other incoming neurotransmitter signals that innervate this brain region. It is possible that such altered responsiveness of NAc neurons to these other synaptic inputs represents one of the major changes in the brain that underlies drug addiction and craving.

Clearly, further experiments are needed to test the validity of the hypothetical model presented above. It will be of particular interest to determine the extent to which these biochemical alterations correlate with behavioral measures of drug addiction. Preliminary studies have indicated that similar intracellular changes are observed in the mesolimbic dopamine system of rats which have chronically self-administered intravenous heroin (D. W. Self, L. Stein, D. Beitner-Johnson, E. J. Nestler, unpublished observations). Other studies are currently underway to identify the precise molecular mechanisms by which opiates and cocaine alter the levels of specific intracellular messenger proteins in the mesolimbic dopamine system. Our findings indicate

---

rate in these cells, as indicated in the figure. This hypothetical decrease in axonal transport may account for the lack of correspondingly increased levels of TH in dopaminergic terminals in the NAc. Decreased TH implies decreased dopamine synthesis, and may result in lower dopaminergic transmission to the NAc. In the NAc of the drug-addicted or drug-preferring state, G_i is *decreased*, and adenylate cyclase and cAMP-dependent protein kinase activities are *increased*, changes that could account for D_1 receptor supersensitivity.[36]

It should be noted that alterations in dopaminergic transmission probably influence many cell types within the NAc, as well as other nerve terminals in the NAc. Similarly, altered local dopaminergic transmission in the VTA could also influence other nerve terminals in this brain region. Thus, biochemical alterations in the mesolimbic dopamine system could potentially lead to altered neuronal function in many other brain regions as well.

that studies of drug-regulated intracellular second messenger systems and individual phosphoproteins in brain reward regions will lead to an improved understanding of the mechanisms underlying addictive processes and the identification of some of the factors that contribute to individual genetic vulnerability to drug addiction.

REFERENCES

1. FIBIGER, H. C. 1978. Drugs and reinforcement mechanisms: A critical review of the catecholamine theory. Ann. Rev. Pharm. and Tox. 18: 37–56.
2. BOZARTH, M. A. 1986. Neural basis of psychomotor stimulant and opiate reward: Evidence suggesting the involvement of a common dopaminergic system. Behav. Brain Res. 22: 107–116.
3. WISE, R. A. & M. A. BOZARTH. 1987. A psychomotor stimulant theory of addiction. Psychol. Rev. 94: 469–492.
4. KOOB, G. F. & F. E. BLOOM. 1988. Cellular and molecular mechanisms of drug dependence. Science 242: 715–723.
5. LIEBMAN, J. M. & S. J. COOPER, Eds. 1989. The Neuropharmacological Basis of Reward. Oxford University Press. New York.
6. LYNESS, W. H., N. M. FRIEDLE & K. E. MOORE. 1979. Destruction of dopaminergic nerve terminals in nucleus accumbens: Effect of d-amphetamine self-administration. Pharmacol. Biochem. Behav. 11: 553–556.
7. ROBERTS, D. C. S. & G. F. KOOB. 1982. Disruption of cocaine self-administration following 6-hydroxydopamine lesions of the ventral tegmental area in rats. Pharmacol. Biochem. Behav. 17: 901–904.
8. SPYRAKI, C., H. C. FIBIGER & A. G. PHILLIPS. 1983. Attenuation of heroin reward in rats by disruption of the mesocorticolimbic dopamine system. Psychopharmacology 79: 278–283.
9. PETTIT, H. O., A. ETTENBERG, F. E. BLOOM & G. F. KOOB. 1984. Destruction of dopamine in the nucleus accumbens selectively attenuates cocaine but not heroin self-administration in rats. Psychopharmacology 84: 167–173.
10. ZITO, K., G. VICKERS & D. C. S. ROBERTS. 1985. Disruption of cocaine and heroin self-administration following kainic acid lesions of the nucleus accumbens. Pharmacol. Biochem. Behav. 23: 1029–1036.
11. BOZARTH, M. A. & R. A. WISE. 1986. Involvement of the ventral tegmental dopamine system in opioid and psychomotor stimulant reinforcement. In Problems of Drug Dependence, 1985. L.S. Harris, Ed., 67: 190–196. US Government Printing Office. Washington, DC.
12. GOEDERS, N. E. & J. E. SMITH. 1983. Cortical dopaminergic involvement in cocaine reinforcement. Science 221: 773–775.
13. DICHIARA, G. & A. IMPERATO. 1988. Drugs abused by humans preferentially increase synaptic dopamine concentrations in the mesolimbic system of freely moving rats. Proc. Natl. Acad. Sci. USA 85: 5274–5278.
14. CHEN, J., W. PAREDES, J. LI, D. SMITHE, J. LOWINSON & E. L. GARDNER. 1990. Δ^9-tetrahydrocannabinol produces naloxone-blockable enhancement of presynaptic basal dopamine efflux in nucleus accumbens of conscious, freely-moving rats as measured by intracerebral microdialysis. Psychopharmacology 102: 156–162.
15. PIAZZA, P. V., J.-M. DEMINIERE, M. LE MOAL & H. SIMON. 1989. Factors that predict individual vulnerability to amphetamine self-administration. Science 245: 1511–1513.
16. LETT, B. T. 1989. Repeated exposures intensify rather than diminish the rewarding effects of amphetamine, morphine, and cocaine. Psychopharmacology (Berlin) 98: 357–362.
17. JAFFE, J. H. 1990. Drug addiction and drug abuse. In The Pharmacological Basis of Therapeutics. A. G. Gilman, T. W. Rall, A. S. Nies & P. Taylor, Eds.: 522–573. Pergamon Press. New York.
18. POST, R. M. & H. ROSE. 1976. Increasing effects of repetitive cocaine administration in the rat. Nature 260: 731–732.

19. KALIVAS, P. W. 1985. Sensitization to repeated enkephalin administration into the ventral tegmental area of the rat. II. Involvement of the mesolimbic dopamine system. J. Pharmacol. Exp. Ther. **235**: 544–550.
20. KALIVAS, P. W. & P. DUFFY. 1988. Effects of daily cocaine and morphine treatment on somatodendritic and terminal field dopamine release. J. Neurochem. **50**: 1498–1504.
21. HENRY, D. J., M. A. GREENE & F. J. WHITE. 1989. Electrophysiological effects of cocaine in the mesoaccumbens dopamine system: Repeated administration. J. Pharmacol. Exp. Ther. **251**: 833–839.
22. PETTIT, H. O., H. PAN, L. H. PARSONS & J. B. JUSTICE, JR. 1990. Extracellular concentrations of cocaine and dopamine are enhanced during chronic cocaine administration. J. Neurochem. **55**: 798–804.
23. STEKETEE, J. D., C. D. STRIPLIN, T. F. MURRAY & P. W. KALIVAS. 1991. Possible role for G-proteins in behavioral sensitization to cocaine. Brain Res. **545**: 287–291.
24. TERWILLIGER, R., D. BEITNER-JOHNSON, K. A. SEVARINO, S. M. CRAIN & E. J. NESTLER. 1991. A general role for adaptations in G-proteins and the cyclic AMP system in mediating the chronic actions of morphine and cocaine on neuronal function. Brain Res. **548**: 100–110.
25. SELF, D. W. & L. STEIN. 1992. Receptor subtypes involved in opioid and stimulant reward. Pharmacol. Toxicol. In press.
26. SHARMA, S. K., W. A. KLEE & M. NIRENBERG. 1975. Dual regulation of adenylate cyclase accounts for narcotic dependence and tolerance. Proc. Natl. Acad. Sci. USA **72**: 3092–3096.
27. NESTLER, E. J. 1990. Adaptive changes in signal transduction systems: Molecular mechanisms of opiate addiction in the rat locus coeruleus. Prog. Cell Res. **1**: 73–88.
28. NESTLER, E. J., J. J. ERDOS, R. TERWILLIGER, R. S. DUMAN & J. F. TALLMAN. 1989. Regulation of G-proteins by chronic morphine in the rat locus coeruleus. Brain Res. **476**: 230–239.
29. NESTLER, E. J. & J. F. TALLMAN. 1988. Chronic morphine treatment increases cyclic AMP-dependent protein kinase activity in the rat locus coeruleus. Mol. Pharmacol. **33**: 127–132.
30. DUMAN, R. S., J. F. TALLMAN & E. J. NESTLER. 1988. Acute and chronic opiate-regulation of adenylate cyclase in brain: Specific effects in locus coeruleus. J. Pharmacol. Exp. Ther. **246**: 1033–1039.
31. GUITART, X. & E. J. NESTLER. 1989. Identification of morphine- and cyclic AMP-regulated phosphoproteins (MARPPs) in the rat locus coeruleus and other regions of the rat brain: Regulation by acute and chronic morphine. J. Neurosci. **9**: 4371–4387.
32. GUITART, X., M. HAYWARD, L. K. NISENBAUM, D. B. BEITNER-JOHNSON, J. W. HAYCOCK & E. J. NESTLER. 1990. Identification of MARPP-58, a morphine- and cyclic AMP-regulated phosphoprotein of 58 kDA, as tyrosine hydroxylase: Evidence for regulation of its expression by chronic morphine in the rat locus coeruleus. J. Neurosci. **10**: 2649–2659.
33. RASMUSSEN, K., D. B. BEITNER-JOHNSON, J. H. KRYSTAL, G. K. AGHAJANIAN & E. J. NESTLER. 1990. Opiate withdrawal and the rat locus coeruleus: Behavioral, electrophysiological, and biochemical correlates. J. Neurosci. **10**: 2308–2317.
34. KOGAN, J. H., E. J. NESTLER & G. K. AGHAJANIAN. 1992. Elevated basal firing rates of rat locus coeruleus neurons in brain slices from opiate-dependent rats: Association with enhanced responses to 8-Br-cAMP. Eur. J. Pharmacol. In press.
35. NESTLER, E. J., R. Z. TERWILLIGER, J. R. WALKER, K. A. SEVARINO & R. S. DUMAN. 1990. Chronic cocaine treatment decreases levels of the G-protein subunits Giα and Goα in discrete regions of rat brain. J. Neurochem. **55**: 1079–1082.
36. HENRY, D. J. & F. J. WHITE. 1991. Repeated cocaine administration causes persistent enhancement of D1 dopamine receptor sensitivity within the rat nucleus accumbens. J. Pharmacol. Exp. Ther. **258**: 882–890.
37. CLOUET, D., K. ASGHAR & R. BROWN, Eds. 1988. Mechanisms of Cocaine Abuse and Toxicity. NIDA Research Monograph **88**. National Institute on Drug Abuse. Rockville, MD.
38. PERIS, J., S. J. BOYSON, W. A. CASS, P. CURELLA, L. P. DWOSKIN, G. LARSON, L.-H. LIN, R. P. YASUDA & N. R. ZAHNISER. 1990. Persistence of neurochemical changes in

dopamine systems after repeated cocaine administration. J. Pharmacol. Exp. Ther. **253:** 38–44.

39. LI, T.-K. & L. LUMENG. 1984. Alcohol preference and voluntary alcohol intakes of inbred rat strains and the NIH heterogeneous stock of rats. Alcoholism: Clin. Exp. Res. **8:** 485–486.

40. SUZUKI, T., F. R. GEORGE & R. A. MEISCH. 1988. Differential establishment and maintenance of oral ethanol reinforced behavior in Lewis and Fischer 344 inbred rat strains. J. Pharmacol. Exp. Ther. **245:** 164–170.

41. GEORGE, F. R. & S. R. GOLDBERG. 1989. Genetic approaches to the analysis of addiction processes. Trends in Pharmacol. Sci. **10:** 78–83.

42. TERWILLIGER, R., C. BRADBERRY, X. GUITART, D. BEITNER-JOHNSON, D. MARBY, T. A. KOSTEN & E. J. NESTLER. 1991. Lewis and Fischer 344 rats and drug addiction: Behavioral and biochemical correlates. Soc. Neurosci. Abst. **17:** 823.

43. BEITNER-JOHNSON, D., X. GUITART & E. J. NESTLER. 1991. Dopaminergic brain reward regions of Lewis and Fischer rats display different levels of tyrosine hydroxylase and other morphine and cocaine-regulated phosphoproteins. Brain Res. **561:** 147–150.

44. NESTLER, E. J. & P. GREENGARD. 1984. Protein Phosphorylation in the Nervous System. Wiley. New York.

45. BEITNER-JOHNSON, D. & E. J. NESTLER. 1991. Morphine and cocaine exert common chronic actions on tyrosine hydroxylase in dopaminergic brain reward regions. J. Neurochem. **57:** 344–347.

46. BROCK, J. W., J. P. NG & J. B. JUSTICE, JR. 1990. Effect of chronic cocaine on dopamine synthesis in the nucleus accumbens as determined by microdialysis with NSD-1015. Neurosci. Lett. **117:** 234–239.

47. ACQUAS, E., E. CARBONI & G. DICHIARA. 1991. Profound depression of mesolimbic dopamine release after morphine withdrawal in dependent rats. Eur. J. Pharmacol. **193:** 133–134.

48. BEITNER-JOHNSON, D., X. GUITART & E. J. NESTLER. 1992. Neurofilament proteins and the mesolimbic dopamine system: Common regulation by chronic morphine and chronic cocaine in the rat ventral tegmental area. J. Neurosci. **12:** 2165–2176.

49. HOFFMAN, P. N. & R. J. LASEK. 1975. Identification of major structural polypeptides of the axon and their generality among mammalian neurons. J. Cell Biol. **66:** 351–366.

50. CHIU, F.-C., E. A. BARNES, K. DAS, J. HALEY, P. SOCOLOW, F. P. MACALUSO & J. FANT. 1989. Characterization of a novel 66 kd subunit of mammalian neurofilaments. Neuron **2:** 1435–1445.

51. FLIENGER, K. H., G. Y. CHING & R. K. H. LIEM. 1990. The predicted amino acid sequence of α-internexin is that of a novel neuronal intermediate filament protein. EMBO J. **9:** 745–759.

52. HOFFMAN, P. N. & R. J. LASEK. 1980. Axonal transport of the cytoskeleton in regenerating motor neurons: Constancy and change. Brain Res. **202:** 317–333.

53. TRONOSCO, J. C., P. N. HOFFMAN, J. W. GRIFFIN, K. M. HESS-KOZLOW & D. L. PRICE. 1985. Aluminum intoxication: A disorder of neurofilament transport in motor neurons. Brain Res. **342:** 172–175.

54. WATSON, D. F., J. W. GRIFFIN, K. O. FITTRO & P. N. HOFFMAN. 1989. Phosphorylation-dependent immunoreactivity of neurofilaments increases during axonal maturation and β,β'-iminodipropionitrile intoxication. J. Neurochem. **53:** 1818–1829.

55. HOFFMAN, P. N., J. W. GRIFFIN & D. L. PRICE. 1984. Control of axonal caliber by neurofilament transport. J. Cell Biol. **99:** 705–714.

56. GOLDSTEIN, M. E., H. S. COOPER, J. BRUCE, M. J. CARDEN, V. M.-Y. LEE & W. W. SCHLAEPFER. 1987. Phosphorylation of neurofilament proteins and chromatolysis following ransection of rat sciatic nerve. J. Neurosci. **7:** 1586–1594.

57. HALL, G. F., V. M.-Y. LEE & K. S. KOSIK. 1991. Microtubule destabilization and neurofilament phosphorylation precede dendritic sprouting after close axotomy of lamprey central neurons. Proc. Natl. Acad. Sci. USA **88:** 5016–5020.

58. GUITART, X., D. BEITNER-JOHNSON & E. J. NESTLER. 1992. Fischer and Lewis rat strains differ in basal levels of neurofilament proteins and their regulation by chronic morphine in the mesolimbic dopamine system. Synapse. In press.

59. MATTHEWS, R. T. & D. C. GERMAN. 1984. Electrophysiological evidence for excitation of rat ventral tegmental area dopamine neurons by morphine. Neuroscience 11: 617–625.
60. EINHORN, L. C., P. A. JOHANSEN & F. J. WHITE. 1988. Electrophysiological effects of cocaine in the mesoaccumbens dopamine system: Studies in the ventral tegmental area. J. Neurosci. 8: 100–112.
61. ROBERTSON, M. W., C. A. LESLIE & J. P. BENNET, JR. 1991. Apparent synaptic dopamine deficiency induced by withdrawal from chronic cocaine treatment. Brain Res. 538: 337–339.
62. NG, J. P., HUBERT, G. W. & J. B. JUSTICE, JR. 1991. Increased stimulated release and uptake of dopamine in nucleus accumbens after repeated cocaine administration as measured by in vivo voltammetry. J. Neurochem. 56: 1485–1492.
63. PAN, H.-T., S. MENACHERRY & J. B. JUSTICE, JR. 1991. Differences in the pharmacokinetics of cocaine in naive and cocaine-experienced rats. J. Neurochem. 56: 1299–1306.
64. CHEN, J., R. MARMUR, W. PAREDES, A. PULLES & E. L. GARDNER. 1991. Systemic cocaine challenge after chronic cocaine treatment yields cocaine sensitization of extracellular dopamine content in nucleus accumbens but direct cocaine perfusion into nucleus accumbens does not–in vivo microdialysis studies. Soc. Neurosci. Abst. 17: 823.
65. BEITNER-JOHNSON, D. & E. J. NESTLER. 1992. Chronic morphine impairs axonal transport in the rat mesolimbic dopamine system. Soc. Neurosci. Abst. 18. In press.
66. REID, L. D., S. H. MARGLIN, M. E. MATTIE & C. L. HUBBEL. 1989. Measuring morphine's capacity to establish a place preference. Pharmacol. Biochem. Behav. 33: 765–775.

Electrophysiological Correlates of Psychomotor Stimulant-induced Sensitization[a]

DOUGLAS J. HENRY AND FRANCIS J. WHITE[b]

Department of Psychiatry
Wayne State University School of Medicine
Neuropsychopharmacology Laboratory
Lafayette Clinic
951 E. Lafayette
Detroit, Michigan 48207

INTRODUCTION

Although a variety of psychological and sociological variables are involved in the voluntary use of psychomotor stimulants, it is the powerful reinforcing (rewarding) properties of these drugs which are primarily responsible for their addictive potential and, thus, their repeated use by humans. Drug self-administration studies in laboratory animals have enabled researchers to identify the neuronal systems involved in this reinforcement process. The evidence clearly indicates that brain dopamine (DA) neurons play an essential role in central reward circuitry.[1,2] More precisely, the DA neurons of the midbrain ventral tegmental area (VTA) innervating the ventral striatal region, known as nucleus accumbens (NAc), have been primarily implicated in reward processes. These same neurons are also intricately involved in the locomotor-stimulating effects of psychomotor stimulants.[3] This commonality of DA system involvement has led to a "psychomotor stimulant theory of addiction" which asserts that a common denominator underlying the addictive qualities of a variety of substances is their ability to cause psychomotor activation.[4] Accordingly, the biological mechanisms underlying locomotor stimulation and positive reinforcement may be the same.

If the psychomotor stimulant theory of addiction is correct, then an understanding of the neural events accompanying repeated psychomotor stimulant administration should be of considerable relevance to the addictive process. One of the best characterized effects of repeated administration of psychomotor stimulants is the development of reverse tolerance or "sensitization" to their ability to cause locomotion.[5,6] Within the past few years, many researchers have addressed the mechanisms underlying the phenomenon of behavioral sensitization to psychomotor stimulants. This chapter will review our recent attempts to define electrophysiological correlates of sensitization, particularly to cocaine. We will present our findings of the effects of repeated cocaine administration on the mesoaccumbens DA system and attempt to synthesize

[a] This work was supported by USPHS Research Grants MH-40832 and DA-04093.
[b] Author to whom all correspondence should be sent; Tel.: (313) 256-9011; Fax: (313) 256-9025.

them with both the pharmacological and neurochemical literatures on sensitization to cocaine and other psychomotor stimulants.

In order to discuss our findings regarding the ways in which the effects of cocaine change as a function of repeated exposure, it is first necessary to describe briefly the acute electrophysiological effects of cocaine within the mesoaccumbens DA system. In these and all other experiments to be described, the subjects are chloral hydrate-anesthetized male rats. Details of single-cell recording procedures can be found in prior publications from our laboratory.[7,8]

ELECTROPHYSIOLOGICAL EFFECTS OF COCAINE IN THE MESOACCUMBENS DA SYSTEM: ACUTE STUDIES

Cocaine is both a local anesthetic agent and an inhibitor of monoamine uptake. The ability of cocaine to inhibit the reuptake of synaptic DA,[9] by binding to a site on the DA transporter, is the action which is most clearly associated with both its locomotor-stimulating and -reinforcing effects.[10,11] This action leads to significant increases in extracellular concentrations of DA and thereby potentiates DA transmission.[12-14]

From a physiological perspective, cocaine-induced increases in extracellular DA concentrations result in enhanced dopaminergic transmission to postsynaptic elements within DA terminal fields.[15] In addition, the ability of cocaine to inhibit DA uptake into the somatodendritic region of DA neurons also results in enhanced extracellular concentrations of DA within the VTA[16] and a decrease in mesoaccumbens DA cell activity[7] due to the presence of impulse-regulating autoreceptors on these cells.[17,18] However, although cocaine causes a dose-dependent (ED_{50} = 0.75 mg/kg) inhibition of the activity of mesoaccumbens DA neurons within the rat VTA, this effect, unlike that of most DA agonists, is usually only partial in that the maximal inhibition (at sublethal doses) seldom exceeds 70% of the basal firing rate.[7] The effect of cocaine is dependent upon endogenous DA since it is attenuated by acute DA depletion[7] and blocked by D_2 DA receptor antagonists.[7,15,19]

Microiontophoretic studies indicate that cocaine only weakly inhibits DA neurons following local application to the VTA. Both in vivo extracellular[7] and in vitro intracellular recordings[19] from DA neurons indicate that simultaneous administration of cocaine and DA significantly enhances the inhibitory and hyperpolarizing effects of DA, indicating further that cocaine acts by blocking the uptake of DA within the VTA. The relatively weak effects of iontophoretic, as compared to systemic, cocaine administration suggest that systemic cocaine might inhibit A_{10} DA neuronal activity by a second mechanism, in addition to potentiation of DA autoreceptor activation. In fact, the inhibition of A_{10} DA cells by cocaine appears to involve a NAc-VTA negative feedback pathway since both excitotoxin lesions of the NAc and acute hemitransections significantly attenuate the partial inhibitory effects of cocaine on A_{10} DA neurons.[7]

Systemic administration of cocaine suppresses the firing of NAc neurons in anesthetized rats with a similar potency (ED_{50} = 0.67) to that obtained with A_{10} DA cells.[15,20] However, iontophoretic cocaine is much more effective at inhibiting NAc neurons as compared to mesoaccumbens A_{10} DA cells.[15] NAc neurons can be divided into at least two subtypes, based primarily on their extracellular waveform.[20] The majority of NAc neurons are referred to as Type I, which exhibit a negative/positive waveform, are seldom spontaneously active and are typically inhibited by 5-HT. In contrast, Type II NAc neurons exhibit positive/negative waveforms, are more often spontaneously active and are usually excited by 5-HT.[15] Iontophoretic administration of the excitatory amino acid glutamate is typically used to "drive" quiescent NAc neurons in chloral hydrate-anesthetized rats.

When applied locally to NAc cells by microiontophoresis, cocaine inhibits neuronal firing.[15,20] Sub-inhibitory currents of cocaine also markedly potentiate the rate-suppressant effects of DA on NAc neurons. Cocaine is considerably more potent on Type I NAc cells as compared to Type II NAc cells.[20] In contrast, DA is equipotent at inhibiting the two subtypes of NAc cells. When directly compared, cocaine is less potent than DA at inhibiting Type II NAc cells but is more potent than DA on Type I NAc cells.[15,20] This latter finding appears to be related to the differential effect of 5-HT on Type I (inhibitory) and II (excitatory) NAc neurons.[20] Since cocaine is a potent inhibitor of both 5-HT and DA reuptake,[10] the enhanced activation of both DA and 5-HT receptors results in a potent inhibition of Type I NAc neurons. In contrast, the typical excitatory effect of 5-HT on Type II neurons results in opposing excitatory 5-HT and inhibitory DA effects following cocaine administration.

In summary, cocaine is more effective at suppressing the firing of postsynaptic cells within the NAc than inhibiting the DA cells themselves, owing, at least in part, to an additive potentiation of DA and 5-HT effects on the majority of NAc cells. By inhibiting NAc neurons, cocaine also activates long-loop feedback inhibitory processes which serve to decrease the firing rate of DA neurons. Yet, even the combination of somatodendritic autoreceptor stimulation and long-loop feedback regulation is apparently insufficient to suppress DA cell firing completely. Thus, the net effect of cocaine on the mesoaccumbens DA system is an initial increase in synaptic levels of DA within the NAc, as a result of blocking DA uptake, followed by continued impulse-dependent release of DA, as a result of incomplete suppression of neuronal activity. Therefore, cocaine causes considerable enhancement of mesoaccumbens DA neurotransmission due to the relatively poor compensatory response of DA cells and the resulting buildup of synaptic DA. We have argued that this poor compensatory inhibition of presynaptic dopaminergic activity might help to explain the powerful reinforcing effects of cocaine as well as other major drugs of abuse.[15] As we will discuss below, this "unbalanced" enhancement of dopaminergic transmission may be further amplified by repeated cocaine administration.

REPEATED COCAINE AND DA AUTORECEPTORS IN THE VTA

One of the earliest hypotheses regarding the mechanisms underlying psychomotor stimulant sensitization was that subsensitivity of DA autoreceptors led to reduced compensatory decreases in DA activity following repeated stimulant administration.[21,22] With respect to impulse-regulating DA autoreceptors, Antelman and Chiodo[23] first demonstrated a subsensitivity of nigral (A9) DA neurons to the rate-suppressant effects of relatively low (i.v.) doses of apomorphine following repeated amphetamine administration. Subsequent studies extended this observation to A10 DA neurons within the VTA.[24,25] Our recent experiments have included an examination of the possible role of A10 DA autoreceptor subsensitivity in sensitization to repeated cocaine administration.

In the first set of experiments, we determined whether repeated cocaine administration alters the sensitivity of impulse-regulating autoreceptors on A10 DA neurons. Cocaine was administered repeatedly (10 mg/kg i.p., twice daily, 14 days), and A10 DA neurons were recorded 12–24 h after the final cocaine injection. In such rats, A10

DA cells are significantly subsensitive to the inhibitory effects of the DA agonist apomorphine, administered i.v. (FIG. 1A). This alteration in sensitivity is not due to an acute effect of cocaine, since a single 10 mg/kg cocaine injection 12–24 h prior to recording failed to alter the response of A_{10} DA neurons to i.v. apomorphine.[8] It also appears unlikely that the local anesthetic effects of cocaine are a factor in the observed results, since repeated administration of procaine does not affect the inhibition of A_{10} DA neurons by apomorphine.[8]

To test the hypothesis of autoreceptor subsensitivity more directly, microiontophoretic experiments were conducted on A_{10} DA neurons from control and cocaine-treated rats. As shown in FIGURE 2, repeated cocaine administration renders impulse-regulating somatodendritic A_{10} DA autoreceptors subsensitive to the inhibitory effects of iontophoretic DA.[8] Therefore, despite the fact that cocaine only weakly enhances the stimulation of A_{10} D_2 autoreceptors by DA (above), this level of stimulation is sufficient to produce desensitized responses to DA and DA agonists after repeated cocaine administration.

Because somatodendritic autoreceptors are important in regulating the basal activity of A_{10} DA neurons, we also conducted cell population analysis of the A_{10} region following repeated cocaine treatment.[8] This was achieved by defining a stereotaxic block of tissue contained within the VTA, and passing a microelectrode 12 times through this area in a fixed pattern while counting both the number of spontaneously active DA neurons encountered and their basal firing rates. As shown in TABLE 1, repeated cocaine administration causes a significant increase in both the number of spontaneously active A_{10} DA neurons encountered per recording track and their average basal firing rate. It is known that a subpopulation of quiescent, hyperpolarized DA neurons exists in chloral-hydrate–anesthetized rats.[26–28] In addition to increasing the basal firing rates of A_{10} DA neurons, desensitization of autoreceptors by chronic psychostimulant administration results in recruitment of a significant portion of normally quiescent DA neurons.[8,25]

Given these findings, autoreceptor subsensitivity would appear to be a plausible substrate for behavioral sensitization to psychostimulants because it results in enhanced DA cell activity. However, sensitization to cocaine and amphetamine is an enduring phenomenon, persisting from weeks to months after the cessation of treatment.[5,29] Thus, we next initiated studies to determine whether cocaine-induced autoreceptor subsensitivity persists more than one day after termination of treatment. In these experiments, rats were tested either 1 day, 4 days, or 8 days after the final injection of cocaine. As shown in FIGURES 1A and 1B, A_{10} DA cells from cocaine-treated rats displayed subsensitive responses to i.v. apomorphine when tested 1 or 4 days after treatment, but by day 8 of withdrawal (FIG. 1C), the overall sensitivity of A_{10} DA neurons to the inhibitory effects of apomorphine was not significantly different from controls.[30] These results are similar to those obtained following withdrawal from repeated amphetamine administration,[25] and argue against a direct involvement of desensitized somatodendritic impulse-regulating autoreceptors in the maintenance of behavioral sensitization to psychomotor stimulants.

REPEATED COCAINE AND NUCLEUS ACCUMBENS DOPAMINE RECEPTORS

The results of our first set of studies indicate that repeated cocaine administration transiently desensitizes impulse-regulating DA autoreceptors within the VTA, de-

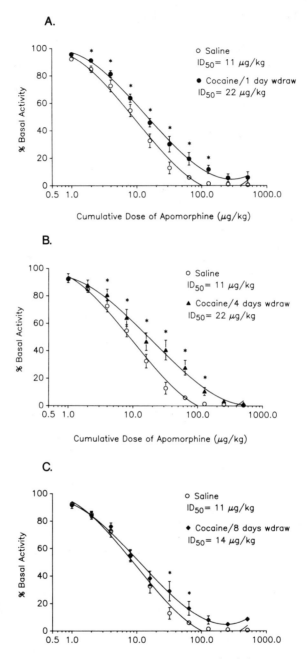

FIGURE 1. Dose-response curves illustrating the effects of intravenous apomorphine on A_{10} DA neurons from rats receiving twice daily injections of cocaine (10 mg/kg, i.p.) or vehicle for 14 days. Animals were tested either: 12–24 h (**A**); 4 days (**B**); or 8 days (**C**) after the final injection of cocaine. Each point represents the mean ± SEM (* $p < .05$, Dunnett's test). (From Ackerman and White,[30] 1990, with permission.)

FIGURE 2. Current-response curves illustrating the effects of iontophoretically applied DA on A₁₀ DA neurons from rats receiving twice daily injections of cocaine (10 mg/kg, i.p.) or vehicle for 14 days. All animals were tested 12–24 h after the final cocaine injection. Each point represents the mean ± SEM (* $p < .01$, Dunnett's test). (From Henry et al.,[8] 1989, with permission.)

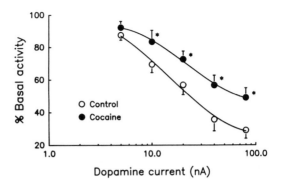

creasing the autoregulation of A₁₀ DA neurons and thereby increasing the DAergic activity of this cell population. We next directed our attention to the NAc, the major projection site of A₁₀ DA neurons, to determine whether DA receptors were desensitized following the same schedule of cocaine injections.[8] In these experiments, animals were tested 16–24 h after the final cocaine injection, unless otherwise noted. Interestingly, our results indicate that NAc neurons from cocaine-treated rats were not subsensitive, but instead were supersensitive to the inhibitory effects of iontophoretic DA (FIG. 3).

Because iontophoretic administration of either D₁ or D₂ agonists results primarily in inhibition of NAc neurons,[31,32] the observed supersensitive response to DA following repeated cocaine could be mediated by alterations in D₁ and/or D₂ receptor sensitivity. In addition, the persistent reduction of DA uptake and an increased effectiveness of cocaine as a DA uptake blocker in the NAc of rats treated repeatedly with cocaine[33] might also lead to apparent increases in the efficacy of iontophoretic DA. Therefore, in the next set of experiments the D₁ agonist SKF 38393 and the D₂ agonist quinpirole were applied iontophoretically onto NAc neurons in control and cocaine-treated rats to determine whether the sensitivity of a specific DA receptor subtype within the NAc was altered by repeated cocaine administration.[34] As seen in FIGURES 4 and 5, NAc neurons from cocaine-treated rats were sensitized to the inhibitory effects of SKF 38393 but not quinpirole. Thus, it appears likely that the observed increase in the inhibitory effects exerted by iontophoretic DA on NAc neurons from cocaine-treated rats was due to an increase in D₁ DA receptor sensitivity. In addition, this D₁ receptor sensitization was relatively persistent in that it was still

TABLE 1. Effects of Repeated Cocaine Administration on the Spontaneous Activity of A₁₀ DA Neurons

	n	Cells/track	Rate (Spikes/sec)
Control	6	1.45 ± 0.09	4.19 ± 0.22
Cocaine-treated	5	2.08 ± 0.14[a]	5.58 ± 0.16[a]

[a] $p < .01$, Student's t-test.

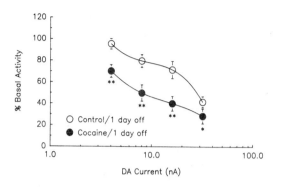

FIGURE 3. Current-response curves illustrating the effects of microiontophoretically applied DA on NAc neurons from rats receiving twice daily injections of cocaine (10 mg/kg, i.p.) or vehicle for 14 days. All animals were tested 16–24 h after the final injection. Each point represents the mean ± SEM (* $p <$ .05, ** $p <$ .01, Dunnett's test). (From Henry and White,[34] 1991, with permission.)

evident following a 1 week or 1 month (but not 2 month) withdrawal from cocaine (FIG. 4).

Because behavioral sensitization to repeated administration of psychomotor stimulants is an enduring phenomenon, lasting for weeks to months following the cessation of drug treatment,[5,35,36] it has been argued that physiological changes proposed

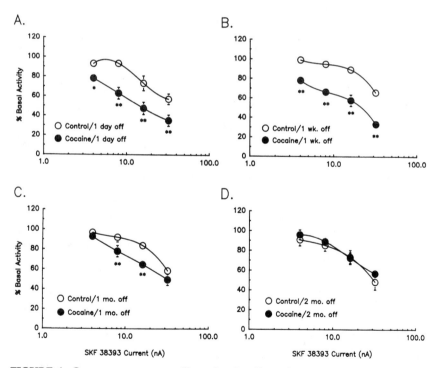

FIGURE 4. Current-response curves illustrating the effects of microiontophoretically applied SKF 38393 on NAc neurons from rats receiving twice daily injections of cocaine (10 mg/kg, i.p.) or vehicle for 14 days, and tested either: 16–24 h (**A**); 1 week (**B**); 1 month (**C**); or 2 months (**D**) after the final injection. Each point represents the mean ± SEM (* $p <$ .05, ** $p <$ .01, Dunnett's test). (From Henry and White,[34] 1991, with permission.)

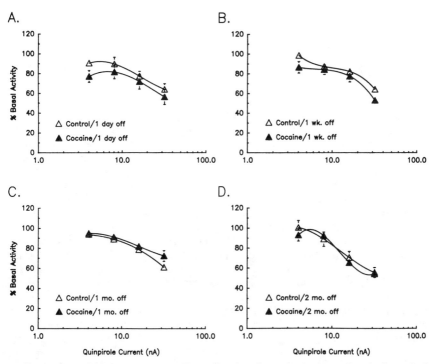

FIGURE 5. Current-response curves illustrating the effects of microiontophoretically applied quinpirole on NAc neurons from rats receiving twice daily injections of cocaine (10 mg/kg, i.p.) or vehicle, and tested either: 16–24 h (**A**); 1 week (**B**); 1 month (**C**); or 2 months (**D**) after the last injection. Each point represents the mean ± SEM. (From Henry and White,[34] 1991, with permission.)

as relevant to this phenomenon should also be of a persistent nature.[5] In our study, the D_1 receptor sensitization within the NAc appeared to be waning somewhat at one month and was no longer evident two months after withdrawal from repeated cocaine administration. Relatively few behavioral studies exist regarding the persistence of sensitization to repeated cocaine injections (as compared to amphetamine), and it is evident that different cocaine treatment schedules can produce varying degrees of both the magnitude of sensitization to cocaine and its persistence following withdrawal. Although various reports indicate sensitization is evident from 7 to 87 days post injection,[37-39] it has also been reported that cocaine-induced horizontal locomotion, typically associated with the NAc,[40] does not remain elevated following a 2 week withdrawal from repeated cocaine administration (3 × 15 mg/kg/day, 3 days).[37] Thus, the persistence of sensitized D_1 responses observed at 1 month, but not 2 months, post injection in the present study may indeed be reflective of the time course of behavioral sensitization under this injection schedule. We are currently conducting behavioral studies using this treatment schedule (10 mg/kg twice daily, 14 days), and preliminary data suggest that cocaine-treated rats displayed sensitized horizontal locomotion in response to cocaine challenge after both a 1 day and 1 week withdrawal period.[41] Experiments using longer withdrawal periods are currently in progress.

Interestingly, this and other studies[42,43] suggest that D_1 DA receptors within the striatum and NAc display enhanced responses to agonists following certain schedules of repeated stimulation. For example, sensitized D_1 responses (hyperpolarizations) in NAc slice preparations have been reported following repeated methamphetamine administration.[43] In addition, repeated injections of the D_1 agonist SKF 38393 enhance the inhibitory responses of striatal[42] and NAc neurons[44] to iontophoretically applied D_1 agonists and also significantly sensitize D_1 agonist-induced grooming responses.[42,45]

Because the D_1 DA receptor is known to enable D_2-mediated functional responses,[32,46–48] we found it somewhat surprising that D_1-sensitized neurons from cocaine-treated rats did not also display enhanced inhibitory responses to iontophoretic quinpirole, as demonstrated in the dorsal striatum following repeated SKF 38393 administration.[42] Because repeated administration of quinpirole results in subsensitive D_2 receptor responses within the NAc,[44] the lack of change in quinpirole responsiveness observed in our cocaine experiments could be due to competing alterations in receptor sensitivity (D_2 subsensitivity vs. D_1 supersensitivity). Alternatively, it is possible that D_2 receptors are relieved of the necessity of concomitant D_1 stimulation when the NAc is sensitized to DA. Such functional "uncoupling" of D_1 and D_2 DA receptors has been reported in previous behavioral and electrophysiological studies of rats with supersensitive D_1 and D_2 receptors. For example, D_1 antagonists block the effects of D_2 agonists in normal rats but not in rats chronically depleted of DA by either selective 6-hydroxydopamine lesions of the ascending DAergic system or repeated reserpine treatment.[49–51] In similarly depleted rats, the electrophysiological effects of D_2 agonists on striatal neurons do not require D_1 receptor stimulation, as is normally the case.[52]

POSSIBLE MECHANISMS OF ENHANCED D_1 RESPONSES

Biochemical studies using similar treatment regimens suggest that the D_1 receptor supersensitivity observed in this study is probably not due to increased densities of D_1 DA receptors within the NAc, as defined by [^{3}H]SCH 23390 binding density. Neither Peris et al.[38] nor Kleven et al.[53] detected an increase in [^{3}H]SCH 23390 binding in the NAc or caudate-putamen of rats following repeated cocaine administration. In fact, transient increases in NAc D_2 receptor density have been observed following such treatments.[38,53,54] However, recent studies indicate that alterations in receptor responsiveness can occur without appreciable changes in the density of binding sites. Dopamine denervation of the striatum produced by 6-hydroxydopamine results in supersensitive inhibitory responses of striatal neurons to SKF 38393 and enhanced behavioral responses to D_1 agonists,[52] yet D_1 receptor density is generally reported to be unchanged or decreased.[55–58] Thus, it appears possible that the D_1 receptor supersensitivity observed in our study results from alterations in D_1 receptor–coupled intracellular transduction mechanisms which are "downstream" from the ligand binding site. This hypothesis is supported by recent work from Nestler and colleagues,[59,60] who have reported increased forskolin-stimulated adenylate cyclase activity, augmented cAMP-dependent protein kinase activity and reduced $G_{i\alpha}$ and $G_{o\alpha}$ levels in the NAc following a repeated cocaine treatment regimen similar to that used in our experiments. However, it should be noted that studies of D_1 receptor–activated transduction events have failed to identify consistent alterations following repeated administration of other psychomotor stimulants.[5] Recent reports indicate a marked, rapid desensitization of D_1 receptor–stimulated adenylate cyclase activity following contin-uous exposure to DA in culture systems of either NS20Y neuroblastoma cells[61] or stri-atal neurons.[62] Repeated amphetamine treatment increases the potency with which amphetamine elicits desensitization of D_1 receptor–coupled adenylate cyclase ac-tivity.[63-65] Thus, it appears that DAergic signal transduction pathways are capable of multiple adaptive responses to perturbations of normal functioning.

IMPORTANCE OF THE VTA AS A COMPONENT OF BEHAVIORAL SENSITIZATION

Although our studies within the NAc have focused on postsynaptic mechanisms of sensitization, other work has made it apparent that the VTA plays a critical role in the development of behavioral sensitization to repeated administration of psychomotor stimulants. For example, repeated intra-VTA[66,67] but *not* intra-NAc[66-70] amphetamine produces sensitized locomotor responses to subsequent agonist challenge. Therefore, although A_{10} DA autoreceptor subsensitivity fails to persist following withdrawal from chronic psychostimulant administration,[25,30] the increased levels of spontaneous do-paminergic activity within the VTA[8] which occur during this period may be a trigger for more persistent alterations, including postsynaptic D_1 receptor supersensitivity. In support of this hypothesis, repeated administration of SKF 38393 produced supersensi-tivity of both striatal neurons[42,44] and behavioral responses to D_1 selective agonists.[42,45] However, these alterations do not endure beyond 8 days post injection.[42] Impor-tantly, D_1 receptor selective agonists do not directly influence impulse-regulating DA autoreceptors, which are exclusively of the D_2 subtype,[18,32] and thus, do not decrease autoreceptor sensitivity following repeated administration.[44]

CONCLUSIONS

Our results demonstrate that repeated cocaine administration (10 mg/kg twice daily, 14 days) results in a significant subsensitivity of impulse-regulating somatodendritic autoreceptors on A_{10} DA neurons. Thus, the characteristic rate-suppressant effects produced by iontophoretic administration of DA or intravenous injection of the DA agonist apomorphine are significantly reduced in cocaine-treated animals, and this al-teration persists for up to 4 days following withdrawal from cocaine. In addition, auto-receptor desensitization results in a significant increase in the percentage of spontane-ously active A_{10} DA neurons and their average basal firing rate (as determined by cells/track analysis), while postsynaptic neurons within the NAc are supersensitive to the inhibitory effects of iontophoretically applied DA and the D_1 agonist SKF 38393. This D_1 receptor supersensitivity persists for at least one month following the last injection of cocaine. Taken together, these findings indicate that repeated cocaine administration may amplify the unbalanced DA neurotransmission (*i.e.*, poor compensatory inhibi-tion of DA neuronal activity) observed following acute cocaine administration,[7,15] in that DA neuronal activity is enhanced, as is the response of postsynaptic NAc neurons to DA.[8] Accordingly, these alterations in mesoaccumbens DA activity may be in-volved in behavioral sensitization to the psychostimulant effects of cocaine.[8,34,71]

We are not proposing that NAc D_1 receptor supersensitivity alone can account for the mechanism of sensitization to psychomotor stimulants. Animals chronically treated with stimulants clearly display a relatively persistent augmentation of DA release in terminal areas in response to challenge with cocaine or amphetamine.[5,14,38,72] In addition, adaptations in the DA uptake processes,[33] in nerve-terminal DA autoreceptor function,[38,73,74] and cocaine disposition within the brain and plasma[75] are also likely to play important roles. Other investigations have suggested that non-dopaminergic systems, perhaps projecting to the NAc, may be altered to influence DA transmission indirectly[29,39,76,77] in sensitized animals. Finally, it appears that amphetamine must act within the VTA to initiate sensitization to peripheral psychostimulant challenge.[66] Thus, it appears that the somewhat simple behavioral phenomenon of sensitization results from a complex cascade of neuronal adaptions, and that some of these alterations (*i.e.*, autoreceptor subsensitivity) may act as triggers for more permanent changes within neuronal DA systems.

ACKNOWLEDGMENTS

The authors thank Vernice Davis for her excellent technical assistance. We also thank Eli Lilly and Company (Indianapolis, IN) for their generous gift of quinpirole HCl.

REFERENCES

1. KOOB, G. F. & F. E. BLOOM. 1988. Science **242:** 715–723.
2. WISE, R. A. & P.-P. ROMPRÉ. 1989. Ann. Rev. Psychol. **40:** 191–225.
3. ROBBINS, T. W., G. MITTLEMAN, J. O'BRIEN & P. WINN. 1990. In Neurobiology of Stereotyped Behavior. S. J. Cooper & C. T. Dourish, Eds.: 25–63. Oxford University Press. New York.
4. WISE, R. A. & M. A. BOZARTH. 1987. Psychol. Rev. **94:** 469–492.
5. ROBINSON, T. E. & J. B. BECKER. 1986. Brain Res. Rev. **11:** 157–198.
6. KALIVAS, P. W. & J. STEWART. 1991. Brain Res. Rev. **16:** 223–244.
7. EINHORN, L. C., P. A. JOHANSEN & F. J. WHITE. 1988. J. Neurosci. **8:** 100–112.
8. HENRY, D. J., M. A. GREENE & F. J. WHITE. 1989. J. Pharmacol. Exp. Ther. **251:** 833–839.
9. HEIKKILA, R. E., H. ORLANSKY & G. COHEN. 1975. Biochem. Pharmacol. **24:** 847–852.
10. RITZ, M. C., R. J. LAMB, S. R. GOLDBERG & M. J. KUHAR. 1987. Science **237:** 1219–1223.
11. REITH, M. E. A. 1988. NIDA Res. Monographs **88:** 23–42.
12. CHURCH, W. H., J. B. JUSTICE, JR. & L. D. BYRD. 1987. Eur. J. Pharmacol. **139:** 345–348.
13. HURD, Y. L., F. WEISS, G. F. KOOB, N.-E. ANDEN & U. UNGERSTEDT. 1989. Brain Res. **498:** 199–203.
14. KALIVAS, P. W. & P. DUFFY. 1990. Synapse **5:** 48–58.
15. WHITE, F. J. 1990. Behavioural Pharmacol. **1:** 303–315.
16. BRADBERRY, C. W. & R. H. ROTH. 1989. Neurosci. Lett. **103:** 97–102.
17. AGHAJANIAN, G. K. & B. S. BUNNEY. 1977. Naunyn-Schmeideberg's Arch. Pharmacol. **297:** 1–7.
18. WHITE, F. J. & R. Y. WANG. 1984. J. Pharmacol. Exp. Ther. **231:** 275–280.
19. LACEY, M. G., N. B. MERCURI & R. A. NORTH. 1990. Br. J. Pharmacol. **99:** 731–735.
20. WHITE, F. J., S. R. WACHTEL, P. A. JOHANSEN & L. C. EINHORN. 1987. In Neurophysiology of Dopaminergic Systems: Current Status and Clinical Perspectives. L. A. Chiodo & A. S. Freeman, Eds.: 317–365. Lakeshore Publishing. Detroit, MI.
21. MARTRES, M. P., J. CONSTENTIN, M. BAUDRY, H. MARCAIS, P. PROTRAIS & J. C. SCHWARTZ. 1977. Brain Res. **136:** 319–337.
22. MULLER, P. & P. SEEMAN. 1979. Eur. J. Pharmacol. **55:** 149–157.
23. ANTELMAN, S. M. & L. A. CHIODO. 1981. Biol. Psychiatry **16:** 717–727.
24. KAMATA, K. & G. V. REBEC. 1984. Life Sci. **34:** 2419–2427.

25. WHITE, F. J. & R. Y. WANG. 1984. Brain Res. 309: 283–292.
26. CHIODO, L. A. & B. S. BUNNEY. 1983. J. Neurosci. 3: 1607–1619.
27. WHITE, F. J. & R. Y. WANG. 1983. Life Sci. 32: 983–993.
28. GRACE, A. A. 1988. In The Mesocorticolimbic Dopamine System. P. W. Kalivas & C. B. Nemeroff, Eds. Ann. N.Y. Acad. Sci. 537: 51–76.
29. POST, R. M. & S. R. B. WEISS. 1988. NIDA Res. Monographs 88: 217–238.
30. ACKERMAN, J. M. & F. J. WHITE. 1990. Neurosci. Lett. 117: 181–187.
31. WHITE, F. J. & R. Y. WANG. 1986. J. Neurosci. 6: 274–280.
32. WACHTEL, S. R., X.-T. HU, M. P. GALLOWAY & F. J. WHITE. 1989. Synapse 4: 327–346.
33. IZENWASSER, S. & B. M. COX. 1990. Brain Res. 531: 338–341.
34. HENRY, D. J. & F. J. WHITE. 1991. J. Pharmacol Exp. Ther. 258: 882–889.
35. POST, R. M. & H. ROSE. 1976. Nature (London) 260: 731–732.
36. POST, R. M. & N. R. CONTEL. 1983. In Stimulants: Neurochemical, Behavioral and Clinical Perspectives. I. Creese, Ed.: 169–203. Raven Press. New York.
37. KALIVAS, P. W., P. DUFFY, L. A. DUMARS & C. SKINNER. 1988. J. Pharmacol. Exp. Ther. 245: 485–492.
38. PERIS, J., S. J. BOYSON, W. A. CASS, P. CURELLA, L. P. DWOSKIN, G. LARSON, L.-H. LIN, R. P. YASUDA & N. R. ZAHNISER. 1990. J. Pharmacol. Exp. Ther. 253: 38–44.
39. POST, R. M., S. R. B. WEISS & A. PERT. 1991. In Cocaine: Pharmacology, Physiology and Clinical Strategies. J. Lakoski, M. P. Galloway & F. J. White, Eds. CRC Press. Boca Raton, In press.
40. DELFS, J. M., L. SCHREIBER & A. E. KELLEY. 1990. J. Neurosci. 10: 303–310.
41. HENRY, D. J. & F. J. WHITE. 1991. Soc. Neurosci. Abstr. 17: In press.
42. WHITE, F. J., X.-T. HU & R. J. BROODERSON. 1990. Eur. J. Pharmacol. 191: 497–499.
43. HIGASHI, H., K. INANAGA, S. NISHI & N. UCHIMURA. 1989. J. Physiol. 408: 587–603.
44. HENRY, D. J. & F. J. WHITE. 1990. Soc. Neurosci. Abstr. 16: 1051.
45. BRAUN, A. R. & T. N. CHASE. 1988. Eur. J. Pharmacol. 147: 441–451.
46. CLARK, D. & F. J. WHITE. 1987. Synapse 1: 347–388.
47. WALTERS, J. R., D. A. BERGSTROM, J. H. CARLSON, T. N. CHASE & A. R. BRAUN. 1987. Science 236: 719–722.
48. WHITE, F. J. 1987. Eur. J. Pharmacol. 135: 101–105.
49. ARNT, J. & J. HYTELL. 1984. Eur. J. Pharmacol. 102: 349–354.
50. ARNT, J. 1985. Eur. J. Pharmacol. 113: 79–88.
51. BREESE, G. R. & R. A. MUELLER. 1985. Eur. J. Pharmacol. 113: 109–114.
52. HU, X.-T., S. R. WACHTEL, M. P. GALLOWAY & F. J. WHITE. 1990. J. Neurosci. 10: 2318–2329.
53. KLEVEN, M. S., B. D. PERRY, W. L. WOOLVERTON & L. S. SEIDEN. 1990. Brain Res. 532: 265–270.
54. GOEDERS, N. E. & M. J. KUHAR. 1987. Alcohol Drug Res. 7: 207–216.
55. ALTAR, C. A. & M. R. MARIEN. 1987. J. Neurosci. 7: 213–222.
56. LESLIE, C. A. & J. P. BENNETT. 1987. Brain Res. 415: 90–97.
57. ARIANO, M. A. 1988. Brain Res. 443: 204–214.
58. MARSHALL, J. F., R. NAVARRETE & J. N. JOYCE. 1989. Brain Res. 493: 247–257.
59. NESTLER, E. J., R. Z. TERWILLIGER, J. R. WALKER, K. A. SEVARINO & R. S. DUMAN. 1990. J. Neurochem. 55: 1079–1082.
60. TERWILLIGER, R. Z., D. BEITNER-JOHNSON, K. A. SEVARINO, S. M. CRAIN & E. J. NESTLER. 1991. Brain Res. 548: 100–110.
61. BARTON, A. C. & D. R. SIBLEY. 1990. Mol. Pharmacol. 38: 531–541.
62. CHNEIWEISS, H., J. GLOWINSKI & J. PREMONT. 1990. Eur. J. Pharmacol.–Mol. Pharmacol. Section 189: 287–292.
63. ROBERTS-LEWIS, J. M., P. H. ROSEBOOM, L. M. IWANIAC & M. E. GNEGY. 1986. J. Neurosci. 6: 2245–2251.
64. BARNETT, J. V., D. S. SEGAL & R. KUCZENSKI. 1987. J. Pharmacol. Exp. Ther. 242: 40–47.
65. ROSEBOOM, P. H., G. H. KEIKILANI HEWLETT & M. E. GNEGY. 1990. J. Pharmacol. Exp. Ther. 255: 197–203.
66. KALIVAS, P. W. & B. WEBER. 1988. J. Pharmacol. Exp. Ther. 245: 1095–1102.
67. VEZINA, P. & J. STEWART. 1990. Brain Res. 516: 99–106.

68. DOUGHERTY, JR., G. G. & E. H. ELLINWOOD. 1981. Life Sci. **28:** 2295–2298.
69. HITZEMANN, R., J. WU, D. HOM & J. LOH. 1980. Psychopharmacol. **72:** 93–101.
70. STEWART, J. & P. VEZINA. 1988. *In* Sensitization in the Nervous System. P. W. Kalivas & C. D. Barnes, Eds.: 207–224. Telford Press. Caldwell, NJ.
71. WHITE, F. J., D. J. HENRY, X.-T. HU, M. JEZIORSKI & J. M. ACKERMAN. 1992. *In* Cocaine: Pharmacology, Physiology and Clinical Strategies. J. Lakoski, M. P. Galloway & F. J. White, Eds.: 261–293. CRC Press. Boca Raton, FL.
72. AKIMOTO, K., T. HAMAMURA & S. OTSUKI. 1989. Brain Res. **490:** 339–344.
73. BROCK, J. W., J. P. NG & J. B. JUSTICE, JR. 1990. Neurosci. Lett. **117:** 234–239.
74. YI, S.-J. & K. M. JOHNSON. 1990. Pharmacol. Biochem. Behav. **36:** 457–461.
75. PETTIT, H. O., H.-T. PAM, L. H. PARSONS & J. B. JUSTICE, JR. 1990. J. Neurochem. **55:** 798–804.
76. KARLER, R., L. D. CALDER, I. A. CHAUDHRY & S. A. TURKANIS. 1989. Life Sci. **45:** 599–606.
77. WOLF, M. E. & M. KHANSA. 1991. Brain Res. **562:** 164–168.

Cortico-Subcortical Interactions in Behavioral Sensitization: Differential Effects of Daily Nicotine and Morphine

JEAN-POL TASSIN, PAUL VEZINA, FABRICE TROVERO,
GÉRARD BLANC, DENIS HERVÉ,
AND JACQUES GLOWINSKI

Chaire de Neuropharmacologie
INSERM U. 114
11, Place Marcelin Berthelot
75005 Paris, France

Acute systemic injections of morphine and nicotine elicit increased locomotion in rats and repeating these injections produces an enhanced or sensitized effect.[1,2] Sensitization of locomotion has also been reported for amphetamine[3,4] and cocaine.[5] Different lines of evidence suggest that mesolimbic dopaminergic (DA) activation underlies the acute locomotor effects of these drugs and that enhanced activity in this system may be responsible for sensitization to their locomotor effects.[4,6–8] Further evidence implicating DA system activation in locomotor sensitization also comes from experiments in which morphine or a μ-opioid receptor agonist was injected directly into the ventral tegmental area (VTA).[9–11] Indeed, this mesencephalic structure contains a high density of DA perikarya[12] innervating cortical and subcortical forebrain areas such as the prefrontal cortex and the nucleus accumbens, one of the main targets of the mesolimbic DA system.[13]

Supporting the view that sensitization of the locomotor hyperactivity induced by repeated enkephalin injections into the VTA is associated with an activation of the mesolimbic DA pathway, an enhanced or sensitized metabolism of DA was found in the nucleus accumbens in response to the drug.[14] However, when morphine or a μ-opioid receptor agonist was repeatedly injected into the nucleus accumbens, no sensitization occurred.[15] Qualitatively similar findings were obtained with amphetamine: repeatedly injecting amphetamine into the VTA produces sensitized locomotor responses to peripheral administrations of either amphetamine, cocaine or morphine, whereas amphetamine repeatedly injected into the nucleus accumbens elicits locomotor hyperactivity but no sensitization.[16,17] It has been proposed therefore, that sensitization involves changes in a local neuronal loop which result in altered modulation of DA neurons in the VTA, rendering them more easily excitable by subsequent pharmacological challenge. A diminished somatodendritic release of DA from mesolimbic DA cell bodies, shown to occur in sensitized animals, could account for the enhanced release of DA in the nucleus accumbens.[15,16,18] Alternatively, but not exclusively, it could be considered that the reason why sensitization occurs only when VTA DA cell bodies are recruited is because it necessitates simultaneous modifications in metabolism in at least two ascending DA systems, the mesolimbic and mesocortical pathways. This latter hypothesis comes from recent data indicating that modulations of rat locomotor activity can be obtained following the differential stimulation of cortical or subcortical DA receptors.[19] To test this hypothesis, we studied the effects of acute and daily treatments of two drugs known to induce behavioral sensitization, morphine and nicotine, on the metabolism of DA in the prefrontal cortex and the nucleus accumbens. Morphine and nicotine were chosen since, in searching for a common mechanism of sensitization, it seemed interesting to test two drugs whose primary effect is not, like amphetamine and cocaine, a modification of the synaptic concentration of DA. Moreover, while the effects of morphine have been extensively studied, relatively little is known about modifications of DA activation following repeated injections of nicotine.

In this chapter, we will first present data showing that changes in rat locomotor activity can be obtained following modifications of a putative cortico-subcortical balance in relation with metabolic activities of the mesolimbic and mesocortical DA pathways. We will then briefly consider the possible anatomical sites of interactions between morphine and nicotine and ascending DA neurons. Finally, the differential modifications of this DA cortico-subcortical balance following acute and repeated injections of morphine and nicotine will be presented. Clear-cut differences between the results obtained with morphine and nicotine suggest that the locomotor sensitization induced by nicotine is DA-independent.

CORTICAL AND SUBCORTICAL MODULATIONS OF LOCOMOTOR ACTIVITY

It is generally agreed that the locomotor activating effects induced by the injection of amphetamine into the nucleus accumbens are related to an increased release of DA in this nucleus.[20] However, bilateral electrolytic lesions of the VTA, which destroy the mesolimbic DA pathway,[21] induce a complex syndrome characterized by the presence of locomotor hyperactivity.[22] Correlational studies obtained in animals rendered hyperactive by such lesions indicate that the amplitude of the locomotor hyperactivity obtained is proportional to the extent of the destruction of the DA fibers innervating the prefrontal cortex.[21] These experiments indicated, therefore, that the cortical DA innervation may play an inhibitory role in locomotor activity. However, this locomotor hyperactivity could not be obtained in animals with cortical DA depletion only,[23] suggesting that a modification in DA transmission in the nucleus accumbens, induced by the VTA lesion, was also necessary to observe the locomotor consequences of the cortical DA denervation.

To test this hypothesis, rats were implanted with chronic bilateral injection cannulae aimed at both the prefrontal cortex and nucleus accumbens. As expected, when amphetamine (1.5 μg/0.5 μl/side) was injected into the nucleus accumbens, a mean increase in locomotor activity of up to 240% compared to the control saline injections was obtained. On the other hand and confirming results obtained with lesions restricted to the cortical DA innervation, there was no significant effect on locomotor activity when amphetamine (2.5 μg/0.5 μl/side) was injected into the prefrontal cortex alone. However, when amphetamine was injected into both sites, prefrontal cortex amphetamine reduced the hyperactivity produced by nucleus accumbens amphetamine injections by a mean of 42% (FIG. 1).[19]

Complementary experiments have indicated that this cortical effect is mediated via D_1 receptors, a subtype of DA receptors positively linked to adenylate cyclase. Indeed, injections of SCH 23390 (0.25 μg/0.5 μl/side), a D_1 antagonist, into the prefrontal cortex increase the locomotor activity induced by nucleus accumbens amphetamine by 110%, while the injection of sulpiride (1 μg/0.5 μl/side), a D_2 antagonist, is without significant effect (FIG. 1). Both of these antagonists, at the doses tested, blocked the locomotor activating effects of amphetamine when co-injected with amphetamine into the nucleus accumbens.[19]

These results suggest that the inhibitory influence on locomotor behavior exerted by the prefrontocortical DA innervation is mediated by D_1 receptors. It is interesting to note that in animals rendered hyperactive with bilateral lesions of the VTA, there is an increase in DA-sensitive adenylate cyclase activity in the prefrontal cortex which parallels the increase in locomotor activity.[24] Modifications in locomotor activity may therefore reflect changes in D_1 cortical transmission if, and only if, DA transmission in the nucleus accumbens has been previously either inhibited (electrolytic lesion of the VTA) or facilitated (local amphetamine injections). As already mentioned, it seemed possible that the locomotor effects induced by repeated morphine and nico-

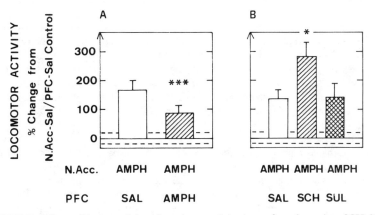

FIGURE 1. Effects of intra-medial prefrontal cortex injections of amphetamine, SCH 23390 and sulpiride on nucleus accumbens amphetamine-induced locomotor activity. Values are the mean ± SEM of total locomotor activity counts obtained in a 30 min test immediately following the combined prefrontal cortex (PFC)–Nucleus Accumbens (N. Acc.) injections. Data are shown as % change from counts obtained after the control saline injection. Doses of amphetamine (AMPH) injected bilaterally in the nucleus accumbens were 4.0 nmol/side. (A) Effects of intra-PFC injections of AMPH. Doses of AMPH injected bilaterally were 6.6 nmol/side. All rats ($n = 9$) received each injection once. *** Significantly different from intra N. Acc. AMPH/intra-PFC saline $p < 0.0005$. (B) Effects of intra-PFC injections of SCH 23390 (SCH) and ± sulpiride (SUL). Doses of SCH and SUL injected bilaterally into the PFC were 0.7 and 2.6 nmol/side, respectively. When injected at these doses into the N. Acc., each of these products blocks the locomotor hyperactivity induced by 4.0 nmol/side of AMPH injected into the N. Acc. Different groups ($n = 7$-15) received different injections. * Significantly different from intra-N. Acc. AMPH/intra-PFC saline, $p < 0.05$. (From ref. 19.)

tine injections might be related to specific modifications in metabolism in both mesocortical and mesolimbic DA pathways.

POSSIBLE SITES OF INTERACTION BETWEEN MORPHINE, NICOTINE AND DA NEURONS

Absence of μ-Opioid Receptors on Ascending DA Neurons

A high density of enkephalin and opiate receptors has been observed in limbic and
forebrain structures.[25,26] Moreover, a close association between the distribution of
enkephalin-containing fibers and DA neurons has been described,[27,28] particularly
high concentrations of enkephalin having been detected in the nucleus accumbens and
the VTA. In 1977, Pollard et al.[29] suggested that a population of μ receptors is located
on DA nerve terminals since they observed a 22–28% reduction in the binding of ³H-
Leu-enkephalin or ³H-naloxone in the striatum of rats following intraventricular
6-OHDA injection or electrocoagulation of the substantia nigra. These same authors
proposed that an even higher proportion (50–70%) of μ receptors in the nucleus accumbens is localized on mesolimbic DA neurons.[30] Similar conclusions were advanced by several other groups who used different ligands and found a substantial depletion of μ binding sites in striatal patches following 6-OHDA lesion of nigrostriatal
DA neurons.[31-33]

In our laboratory, we have observed that both μ and δ agonists stimulate the release
of DA when applied locally into the cat caudate nucleus. However, the pattern of the
response induced by μ agonists differed from that produced by δ agonists.[34] Further
studies performed on rat striatal slices, strongly suggested that δ but not μ receptors
are located on DA nerve terminals. Specific ligands of δ receptors were found to stimulate the release of newly synthesized ³H-DA while morphine (even when used at a
high concentration), or specific μ agonists, such as DAGO, were devoid of activity, indicating that μ agonists act indirectly in vivo.[35]

The decrease in ³H-naloxone binding following DA denervation of the striatum
or the nucleus accumbens, described by different authors, might therefore be due to
a down-regulation of μ receptors postsynaptic to DA nerve terminals. The density of
these receptors would be regulated by DA release. In order to explore this possibility,
we compared by quantitative autoradiography the modifications of ³H-naloxone
binding in rat striatum and nucleus accumbens produced by interrupting DA transmission, either with long-term neuroleptic treatment with palmitate of pipotiazine,
or with a unilateral injection of 6-OHDA into the medial forebrain bundle.[36] As illustrated in FIGURE 2, ³H-naloxone binding was distributed heterogeneously in the striatum and the anterior nucleus accumbens. The densely labeled areas in the striatum
correspond to striosomes.[37] In agreement with previous observations, the 6-OHDA
lesions significantly reduced ³H-naloxone binding in the ipsilateral striatum and anterior nucleus accumbens (FIG. 2), while no modification was seen on the contralateral
side when compared to controls.[36] In these lesioned rats, the mean reduction in ³H-
naloxone binding was 35 and 42% for the striatum and the anterior nucleus accumbens, respectively. The surface of μ-opiate binding site patches in the striatum was
decreased by about 36% when compared to controls.

The prolonged interruption of DA transmission by the long-acting neuroleptic reduced ³H-naloxone binding and striosomal surface in the striatum in a way similar to

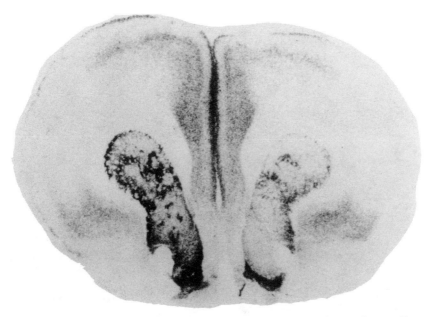

FIGURE 2. Autoradiogram of ³H-naloxone binding in the anterior striatum of a rat unilaterally lesioned with 6-OHDA in the medial forebrain bundle. The 6-OHDA lesioned hemisphere is on the right side of the autoradiogram. The anteriority level corresponds to the 9760 μm plane of the Atlas of König and Klippel.[74] Note the important decrease of ³H-naloxone binding in the right nucleus accumbens. (From ref. 36.)

that observed in 6-OHDA lesioned rats.[36] Similarly, a decrease of 33% in ³H-naloxone binding was obtained in the anterior nucleus accumbens of rats treated with the long-term neuroleptic when compared to control values. These results together with those above indicate not only that the density of μ-opiate receptors is controlled by DA transmission but also that μ-opiate receptors in the striatum and in the anterior nucleus accumbens are exclusively post-synaptic to DA neurons.

Interestingly, μ-opiate receptors labeled by ³H-naloxone in the posterior nucleus accumbens were not modified by the unilateral 6-OHDA lesion of the medial forebrain bundle (FIG. 3). Initially, it was Zaborszky et al. who defined two regions in the nucleus accumbens, the core and the shell.[38] The postero-medial part of the nucleus accumbens, which corresponds to the shell, receives mixed cholecystokinin/DA afferent fibers originating in the VTA.[39,40] Specificities exist in the projection patterns of the core and the shell[41] as well as different reactivities to behavioral consequences of anterior or postero-medial injections of cholecystokinin.[42] In addition, sulfated cholecystokinin has been shown to exert opposite effects on DA-sensitive adenylate cyclase activity in the anterior and the postero-medial nucleus accumbens.[43] Our lesion experiments indicate that the receptors labeled by low concentrations of ³H-naloxone in the shell are not affected by DA denervation, whereas μ-opiate receptor density is decreased at the same anteriority in the striatum (FIG. 3) and in the core of the nucleus accumbens in more rostral slices (FIG. 2). This observation may explain the paradoxical

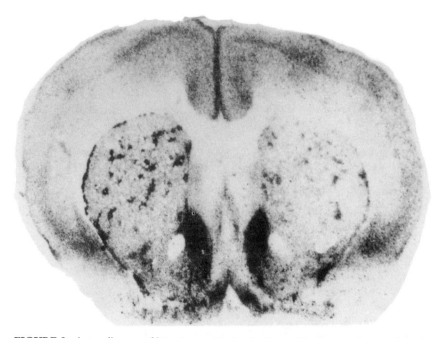

FIGURE 3. Autoradiogram of ^{3}H-naloxone binding in the caudal striatum of a rat unilaterally lesioned with 6-OHDA in the medial forebrain bundle. This coronal slice is taken from the same rat as FIGURE 2, the 6-OHDA lesioned hemisphere being on the right side of the autoradiogram. The anteriority level corresponds to the 8800 μm plane of the atlas of König and Klippel.[74] Note the decrease of ^{3}H-naloxone binding in the lesioned striatum, whereas there is no change of optical density in the lesioned nucleus accumbens. (From ref. 36.)

findings that DA denervation of the nucleus accumbens or chronic neuroleptic treatment induce a behavioral supersensitivity to the injection of opioid agonists or morphine into this site.[44] Indeed, as it has just been shown, these treatments modify the relative densities of opiate receptors between the core and the shell of the nucleus accumbens and may therefore induce a hyperreactivity to intra-accumbens opiate infusion.

Two other observations suggest that μ-opiate receptors are not located on ascending DA neurons. First, Dilts and Kalivas showed that injections of 6-OHDA into the ventral mesencephalon did not decrease the density of μ-opiate receptors in the VTA.[45] This difference with what is observed at the level of the DA nerve terminals can be explained if we assume that, in the VTA, μ-opiate receptors density is not regulated by DA release. Second, the close examination of the topographical distribution of μ-opiate receptors in the VTA indicates that they are not co-localized with DA cell bodies. This can be seen, for example, in the work of Mansour et al.[46] where autoradiograms of mesencephalic μ-opiate receptors clearly show that they are located in a zone more medial and dorsal than that of tyrosine hydroxylase–containing cell bodies.[47]

In any case, the main consequence of these observations is that μ-opiate receptors located in the striatum and the nucleus accumbens are post-synaptic to DA neurons.

It must therefore be assumed that morphine is activating ascending DA neurons via the inhibition of μ-opiate-receptor–bearing, probably GABAergic,[48] VTA interneurons. This hypothesis lends itself more easily to the definition of a mechanism that would differentially activate mesolimbic and mesocortical DA neurons.

Presence of Nicotinic Receptors on Some DA Ascending Neurons

There are at least two classes of molecules that might be candidates for the nicotine-binding site(s) associated with nicotine's action in the central nervous system: the nicotine acetylcholine receptors and the α-bungarotoxin/nicotine binding molecules present on some neuronal populations.

The nicotinic acetylcholine receptors are found on muscle and on neurons. Alpha-bungarotoxin blocks activation of the muscle nicotinic acetylcholine receptors but does not block activation of mammalian neuronal nicotinic acetylcholine receptors.[49,50] Alpha-bungarotoxin, however, has a specific binding site on neurons, and its binding to this site can be blocked by nicotine.

The topographical distribution of the neuronal binding sites has been studied by quantitative autoradiography using either ^{3}H-acetylcholine (in the presence of atropine) and ^{3}H-nicotine (first site) or ^{125}I-α-bungarotoxin (second site).[51] The highest densities of the first site were found in the interpeduncular nucleus, most thalamic nuclei, superior colliculus, medial habenula, presubiculum and molecular layer of the dentate gyrus. Binding was also prominent in the substantia nigra of the zona compacta, VTA and certain laminae of the cerebral cortex. Labeling was only moderate in the neostriatum and the nucleus accumbens. The second site, labeled by ^{125}I-α-bungarotoxin, had a strikingly different distribution. The only significant overlap with the first site occurred in the cerebral cortex and the superior colliculus. Most notably, the striatum, nucleus accumbens and mesencephalic regions such as the substantia nigra and the VTA were devoid of ^{125}I-α-bungarotoxin labeling.

The topographical distribution of the second ^{125}I-α-bungarotoxin–labeled site suggests that there is no relation between it and the ascending DA neurons. At the opposite, the first site, labeled by ^{3}H-nicotine and present in the ventral mesencephalon at the level of the substantia nigra and the VTA could be localized on DA neurons. This was in fact demonstrated by Clarke and Pert[52] who showed that a unilateral 6-OHDA injection into the ascending DA fiber bundle, which resulted in a near total depletion of DA in the ipsilateral striatum and the disappearance of DA cell bodies in the substantia nigra and the VTA, was accompanied by a reduction of ^{3}H-nicotine labeling in terminal areas of the nigrostriatal and mesolimbic systems and a virtual disappearance of specific labeling in the corresponding DA cell body regions.

These data are in agreement with previous experiments, performed in our laboratory, which suggested the presence of nicotinic receptors on presynaptic DA nerve terminals by showing a nicotinic effect of acetylcholine on the release of ^{3}H-DA from rat striatal slices or from cat caudate nucleus.[53] Moreover, Lichtensteiger *et al.*, using extracellular single unit recording procedures, demonstrated that subcutaneously administered nicotine increases the firing rate of zona compacta cells in the substantia nigra.[54]

The neuronal nicotinic receptor family has been further studied with molecular approaches. This was based on the experimentally supported hypothesis[55] that although the primary structures of the electric organ and muscle nicotinic receptors are likely to be distinct from their neuronal counterparts, they are encoded by homologous genes. In fact, five different α and four different β subunits of the neuronal nicotinic receptors have been demonstrated in the rat brain.[56] It is likely that the different possible combinations of these subunits will give rise to different receptors with pharmacological and functional diversity. It seems, however, that there exists a majority of α_4 and β_2 combinations which constitute the predominant α-bungarotoxin-insensitive nicotinic receptor in adult vertebrate brain. These receptors are sensitive to a "neuronal bungarotoxin" or toxin F.

In 1987, Deutch et al., using an antibody raised against purified acetylcholine receptor from *Torpedo*, were able to show a cross-reactivity with neuronal acetylcholine receptor.[57] Regions of the rat brain stained with this antibody paralleled those areas of the brain exhibiting ^{3}H-nicotine binding sites and corresponded to areas in which mRNAs encoding for α subunits of the neuronal nicotinic receptor are present. Labeled neuronal cell bodies in the substantia nigra compacta and VTA were clearly shown. These neurons correspond in both position and morphology to the DA neurons of the A_{10}, A_9 and A_8 cell groups of the ventral midbrain. However, although these immunohistochemical data are in agreement with those of autoradiographic studies, they also indicated that only a part of these probably DA ventral midbrain neurons of the VTA/substantia nigra/retrorubral field synthetize a nicotinic receptor. Moreover, a relatively weak immunostaining of the striatum and nucleus accumbens was found. This observation, consistent with autoradiographic localization of ^{3}H-nicotine binding sites, may indicate that relatively little nicotinic receptor is axonally transported to the striatum or that only a part of the nigro-striatal DA neurons possess it.

Thus, the presence of a subtype of nicotinic receptors on DA neurons of the ventral mesencephalon has been clearly demonstrated by various technics. These neuronal receptors can be labeled by ^{3}H-nicotine or by antibodies raised against the α subunit of the nicotinic receptor and correspond to the neuronal subtype insensitive to α-bungarotoxin. Given that immunohistochemical experiments have indicated that not all the DA neurons of the ventral mesencephalon synthetize nicotinic receptors, it is possible that nicotine may differentially regulate sub-groups of ascending DA neurons. It is not yet known, however, whether nicotinic receptors are homogeneously distributed among the different ascending DA systems or whether they are borne by specific DA neurons and correspond to functional subdivisions.

DIFFERENTIAL ACTIVATIONS OF MESOCORTICAL AND MESOLIMBIC DA NEURONS BY MORPHINE AND NICOTINE

To test the effects of morphine and nicotine on ascending DA neurons, Sprague-Dawley rats were treated acutely or chronically with systemic injections of either drug and the dihydroxy phenylacetic acid (DOPAC)/DA ratios were measured in the prefrontal cortex, the nucleus accumbens and, in some cases, in antero-medial and latero-dorsal striatum.

Morphine Effects

Acute morphine hydrochloride (5.0 mg/kg, base, s.c.) produced large increases in the DOPAC/DA ratio in the nucleus accumbens ($+59\%$) and in the prefrontal cortex

(+61%). Repeating these injections (10.0 mg/kg every day for 12 days and 5 mg/kg at test, base, s.c.) substantially enhanced the effect of morphine in the nucleus accumbens (+96%) but slightly reduced it in the prefrontal cortex (+52%) (FIG. 4).[58] These doses have been shown to produce behavioral sensitization to morphine[8] and it was indeed verified that the chronically injected animals had become sensitized.

These findings are consistent with the induction of sensitization by repeated morphine exposure. We mentioned, in the first part of this chapter, that an activation of the mesocortical DA pathway may have an inhibitory role on locomotor activity. We find here that repeated morphine treatments increase the ratio between the activation of the mesolimbic versus the mesocortical DA pathways. This latter result would then be consistent with a hyperactive locomotor response to morphine in animals chronically injected with morphine.

Nicotine Effects

Acute injections of (–)-nicotine bitartrate (0.4–0.8 mg/kg, base, s.c.) produce substantial increases (+39%) in the DOPAC/DA ratio in the nucleus accumbens and more moderate increases (+29%) in the antero-medial striatum.[58] These increases in DOPAC/DA were linked to significant increases in levels of DOPAC while DA levels were unaffected. No modification of the DOPAC/DA ratio was observed in the latero-dorsal striatum.

After repeated injections, however, nicotine no longer produced significant increases either in DOPAC/DA or in DOPAC levels in the nucleus accumbens and the

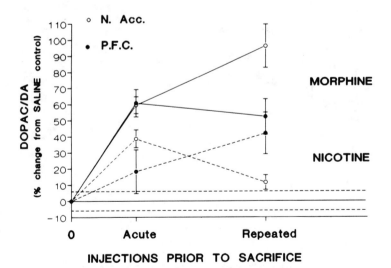

FIGURE 4. Effects of acute and repeated injections of nicotine and morphine on DA utilization in the nucleus accumbens and the prefrontal cortex. Animals received a test injection of nicotine or morphine and were sacrificed 30 or 60 min later, respectively. Repeated group animals received 12 drug injections prior to test. Data are the mean DOPAC/DA ratios for the nucleus accumbens and the prefrontal cortex shown as % changes from ratios obtained for saline control animals. (From ref. 58.)

antero-medial striatum. The DOPAC/DA ratio in the latero-dorsal striatum remained unaffected.

Interestingly, in the prefrontal cortex, acute nicotine did not significantly increase the DOPAC/DA ratio. Repeating the nicotine injections, however, produced a significant increase in this ratio (+42%) (FIG. 4).[58]

Thus, repeated nicotine decreased its acute DA activating effect in the nucleus accumbens and increased it in the prefrontal cortex, while repeated morphine increased this effect in the nucleus accumbens and produced a small decrease in the prefrontal cortex. FIGURE 5 illustrates these opposing effects of nicotine and morphine by plotting (nucleus accumbens DOPAC/DA)/(prefrontal cortex DOPAC/DA) as a function of drug exposure.

From these data, it is clear that the behavioral sensitizations produced by morphine and nicotine cannot both be accounted for by similar changes in reactivity to the drug of DA cortical and subcortical neurons. The possibility that these two examples of behavioral sensitization arise from different substraits was further tested by a cross-sensitization procedure.

Lack of Behavioral Sensitization between Nicotine and Morphine

Two groups of rats received daily injections of nicotine or saline for 12 days. The locomotor sensitizing effects of nicotine became apparent only on the fourth day of injection and were clearly visible, although small (+57%), on the 12th day.[58]

On the following day, all animals were injected with morphine (5 mg/kg). We found that preexposure to nicotine did not enhance the locomotor activating effects of mor-

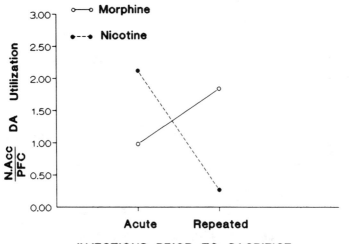

FIGURE 5. Illustration of the opposite effects of nicotine and morphine on the cortico-subcortical balance. Subcortical and prefrontocortical DA activations are shown by plotting (nucleus accumbens DOPAC/DA)/(prefrontal cortex DOPAC/DA) as a function of exposure to the drug. (From ref. 58.)

phine. Both groups of animals (nicotine and saline pre-exposed) responded to morphine with similar levels of locomotion. These were significantly greater than the locomotor response to saline (+180%).

CONCLUDING REMARKS

In the first part of this paper, we have presented some evidence that the stimulations of ascending mesocortical and mesolimbic DA pathways have antagonistic effects on locomotor behavior. An activation of the mesolimbic DA pathway would increase locomotor activity, whereas the stimulation of the mesocortical DA system would inhibit this increased locomotor activity.

Given the earlier reports indicating that locomotor sensitization is obtained only when the drug has access to the VTA, we have proposed that locomotor sensitization could be the result of the differential effects of sensitizing drugs on mesolimbic *and* mesocortical DA pathways. To test this hypothesis, we have studied the effect of morphine and nicotine, two drugs which induce behavioral sensitization, on the metabolism of ascending DA neurons.

First, it was demonstrated that morphine does not interact directly with DA cells, since these latter do not possess μ-opiate receptors. In the VTA, it is likely that morphine inhibits interneurons which, in turn, may influence ascending DA neurons. Mesencephalic DA cells, however, possess nicotinic receptors that are insensitive to α-bungarotoxin but sensitive to neuronal bungarotoxin. Interestingly, only a part of the tyrosine-hydroxylase containing cell bodies synthetizes nicotinic receptors.

Repeating the morphine injections increases the activity of mesolimbic DA neurons more than that of mesocortical DA neurons. This could be related to the fact that the control of DA neurons by VTA interneurons which possess μ-opiate receptors is preferentially directed towards mesolimbic DA neurons rather than towards mesocortical DA neurons. In any case, as previously mentioned, the differential regulation of both subtypes of DA neurons by chronic morphine treatment is consistent with the development of locomotor sensitization. On the other hand, repeated nicotine injections appear to desensitize mesolimbic DA neurons and to increase the activation of mesocortical DA cells. The finding that the ratio between the activation of mesolimbic and mesocortical DA neurons decreased when nicotine was administered repeatedly suggests that this drug's emerging locomotor effects are due to actions on other neurotransmitter systems.

The effects of nicotine on mesolimbic DA neurons has already been studied by different technics that have given somewhat different results. Mitchell *et al.*,[59] using the dihydroxyphenylalanine (DOPA) accumulation method, found no difference in the nucleus accumbens between acutely and chronically treated animals. Using *in vivo* microdialysis, Imperato *et al.*[60] showed that an acute systemic injection of nicotine enhanced DA overflow in the nucleus accumbens and Damsa *et al.*[61] obtained similar levels of nucleus accumbens DA overflow in this site following a systemic nicotine injection in acutely or repeatedly treated animals. Finally, when the DOPAC/DA ratio was used as an index of the modifications of DA metabolism in the nucleus accumbens, two other teams found results similar to ours, that is an attenuation of the increased DA metabolism induced by nicotine in chronically treated animals when compared with naïve rats.[62,63] Results seem, therefore, dependent on the techniques employed. There is some possibility that the DOPA accumulation method not only estimates modifications of DA but also of noradrenaline metabolism.[64] Concerning the differences observed between the microdialysis and the DOPAC/DA ratio methods, it cannot be excluded that the estimate of DA overflow provided by the former reflects more the effects of nicotine on DA presynaptic receptors than the chronic modifications of neuronal metabolism which may be better estimated by the DOPAC/DA ratio method. In any case, the fact that there is no behavioral cross-sensitization between nicotine and morphine strongly suggests that chronic nicotine has not induced any sensitization of mesolimbic DA neurons.

One of the most interesting aspects of our results concerns the increased reactivity of *mesocortical* DA neurons to nicotine, observed on animals repeatedly exposed to the drug. As demonstrated in this chapter, our results obtained with DA utilization in the nucleus accumbens suggest that locomotor sensitization to nicotine is a non-DA dependent event. Furthermore, given that drug abuse necessarily involves repeated exposure to the drug and that such exposure to the nicotine was found to reduce its stimulatory effects on DA utilization in the nucleus accumbens, these same results suggest that nicotine differs importantly from other abused drugs such as opiates and psychomotor stimulants which are generally accepted to achieve their rewarding properties by activating mesolimbic DA neurons.[65-67] On the other hand, the significance of nicotine's activation of mesocortical DA neurons remains to be explored. It has been demonstrated, for example, that the prefrontal cortex supports self-administration of cocaine.[68] Although our findings indicate an opposing relationship between mesolimbic and mesocortical DA neuron influences on locomotor activity, this does not exclude the possibility that prefrontal cortex is, in addition to nucleus accumbens,[65-67] a site involved in drug reward. Indeed, it should be remembered that mesocortical DA neurons have been shown to play a major role in cognitive processes.[69-71] It can be proposed, therefore, that the activation of these neurons by nicotine represents the physiological basis of tobacco smoking's facilitatory effects on learning and increased attention.[72,73] Such effects may be an important basis for the pursuit of nicotine.

REFERENCES

1. BABINI, M. & W. M. DAVIS. 1972. Time-dose relationships for locomotor activity effects of morphine after acute or repeated treatment. Br. J. Pharmacol. 46: 213–224.
2. KSIR, C., R. L. HAKAN & K. J. KELLAR. 1987. Chronic nicotine and locomotor activity: Influences of exposure dose and test dose. Psychopharmacology 92: 25–29.
3. TILSON, H. A. & R. H. RECH. 1973. Conditioned drug effects and absence of tolerance to *d*-amphetamine induced motor activity. Pharmacol. Biochem. Behav. 1: 149–153.
4. ROBINSON, T. E. & J. B. BECKER. 1986. Enduring changes in brain and behavior produced by chronic amphetamine administration: A review and evaluation of animals models of amphetamine psychosis. Brain Res. Rev. 11: 157–198.
5. POST, R. M., A. LOCKFELD, K. M. SQUILLACE & N. R. CONTEL. 1981. Drug-environment interaction: Context dependency of cocaine-induced behavioral sensitization. Life Sci. 28: 755–760.
6. CLARKE, P. B. S., D. S. FU, A. JAKUBOVIC & H. C. FIBIGER. 1988. Evidence that mesolimbic dopaminergic activation underlies the locomotor stimulant action of nicotine in rats. J. Pharmacol. Exp. Ther. 246: 701–708.
7. KALIVAS, P. W. & P. DUFFY. 1987. Sensitization to repeated morphine injection in the rat: Possible involvement of A10 dopamine neurons. J. Pharmacol. Exp. Ther. 241: 204–212.
8. KALIVAS, P. W., P. DUFFY, L. A. DUMARS & C. SKINNER. 1988. Behavioral and neuro-

chemical effects of acute and daily cocaine administration in rats. J. Pharmacol. Exp. Ther. 245: 485–492.
9. JOYCE, E. M. & S. D. IVERSEN. 1979. The effects of morphine applied locally to mesencephalic dopamine cell bodies on spontaneous locomotor activity in the rat. Neurosci. Lett. 14: 207–212.
10. VEZINA, P. & J. STEWART. 1984. Conditioning and place-specific sensitization of increases in activity induced by morphine in the VTA. Pharmacol. Biochem. Behav. 20: 925–934.
11. KALIVAS, P. W., S. TAYLOR & J. S. MILLER. 1985. Sensitization to repeated enkephalin administration into the ventral tegmental area of the rat. I. Behavioral characterization. J. Pharmacol. Exp. Ther. 235: 537–543.
12. DAHLSTRÖM, A. & K. FUXE. 1964. Evidence for the existence of monoamine-containing neurons in the central nervous system. II. Demonstration of monoamines in the cell bodies of brain stem neurons. Acta Physiol. Scand. 62: 1–55.
13. BJÖRKLUND, A. & O. LINDVALL. 1984. Dopamine-containing systems in the CNS. In Handbook of Chemical Neuroanatomy. A. Björklund & T. Hökfelt, Eds.: 55–122. Elsevier. Amsterdam.
14. KALIVAS, P. W. 1985. Sensitization to repeated enkephalin administration into the ventral tegmental area of the rat. II. Involvement of the mesolimbic DA system. J. Pharmacol. Exp. Ther. 235: 544–550.
15. VEZINA, P., P. W. KALIVAS & J. STEWART. 1987. Sensitization occurs to the locomotor effects of morphine and the specific μ opioid receptor agonist, DAGO, administered repeatedly to the ventral tegmental area but not to the nucleus accumbens. Brain Res. 417: 51–58.
16. VEZINA, P. & J. STEWART. 1990. Amphetamine administered to the ventral tegmental area but not to the nucleus accumbens sensitizes rats to systemic morphine: Lack of conditioned effects. Brain Res. 516: 99–106.
17. KALIVAS, P. W. & B. WEBER. 1988. Amphetamine injection into the ventral mesencephalon sensitizes rats to peripheral amphetamine and cocaine. J. Pharmacol. Exp. Ther. 245: 1095–1102.
18. KALIVAS, P. W. & P. DUFFY. 1988. Effects of daily cocaine and morphine treatment on somatodendritic and terminal field dopamine release. J. Neurochem. 50: 1498–1504.
19. VEZINA, P., G. BLANC, J. GLOWINSKI & J. P. TASSIN. 1991. Opposed behavioural outputs of increased dopamine transmission in prefrontocortical and subcortical areas: A role for cortical D1 receptor. Eur. J. Neurosci. 3: 1001–1007.
20. KELLY, P. H., P. W. SEVIOUR & S. D. IVERSEN. 1975. Amphetamine and apomorphine responses in the rat following 6-OHDA lesion of the nucleus accumbens septi and corpus striatum. Brain Res. 94: 507–523.
21. TASSIN, J. P., L. STINUS, H. SIMON, G. BLANC, A. M. THIERRY, M. LE MOAL, B. CARDO & J. GLOWINSKI. 1978. Relationship between the locomotor hyperactivity induced by A10 lesions and the destruction of fronto-cortical DA innervation in the rat. Brain Res. 141: 267–281.
22. LE MOAL, M., L. STINUS & D. GALEY. 1976. Radio-frequency lesions of the ventral mesencephalic tegmentum: Neurological and behavioural considerations. Exp. Neurol. 50: 521–535.
23. JOYCE, E. M., L. STINUS & S. D. IVERSEN. 1983. Effect of injections of 6-OHDA into either nucleus accumbens septi or frontal cortex on spontaneous and drug-induced activity. Neuropharmacology 22: 1141–1145.
24. TASSIN, J. P., H. SIMON, J. GLOWINSKI & J. BOCKAËRT. 1982. Modulations of the sensitivity of dopaminergic receptors in the prefrontal cortex and the nucleus accumbens: Relationship with locomotor activity. In Brain Peptides and Hormones. R. Collu, J. R. Ducharme, A. Barbeau & G. Tobis, Eds.: 17–30. Raven Press. New York.
25. ATWEH, S. E. & M. J. KUHAR. 1977. Autoradiographic localization of opiate receptors in rat brain. III. The telencephalon. Brain Res. 134: 393–450.
26. LA MOTTE, C. C., A. SNOWMAN, C. C. PERT & S. H. SNYDER. 1978. Opiate receptor binding in rhesus monkey brain: Association with limbic structures. Brain Res. 155: 374–379.

27. IWATSUBO, K. & D. H. CLOUET. 1977. Effects of morphine and haloperidol on the electrical activity of rat nigrostriatal neurons. J. Pharmacol. Exp. Ther. 202: 429–436.
28. JOHNSON, R. P., M. SAR & W. E. STUMP. 1981. A topographical localization of enkephalin on the dopamine neurons of the rat substantia nigra and ventral tegmental area are demonstrated by combined histofluorescence-immunohistochemistry. Brain Res. 194: 566–571.
29. POLLARD, H., C. LLORENS-CORTES & J. C. SCHWARTZ. 1977. Enkephalin receptors on dopaminergic neurones in rat striatum. Nature 268: 745–747.
30. POLLARD, H., C. LLORENS-CORTES, J. J. BONNET, J. COSTENTIN & J. C. SCHWARTZ. 1977. Opiate receptors on mesolimbic dopaminergic neurons. Neurosci. Lett. 7: 295–299.
31. BOWEN, W. D., C. B. PERT & A. PERT. 1982. Nigral 6-OHDA equally decreases μ and δ opiate binding to striatal patches: Further evidence for a conformationally malleable distinct type 1 opiate receptor. Life Sci. 31: 1679–1685.
32. EGHBALI, M., C. SANTORO, W. PAREDES, E. GARDNER & R. S. ZUKIN. 1987. Visualization of multiple opioid-receptor types in rat striatum after specific mesencephalic lesions. Proc. Natl. Acad. Sci. USA 84: 6582–6586.
33. WAKSMAN, G., E. HAMEL, P. DELAY-GOYET & B. P. ROQUES. 1987. Neutral endopeptidase-24.11, μ and δ opioid receptors after selective brain lesions: An autoradiographic study. Brain Res. 436: 205–216.
34. CHESSELET, M. F., A. CHÉRAMY, T. D. REISINE, C. LUBETZKI, J. GLOWINSKI, M. C. FOURNIÉ-ZALUSKI & B. ROQUES. 1982. Effects of various opiates including specific δ and μ agonists on dopamine release from nigrostriatal dopaminergic neurons in vitro in the rat and in vivo in the cat. Life Sci. 31: 2291–2294.
35. LUBETZKI, C., M-F. CHESSELET & J. GLOWINSKI. 1982. Modulation of dopamine release in rat striatal slices by delta opiate agonist. J. Pharmacol. Exp. Ther. 222: 435–440.
36. TROVERO, F., D. HERVÉ, M. DESBAN, J. GLOWINSKI & J. P. TASSIN. 1990. Striatal opiate μ-receptors are not located on dopamine nerve endings in the rat. Neuroscience 39: 313–321.
37. HERKENHAM, M. & C. B. PERT. 1981. Mosaic distribution of opiate receptors, parafascicular projections and acetylcholinesterase in the striatum. Nature 291: 415–418.
38. ZABORSZKY, L., G. F. ALHEID, M. C. BEINFELD, L. E. EIDEN, L. HEIMER & M. PALKOVITS. 1985. Cholecystokinin innervation of the ventral striatum: A morphological and radioimmunological study. Neuroscience 14: 427–453.
39. HÖKFELT, T., L. SKIRBOLL, J. F. REHFELD, M. GOLDSTEIN, K. MARKEY & O. DANN. 1980. A subpopulation of mesencephalic dopamine neurons projecting to limbic areas contains a cholecystokinin-like peptide: Evidence from immunohistochemistry combined with retrograde tracing. Neuroscience 5: 2093–2124.
40. STUDLER, J. M., H. SIMON, F. CESSELIN, J. C. LEGRAND, J. GLOWINSKI & J. P. TASSIN. 1981. Biochemical investigation on the localization of the cholecystokinin octapeptide in dopaminergic neurons originating from the ventral tegmental area of the rat. Neuropeptide 2: 131–139.
41. HEIMER, L., D. S. ZAHM, L. CHURCHILL, P. W. KALIVAS & C. WOHLTMANN. 1991. Specificity in the projection patterns of accumbal core and shell in the rat. Neuroscience 41: 89–125.
42. CRAWLEY, J. N., J. A. STIVERS, L. K. BLUMSTEIN & S. M. PAUL. 1985. Cholecystokinin potentiates dopamine-mediated behaviors: Evidence for a modulation specific to a site of coexistence. J. Neurosci. 5: 1972–1983.
43. STUDLER, J. M., M. REIBAUD, D. HERVÉ, J. GLOWINSKI & J. P. TASSIN. 1986. Opposite effects of sulfated cholecystokinin on DA-sensitive adenylate cyclase in two areas of the rat nucleus accumbens. Europ. J. Pharmacol. 126: 125–128.
44. STINUS, L., M. WINNOCK & A. E. KELLEY. 1985. Chronic neuroleptic treatment and mesolimbic dopamine denervation induce behavioural supersensitivity to opiates. Psychopharmacology 85: 323–328.
45. DILTS, R. P. & P. W. KALIVAS. 1988. Localization of μ opioid and neurotensin receptors within the A10 region of the rat. Ann. NY Acad. Sci. 537: 472–474.
46. MANSOUR, A., H. KHACHATURIAN, M. E. LEWIS, H. AKIL & S. J. WATSON. 1987. Autoradiographic differentiation of Mu, Delta, and Kappa opioid receptors in the rat forebrain and midbrain. J. Neurosci. 7: 2445–2464.

47. HERVÉ, D. 1988. La transmission dopaminergique dans le système nerveux central du rat: Modulation de l'activité nerveuse et régulation des récepteurs par des afférences hétérologues. Ph.D. Thesis. University of Paris VII, France.
48. NORTH, R. A. 1992. Cellular actions of opiates and cocaine. Ann. NY Acad. Sci. **654**: 1–6. This volume.
49. MORLEY, B. J. & G. E. KEMP. 1981. Characterization of a putative nicotinic acetylcholine receptor in mammalian brain. Brain Res. Rev. **3**: 81–104.
50. LORING, R. H., V. A. CHIAPPINELLI, R. E. ZIGMOND & J. B. COHEN. 1984. Characterization of a snake venom neurotoxin which blocks nicotinic transmission in the avian ciliary ganglion. Neuroscience **11**: 989–999.
51. CLARKE, P. B. S., R. D. SCHWARTZ, S. M. PAUL, C. B. PERT & A. PERT. 1985. Nicotine binding in rat brain: Autoradiographic comparison of ^{3}H-acetylcholine, ^{3}H-nicotine and ^{125}I-alpha-bungarotoxin. J. Neurosci. **5**: 1307–1315.
52. CLARKE, P. B. S. & A. PERT. 1985. Autoradiographic evidence for nicotine receptors on nigrostriatal and mesolimbic dopaminergic neurons. Brain Res. **348**: 355–358.
53. GIORGUIEFF, M. F., M. L. LE FLOC'H, T. C. WESTFALL, J. GLOWINSKI & M. J. BESSON. 1976. Nicotinic effect of acetylcholine on release of newly synthesized ^{3}H-DA in rat striatal slices and cat caudate nucleus. Brain Res. **106**: 117–131.
54. LICHTENSTEIGER, W., D. FELIX, R. LIENHART & F. HEFTI. 1976. A quantitative correlation between single unit activity and fluorescence intensity of dopamine neurons in zona compacta of substantia nigra, as demonstrated under the influence of nicotine and physostigmine. Brain Res. **117**: 85–103.
55. SWANSON, L. W., J. LINDSTROM, S. TZARTOS, L. C. SCMUED, D. D. M. O'LEARY & W. M. COWAN. 1983. Immunohistochemical localization of monoclonal antibodies to the nicotinic acetylcholine receptor in chick midbrain. Proc. Natl. Acad. Sci. USA **80**: 4532–4536.
56. DENERIS, E. S., J. CONNOLLY, S. W. ROGERS & R. DUVOISIN. 1991. Pharmacological and functional diversity of neuronal nicotinic acetylcholine receptors. Trends Pharmacol. Sci. **12**: 34–40.
57. DEUTCH, A. Y., J. HOLLIDAY, R. R. ROTH, L. L. Y. CHUN & E. HAWROT. 1987. Immunohistochemical localization of a neuronal nicotinic acetylcholine receptor in mammalian brain. Proc. Natl. Acad. Sci. USA **84**: 8697–8701.
58. VEZINA, P., G. BLANC, J. GLOWINSKI & J. P. TASSIN. 1992. Nicotine and morphine differentially activate brain dopamine in prefrontocortical and subcortical terminal fields: Effects of acute and repeated injections. J. Pharmacol. Exp. Ther. In press.
59. MITCHELL, S. N., M. P. BRAZELL, M. H. JOSEPH, M. S. ALAVIJEH & J. A. GRAY. 1989. Regionally specific effects of acute and chronic nicotine on rates of catecholamine and 5-hydroxytryptamine synthesis in rat brain. Eur. J. Pharmacol. **167**: 311–322.
60. IMPERATO, A., A. MULAS & G. DI CHIARA. 1986. Nicotine preferentially stimulates dopamine release in the limbic system of freely moving rats. Eur. J. Pharmacol. **132**: 337–338.
61. DAMSMA, G., J. DAY & H. C. FIBIGER. 1989. Lack of tolerance to nicotine-induced dopamine release in the nucleus accumbens. Eur. J. Pharmacol. **168**: 363–368.
62. LAPIN, E. P., H. S. MAKER, H. SERSHEN & A. LAJTHA. 1989. Action of nicotine on accumbens dopamine and attenuation with repeated administration. Eur. J. Pharmacol. **160**: 53–59.
63. GRENHOFF, J. & T. H. SVENSSON. 1989. Acute and chronic effects of nicotine on rat brain dopaminergic systems. European Winter Conference on Brain Research. Abstract, p. 44.
64. MITCHELL, S. N., M. P. BRAZELL, M. M. SCHUGENS & J. A. GRAY. 1990. Nicotine-induced catecholamine synthesis after lesions to the dorsal or ventral noradrenergic bundle. Eur. J. Pharmacol. **179**: 383–391.
65. DI CHIARA, G. & A. IMPERATO. 1988. Drugs abused by humans preferentially increase synaptic dopamine concentrations in the mesolimbic system of freely moving rats. Proc. Natl. Acad. Sci. **85**: 5274–5278.
66. KOOB, G. F. & F. E. BLOOM. 1988. Cellular and molecular mechanisms of drug dependence. Science **242**: 715–723.
67. WISE, R. A. & M. A. BOZARTH. 1987. A psychomotor stimulant theory of addiction. Psychol. Rev. **94**: 469–492.

68. GOEDERS, N. E. & J. E. SMITH. 1983. Cortical dopaminergic involvement in cocaine reinforcement. Science **221:** 773–775.
69. BROZOSKI, T. J., R. MCBROWN, H. E. ROSVOLD & P. S. GOLDMAN-RAKIC. 1979. Cognitive deficit caused by regional depletion of dopamine in prefrontal cortex of rhesus monkey. Science **205:** 929–932.
70. SIMON, H., B. SCATTON & M. LE MOAL. 1980. Dopaminergic A10 neurons are involved in cognitive functions. Nature **286:** 150–151.
71. SAWAGUCHI, T. & P. S. GOLDMAN-RAKIC. 1991. D1 receptors in prefrontal cortex: Involvement in working memory. Science **251:** 947–950.
72. EDWARDS, J. A., K. WESNES, D. WARBURTON & A. GALE. 1985. Evidence of more rapid stimulus evaluation following cigarette smoking. Addictive Behav. **10:** 113–126.
73. WARBURTON, W., K. WESNES, K. SHERGOLD & M. JAMES. 1986. Facilitation of learning and state dependency with nicotine. Psychopharmacology **89:** 55–59.
74. KÖNIG, S. F. R. & R. A. KLIPPEL. 1963. A stereotaxic atlas of forebrain and lower parts of the brain stem. Williams & Wilkins. Baltimore.

Serotonin Neurotransmission in Cocaine Sensitization[a]

KATHRYN A. CUNNINGHAM[b]
AND JOSEPH M. PARIS

Department of Pharmacology and Toxicology
University of Texas Medical Branch
Galveston, Texas 77550

NICK E. GOEDERS

Department of Pharmacology and Therapeutics
Louisiana State University School of Medicine
Shreveport, Louisiana 71130

INTRODUCTION

Cocaine binds to neuronal transporter molecules[1] and inhibits uptake processes for dopamine (DA), serotonin (5-hydroxytryptamine; 5-HT) and norepinephrine (NE). As a consequence of this action, cocaine potentiates DA, 5-HT and NE neurotransmission,[2] although cocaine has little affinity for monoamine receptors,[1] except 5-HT$_3$ receptors.[3] The inhibition of DA uptake processes appears to play a prominent role in the behavioral effects of cocaine. Thus, antagonists of DA systems and destruction of DA pathways disrupt cocaine-induced locomotor activation and stereotypy[4] as well as the reinforcing efficacy[5,6] and discriminative stimulus properties of this psychotropic agent.[7,8] However, not all studies point to a unitary role for DA in these effects of cocaine[9-12] and the multiplicity of its monoaminergic actions suggests that the behavioral and physiological effects of cocaine cannot be explained solely on the basis of interactions with one biogenic amine system. Cocaine also inhibits 5-HT uptake[2] as well as the uptake of the 5-HT precursor tryptophan and the activity of tryptophan hydroxylase,[13] all of which probably contribute to its ability to suppress 5-HT synthesis.[14] ^{3}H-Cocaine labels sites on 5-HT terminals which are probably recognition sites associated with 5-HT reuptake.[15] In fact, the affinity of cocaine is higher for the 5-HT transporter than for either the DA or NE transporter.[1] Classical pharmacological studies have also shown that cocaine antagonizes 5-HT$_3$-mediated responses in the periphery[16] and inhibits 5-HT$_3$ binding in the brain.[3] While there are mixed results with regard to the importance of 5-HT$_3$ receptors in the behavioral effects of cocaine,[17-20] the significant effects of cocaine on the 5-HT system appear to have behavioral relevance since 5-HT synthesis or receptor blockade potentiates,[4] while the

[a] This work was supported by the National Alliance for Schizophrenia and Affective Disorders and USPHS Grants DA 05708 and DA 06511 (KAC), DA 05381 (JMP) and DA 04293 (NEG) from the National Institute on Drug Abuse (NIDA).

[b] Author to whom all correspondence should be addressed; Tel.: (409) 772-9629.

117

5-HT precursor 5-hydroxytryptophan antagonizes,[21] cocaine-induced locomotor activity. Thus, these studies suggest that a comprehensive understanding of the mechanisms of action of cocaine should not overlook interactions between cocaine and 5-HT.

EFFECTS OF ACUTE COCAINE ADMINISTRATION ON 5-HT NEURONS

Serotonin neurons which provide innervation for the forebrain are predominantly localized to the dorsal (DR) and median (MR) raphe nuclei of the midbrain.[22] These 5-HT neurons possess a high density of 5-HT transporters[23] and 5-HT$_{1A}$ receptors[24] which appear to function as impulse-modulating autoreceptors.[25] Single unit extracellular recordings have demonstrated that the intravenous administration of (−)-cocaine, but not the local anesthetic procaine, potently and reversibly depresses the activity of 5-HT neurons in the DR of the rat (FIG. 1).[26-28] Interestingly, while cocaine is relatively equipotent as an inhibitor of DA, 5-HT and NE uptake[2] as well as ligand binding to DA, 5-HT and NE transporter sites,[1] cocaine is a more efficacious and potent inhibitor of the impulse activity of 5-HT neurons (TABLE 1)[26-28] than that of either DA[29] or NE neurons.[30] Microiontophoretic application of cocaine depresses the activity of 5-HT neurons, with prolonged application resulting in a progressive increase in the magnitude of the drug-induced depression; cocaine also potentiates the inhibitory effects of iontophoretically applied 5-HT in the DR.[26] Thus, not only does administration of cocaine significantly modify the functional activity of 5-HT neurons, but cocaine also directly alters the activity of the 5-HT neurons located in the DR.

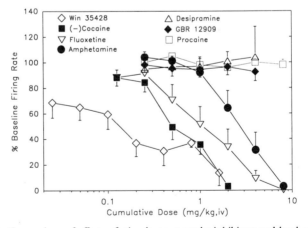

FIGURE 1. Comparison of effects of stimulants, reuptake inhibitors and local anesthetics on the spontaneous activity of 5-HT DR neurons. Drugs were administered (i.v.) at 2 min intervals such that each dose doubled the previously administered dose (*abscissa*). Symbols represent the mean (± SEM) percentage of baseline firing rate observed at each dose of the test compound (*ordinate*). The effects of each drug were tested on 7–12 5-HT cells. The potency order to completely inhibit cell firing is as follows: Win 35428 > (−)-cocaine > fluoxetine > amphetamine. The uptake inhibitor for NE (desipramine) and DA (GBR 12909) as well as the local anesthetic procaine were ineffective. (Adapted from ref. 26).

TABLE 1. Cocaine: Inhibition of Somal Activity

	Dopamine[a]	Serotonin[b]	Norepinephrine[c]
ID$_{50}$ (mg/kg)	2.2	0.6	0.8
Maximum % inhibition	60%	100%	70%

Data derived from [a] Einhorn *et al.* (1988); [b] Cunningham & Lakoski (1990); [c] Pitts & Marwah (1987).

To assess the role of monoamine reuptake processes in the cocaine-induced inhibition of 5-HT DR neurons, the effects of reuptake inhibitors selective for DA (GBR 12909), NE (desipramine) and 5-HT (fluoxetine) were compared.[27] Neither GBR 12909 nor desipramine (FIG. 1) suppressed 5-HT DR firing at doses previously shown to inhibit the unit activity of DA[29] and NE somata,[31] respectively. However, fluoxetine inhibited neuronal activity in a dose-related fashion. Although fluoxetine is a *more* potent inhibitor of 5-HT reuptake *in vitro*,[2] this compound exhibited one-third the potency of cocaine to suppress 5-HT DR activity.[26] The phenyltropane analog Win 35428, which shares the ability of cocaine to block monoamine uptake, also inhibited impulse flow in 5-HT neurons (FIG. 1). The catecholamine releaser and stimulant amphetamine inhibited 5-HT cell firing in most (87%) of the cells tested (FIG. 1). The complete suppression induced by amphetamine was observed at 4× the dose of cocaine which is the reverse potency order typically seen in behavioral studies.

To determine the relative role of specific monoamine receptors in mediating the systemic effects of cocaine, attempts were made to reverse the cocaine-induced suppression of 5-HT DR activity with neurotransmitter antagonists. The DA antagonist haloperidol, the γ-aminobutyric acid antagonist picrotoxin and the 5-HT$_2$ antagonist ketanserin were inactive in this regard. Methiothepin, which is an antagonist for both DA receptors and 5-HT terminal autoreceptors, did not alter the response to cocaine. On the other hand, spiperone which has been shown to block 5-HT$_{1A}$-mediated inhibitory responses of 5-HT DR neurons,[32] reversed cocaine-induced (1 mg/kg) suppression. Although spiperone is also a potent DA antagonist, the complete lack of effect of the DA antagonist haloperidol suggests that DA blockade by spiperone is not relevant to the observed cocaine antagonism. In rats depleted of 5-HT with the synthesis inhibitor *p*-chlorophenylalanine, the sensitivity to cocaine-induced depression was significantly reduced as compared to control which suggests that the effects of cocaine are dependent in part on endogenous 5-HT stores.

In summary, the comparative and pharmacological research reviewed here supports the hypothesis that autoregulatory feedback mechanisms recruited by the increased availability of 5-HT and subsequent stimulation of impulse-modulating 5-HT$_{1A}$ autoreceptors on 5-HT cell bodies probably accounts for this cocaine-induced inhibitory response.[26,27]

EFFECTS OF REPEATED COCAINE ADMINISTRATION ON 5-HT NEUROTRANSMISSION

Serotonin has been implicated in a number of psychiatric disorders (anxiety, depression, psychosis) experienced by chronic cocaine abusers.[33,34] Furthermore, the significant effects of cocaine on 5-HT systems illustrated by the electrophysiological findings (above) suggest the possibility that alterations in 5-HT function may account for the consequences of long-term cocaine abuse. Repeated exposure to cocaine (and other stimulants) can result in a progressive enhancement of behaviors including loco-motor activity, stereotypy and convulsions ("sensitization").[35,36] This phenomenon is paralleled in humans whereupon continued use or abuse of high doses of cocaine changes the nature of the stimulant experience and psychiatric disorders such as anxiety, panic attacks, depression and paranoid psychosis as well as toxic physiological reactions often occur.[33,34] In fact, cocaine sensitization has been proposed as an animal model for paranoid psychosis.[35] The focus of numerous studies has been to as-certain alterations in DA function after chronic treatment with cocaine, whether be-havioral sensitization was measured or not. In this light, a number of alterations in DA release,[37-39] the numbers and/or affinity of DA receptors[37,40,41] or electrophysio-logical sensitivity of DA pre-or post-synaptic receptors[42,43] has been measured. Behav-ioral studies suggest that dopamine antagonists may also block the development, but not the expression, of cocaine-induced behavioral sensitization.[35,36] However, there have been few attempts to investigate alterations in 5-HT function associated with co-caine sensitization, although an enhanced behavioral responsiveness to 5-HT agonists occurs in cocaine-[44] and amphetamine-sensitized rats.[45]

To characterize more fully whether alterations in 5-HT function are associated with cocaine sensitization, electrophysiologic and autoradiographic assays[46] were utilized to

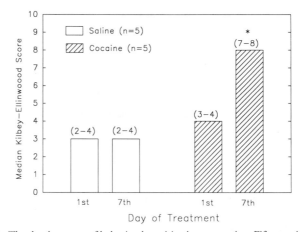

FIGURE 2. The development of behavioral sensitization to cocaine. Fifteen min after the first (Day 1) and last (Day 7) injection, the behaviors of rats treated with saline or cocaine were rated in their home cage using the Kilbey-Ellinwood scale.[47] The animals were assigned a score of 1–9 based upon the following behavioral characteristics: 1–asleep, lying down, eyes closed; 2–inactive, lying down, eyes open; 3–in-place activities, normal grooming, chewing cage litter, eating, or drinking; 4–normal, alert, active, moving about cage, sniffing, rearing; 5–hyperactive with rapid changes in position; 6–slow-patterned, repetitive exploration of the cage at normal levels of activity; 7–fast-patterned, repetitive exploration of the cage with hyperactivity; 8–restricted, remaining in same place in cage with fast, repetitive head and/or forelimb move-ment (includes licking, chewing, and gnawing stereotypies); and 9–dyskinetic-reactive with backing up, jumping, seizures and abnormally maintained postures. Data are represented as median scores. Stereotypy scores on Day 1 did not differ between treatment groups. Cocaine-treated rats exhibited stereotypy scores which differed significantly between Day 1 and Day 7 (* $p < 0.005$) which suggested that behavioral sensitization had developed. Numbers (above bars) represent the range of scores recorded for each treatment group on Day 1 and Day 7.

investigate the 5-HT system in rats exposed to a cocaine treatment regimen (15 mg/kg, b.i.d. for 7 days) which elicited behavioral sensitization as measured on a 9-point scale.[47,48] This enhanced behavioral response was characterized by hyperactivity as well as repetitive head and forelimb movements and indicated that sensitization had developed (FIG. 2).[47,48] Within 18 to 24 h following the final injection of cocaine or saline, rats were anesthetized with urethane (1.5 g/kg, i.p.) and prepared for single unit recordings of DR 5-HT neurons.[26,27] Although mean baseline firing rates of recorded 5-HT cells did not differ significantly between cocaine- and saline-treated rats, the ability of (−)-cocaine (FIG. 3) and fluoxetine (FIG. 4) to inhibit the activity of 5-HT DR neurons was significantly enhanced in rats that were behaviorally sensitized to cocaine.

Using autoradiographic techniques, the density of 5-HT uptake sites labeled by [³H]-imipramine and 5-HT_{1A} receptors labeled by [³H]-8-hydroxy-2-[di-N-propyl-amino]tetralin ([³H]-8-OHDPAT) was measured in cocaine-sensitized and control rats. In addition to the DR and MR which contain 5-HT somata, cortical and subcortical 5-HT terminal fields were also investigated.[46] These included several limbic nuclei, such as the amygdala, nucleus accumbens and medial prefrontal cortex, which have been implicated as important in the behavioral effects of cocaine.[5,35,38,49,50] Significant increases in the labeling of 5-HT uptake sites were observed in the DR (but not MR) nucleus and in several cortical areas (frontal cortex, medial and sulcal prefrontal cortex) of cocaine-treated rats (FIG. 5). On the other hand, with the exception of a decrease in the density of labeling in the central medial amygdala in cocaine-sensitized rats, no other changes in 5-HT_{1A} binding sites were observed (FIG. 6).

Behavioral sensitization to cocaine is, therefore, associated with an enhancement in the electrophysiologic sensitivity of 5-HT DR neurons to subsequent challenge with (−)-cocaine or the 5-HT uptake inhibitor fluoxetine; concomitantly, [³H]-imipramine

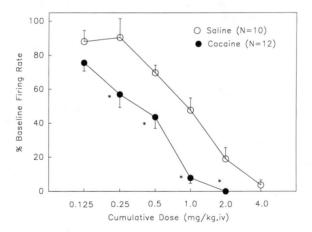

FIGURE 3. Dose-response curves for the inhibition of 5-HT DR neurons induced by (−)-cocaine challenge after repeated cocaine or saline exposure. Drugs were administered i.v. at 2 min intervals such that each dose doubled the previously administered dose (*abscissa*). Circles represent the mean (± SEM) percentage of baseline firing rate observed at each dose of (−)-cocaine (*ordinate*); closed and open circles denote the percent inhibition from baseline firing rate observed in response to i.v. (−)-cocaine challenge in animals exposed to either cocaine or saline treatment, respectively. Asterisks represent doses at which cocaine- and saline-treated rats differed ($p < 0.05$).

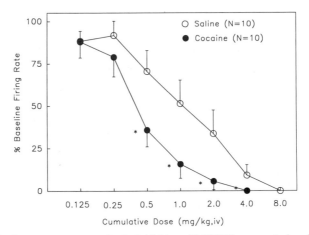

FIGURE 4. Dose-response curves for the inhibition of 5-HT DR neurons induced by fluoxetine challenge after repeated cocaine or saline exposure. Symbols as in FIGURE 3.

binding was selectively increased in the DR.[46] Under the assay conditions used here, [³H]-imipramine is known to label high affinity recognition sites functionally relevant to 5-HT uptake processes.[51,52] This increase in [³H]-imipramine binding suggests that chronic cocaine treatment resulted in a compensatory up-regulation of 5-HT transporter sites in somal DR as well as specific terminal regions. Thus, the enhancement in the electrophysiologic sensitivity of 5-HT systems in cocaine-sensitized rats may be attributed to a functionally relevant increase in the number or affinity of 5-HT uptake sites in the DR. These changes in 5-HT uptake sites occur in the absence of overt cocaine-induced neurotoxicity of 5-HT systems, as measured *ex vivo* by immunohisto-chemical[48] or neurochemical assays.[53,54]

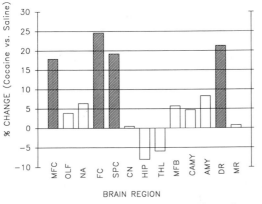

FIGURE 5. Effects of repeated cocaine exposure on 5-HT transporters labeled by [³H]-imipramine using quantitative autoradiography. Values are the differences in 5-HT transporter binding obtained between the treatment groups. Shaded bars represent significant changes in receptor densities (ANOVA, Tukey's, $p < 0.05$). Cocaine-sensitized rats ($n = 6$) exhibited significant increases in [³H]-imipramine binding in the MFC, FC, SPC and DR when compared to saline-treated rats ($n = 6$).

Abbreviations: MPC, medial prefrontal cortex; OLF, olfactory tubercle; NA, nucleus accumbens; FC, frontal cortex; SPC, sulcal prefrontal cortex; CN, caudate nucleus; GP, globus pallidus; HYP, hypothalamus; HIP, hippocampus; THL, thalamus; MFB, medial forebrain bundle; CAMY, central medial amygdala; AMY, amygdala; DR, dorsal raphe nucleus; MR, median raphe nucleus; SN, substantia nigra; VTA, ventral tegmental nucleus.

FIGURE 6. Effects of repeated cocaine exposure on 5-HT$_{1A}$ transporters labeled by [^{3}H]-8-OHDPAT using quantitative autoradiography. Values are the differences in 5-HT$_{1A}$ receptors obtained between the treatment groups. Shaded bars represent significant changes in receptor densities (ANOVA, Tukey's, $p < 0.05$). Cocaine-sensitized rats ($n = 6$) exhibited a significant decrease in [^{3}H]-8-OHDPAT binding only in the CAMY when compared to saline-treated rats ($n = 6$). Abbreviations as in FIGURE 5.

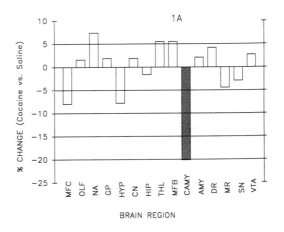

The alterations in DR sensitivity and somal uptake sites seen with cocaine exposure tend to be opposite to those observed after repeated exposure to much more selective 5-HT reuptake inhibitors.[52,55-59] Thus, while long-term treatment with 5-HT uptake inhibitors has been hypothesized to result in a net *increase* in 5-HT neurotransmission, in part by decreasing 5-HT autoreceptor sensitivity,[55,56,58] a net *decrease* in 5-HT neurotransmission may have developed in cocaine-sensitized rats as a consequence of enhanced 5-HT autoregulatory mechanisms.[46] Serotonin neurotransmission is largely inhibitory and effectively regulated by somal automodulatory processes *in vivo*.[60-64] Serotonin neurons of raphe nuclei innervate midbrain DA neurons and their limbic targets,[65,66] which have been implicated in the behavioral effects of cocaine.[5,35,38,49,50] Thus, enhancement of 5-HT autoregulation after repeated cocaine exposure might be expected to result in decreased inhibitory 5-HT tone in terminal areas such as meso-corticolimbic DA regions. This hypothesis is supported by the recent finding that the inhibitory response of nucleus accumbens neurons to microiontophoretic 5-HT is enhanced in cocaine-treated rats.[43] Since repeated cocaine treatment is also associated with supersensitive DA responses in the nucleus accumbens,[42,43] the normal balance of DA and 5-HT neurotransmission in this mesolimbic region appears to be disrupted and this imbalance could contribute to the development of cocaine sensitization.

The prefrontal cortex which is believed to be critically involved in the behavioral response to stressors (including cocaine),[67,68] the initiation of cocaine self-administration,[50] and cocaine-conditioned place preferences[69] also exhibited an increase in 5-HT uptake recognition sites. The action of cocaine on prefrontal cortical 5-HT systems could contribute, therefore, to both the anxiety and panic attacks experienced by cocaine users[70,71] as well as the potent reinforcing properties of the drug. In fact, the apparent reinforcing efficacy of cocaine was increased after 5,7-dihydroxytryptamine lesions,[72] while the 5-HT uptake inhibitor fluoxetine[73] and the 5-HT precursor *l*-tryptophan reduced the rate of cocaine self-administration.[74]

CONCLUSIONS

Acute cocaine administration results in a profound suppression of the activity of 5-HT neurons which appears to be related to its ability to inhibit the reuptake of 5-HT and subsequently activate 5-HT$_{1A}$ impulse-regulating autoreceptors.[26,27] The development of behavioral sensitization to cocaine is also associated with the development of supersensitivity of these 5-HT autoregulatory mechanisms as well as selective increases in 5-HT transporters (DR and cortical regions).[46] These findings raise the possibility that some of the psychological consequences of chronic cocaine abuse may be attributable to modifications in 5-HT function. Thus, medications which counteract cocaine-induced alterations of 5-HT systems may prove useful as pharmacotherapies in the treatment of the myriad of physiological and psychological problems exhibited by cocaine abusers. Such clinical studies are currently underway, and, with a further understanding of the interaction of cocaine with 5-HT systems, the rationale for 5-HT pharmacotherapy of cocaine abusers can be more fully developed.

ACKNOWLEDGMENTS

We extend our thanks to Ms. Marcia McNulty and Ms. Ann Guidroz for their expert technical assistance. (−)-Cocaine and fluoxetine were graciously supplied by NIDA and Eli Lilly and Co, respectively.

REFERENCES

1. RITZ, M. C., E. J. CONE & M. J. KUHAR. 1990. Cocaine inhibition of ligand binding at dopamine, norepinephrine and serotonin transporters: A structure-activity study. Life Sci. **46:** 635–645.
2. KOE, B. K. 1976. Molecular geometry of inhibitors of the uptake of catecholamines and serotonin in synaptosomal preparations of rat brain. J. Pharmacol. Exp. Ther. **199:** 649–661.
3. KILPATRICK, G. J., B. J. JONES & M. B. TYERS. 1989. Binding of the 5-HT₃ ligand GR65630, to rat area postrema vagus nerve and the brain of several species. Eur. J. Pharmacol. **159:** 157–164.
4. SCHEEL-KRUGER, J., C. BRAESTRUP, M. NIELSON, K. GOLEMBIOWSKA & E. MOGILNICKA. 1976. Cocaine: Discussion on the role of dopamine in the biochemical mechanism of action. *In* Cocaine and Other Stimulants. E. H. Ellinwood & M. M. Kilbey, Eds.: 373–407. Plenum Press. New York.
5. ROBERTS, D. C. S., M. E. CORCORAN & H. C. FIBIGER. 1977. On the role of ascending catecholamine systems in intravenous self-administration of cocaine. Pharmacol. Biochem. Behav. **6:** 615–620.
6. DE WIT, H. & R. A. WISE. 1977. Blockade of cocaine reinforcement in rats with the dopamine receptor blocker pimozide, but not with the noradrenergic blockers phentolamine or phenoxybenzamine. Can. J. Psychol. **31:** 195–203.
7. CALLAHAN, P. M., J. B. APPEL & K. A. CUNNINGHAM. 1991. Dopamine D₁ and D₂ mediation of the discriminative stimulus properties of *d*-amphetamine and cocaine. Psychopharmacology **103:** 50–55.
8. COLPAERT, F. C., C. J. E. NIEMEGEERS & P. A. J. JANSSEN. 1979. Discriminative stimulus properties of cocaine: Neuropharmacological characteristics as derived from stimulus generalization experiments. Pharmacol. Biochem. Behav. **10:** 535–546.
9. CUNNINGHAM, K. A. & J. B. APPEL. 1982. Discriminative stimulus properties of cocaine and phencyclidine: Similarities in mechanism of action. *In* Drug Discrimination: Applications in CNS Pharmacology. F. C. Colpaert & J. L. Slangen, Eds.: 181–192. Elsevier/North Holland Biomedical Press. Amsterdam.
10. CUNNINGHAM, K. A. & P. M. CALLAHAN. 1991. Monoamine reuptake inhibitors potentiate the discriminative state induced by cocaine in the rat. Psychopharmacology **104:** 177–180.

11. GALE, K. 1984. Catecholamine-independent behavioral and neurochemical effects of cocaine in rats. *In* Mechanisms of Tolerance and Dependence, NIDA Monograph 54. C. W. Sharp, Ed.: 323–332. U. S. Government Printing Office, Washington, D.C.

12. SPYRAKI, C., H. C. FIBIGER & A. G. PHILLIPS. 1982. Cocaine-induced place preference conditioning: Lack of effects of neuroleptics and 6-hydroxydopamine lesions. Brain Res. 253: 195–203.

13. KNAPP, S. & A. J. MANDELL. 1972. Narcotic drugs: Effects on the serotonin biosynthetic systems of the brain. Science 177: 1209–1211.

13. GALLOWAY, M. P. 1990. Regulation of dopamine and serotonin synthesis by acute administration of cocaine. Synapse 6: 63–72.

15. REITH, M. E. A., H. SERSHEN, D. L. ALLEN & A. LAJTHA. 1983. A portion of ³H-cocaine binding in brain is associated with serotonergic neurons. Mol. Pharmacol. 23: 600–606.

16. FOZARD, J. R., A. T. M. MOBAROK ALI & G. NEWGROSH. 1979. Blockade of serotonin receptors on autonomic neurones by (−)-cocaine and some related compounds. Eur. J. Pharmacol. 59: 195–210.

17. COSTALL, B., A. M. DOMENEY, R. J. NAYLOR & M. B. TYERS. 1987. Effects of the 5-HT₃ receptor antagonist, GR38032F, on raised dopaminergic activity in the mesolimbic system of the rat and marmoset brain. Br. J. Pharmacol. 92: 881–894.

18. PARIS, J. M. & K. A. CUNNINGHAM. 1991. Serotonin 5-HT₃ antagonists do not alter the discriminative stimulus properties of cocaine. Psychopharmacology 104: 475–478.

19. PELTIER, R. & S. SCHENK. 1991. GR38032F, a serotonin 5-HT₃ antagonist, fails to alter cocaine self-administration in rats. Pharmacol. Biochem. Behav. 39: 133–136.

20. VAN DER HOEK, G. A. & S. J. COOPER. 1990. Evidence that ondansetron, a selective 5-HT₃ antagonist, reduces cocaine's psychomotor stimulant effects in the rat. Psychopharmacology 101: S59.

21. PRADHAN, S. N., A. K. BATTACHARYYA & S. PRADHAN. 1978. Serotonergic manipulation of the behavioral effects of cocaine in rats. Commun. Psychopharmacol. 2: 481–486.

22. STEINBUSCH, H. W. M. 1984. 3: Serotonin-immunoreactive neurons and their projections in the CNS. *In* Handbook of Chemical Neuroanatomy: Classical Transmitters and Transmitter Receptors in the CNS. A. Björklund, T. Hökfelt & M. J. Kuhar, Eds.: 68–125. Elsevier Science Publishers. Amsterdam.

23. GOBBI, M., L. CERVO, C. TADDEI & T. MENNINI. 1990. Autoradiographic localization of [³H]paroxetine specific binding in the rat brain. Neurochem. Int. 16: 247–251.

24. RADJA, F., A.-M. LAPORTE, G. DAVAL, D. VERGE, H. GOZLAN, M. HAMON, J. M. PALACIOS. C. WAEBER, G. MENGOD & D. HOYER. 1991. Autoradiography of serotonin receptor subtypes in the central nervous system. Neurochem. Int. 18: 1–15.

25. SPROUSE, J. S. & G. K. AGHAJANIAN. 1987. Electrophysiological responses of serotoninergic dorsal raphe neurons to 5-HT₁A and 5-HT₁B agonists. Synapse 1: 3–9.

26. CUNNINGHAM, K. A. & J. M. LAKOSKI. 1988. Electrophysiological effects of cocaine and procaine on dorsal raphe serotonin neurons. Eur. J. Pharmacol. 148: 457–462.

27. CUNNINGHAM, K. A. & J. M. LAKOSKI. 1990. The interaction of cocaine with serotonin dorsal raphe neurons: Single unit extracellular recording studies. Neuropsychopharmacology 3: 41–50.

28. PITTS, D. K. & J. MARWAH. 1987. Cocaine modulation of central monoaminergic neurotransmission. Pharmacol. Biochem. Behav. 26: 453–461.

29. EINHORN, L. C., P. A. JOHANSEN & F. J. WHITE. 1988. Electrophysiological effects of cocaine in the mesoaccumbens dopamine system: Studies in the ventral tegmental area. J. Neurosci. 8: 100–112.

30. PITTS, D. K. & J. MARWAH. 1987. Electrophysiological actions of cocaine on noradrenergic neurons in rat locus coeruleus. J. Pharmacol. Exp. Ther. 240: 345–351.

31. NYBACK, H. V., J. R. WALTERS, G. K. AGHAJANIAN & R. H. ROTH. 1975. Tricyclic antidepressants: Effects on the firing rate of noradrenergic neurons. Eur. J. Pharmacol. 32: 302–312.

32. LUM, J. R. & M. F. PIERCEY. 1988. Electrophysiological evidence that spiperone is an antagonist of 5-HT₁A receptors in the dorsal raphe nucleus. Eur. J. Pharmacol. 149: 9–15.

33. LOWENSTEIN, D. H., S. M. MASSA, M. C. ROWBOTHAM, S. D. COLLINS, H. E.

McKinney & R. P. Simon. 1987. Acute neurologic and psychiatric complications associated with cocaine abuse. Am. J. Med. **83:** 841–846.

34. Post, R. M. 1975. Cocaine psychoses: A continuum model. Am. J. Psychiatry **132:** 225–230.

35. Post, R. M., S. R. B. Weiss, A. Pert & T. W. Uhde. 1987. Chronic cocaine administration: Sensitization and kindling effects. *In* Cocaine: Clinical and Biobehavioral Aspects. S. Fisher, A. Raskin & E. H. Uhlenhuth, Eds.: 109–173. Oxford University Press. New York.

36. Robinson, T. E. & J. B. Becker. 1986. Enduring changes in brain and behavior produced by chronic amphetamine administration: A review and evaluation of animal models of amphetamine psychosis. Brain Res. Rev. **11:** 157–198.

37. Peris, J., S. J. Boyson, W. A. Cass, P. Curella, L. P. Dwoskin, G. Larson, L.-H. Lin, R. P. Yasuda & N. R. Zahniser. 1990. Persistence of neurochemical changes in dopamine systems after repeated cocaine administration. J. Pharmacol. Exp. Ther. **253:** 38–44.

38. Pettit, H. O., H.-T. Pan, L. H. Parsons & J. B. Justice, Jr. 1990. Extracellular concentrations of cocaine and dopamine are enhanced during chronic cocaine administration. J. Neurochem. **55:** 798–804.

39. Yi, S. J. & K. M. Johnson. 1990. Effects of acute and chronic administration of cocaine on striatal uptake, compartmentalization and release [3H]dopamine. Neuropharmacology **29:** 475–486.

40. Goeders, N. E. & M. J. Kuhar. 1987. Chronic cocaine administration induces opposite changes in dopamine receptors in the striatum and nucleus accumbens. Alc. Drug Res. **7:** 207–216.

41. Kleven, M. S., B. D. Perry, W. L. Woolverton & L. S. Seiden. 1990. Effects of repeated injections of cocaine on D1 and D2 dopamine receptors in rat brain. Brain Res. **532:** 265–270.

42. Henry, D. J., M. A. Greene & F. J. White. 1989. Electrophysiological effects of cocaine in the mesoaccumbens dopamine system: Repeated administration. J. Pharmacol. Exp. Ther. **251:** 833–839.

43. Henry, D. J. & F. J. White. 1989. Effects of repeated cocaine administration on the sensitivity of D1 and D2 receptors in the nucleus accumbens. Soc. Neurosci. Abst. **15:** 1013.

44. Cunningham, K. A. 1988. Cocaine: Behavioral sensitization and the serotonin syndrome. Soc. Neurosci. Abst. **14:** 659.

45. Karler, R., L. D. Calder & S. A. Turkanis. 1990. Reverse tolerance to amphetamine evokes reverse tolerance to 5-hydroxytryptophan. Life Sci. **46:** 1773–1780.

46. Cunningham, K. A., J. M. Paris & N. E. Goeders. Chronic cocaine enhances serotonin autoregulation and serotonin uptake binding. Synapse. In press.

47. Kilbey, M. M. & E. H. Ellinwood. 1976. Chronic administration of stimulant drugs: Response modification. *In* Cocaine and Other Stimulants. E. H. Ellinwood & M. M. Kilbey, Eds.: 409–429. Plenum Press. New York.

48. Paris, J. M., P. M. Callahan, J. M. Lee & K. A. Cunningham. 1991. Behavioral sensitization to cocaine is not associated with changes in serotonin (5-HT) immunoreactivity in rat forebrain. Brain Res. Bull. **27:** 843–847.

49. Delfs, J. M., L. Schreiber & A. E. Kelley. 1990. Microinjection of cocaine into the nucleus accumbens elicits locomotor activation in the rat. J. Neurosci. **10:** 303–310.

50. Goeders, N. E. & J. E. Smith. 1983. cortical dopaminergic involvement in cocaine reinforcement. Science **221:** 773–775.

51. Conway, P. G. & D. J. Brunswick. 1985. High- and low-affinity binding components for [3H]imipramine in rat cerebral cortex. J. Neurochem. **45:** 206–209.

52. Hrdina, P. D. 1987. Regulation of high- and low-affinity [3H]imipramine recognition sites in rat brain by chronic treatment with antidepressants. Eur. J. Pharmacol. **138:** 159–168.

53. Kleven, M. S., W. L. Woolverton & L. S. Seiden. 1988. Lack of long-term monoamine depletions following repeated or continuous exposure to cocaine. Brain Res. Bull. **21:** 233–237.

54. Yeh, S. Y. & E. B. De Souza. 1991. Lack of neurochemical evidence for neurotoxic effects of repeated cocaine administration in rats on brain monoamine neurons. Drug Alcohol Depend. **27:** 51–61.

55. BLIER, P., C. DE MONTIGNY & D. TARDIF. 1984. Effects of the two antidepressant drugs mianserin and indalpine on the serotonergic system: Single-cell studies in the rat. Psychopharmacology **84:** 242–249.
56. BLIER, P., Y. CHAPUT & C. DE MONTIGNY. 1988. Long-term 5-HT reuptake blockade, but not monoamine oxidase inhibition, decreases the function of terminal 5-HT autoreceptors: An electrophysiological study in the rat brain. Naunyn-Schmiedeberg's Arch. Pharmacol. **337:** 246–254.
57. BRUNELLO, N., M. RIVA, A. VOLTERRA & G. RACAGNI. 1987. Effect of some tricyclic and nontricyclic antidepressants on [³H]imipramine binding and serotonin uptake in rat cerebral cortex after prolonged treatment. Fundam. & Clin. Pharmacol. **1:** 327–333.
58. CHAPUT, Y., C. DE MONTIGNY & P. BLIER. 1986. Effects of a selective 5-HT reuptake blocker, citalopram, on the sensitivity of 5-HT autoreceptors: Electrophysiological studies in the rat brain. Naunyn-Schmiedeberg's Arch. Pharmacol. **333:** 342–348.
59. MONTERO, D., M. L. DE CEBALLOS & J. DEL-RIO. 1990. Down-regulation of [³H]imipramine binding sites in rat cerebral cortex after prenatal exposure to antidepressants. Life Sci. **46:** 1619–1626.
60. HILLEGAART, V., S. HJORTH & S. AHLENIUS. 1990. Effects of 5-HT and 8-OHDPAT on forebrain monoamine synthesis after local application into the median and dorsal raphe nuclei of the rat. J. Neural Transm. **81:** 131–145.
61. MANTZ, J., R. GODBOUT, J.-P. TASSIN, J. GLOWINSKI & A.-M. THIERRY. 1990. Inhibition of spontaneous and evoked unit activity in the rat medial prefrontal cortex by mesencephalic raphe nuclei. Brain Res. **524:** 22–30.
62. SHARP, T., S. R. BRAMWELL, D. CLARK & D. G. GRAHAME-SMITH. 1989. In vivo measurement of extracellular 5-hydroxytryptamine in hippocampus of the anaesthetized rat using microdialysis: Changes in relation to 5-hydroxytryptaminergic neuronal activity. J. Neurochem. **53:** 234–240.
63. WANG, R. Y. & G. K. AGHAJANIAN. 1977. Inhibition of the neurons of the amygdala by dorsal raphe stimulation: Mediation through direct serotonergic pathway. Brain Res. **120:** 85–102.
64. WHITE, F. J. 1986. Comparative effects of LSD and lisuride: Clues to specific hallucinogenic drug actions. Pharmacol. Biochem. Behav. **24:** 365–379.
65. FIBIGER, H. C. & J. J. MILLER. 1977. An anatomical and electrophysiological investigation of the serotonergic projection from the dorsal raphe nucleus to the substantia nigra in the rat. Neuroscience **2:** 975–987.
66. MOORE, R. Y., A. E. HALARIS & B. E. JONES. 1978. Serotonin neurons of the midbrain raphe: Ascending projections. J. Comp. Neurol. **180:** 417–438.
67. KALIVAS, P. W. & P. DUFFY. 1988. Effects of daily cocaine and morphine treatment on somatodendritic and terminal field dopamine release. J. Neurochem. **50:** 1498–1504.
68. THIERRY, A. M., J. P. TASSIN, G. BLANC & J. GLOWINSKI. 1976. Selective activation of the mesocortical dopaminergic system by stress. Nature **263:** 242–244.
69. ISAAC, W. L., A. J. NONNEMAN, J. NEISEWANDER, T. LANDERS & M. T. BARDO. 1989. Prefrontal cortical lesions differentially disrupt cocaine-reinforced conditioned place preference but not conditioned taste aversion. Behav. Neurosci. **103:** 345–355.
70. ANTHONY, J. C., A. Y. TIEN & K. R. PETRONIS. 1989. Epidemiologic evidence on cocaine use and panic attacks. Am. J. Epidemiology **129:** 543–549.
71. ARONSON, T. A. & T. J. CRAIG. 1986. Cocaine precipitation of panic disorder. Am. J. Psychiatry **143:** 643–645.
72. LOH, E. A. & D. C. S. ROBERTS. 1990. Break points on a progressive ratio schedule reinforced by intravenous cocaine increase following depletion of forebrain serotonin. Psychopharmacology **101:** 262–266.
73. CARROLL, M. E., S. T. LAC, M. ASENCIO & R. KRAGH. 1990. Fluoxetine reduces intravenous cocaine self-administration in rats. Pharmacol. Biochem. Behav. **35:** 237–244.
74. CARROLL, M. E., S. T. LAC, M. ASENCIO & R. KRAGH. 1990. Intravenous cocaine self-administration in rats is reduced by dietary L-tryptophan. Psychopharmacology **100:** 293–300.

Cellular Mechanisms of Behavioral Sensitization to Drugs of Abuse[a]

PETER W. KALIVAS, CARYN D. STRIPLIN,
JEFFERY D. STEKETEE, MARK A. KLITENICK,
AND PATRICIA DUFFY

Alcoholism and Drug Abuse Program
Washington State University
Pullman, Washington 99164-6530

INTRODUCTION

When administered repeatedly the motor stimulant effect of amphetamine-like psychostimulants augments (see refs. 1 and 2 for reviews). A similar sensitization of motor activity occurs following repeated opioid administration in rodents, and for both classes of motor stimulants the behavioral sensitization is long-lasting or permanent (see refs. 1 and 2 for reviews). Because acute motor stimulation produced by both opioids and amphetamine-like psychostimulants is, at least in part, the result of enhanced dopamine transmission in the nucleus accumbens and striatum, the possibility that the sensitized motor behavior after repeated administration may result from augmented dopamine transmission has been evaluated. Using *in vivo* microdialysis, many laboratories have demonstrated that behavioral sensitization to repeated administration of amphetamine,[3] methamphetamine,[4] methylphenidate, cocaine,[5-7] and morphine[2] is associated with enhanced extracellular dopamine levels in the nucleus accumbens and/or striatum (however, see refs. 8 and 9). These findings complement many studies showing that the amphetamine or depolarization-induced release of dopamine from striatal tissue slices or synaptosomes is enhanced in rats pretreated with repeated amphetamine (see ref. 1 for review).

While the majority of reports support a role for augmented axonal dopamine release in drug-induced behavioral sensitization, for alterations in the axon terminals to be long lasting a change in protein synthesis is likely. Correspondingly, Robinson[10] recently demonstrated that pretreatment with the protein synthesis inhibitor, anisomycin, prevented the development of behavioral sensitization to amphetamine. The most likely site of a change in protein synthesis which would affect axonal dopamine release is the dopamine neurons in the ventromedial mesencephalon (VM). Many recent studies support an hypothesis that behavioral sensitization to amphetamine-like psychostimulants and opioids results from an action of these drugs in the ventromedial mesencephalon (see ref. 2 for review). Directly testing this hypothesis, amphetamine or μ opioids were microinjected into the VM or dopamine axon terminal fields, in-

[a] The research reported was supported in part by U.S.P.H.S. grants MH-40817, DA-03906, a Research Career Development Award DA-00158 (PWK), and National Research Service Award DA-05391 (MAK), DA-05498 (CDS).

128

cluding the nucleus accumbens and striatum.[11-16] These studies revealed that the repeated administration of these drugs into the VM, but not into the axon terminal fields results in an augmented motor response to a subsequent drug challenge. Furthermore, it has been shown in the case of μ opioids that the augmented motor response to daily injection into the VM was associated with an enhanced increase in extracellular dopamine in the nucleus accumbens.[17]

While the VM has been identified as a site of action in the brain where amphetamine-like psychostimulants and opioids act to initiate behavioral sensitization, the sequelae of cellular and molecular events underlying the enduring behavioral change remains to be elucidated. Recently, Stewart and coworkers demonstrated that pretreatment of the VM with the D_1 receptor antagonist, SCH-23390, prevents the development of behavioral sensitization to repeated systemic amphetamine or morphine administration.[2,18] Furthermore, Ujike *et al.*[19] found that repeated administration with methamphetamine produced an upregulation in D_1 binding density in the lateral substantia nigra. These findings pose the possibility that stimulation of D_1 receptors in the VM by somatodendritically released dopamine is critical in the initiation of behavioral sensitization. This further presupposes that an increase in somatodendritic dopamine release may be produced in rats pretreated with daily amphetamine or morphine. Below are outlined recent data indicating that an elevation in somatodendritically released dopamine does occur in the VM of rats behaviorally sensitized to cocaine, and that this may result from an uncoupling of D_2 autoreceptors. Furthermore, an effort is made to integrate this sequence of events with the long-term changes produced in dopamine terminal field release in behaviorally sensitized rats.

CHANGES IN SOMATODENDRITICALLY RELEASED DOPAMINE

FIGURE 1 shows that rats pretreated with daily cocaine (15 mg/kg, i.p. × 1 day followed by 30 mg/kg, i.p. × 5 days) demonstrate an increase in extracellular dopamine in the VM if challenged 24 h later with cocaine (15 mg/kg, i.p.). However, if the rats were challenged two wks after the last daily injection of cocaine, the augmentation in somatodendritic extracellular dopamine was absent even though behavioral sensitization remained intact. In contrast, this cocaine pretreatment regimen produced opposite effects on extracellular dopamine content in the nucleus accumbens. FIGURE 1 shows that at 24 h after the last daily cocaine injection there was not a significant elevation in extracellular dopamine. In contrast, after 11 to 15 days of withdrawal the cocaine-induced increase in extracellular dopamine was augmented. In all treatment groups behavioral sensitization was observed (data not shown).

Since somatodendritic dopamine release is under regulatory control by D_2 dopamine autoreceptors[20,21] one mechanism whereby dopamine release in the VM may be augmented in cocaine-sensitized rats is via a decrease in D_2 receptor autoinhibition. It is well established that daily treatment with amphetamine or cocaine results in a desensitization of the capacity of the D_2 receptor to inhibit dopamine impulse generation.[22-26] Furthermore, similar to the effect of withdrawal time on augmented somatodendritic dopamine release, the desensitization of D_2 receptors persists for less than eight days following the last daily injection of cocaine.[27] While these data support the hypothesis that desensitization of the D_2 receptor may mediate the augmentation in somatodendritic dopamine release, there is no evidence for a downregulation in D_2 receptor density in the VM of rats treated with daily cocaine.[28] Hyperpolariza-

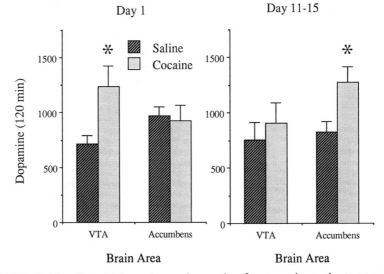

FIGURE 1. The effect of daily cocaine on the capacity of acute cocaine to elevate extracellular dopamine in the VM and nucleus accumbens. Two groups of rats were used, one receiving daily cocaine injections (15 mg/kg, i.p. × 1 day followed by 30 mg/kg, i.p. × 5 days) and one group receiving daily saline (1 ml/kg, i.p. × 6 days). One day later, the rats were examined in a dialysis/photocell chamber for their behavioral response and levels of extracellular dopamine in the VM or nucleus accumbens after an acute injection of cocaine (15 mg/kg, i.p.). Another group of rats were allowed 11 to 15 day withdrawal from daily cocaine or saline prior to an acute injection of cocaine in the photocell/dialysis chamber. (See Kalivas and Duffy[17] for methodological details of the dialysis study.) The dopamine levels were determined from the area under the curve for 120 min after cocaine injection following normalization of the data to percent change from the baseline measurements obtained prior to injecting cocaine. * $p < 0.05$, comparing daily cocaine to daily saline treatment using a two-tailed Student's t-test.

tion by stimulation of D_2 receptors results from a pertussis toxin–sensitive G protein–coupled increase in potassium conductance.[29,30] Since the receptors are not altered, it is possible that an uncoupling of the receptor from the potassium channel may mediate desensitization of the D_2 receptor.

CHANGES IN G PROTEINS

Recently, Nestler et al.[31] demonstrated that daily cocaine pretreatment produced a decrease in the *in vitro* pertussis-toxin catalyzed ADP-ribosylation of G proteins and a decrease in the immunoprecipitation of G_i and G_o in the VM at one h after the last daily injection of cocaine. Interestingly, the decrease was observed only in the ventral tegmental area and not the substantia nigra, indicating that the medial dopamine cells in the VM are more affected. FIGURE 2 shows that the *in vitro* pertussis toxin-catalyzed ADP-ribosylation of G proteins in the VM was decreased at one h after the last daily treatment of cocaine (15 mg/kg, i.p. × 5 days). In contrast, when rats were challenged with cocaine two wks after discontinuing the daily treatments, there was no decrease

FIGURE 2. The effect of daily co-caine on the level of *in vitro* pertussis toxin–catalyzed ADP-ribosylation of G proteins or the content of G_i in the ventral tegmental area. The rats were treated with either saline (1 ml/kg, i.p. × 5 days) or cocaine (30 mg/kg, i.p. × 5 days) and killed 1 h or two wks after the last injection. (See Steketee et al.[33] for methodological details of pertussis toxin–catalyzed ADP-ribosylation.) Western blots were used to quantify G_i content using a modification of the methods described by Nestler et al.[31] The data from one h were obtained using pertussis toxin-catalyzed ADP-ribosylation of G_i/G_o, and the data from two wks were obtained with Western blot analysis. The data are shown as the mean ± SEM change from the saline-treated group. * $p < 0.05$, comparing daily cocaine to daily saline using a one-way ANOVA followed by a Dunnett's test for multiple comparisons to saline.

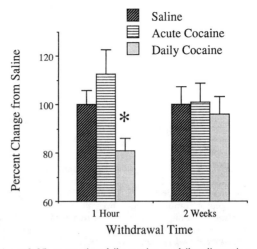

in the immunoprecipitation of G_i in the VM compared to daily saline-treated animals (FIG. 2). Likewise, no alteration in the content of G_s, G_o or G_B was measured (data not shown). Thus, similar to the augmentation in somatodendritic dopamine release and the desensitization of the D_2 receptor, the capacity of cocaine to reduce G_i and G_o in the VM persists for less than two wks after discontinuing the daily drug treatments.

Steketee and coworkers[32,33] recently evaluated a potential role for G proteins in sensitization to cocaine by pretreating the VM with pertussis toxin. Two weeks later the rats were administered an acute systemic injection of cocaine. Pertussis toxin–pretreated rats demonstrated an augmentation in cocaine-induced motor activity and extracellular dopamine content in the nucleus accumbens. These data indicate that reducing pertussis toxin–sensitive G proteins, G_i and G_o, in the VM produces sensitization to acute cocaine that is behaviorally and neurochemically similar to that resulting from repeated cocaine injections.

DISCUSSION

FIGURE 3 shows a model whereby rats receiving daily cocaine treatments demonstrate augmented release of somatodendritic dopamine in the VM, and thereby, hyperstimulation of D_1 receptors. It is proposed that the increase in somatodendritic dopamine release results from a reduction in G_i and/or G_o content, which causes a decrease in the coupling of D_2 autoreceptors to ATP-sensitive potassium channels.[31] The D_1 receptors are shown on nondopaminergic neurons and terminals since dopamine depletions do not reduce D_1 receptor density in the VM, but transection of the striato-nigral pathway produces a marked reduction.[34,35]

While the data outlined above adequately describe how hyperstimulation of the D_1 receptor might occur to initiate behavioral sensitization after repeated drug treatment, they do not address how enhanced stimulation of D_1 receptors in the VM

Control   Sensitized

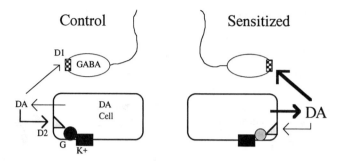

FIGURE 3. A model of the VM dopamine cell illustrating how repeated drug administration may uncouple the D_2 receptor via a reduction in G_i/G_o (G), thereby increasing somatodendritic dopamine release and hyperstimulating D_1 receptors. By decreasing the concentration of G_i/G_o, D_2 receptor stimulation less effectively increases K+ conductance. The decrease in membrane hyperpolarization results in augmented somatodendritic dopamine release which produces a hyperstimulation of D_1 receptors located presynaptically on GABAergic terminals. It is postulated that altered D_1 regulation of GABA release in the VM is critical in the initiation of behavioral sensitization.

leads to long-lasting changes in dopamine function. Considering that D_1 receptors are not located on dopamine neurons it is possible that the permanent alteration corresponding to enduring behavioral sensitization may reside in the afferent regulation of dopamine perikarya, and not in the dopamine cells themselves. A likely candidate for the location of D_1 receptors is on GABAergic afferents to the dopamine cells. Along these lines, Waszczak[36] found that the firing frequency of nondopaminergic, presumably GABAergic, neurons in the substantia nigra, pars reticulata was elevated by stimulation of D_1 receptors.

To evaluate a role for GABAergic neurons in the VM in sensitization to cocaine, mRNA content of the GABA synthetic enzyme, glutamic acid decarboxylase (GAD), was measured using *in situ* hybridization (see ref. 37 for methods used). The distribution of GAD mRNA expressing cells in the VM was evaluated 24 h after discontinuing daily cocaine (15 mg/kg, i.p. × 5 days). FIGURE 4 shows that the number of cells

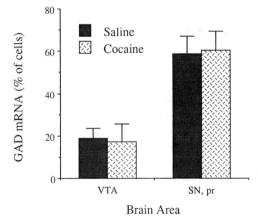

FIGURE 4. Effect of daily cocaine treatment (15 mg/kg, i.p. × 5 days) on GAD mRNA in the VM. Data are shown as mean ± SEM neurons containing GAD mRNA in the ventral tegmental area (VTA) and substantia nigra, pars reticulata (SN,pr), $n = 3$ for daily saline, $n = 3$ for daily cocaine. Hybridization was performed as described by Churchill *et al.*,[32] and integrated cell density, calibrated to grain counts/unit area, was used to estimate the density of hybridized mRNA. A cell was considered to contain GAD mRNA if the density was 5× background.

expressing GAD mRNA was unaltered in cocaine- versus saline-treated animals. Likewise, the mean density of GAD mRNA/cell was not altered in the VM or substantia nigra, pars reticulata of daily cocaine-pretreated rats (data not shown). Although GAD mRNA in the VM was not altered, other modifications of GABA transmission in the VM may be produced in behaviorally sensitized rats. For example, morphine-induced behavioral sensitization results from an action in the VM,[14] and it was recently shown that acute morphine markedly reduces basal extracellular GABA content in the VM.[38] Furthermore, many of the D_1 receptors are on terminals originating in the striatum and pallidum. Therefore, alterations in GAD mRNA capable of influencing GABA transmission in the VM need to be evaluated in the striatal/pallidal cell bodies.

CONCLUSIONS

It is postulated that sensitization is initiated in the VM by an augmentation in somatodendritic dopamine release following cocaine administration. This may result from an uncoupling of D_2 autoreceptor-induced hyperpolarization via a reduction in G protein content. The augmented somatodendritic dopamine release then hyperstimulates D_1 receptors which has been shown critical in the initiation of behavioral sensitization.[18] How these short term changes in the VM lead to the enduring alterations observed on dopamine transmission in the nucleus accumbens is uncertain. However, Beinter-Johnson *et al.*[39] observed that neurofilament content in the VM is altered by repeated cocaine administration. Since neurofilaments are involved in axonal transport, this may indicate a modification of protein transport to the dopamine terminals in the nucleus accumbens. This is suggested by the observation that while tyrosine hydroxylase phosphorylation is elevated in the VM after repeated cocaine, it is reduced in the nucleus accumbens.[40]

ACKNOWLEDGMENTS

We would like to thank Jenny Baylon for her assistance in preparing this manuscript.

REFERENCES

1. ROBINSON, T. E. & J. B. BECKER. 1986. Enduring changes in brain and behavior produced by chronic amphetamine administration: A review and evaluation of animal models of amphetamine psychosis. Brain Res. Rev. **11:** 157–198.
2. KALIVAS, P. W. & J. STEWART. 1991. Dopamine transmission in the initiation and expression of drug- and stress-induced sensitization of motor activity. Brain Res. Rev. **16:** 223–244.
3. ROBINSON, T. E., P. A. JURSON, J. A. BENNETT & K. M. BENTGEN. 1988. Persistent sensitization of dopamine neurotransmission in ventral striatum (nucleus accumbens) produced by prior experience with (+)-amphetamine: A microdialysis study in freely moving rats. Brain Res. **462:** 211–222.
4. AKIMOTO, K., T. HAMAMURA, Y. KAZAHAYA, K. AKIYAMA & S. OTSUKI. 1990. Enhanced extracellular dopamine level may be the fundamental neuropharmacological basis of cross-behavioral sensitization between methamphetamine and cocaine–An in vivo dialysis study in freely moving rats. Brain Res. **507:** 344–346.
5. AKIMOTO, K., T. HAMAMURA & S. OTSUKI. 1989. Subchronic cocaine treatment enhances

cocaine-induced dopamine efflux, studies by in vivo intracerebral dialysis. Brain Res. **490:** 339–344.
6. KALIVAS, P. W. & P. DUFFY. 1990. The effect of acute and daily cocaine treatment on extracellular dopamine in the nucleus accumbens. Synapse **5:** 48–58.
7. PETTIT, H. O., H.-T. PAN, L. H. PARSONS & J. B. JUSTICE, JR. 1990. Extracellular concentrations of cocaine and dopamine are enhanced during chronic cocaine administration. J. Neurochem. **55:** 798–804.
8. HURD, Y. L., F. WEISS, G. F. KOOB & N.-E. U. UNGERSTEDT. 1989. Cocaine reinforcement and extracellular dopamine overflow in rat nucleus accumbens: An in vivo microdialysis study. Brain Res. **498:** 199–203.
9. KUCZENSKI, R. & D. S. SEGAL. 1990. In vivo measures of monoamines during amphetamine-induced behavior in rat. Prog. Neuropsychopharmacol. Biol. Psychiatr. **14:** S37–S50.
10. ROBINSON, T. E. 1991. In Taniguchi Symposia on Brain Sciences, Vol. 14, Biological Basis of Schizophrenic Disorders. T. Nakazawa, Ed.: 185–201. Japan Scientific Societies Press. Tokyo.
11. DOUGHERTY, G. G., JR. & E. H. ELLINWOOD, JR. 1981. Chronic d-amphetamine in nucleus accumbens: Lack of tolerance or reverse tolerance of locomotor activity. Life Sci. **28:** 2295–2298.
12. HITZEMANN, R., J. WU, D. HOM & H. LOH. 1980. Brain locations controlling the behavioral effects of chronic amphetamine intoxication. Psychopharmacology **72:** 93–101.
13. KALIVAS, P. W. & B. WEBER. 1988. Amphetamine injection into the A10 dopamine region sensitizes rats to peripheral amphetamine, and cocaine. J. Pharmacol. Exp. Ther. **245:** 1095–1102.
14. VEZINA, P., P. W. KALIVAS & J. STEWART. 1987. Sensitization occurs to the locomotor effects of morphine and the specific mu opioid receptor agonist, DAGO, administered repeatedly to the VTA but not to the nucleus accumbens. Brain Res. **417:** 51–58.
15. VEZINA, P. & J. STEWART. 1990. Amphetamine administered to the ventral tegmental area but not to the nucleus accumbens sensitizes rats to systemic morphine: Lack of conditioned effects. Brain Res. **516:** 99–106.
16. HOOKS, M. S., G. H. JONES, C. B. NEILL & J. B. JUSTICE. 1992. Sensitization and individual differences to systemic amphetamine, cocaine or caffeine following repeated intracranial amphetamine infusions. Pharmacol. Biochem. Behav. In press.
17. KALIVAS, P. W. & P. DUFFY. 1990. Effect of acute and daily neurotensin and enkephalin treatments on extracellular dopamine in the nucleus accumbens. J. Neurosci. **10:** 2940–2949.
18. STEWART, J. & P. VEZINA. 1989. Microinjections of SCH-23390 into the ventral tegmental area and substantia nigra pars reticulata attenuate the development of sensitization to the locomotor activating effects of systemic amphetamine. Brain Res. **495:** 401–406.
19. UJIKE, H., K. AKIYAMA, H. NISHIKAWA, T. ONOUE & S. OTSUKI. 1991. Lasting increase in D1 dopamine receptors in the lateral part of the substantia nigra pars reticulata after subchronic methamphetamine administration. Brain Res. **540:** 159–163.
20. KALIVAS, P. W. & P. DUFFY. 1990. Comparison of somatodendritic and axonal mesolimbic dopamine release using in vivo dialysis. J. Neurochem. **56:** 961–967.
21. ROBERTSON, G. S., G. DAMSMA & H. C. FIBIGER. 1991. Characterization of dopamine release in the substantia nigra by in vivo microdialysis in freely moving rats. J. Neurosci. **11:** 2209–2216.
22. ANTELMAN, S. M. & L. A. CHIODO. 1981. Dopamine autoreceptor subsensitivity: A mechanism common to the treatment of depression and the induction of amphetamine psychosis. Biol. Psychiatr. **16:** 717–727.
23. HENRY, D. J., A. G. MARGARET & F. J. WHITE. 1989. Electrophysiological effects of cocaine in the mesoaccumbens dopamine system: Repeated administration. J. Pharmacol. Exp. Ther. **251:** 833–839.
24. KAMATA, K. & G. V. REBEC. 1984. Nigra dopaminergic neurons: Differential sensitivity to apomorphine following long-term treatment with low and high doses of amphetamine. Brain Res. **32:** 147–150.
25. LEE, T. H., E. H. ELLINWOOD, JR. & J. K. NISHITA. 1988. Dopamine receptor sensitivity changes with chronic stimulants. Ann. N. Y. Acad. Sci. **537:** 324–329.

KALIVAS *et al.*: CELLULAR MECHANISMS

135

26. WHITE, F. J. & R. Y. WANG. 1984. Electrophysiological evidence for A10 dopamine auto-receptor sensitivity following chronic *d*-amphetamine treatment. Brain Res. **309:** 283–292.
27. ACKERMAN, J. M. & F. J. WHITE. 1990. A10 somatodendritic dopamine autoreceptor sensitivity following withdrawal from repeated cocaine treatment. Neurosci. Lett. **117:** 181–187.
28. PERIS, J., S. J. BOYSON, W. A. CASS, P. CURELLA, L. P. DWOSKIN, G. LARSON, L.-H. LIN, R. P. YASUDA & N. R. ZAHNISER. 1990. Persistence of neurochemical changes in dopamine systems after repeated cocaine administration. J. Pharmacol. Exp. Ther. **253:** 38–44.
29. INNIS, R. B. & G. K. AGHAJANIAN. 1987. Pertussis toxin blocks autoreceptor-mediated inhibition of dopaminergic neurons in rat substantia nigra. Brain Res. **411:** 139–143.
30. LACEY, M. G., N. B. MERCURI & R. A. NORTH. 1987. Dopamine acts at D2 receptors to increase potassium conductance in neurons of the rat substantia nigra. J. Physiol. (Lond.) **392:** 397–416.
31. NESTLER, E. J., R. Z. TERWILLIGER, J. R. WALKER, K. A. SEVARINO & R. S. DUMAN. 1990. Chronic cocaine treatment decreases levels of the G protein subunits G_{ia} and G_{oa} in discrete regions of rat brain. J. Neurochem. **55:** 1079–1082.
32. STEKETEE, J. D., T. F. MURRAY & P. W. KALIVAS. 1990. Possible role for G proteins in behavioral sensitization. Brain Res. **545:** 287–291.
33. STEKETEE, J. D. & P. W. KALIVAS. 1991. Sensitization to psychostimulants and stress following injection of pertussis toxin into the A10 dopamine region. J. Pharmacol. Exp. Ther. **259:** 916–924.
34. ALTAR, C. A. & K. HAUSER. 1987. Topography of substantia nigra innervation by D1 receptor-containing striatal neurons. Brain Res. **410:** 1–11.
35. BECKSTEAD, R. M. 1988. Association of dopamine D1 and D2 receptors with specific cellular elements in the basal ganglia of the cat: The uneven topography of dopamine receptors in the striatum is determined by intrinsic striatal cells, not nigrostriatal axons. Neuroscience **27:** 851–863.
36. WASZCZAK, B. L. 1990. Differential effects of D1 and D2 dopamine receptor agonists on substantia nigra pars reticulata neurons. Brain Res. **513:** 125–135.
37. CHURCHILL, L., A. BOURDELAIS, M. C. AUSTIN, S. J. LOLAIT, L. C. MAHAN, A.-M. O'CARROLL & P. W. KALIVAS. 1991. GABA_A receptors containing α_1 and β_2 subunits are mainly localized on neurons in the ventral pallidum. Synapse **8:** 75–85.
38. KLITENICK, M. A., P. DEWITTE & P. W. KALIVAS. 1992. Regulation of dopamine and GABA release in the ventral tegmental area by opioids and GABA. J. Neurosci. In press.
39. BEITNER-JOHNSON, D., X. GUITART & E. J. NESTLER. 1992. Common intracellular actions of chronic morphine and cocaine in dopaminergic brain reward areas. Ann. NY Acad. Sci. **654:** 70–87. This volume.
40. BEITNER-JOHNSON, D. & E. J. NESTLER. 1991. Morphine and cocaine exert common chronic actions on tyrosine hydroxylase in dopaminergic brain reward regions. J. Neurochem. **57:** 344–347.

Mesocorticolimbic Dopamine Systems: Cross-Sensitization between Stress and Cocaine

BARBARA A. SORG

Department of Veterinary and Comparative Anatomy,
Pharmacology, and Physiology
Washington State University
Pullman, Washington 99164-6520

INTRODUCTION

The mesocortical and mesolimbic pathways implicated in the reinforcing effects of cocaine include projections from the A_{10} dopamine perikarya in the ventral mesencephalon to the medial prefrontal cortex (mPFC) and the nucleus accumbens (NAc).[1,2] A number of studies using the *in vivo* microdialysis method have shown that cocaine increases extracellular dopamine levels in the NAc,[3,4] and that the magnitude of this response is greater in animals given repeated cocaine.[5,6] The increase in dopamine levels in the NAc is believed to be the primary mediator of the locomotor response to cocaine,[7–9] and the enhanced dopamine levels are correlated with the augmented locomotor response (behavioral sensitization) following repeated cocaine treatment.[5] The role of dopamine transmission in the medial prefrontal cortex in cocaine-induced behavioral sensitization has not been examined, but several studies support a role for mPFC dopamine in modulating dopamine release in the NAc by a transsynaptic mechanism, resulting in a partial regulation of locomotor activity.[10,11]

Increased activation of dopamine transmission in the mPFC and NAc also occurs in response to stressful stimuli.[12–15] Moreover, animals demonstrate behavioral cross-sensitization between environmental stress and stimulant drugs such as amphetamine[16–18] and cocaine.[19–21] This interchangeability has been widely documented using a variety of behavioral endpoints, but *in vivo* neurochemical analysis has been limited to indirect measures.[19,22,23]

The goal of this work was to examine the effects of cross-sensitization paradigms on extracellular dopamine levels in the mPFC and NAc using footshock stress and cocaine. Evaluation of these sensitizing treatments in producing differential effects between the mPFC and NAc is considered in light of the known interaction between psychostimulants and stress in producing paranoid psychosis in humans.

EXPERIMENTAL DESIGN

Male Sprague-Dawley rats weighing 250–350 g were anesthetized, and unilateral chronic guide cannulae were placed 3 mm dorsal to the NAc at A/P 8.6 mm, M/L 1.5 mm, D/V 0.0 mm relative to the interaural line.[24] Guide cannulae were placed 4 mm dorsal to the mPFC at 3.2 mm from bregma, 0.6 mm from midline, and 1.5

mm from the skull.[25] All rats were housed individually at least five days following surgery before beginning experimentation.

The footshock and sham shock apparatus and photocell cages coupled to the *in vivo* microdialysis system used were as described previously.[21]

Two types of cross-sensitization experiments were performed. In the first experiment, rats were given five daily injections of cocaine (15 mg/kg, i.p.) or saline (1 ml/kg, i.p.) in the home cage. A separate group of animals received no prior handling (naive group). Five to seven days after the last injection, animals were placed in the footshock or sham shock apparatus and four 20 min dialysis samples were collected prior to shock or sham shock followed by at least two hours of post-shock sample collection. The shock administered was 0.45 mA/200msec/sec for 20 min.

In the second experiment, rats were placed either in the footshock or sham shock apparatus and footshock was delivered (as described above) once daily for five days. Following a five to seven day period of no treatment, *in vivo* dialysis was carried out in the photocell cages. After four baseline sample collections, animals were given a cocaine (15 mg/kg, i.p.) or saline (1 ml/kg, i.p.) injection, and sample collection was continued for at least two hours. In both experiments dialysis probes were implanted the evening before the experiment and buffer [21] was allowed to perfuse through the probes at least two hours before baseline sample collection. Extracellular levels of dopamine and the metabolites, 3,4-dihydroxyphenylacetic acid (DOPAC) and homovanillic acid (HVA), were measured by HPLC with coulometric electrochemical detection as described previously.[21]

ACUTE RESPONSE TO COCAINE AND FOOTSHOCK STRESS IN mPFC AND NAc

Several laboratories have shown that a variety of stressors preferentially leads to increased dopamine transmission in the mPFC, while NAc dopamine is altered only

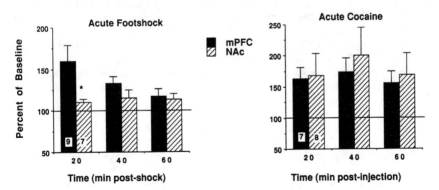

FIGURE 1. Effect of acute footshock stress and acute cocaine treatment on extracellular dopamine concentrations in the mPFC and NAc. Data are mean ± SEM percent change from baseline values at 20, 40 and 60 min after initiation of footshock. * $p < .05$, comparing NAc to mPFC dopamine levels using a two-way ANOVA followed by a least squares difference analysis. Animals receiving acute footshock stress were non-handled prior to microdialysis; animals receiving acute cocaine had received five daily sham shock pretreatments, as described for experiment 1 in EXPERIMENTAL DESIGN.

slightly or not at all.[26,27] Specificity of the stress-evoked mPFC dopamine release appears to result from a preferential increase in the firing rate of mesoprefrontal cortical dopamine neurons.[28] In agreement with these reports, FIGURE 1 shows the significant increase in extracellular dopamine concentrations in the mPFC compared to NAc in response to an acute 20 min footshock. The effect of acute cocaine administration on mPFC and NAc dopamine concentrations is also shown in FIGURE 1. A previous report has shown that cocaine is less effective in increasing extracellular dopamine in the mPFC compared to the NAc in anesthetized rats[29]; however, the present results show no significant differences in the dopamine response between mPFC and NAc. These cocaine and shock parameters were used for all cross-sensitization experiments because 1) although a higher intensity of footshock increases dopamine levels in the NAc as well as the mPFC,[21] this intensity produces overt escape behavior and was thus avoided, and 2) repeated administration of the cocaine dosage shown in FIGURE 1 has previously been shown to produce a sensitized motor-stimulant response to subsequent cocaine.[5]

CROSS-SENSITIZATION BETWEEN COCAINE AND FOOTSHOCK STRESS

Cross-sensitization studies typically have employed paradigms which administer repeated daily stress followed by a delay of one to several days and a subsequent amphetamine or cocaine challenge. The primary emphasis has been on behavioral activity such as locomotor or stereotypic responses as measures of sensitization, and in general, animals display an enhanced behavioral response to amphetamine or cocaine following repeated stress.[16–18,20,21] Less common is the converse experiment, in which repeated daily psychostimulants are administered followed by an acute stress challenge. Little is known about alterations in dopamine transmission following either type of cross-sensitization paradigm. Indices of *in vivo* dopamine release have thus far been limited to indirect measures, including analysis of dopamine metabolite levels,[19,23] and assessment of dopamine depletion following administration of a dopamine synthesis inhibitor.[22]

The *in vivo* microdialysis technique was used to re-examine the dopamine response in the mPFC and NAc following the two types of cross-sensitization paradigms. In addition, concurrent measures of the motor-stimulant response to acute cocaine were obtained to determine if this response was augmented in repeatedly stressed rats.

Repeated Footshock Stress and Acute Cocaine

FIGURE 2 shows the dopamine response to an acute cocaine challenge in animals that received repeated daily footshock or sham shock. Dopamine levels in the NAc were significantly augmented in shock pretreated rats during the first 20 min after cocaine injection. These animals also demonstrated a corresponding increase in locomotor activity (data not shown), which is in line with the well-established role of the NAc in mediating the psychostimulant-induced enhancement in locomotor activity.[5,7,30] In contrast, in the mPFC, pretreatment with footshock stress failed to evoke a sensitized dopamine response to a challenge cocaine injection. In addition, no significant differences were found between shock and sham shock groups in locomotor

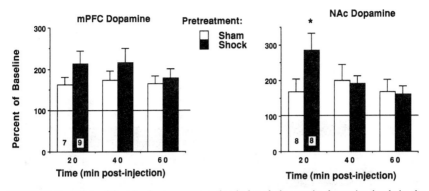

FIGURE 2. Effect of footshock stress on cocaine-induced changes in dopamine levels in the mPFC and NAc. Values are mean ± SEM percent change from baseline levels at 20, 40, and 60 min post-injection. * $p < .05$, comparing to sham shock–pretreated animals, using the analysis described for FIGURE 1.

activity, suggesting that when dialysis probes are placed in the mPFC, animals may not be capable of responding to cocaine with behavioral sensitization.

Repeated Cocaine and Acute Footshock Stress

FIGURES 3A and B show acute footshock-induced changes in extracellular dopamine, DOPAC and HVA in the mPFC and NAc in daily saline- or cocaine-pretreated rats. In the mPFC, daily cocaine treatment prevented the large footshock-induced increase in extracellular dopamine observed in the saline controls, and attenuated the increase in DOPAC and HVA levels. Dopamine levels in the NAc showed changes in the opposite direction from the mPFC. In this region, there was a nonsignificant trend towards enhanced extracellular dopamine and metabolite levels in cocaine-pretreated rats after acute footshock. Based on a previous study examining various doses of amphetamine challenge in amphetamine-sensitized rats,[31] it is likely that a more robust sensitized response may have been observed in the NAc following a higher intensity of footshock challenge.

Previous cross-sensitization studies have demonstrated a complexity in the dynamics of dopamine turnover in the mPFC and NAc following acute footshock stress.[19,23] These studies showed a time-dependent relationship between dopamine and the initiation of footshock such that, in general, amphetamine- or cocaine-pretreated animals showed higher post-mortem tissue metabolite levels early (5–10 min) after footshock but equal or lower levels than saline controls after continued application of footshock. In a dopamine depletion study, Robinson et al.[22] reported that a 20 min footshock prevented an increase in dopamine utilization in the mPFC in rats given repeated amphetamine, which they attributed to enhanced basal levels of utilization prior to the footshock. These studies taken together with the present results suggest that in cocaine pretreated rats, dopamine may not be released in response to stress, and that the increase in metabolite levels may occur independently of dopamine release. Metabolism of dopamine to DOPAC in the absence of release and reuptake has previously been reported.[32,33] Further support for this hypothesis is the finding that DOPAC and (to

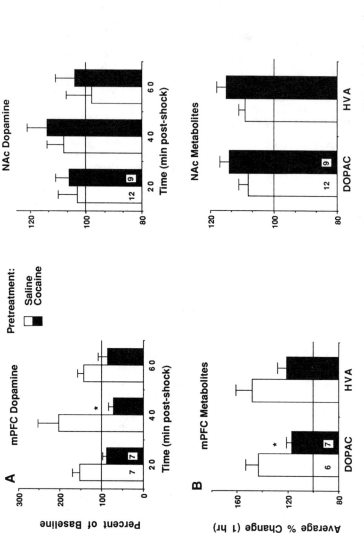

FIGURE 3. Effect of cocaine on footshock stress-induced changes in dopamine, DOPAC and HVA. Data are mean ±SEM percent change from baseline levels 20, 40 and 60 min after the start of the 20 min footshock (dopamine) and average percent change over a one hour period post-shock (DOPAC and HVA). * $p < .05$, comparing to saline pretreated group using the analysis described for FIGURE 1 (dopamine) and a one-way ANOVA followed by a least squares differences analysis (DOPAC and HVA).

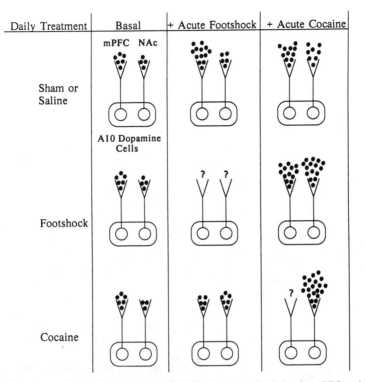

FIGURE 4. Schematic diagram showing extracellular dopamine levels in the mPFC and NAc in response to cocaine and stress administration. Black dots represent levels of extracellular dopamine.

some extent) HVA levels were elevated more rapidly in cocaine than in saline-pretreated rats (data not shown). This may be indicative of the time necessary for release and re-uptake of dopamine prior to metabolism in saline controls, while this pathway is by-passed in cocaine-pretreated animals.

SUMMARY MODEL AND RELEVANCE TO PSYCHOSTIMULANT-INDUCED PSYCHOSIS

The diagram shown in FIGURE 4 is a summary of the dopamine response in the mPFC and NAc following cross-sensitizing treatments. Previous evidence indicates that dopamine turnover is greater in the mPFC than in the NAc.[34,35] This is depicted in the far left panel showing higher levels of basal dopamine molecules released per terminal in the mPFC than in NAc in sham shock, footshock and saline-pretreated animals. These pretreatments are presumed not to alter basal levels of extracellular dopamine. Some evidence has been presented to suggest that basal levels of extracellular dopamine are decreased in the NAc in animals given repeated cocaine,[36] which is represented by a decrease in extracellular dopamine levels in the left panel.

In the center panel is shown the changes that occur in response to acute footshock. In saline-pretreated animals, footshock induces a large increase in mPFC dopamine levels but only a slight elevation in NAc dopamine. However, pretreatment with cocaine completely abolishes the footshock-induced increase in mPFC dopamine, with a slight, nonsignificant increase in dopamine and metabolite levels in the NAc. The effect of prior footshock treatment on the capacity of acute footshock to alter extracellular dopamine levels has not been tested.

Shown in the top of the third panel is the effect of acute cocaine in sham shock–pretreated rats. Acute cocaine produces a robust dopamine response in both the mPFC and NAc. Pretreatment with daily footshock does not significantly alter this dopamine response in the mPFC but produces an augmentation in dopamine levels in the NAc. The sensitized dopamine response in the NAc is very similar to what is observed in animals pretreated with daily cocaine,[5,6] while the effect of a challenge cocaine treatment on mPFC dopamine levels in cocaine-pretreated rats is not known.

In summary, the cross-sensitization studies show that the dopamine response is differentially affected in the mPFC and NAc. Much evidence has emerged supporting an inhibitory role for dopamine in the mPFC on glutamatergic neurons projecting to subcortical sites, including the NAc.[27,37] Glutamate release in the NAc and striatum is believed to regulate dopamine release through a pre-synaptic mechanism,[38-40] and therefore a depletion of dopamine levels in the mPFC leads to enhanced basal and/or pharmacologically or stress-induced dopamine and metabolite levels in the NAc.[10,11,27,37,41] However, while the present studies show that the mPFC and NAc are affected differently from each other by cocaine and stress, they do not give strong support for a major role of glutamatergic projections from the mPFC in modulating NAc dopamine levels.

The development of behavioral sensitization in rodents resembles the progressive onset of behaviors associated with paranoid schizophrenia and panic disorder in humans.[42,43] Furthermore, repeated use of amphetamine or cocaine in humans leads to the development of symptoms that are similar to those observed in paranoid schizophrenia[44] and panic disorder.[43] Cross-sensitization studies are relevant to these disorders in that during abstinence from the drug, individuals can remain stable for extended periods until the condition is reinstated by stressful life events.[42] Neurochemical evidence in schizophrenic individuals shows that there is a decrease in prefrontal cortical activity, and that this may be an important factor in disruption of physiological and cognitive adaption to stress.[45] It is perhaps the presence of a sensitized response to cocaine or a stress-induced increase in dopamine in the mPFC that is important in providing the normal adaptive response to pharmacological or environmental stressors. Therefore, in the cocaine- or stress-sensitized organism, prevention of an appropriate mPFC dopamine response to further stressful stimuli may in part explain reinstatement of the paranoid psychotic state following perturbation by stress or psychostimulants.

REFERENCES

1. GOEDERS, N. E. & J. E. SMITH. 1983. Cortical dopaminergic involvement in cocaine reinforcement. Science 221: 773–775.
2. PETTIT, H. O., A. ETTENBERG, F. E. BLOOM & G. F. KOOB. 1984. Destruction of dopamine in the nucleus accumbens selectively attenuates cocaine but not heroin self-administration in rats. Psychopharmacology 84: 167–173.
3. BRADBERRY, C. W. & R. H. ROTH. 1989. Cocaine increases extracellular dopamine in rat

nucleus accumbens and ventral tegmental area as shown by in vivo microdialysis. Neurosci. Lett. **103**: 97–102.

4. HURD, Y. L., F. WEISS, G. F. KOOB, N.-E. ANDEN & U. UNGERSTEDT. 1989. Cocaine reinforcement and extracellular dopamine overflow in rat nucleus accumbens: An in vivo microdialysis study. Brain Res. **498**: 199–203.

5. KALIVAS, P. W. & P. DUFFY. 1990. Effect of acute and daily cocaine treatment on extracellular dopamine in the nucleus accumbens. Synapse **5**: 48–58.

6. PETTIT, H. O., H.-T. PAN, L. H. PARSONS & J. B. JUSTICE, JR. 1990. Extracellular concentrations of cocaine and dopamine are enhanced during chronic cocaine administration. J. Neurochem. **55**: 798–804.

7. DELFS, J. M., L. SCHREIBER & A. E. KELLY. 1990. Microinjection of cocaine into the nucleus accumbens elicits locomotor activation in the rat. J. Neurosci. **10**: 303–310.

8. KELLY, P. & S. D. IVERSEN. 1976. Selective 6-OHDA-induced destruction of mesolimbic dopamine neurons: Abolition of psychostimulant-induced locomotor activities in rats. Eur. J. Pharmacol. **40**: 45–56.

9. SCHEEL-KRUGER, J., C. BRAESTRUP, M. MIELSON, K. GOLEMBIOWSKA & E. MOGLINICKA. 1977. Cocaine: Discussion on the role of dopamine in the biochemical mechanism of action. In Cocaine and Other Stimulants, Advances in Behavioral Biology. E. H. Ellinwood, Jr. & M. M. Kilbey, Eds.: 373–407. Plenum Press. New York.

10. DEUTCH, A. Y., W. A. CLARK & R. H. ROTH. 1990. Prefrontal cortical dopamine depletion enhances the responsiveness of mesolimbic dopamine neurons to stress. Brain Res. **521**: 311–315.

11. LOUILOT, A., M. LE MOAL & H. SIMON. 1989. Opposite influences of dopaminergic pathways to the prefrontal cortex or the septum on the dopaminergic transmission in the nucleus accumbens. An in vivo voltammetric study. Neuroscience **29**: 45–56.

12. ABERCROMBIE, E. D., K. A. KEEFE, D. S. DIFRISCHIA & M. J. ZIGMOND. 1989. Differential effect of stress on in vivo dopamine release in striatum, nucleus accumbens, and medial frontal cortex. J. Neurochem. **52**: 1655–1658.

13. DUNN, A. J. 1988. Stress-related activation of cerebral dopaminergic systems. Ann. NY Acad. Sci. **537**: 188–205.

14. FADDA, F., A. ARGIOLIS, M. R. MELIS, A. H. RISSARI, P. C. ONALI & G. L. GESSA. 1978. Stress-induced increase in 3,4-dihydroxyphenylacetic acid (DOPAC) levels in the cerebral cortex and in nucleus accumbens: Reversal by diazepam. Life Sci. **23**: 2219–2224.

15. HERMAN, J.-P., D. GUILLONNEAU, R. DANTZER, B. SCATTON, L. SEMERDJIAN-ROUQUIER & M. LE MOAL. 1982. Differential effects of inescapable footshocks on dopamine turnover in cortical and limbic areas of the rat. Life Sci. **30**: 2207–2214.

16. ANTELMAN, S. M., A. J. EICHLER, C. A. BLACK & D. KOCAN. 1980. Interchangeability of stress and amphetamine in sensitization. Science **207**: 329–331.

17. HERMAN, J.-P., L. STINUS & M. LE MOAL. 1984. Repeated stress increases locomotor response to amphetamine. Psychopharmacology **84**: 431–435.

18. ROBINSON, T. E., A. L. ANGUS & J. B. BECKER. 1985. Sensitization to stress: The enduring effects of prior stress on amphetamine-induced rotational behavior. Life Sci. **37**: 1039–1042.

19. KALIVAS, P. W. & P. DUFFY. 1989. Similar effects of daily cocaine and stress on mesocorticolimbic dopamine neurotransmission in the rat. Biol. Psychiatr. **25**: 913–928.

20. MACLENNAN, A. J. & S. F. MAIER. 1983. Coping and the stress-induced potentiation of stimulant stereotypy in the rat. Science **219**: 1091–1093.

21. SORG, B. A. & P. W. KALIVAS. 1991. Effects of cocaine and footshock stress on extracellular dopamine levels in the ventral striatum. Brain Res. **559**: 29–36.

22. ROBINSON, T. E., J. B. BECKER, C. J. MOORE, E. CASTANEDA & G. MITTLEMAN. 1985. Enduring enhancement in frontal cortex dopamine utilization in an animal model of amphetamine psychosis. Brain Res. **343**: 374–377.

23. ROBINSON, T. E., J. B. BECKER, E. A. YOUNG, H. AKIL & E. CASTANEDA. 1987. The effects of footshock stress on regional brain dopamine metabolism and pituitary β-endorphin release in rats previously sensitized to amphetamine. Neuropharmacology **26**: 679–691.

24. PELLEGRINO, L. K., A. S. PELLEGRINO & A. J. CUSHMAN. 1979. A Stereotaxic Atlas of the Rat Brain. Plenum Press. New York.

25. PAXINOS, G. & C. WATSON. 1986. The Rat Brain in Stereotaxic Coordinates. Plenum Press. New York.
26. THIERRY, A. M., J. P. TASSIN, G. BLANC & J. GLOWINSKI. 1976. Selective activation of the mesocortical DA system by stress. Nature 263: 242–243.
27. DEUTCH, A. Y. & R. H. ROTH. 1990. The determinants of stress-induced activation of the prefrontal cortical dopamine system. Prog. Brain Res. 85: 357–393.
28. MANTZ, J., A. M. THIERRY & J. GLOWINSKI. 1989. Effect of noxious tail pinch on the discharge rate of mesocortical and mesolimbic dopamine neurons. Selective activation of the mesocortical system. Brain Res. 476: 377–381.
29. MOGHADDAM, B. & B. S. BUNNEY. 1989. Differential effect of cocaine on extracellular dopamine levels in rat medial prefrontal cortex and nucleus accumbens: Comparison to amphetamine. Synapse 4: 156–161.
30. SESSIONS, G., J. MEYERHOFF, G. J. KANT & G. F. KOOB. 1980. Effects of lesions of the ventral medial tegmentum on locomotor activity, biogenic amines and response to amphetamine in rats. Pharmacol. Biochem. Behav. 12: 603–608.
31. CASTANEDA, E., J. B. BECKER & T. E. ROBINSON. 1988. The long-term effects of repeated amphetamine treatment in vivo on amphetamine, KCl and electrical stimulation evoked striatal dopamine release in vitro. Life Sci. 42: 2447–2456.
32. SOARES-DA-SILVA, P. & M. C. GARRETT. 1990. A kinetic study of the rate of formation of dopamine, 3,4-dihydroxyphenylacetic acid (DOPAC) and homovanillic acid (HVA) in the brain of the rat: Implications for the origin of DOPAC. Neuropharmacology 29: 869–874.
33. ZETTERSTROM, T., T. SHARP, A. K. COLLIN & U. UNGERSTEDT. 1988. In vivo measurement of extracellular dopamine and DOPAC in rat striatum after various dopamine-releasing drugs: Implications for the origin of extracellular DOPAC. Eur. J. Pharmacol. 148: 327–334.
34. BANNON, M. J. & R. ROTH. 1983. Pharmacology of mesocortical dopamine neurons. Pharmacol. Rev. 35: 53–68.
35. BANNON, M. J., E. B. BUNNEY & R. H. ROTH. 1981. Mesocortical dopamine neurons: Rapid neurotransmitter turnover compared to other brain catecholamine systems. Brain Res. 218: 376–382.
36. PARSONS, L. H., A. D. SMITH & J. B. JUSTICE, JR. 1991. Basal extracellular dopamine is decreased in the rat nucleus accumbens during abstinence from chronic cocaine. Synapse 9: 60–65.
37. CARTER, C. J. & C. J. PYCOCK. 1980. Behavioural and biochemical effects of dopamine and noradrenaline depletion within the medial prefrontal cortex of the rat. Brain Res. 192: 163–176.
38. CARTER, C. J. 1980. Glutamatergic pathways from the medial prefrontal cortex to the anterior striatum, nucleus accumbens and substantia nigra. Br. J. Pharmacol. 70: 50P–51P.
39. GIRAULT, J. A., L. BARBEITO, U. SPAMPINATO, H. GOZLAN, J. GLOWINSKI & M. J. BESSON. 1986. In vivo release of endogenous amino acids from the rat striatum: Further evidence for a role of glutamate and aspartate in corticostriatal transmission. J. Neurochem. 47: 98–106.
40. GLOWINSKI, J., A. CHERAMY, R. ROMO & L. BARBEITO. 1988. Presynaptic regulation of dopaminergic transmission in the striatum. Cell. Mol. Neurobiol. 8: 7–17.
41. PYCOCK, C. J., C. J. CARTER & R. W. KERWIN. 1980. Effect of 6-hydroxydopamine lesions of the medial prefrontal cortex on neurotransmitter systems in subcortical sites in the rat. J. Neurochem. 34: 91–99.
42. LIEBERMAN, J. A., B. J. KINON & A. D. LOEBEL. 1990. Dopaminergic mechanisms in idiopathic and drug-induced psychoses. Schiz. Bull. 16: 97–110.
43. POST, R. M. & S. R. B. WEISS. 1988. Sensitization and kindling: Implications for the evolution of psychiatric symptomatology. In Sensitization in the Nervous System. P. W. Kalivas & C. D. Barnes, Eds.: 257–292. Telford Press. New Jersey.
44. ROBINSON, T. E. & J. B. BECKER. 1986. Enduring changes in brain and behavior produced by chronic amphetamine administration: A review and evaluation of animal models of amphetamine psychosis. Brain Res. 11: 157–198.
45. WEINBERGER, D. R. 1987. Implications of normal brain development for the pathogenesis of schizophrenia. Arch. Gen. Psychiat. 44: 660–669.

Effects of Chronic Ethanol and Benzodiazepine Treatment and Withdrawal on Corticotropin-releasing Factor Neural Systems[a]

M. ADRIANA VARGAS,[b] GARTH BISSETTE,[b]
MICHAEL J. OWENS,[c] CINDY L. EHLERS,[d]
AND CHARLES B. NEMEROFF[c,e]

[b]Department of Psychiatry
Duke University Medical Center
Durham, North Carolina 27710

[c]Department of Psychiatry
Emory University Medical School
Atlanta, Georgia 30322

[d]Research Institute of the Scripps Clinic
La Jolla, California 92037

Corticotropin-releasing factor (CRF) is the major physiological regulator of adrenocorticotropin (ACTH) and β-endorphin release from the anterior pituitary gland.[1-4] Immunohistochemical and radioimmunoassay studies have revealed that CRF is heterogeneously distributed throughout the mammalian central nervous system (CNS). High concentrations of CRF are found in the hypothalamus, certain autonomic brainstem nuclei, and several limbic areas.[5-7] Similarly, biochemical and autoradiographic studies have identified specific CRF receptors in the CNS.[8-10]

When administered directly into the CNS, CRF produces a variety of behavioral[11,12] and physiological effects[13,14] that are independent of the hypothalamic-pituitary-adrenal (HPA) axis, and closely approximate a laboratory animal's response to stress as well as many of the symptoms of both affective and anxiety disorders in humans. These findings strongly suggest that CRF, acting as a neurotransmitter, may ultimately be responsible for integrating the endocrine, as well as the autonomic and behavioral responses, of an organism to stress.

Although there is substantial evidence that CRF is hypersecreted in patients with major depression,[15,16] there are also considerable data that support a role for CRF in anxiety disorders.[17] For example, direct microinjection of CRF into the locus coeruleus produces profound anxiogenic effects in rats[18] and intraventricularly administered CRF has a similar effect.[11,19] Like depressed patients, patients with two DSM-

[a] Supported by NIMH MH-42088 to CBN, NIAAA 06059 and 00098 to CLE, and the John A. and Catherine T. McArthur Foundation.
[e] Author to whom all correspondence and requests for reprints should be addressed.

IIIR anxiety disorders, panic disorder[20] and post-traumatic stress disorder,[21] exhibit a blunted ACTH response to CRF. This neuroendocrine abnormality is likely due to CRF hypersecretion and resultant CRF receptor down-regulation in the anterior pituitary. Moreover, our laboratory has previously reported that acute and chronic stress alter the concentrations of CRF in a number of discrete brain regions of the rat, several of which have been postulated to play a role in the etiology of human affective and anxiety disorders (FIG. 1).[22] These results suggest that CRF of both hypothalamic and extrahypothalamic origin is altered by stress and these alterations may mediate some of the signs and symptoms observed in anxiety disorders.

This concatenation of findings led to the hypothesis that the anxiolytic properties of benzodiazepines may be related, in part, to their actions on CRF-containing neurons in the CNS. Because CRF neurons of both hypothalamic and extrahypothalamic origin may be involved in the pathophysiology of anxiety disorders, we examined the actions of a single acute injection of alprazolam or adinazolam on CRF concentrations in eighteen rat brain regions.[23] Alprazolam and its dimethylamino analog, adinazolam, are atypical triazolobenzo-diazepines[24-27] that possess the anxiolytic properties typical of benzodiazepines and have been reported to possess clinical antidepressant and anti-panic activities that are apparently unique to these benzodiazepines.[28-32] One hour following acute injection, CRF concentrations were decreased in the locus coeruleus, amygdala, piriform cortex, and cingulate cortex in both alprazolam- and adinazolam-treated rats, and increased concentrations of the peptide were observed in the hypothalamus/median eminence. These effects are opposite to those observed following exposure of rats to acute or chronic stress.[22] Both these drugs effectively decreased plasma ACTH concentrations compared to controls. In agreement with this observed decrease in HPA axis activity, Kalogeras et al.[33] reported that alprazolam dose-dependently decreases plasma ACTH concentrations in nonrestrained rhesus monkeys. This decrease was attributed to inhibition of median eminence CRF secretion, because alprazolam was also found to potently inhibit 5-HT-stimulated CRF release from isolated rat hypothalamic explants in vitro. In addition, Grigoriadis et al.[34] found that chronic benzodiazepine treatment decreased CRF receptor binding in a number of cortical and subcortical brain areas. However, these receptor decreases were statistically significant only in the frontal cortex and hippocampus. In a recent study,[35] we studied the time course of the alprazolam-induced decrease in locus coeruleus CRF concentrations. The effect persisted for 180 min postinjection. The 180 min time-course corresponds very closely with the bioavailability and metabolism of alprazolam. Moreover, CRF concentrations in the locus coeruleus remained decreased over the course of 13 days of continuous administration, indicative of a lack of tolerance to this effect of the drug. In addition, CRF concentrations in the dorsal vagal complex were decreased 24 h following abrupt alprazolam withdrawal (FIG. 1). These changes during drug withdrawal are similar to those observed following acute or chronic stress.[22]

Of particular interest is the finding of decreased CRF concentrations in the locus coeruleus following acute or chronic alprazolam treatment, which is opposite to that observed following exposure of rats to either acute or chronic stress. Iontophoretically applied CRF has been shown to increase the firing rate of neurons in several CNS regions, including the locus coeruleus (the A_6 noradrenergic cell group)[36]; which has been implicated in the pathophysiology of stress, anxiety and depression.[37-39] It remains unclear at present whether other classical benzodiazepines alter regional CRF

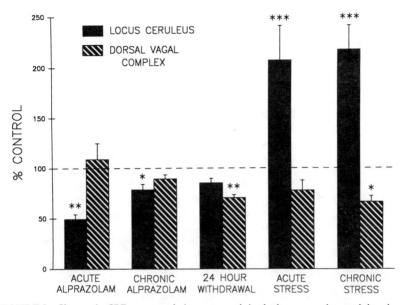

FIGURE 1. Changes in CRF content relative to controls in the locus coeruleus and dorsal vagal complex after acute (1 h) alprazolam (1 mg/kg),[23] chronic (14 days) alprazolam in liquid diet or 24 h after withdrawal from chronic alprazolam,[35] or after a regimen of acute or chronic stress.[22] Statistical analysis by two-way ANOVA and Student-Newman-Keuls. * $p \leqslant 0.05$ compared to controls; ** $p \leqslant 0.01$ compared to controls; *** $p \leqslant 0.001$ compared to controls.

immunoreactivity, or whether treatment with anxiolytics or antidepressants abolish stress-induced changes in CRF neurons.

Both human and animal studies have demonstrated a stimulatory effect of ethanol on the HPA axis.[40] In animal studies, acutely administered ethanol produces a dose-related increase in plasma corticosterone concentrations, which parallel increases in blood alcohol concentrations.[41-44] Because hypophysectomy abolishes ethanol-induced corticosteroid secretion,[41] a primary role for CRF in the modulation of these actions has been inferred. These increases in HPA activity have been reported to persist during repeated exposure to alcohol by some investigators,[41,42] whereas others have observed the development of tolerance.[44] In humans, acute and chronic ethanol exposure produces hypercortisolemia[45,46] which sometimes results in pseudo-Cushing's syndrome.[47-50] Some alcohol-treated subjects may even display non-suppression of plasma cortisol in response to the synthetic glucocorticoid, dexamethasone.[51-57] This suggests the possibility that either chronic hypersecretion of CRF may develop in alcoholic patients, or alternatively they may lose the ability of circulating glucocorticoids to inhibit activation of the HPA axis via negative feedback.

Rivier *et al.*[58] were the first to demonstrate that the acute administration of alcohol to non-anesthetized rats caused dose-related increases in plasma ACTH levels and that this release of ACTH is highly dependent on CRF production. They also observed that chronic exposure to alcohol vapors results in a slight, but significant, decrease in hypothalamic CRF content. Moreover, the stimulatory effect of ethanol on ACTH is totally abolished by immunoneutralization of endogenous CRF, indicating that CRF is an essential intermediate. In addition to changes in CRF production, the authors reported that chronic *in vivo* exposure to ethanol vapors may be accompanied by varying degrees of diminished pituitary responsiveness to CRF. Whether this loss of pituitary sensitivity is the mechanism(s) responsible for the development of ethanol tolerance, as reported by some investigators,[44] is presently unclear.

The precise mechanism(s) whereby chronic ethanol exposure induces hypothalamic CRF secretion have not been elucidated, though it is likely similar to the acute. It has been suggested that ethanol administration may act as a nonspecific stressor. We have evaluated[59] the effect of intraventricular infusions of CRF on certain behavioral measures in rats chronically exposed to ethanol vapors. The results suggest that chronic ethanol can potentiate the locomotor-activating effects of centrally administered CRF in rats. The greatest difference in CRF response between ethanol-treated and control rats was observed in the acutely withdrawn group. Following two weeks of withdrawal of ethanol vapors, the CRF-induced locomotor responses of rats treated chronically with ethanol were again similar to controls. These data are consistent with those provided by Mendelson and Stein[60] who showed that human alcoholic subjects had their peak plasma cortisol levels during ethanol withdrawal.

In humans, it has also been suggested that alcohol may also increase cortisol levels through alternate mechanisms. During acute stress, cortisol levels are increased but the normal diurnal variation remains intact. Even during chronic stress, inhibition of cortisol by dexamethasone remains normal and no Cushing-like features appear, while after stress glucocorticoid levels eventually return to normal regardless of the duration of the stressful stimuli.[40] However, in chronic alcoholism, glucocorticoid levels often remain high, Cushing-like features may appear,[47,48,50] and escape from dexamethasone-suppression of ACTH may occur.[52,53] In addition, Rivier *et al.*[58] have demonstrated in rats that although CRF antiserum can completely abolish ethanol-induced ACTH secretion, it can only partially block the ACTH response to ether stress.[61] Taken together, these studies suggest that certain aspects of stress-induced HPA axis activation occur through different mechanisms than those produced by chronic ethanol exposure.

In addition to its HPA axis effects, ethanol may act through its now widely recognized interaction with GABA receptors.[62-64] It has been well established that some of the effects of ethanol are mediated by the stimulation of GABA receptors. Both behavioral and electrophysiological studies suggest that low doses of ethanol can potentiate GABAergic neurotransmission,[62-65] although some negatives results have also been reported.[66] In contrast, at pharmacologically relevant concentrations, ethanol has been shown to have little or no effect on the binding of the benzodiazepine, GABA, or barbiturate receptor ligands to their respective receptor sites in brain.[67,68] Ethanol shares many of the pharmacologic actions of barbiturates and benzodiazepines such as anxiolytic, sedative and hypnotic activity.[69,70] Some studies have documented the development of cross-tolerance between ethanol, barbiturates and benzodiazepines[71] and also cross-dependence, suggesting that three drugs may share a common mechanism of action.[72] Further, both benzodiazepines and barbiturates bind to specific recognition sites associated with postsynaptic GABA receptors and possess affinities that are highly correlated with their respective anxiolytic, sedative and hypnotic effects.[73,74] Recent studies have reported that ethanol stimulates GABA receptor-mediated chloride uptake into brain vesicles.[75] Interactions with GABAergic systems in the secretion of CRF in the rat have also been reported. These studies suggest that the GABA/benzodiazepine system is involved in the regulation of hypothalamic CRF secretion. It appears that both GABA$_A$ and GABA$_B$ receptors mediate the suppressive effects of GABA upon 5-HT induced CRF secretion from the median eminence.[76]

In summary, the effects of stress and ethanol abuse and withdrawal have certain similarities in their effects on the HPA axis and the secretion of CRF. However, these similarities are in many cases due to distinctly different mechanisms that eventually converge and result in activation of the HPA axis. Further research will be required to fully understand the way in which these qualitatively different stimuli elicit this response.

REFERENCES

1. VALE, W., J. SPIESS, C. RIVIER & J. RIVIER. 1981. Characterization of a 41-residue ovine hypothalamic peptide that stimulates secretion of corticotropin and β-endorphin. Science 213: 1394–1397.

2. VALE, W., J. VAUGHAN, M. SMITH, G. YAMAMOTO, J. RIVIER & C. RIVIER. 1983. Effects of synthetic ovine corticotropin-releasing factor, glucocorticoids, catecholamines, neurohypophysial peptides, and other substances on cultured corticotropic cells. Endocrinology 113: 1121–1131.

3. RIVIER, C., J. RIVIER & W. VALE. 1982. Inhibition of adrenocorticotropic hormone secretion in the rat by immunoneutralization of corticotropin-releasing factor. Science 218: 377–379.

4. RIVIER, C., M. BROWNSTEIN, J. SPIESS, J. RIVIER & W. VALE. 1982. In vivo corticotropin-releasing factor-induced secretion of adrenocorticotropin, β-endorphin and corticosterone. Endocrinology 110: 272–278.

5. SWANSON, L. W., P. E. SAWCHENKO, J. RIVIER & W. W. VALE. 1983. Organization of ovine corticotropin-releasing factor immunoreactive cells and fibers in the rat brain: An immunohistochemical study. Neuroendocrinology 36: 165–186.

6. CUMMINGS, S., R. ELDE, J. ELLS & A. LINDALL. 1983. Corticotropin-releasing factor immunoreactivity is widely distributed within the central nervous system of the rat: An immunohistochemical study. J. Neurosci. 3: 1355–1368.

7. SAKANAKA, M., T. SHIBASAKI & K. LEDERIS. 1987. Corticotropin-releasing factor-like immunoreactivity in the rat brain as revealed by a modified cobalt-glucose oxidase-diaminobenzidine method. J. Comp. Neurol. 260: 256–298.

8. DE SOUZA, E. B., T. R. INSEL, M. H. PERRIN, J. RIVIER, W. W. VALE & M. J. KUHAR. 1985. Corticotropin-releasing factor receptors are widely distributed within the rat central nervous system: An autoradiographic study. J. Neurosci. 5: 3189–3203.

9. DE SOUZA, E. B. 1987. Corticotropin-releasing factor receptors in the rat central nervous system: Characterization and regional distribution. J. Neurosci. 7: 88–100.

10. HAUGER, R. L., M. MILLAN, M. LORANG, J. HARWOOD & G. AGUILERA. 1988. Corticotropin-releasing factor receptors and pituitary adrenal responses during immobilization stress. Endocrinology 123: 396–405.

11. BRITTON, K. T., M. VARELA, A. GARCIA & M. ROSENTHAL. 1986. Dexamethasone suppresses pituitary-adrenal but not behavioral effects of centrally administered CRF. Life Sci. 38: 211–216.

12. BRITTON, K. T., G. LEE, W. VALE & G. F. KOOB. 1986. Corticotropin-releasing factor (CRF) receptor antagonist blocks activating and "anxiogenic" actions of CRF in the rat. Brain Res. 369: 303–306.

13. BROWN, M. R., L. A. FISHER, J. SPIESS, C. RIVIER, J. RIVIER & W. VALE. 1982. Corticotropin-releasing factor: Actions on the sympathetic nervous system and metabolism. Endocrinology 111: 928–931.

14. FISHER, L. A. 1989. Corticotropin-releasing factor: Endocrine and autonomic integration of responses to stress. Trends Pharmacol. Sci. 10: 189–193.

15. NEMEROFF, C. B., M. J. OWENS, G. BISSETTE, A. C. ANDORN & M. STANLEY. 1988. Reduced corticotropin-releasing factor binding sites in the frontal cortex of suicide victims. Arch. Gen. Psychiatry 45: 577–579.

16. NEMEROFF, C. B. & M. J. OWENS. 1989. Preclinical and clinical investigations of corticotropin-releasing factor: Assessment of its role in depressive disorders. *In* New Directions in Affective Disorders. B. Lerer & S. Gershon, Eds.: 262–266. Springer-Verlag. New York.

17. BUTLER, P. & C. B. NEMEROFF. 1988. Corticotropin-releasing factor as a possible cause of comorbidity in anxiety and depressive disorders. *In* Comorbidity of Mood and Anxiety Disorders. J. D. Maser & C. R. Cloninger, Eds.: 413–435. American Psychiatry Press, Inc. Washington, D.C.

18. BUTLER, P., J. M. WEISS, J. C. STOUT & C. B. NEMEROFF. 1990. Corticotropin-releasing factor produces fear-enhancing and behavioral activating effects following infusion into the locus coeruleus. J. Neurosci. **10:** 176–183.

19. BRITTON, K. T., J. MORGAN, J. RIVIER, W. VALE & G. F. KOOB. 1985. Chlordiazepoxide attenuates response suppression induced by corticotropin-releasing factor in the conflict test. Psychopharmacology **86:** 170–174.

20. ROY-BYRNE, P. P., T. W. UHDE, R. M. POST, W. GALLUCCI, G. P. CHROUSOS & P. W. GOLD. 1986. The corticotropin-releasing hormone stimulation test in patients with panic disorder. Am. J. Psychiatry **143:** 896–899.

21. SMITH, M. A., J. DAVIDSON, J. C. RITCHIE, H. KUDLER, S. LIPPER, P. CHAPPELL & C. B. NEMEROFF. 1989. The corticotropin-releasing hormone test in patients with post-traumatic stress disorder. Biol. Psychiatry **26:** 349–355.

22. CHAPPELL, P. B., M. A. SMITH, C. D. KILTS, G. BISSETTE, J. RITCHIE, C. ANDERSON & C. B. NEMEROFF. 1986. Alterations in corticotropin-releasing factor-like immunoreactivity in discrete rat brain regions after acute and chronic stress. J. Neurosci. **6:** 2908–2914.

23. OWENS, M. J., G. BISSETTE & C. B. NEMEROFF. 1989. Acute effects of alprazolam and adinazolam on the concentrations of corticotropin-releasing factor in the rat brain. Synapse **4:** 196–202.

24. HESTER, J. B., JR., A. D. RUDZIK & B. V. KAMDAR. 1971. 6-Phenyl-^{4}H-s-triazolo[4,3-a] [1,4]benzodiazepines which have central nervous system depressant activity. J. Med. Chem. **14:** 1078–1081.

25. HESTER, J. B. & P. VOIGTLANDER. 1979. 6-Aryl-^{4}H-s-triazolo[4,3-a][1,4] benzodiazepines. Influences of 1-substitution on pharmacological activity. J. Med. Chem. **22:** 1390–1398.

26. HESTER, J. B., JR., A. D. RUDZIK & P. F. VON VOIGTLANDER. 1980. 1-(Aminoalkyl)-6-aryl-^{4}H-s-triazolo[4,3-a][1,4]benzodiazepines with antianxiety and antidepressant activity. J. Med. Chem. **23:** 392–402.

27. LATHI, R. A., V. H. SETHY, C. BARSUHN & J. B. HESTER. 1983. Pharmacological profile of the antidepressant adinazolam, a triazolobenzodiazepine. Neuropharmacology **22:** 1277–1282.

28. AMSTERDAM, J. D., M. KAPLAN, L. POTTER, L. BLOOM & K. RICKELS. 1986. Adinazolam, a new triazolobenzodiazepine, and imipramine in the treatment of major depressive disorder. Psychopharmacology **88:** 484–488.

29. DUNNER, D., J. MYERS, A. KHAN, D. AVERY, D. ISHIKI & R. PYKE. 1987. Adinazolam—a new antidepressant: Findings of a placebo-controlled, double-blind study in outpatients with major depression. J. Clin. Psychopharmacol. **7:** 170–172.

30. FAWCETT, J., J. H. EDWARDS, H. M. KRAVITZ & H. JEFFRIESS. 1987. Alprazolam: An antidepressant? Alprazolam, desipramine, and alprazolam-desipramine combination in the treatment of adult depressed outpatients. J. Clin. Psychopharmacol. **7:** 295–310.

31. FEIGHNER, J. P., G. C. ADEN, L. F. FABRE, K. RICKELS & W. T. SMITH. 1983. Comparison of alprazolam, imipramine, and placebo in the treatment of depression. J. Am. Med. Assoc. **249:** 3057–3064.

32. RICKELS, K., H. R. CHUNG, I. B. CSANALOSI, A. M. HUROWITZ, J. LONDON, K. WISEMAN, M. KAPLAN & J. D. AMSTERDAM. 1987. Alprazolam, diazepam, imipramine, and placebo in outpatients with major depression. 1987. Arch. Gen. Psychiatry **44:** 862–866.

33. KALOGERAS, K. T., A. E. CALOGERO, T. KURIBAYIASHI, I. KHAN, W. T. GALLUCCI, M. A. KLING, G. P. CHROUSOS & P. W. GOLD. 1990. In vitro and in vivo effects of

the triazolobenzodiazepine alprazolam on hypothalamic-pituitary-adrenal function: Pharmacological and clinical implications. J. Clin. Endocrinol. Metab. **70**: 1462–1471.
34. GRIGORIADIS, D. E., D. PEARSALL & E. B. DE SOUZA. 1989. Effects of chronic antidepressant and benzodiazepine treatment on corticotropin-releasing factor receptors in rat brain and pituitary. Neuropsychopharmacology **2**: 53–60.
35. OWENS, M. J., M. A. VARGAS, D. L. KNIGHT & C. B. NEMEROFF. 1991. The effects of alprazolam on corticotropin-releasing factor neurons in the rat brain: Acute time course, chronic treatment and abrupt withdrawal. J. Pharmacol. Exp. Ther. **258**: 349–356.
36. VALENTINO, R. J., S. L. FOOTE & G. ASTON-JONES. 1983. Corticotropin-releasing factor activates noradrenergic neurons on the locus coeruleus. Brain Res. **270**: 363–367.
37. BLOOM, F. E. 1979. Norepinephrine mediated synaptic transmission and hypotheses of psychiatric disorders. *In* Research in the Psychobiology of Human Behavior. E. Meyer III & J. Brady, Eds.: 1–11. The Johns Hopkins University Press. Baltimore.
38. KLEIN, D. F. 1987. Anxiety reconceptualized. Gleaning from pharmacological dissection – Early experience with imipramine and anxiety. *In* Anxiety. D. F. Klein, Ed.: 1–35. Karger. Basel.
39. REDMOND, D. E., JR. 1987. Studies of the nucleus locus coeruleus in monkeys and hypotheses for neuropsychopharmacology. *In* Psychopharmacology: The Third Generation of Progress. H. Y. Meltzer, Ed.: 967–976. Raven Press. New York.
40. VAN THIEL, D. 1983. Adrenal response to ethanol: A stress response. *In* Stress and Alcohol Use. L. A. Pohorecky & J. Brick, Eds.: 23–27. Elsevier. Amsterdam.
41. ELLIS, F. W. 1966. Effect of ethanol on plasma corticosterone levels. J. Pharmacol. Exp. Ther. **153**: 121–127.
42. TABAKOFF, B., R. C. JAFFE & R. F. RITZMANN. 1978. Corticosterone concentrations in mice during ethanol drinking and withdrawal. J. Pharm. Pharmacol. **30**: 371–374.
43. KAKIHANA, R. & J. A. MOORE. 1976. Circadian rhythm of corticosterone in mice: The effect of chronic consumption of alcohol. Psychopharmacology (Berlin) **46**: 301–305.
44. KNYCH, E. T. & J. R. PROHASKA. 1981. Effect of chronic intoxication and naloxone on the ethanol-induced increase in plasma corticosterone. Life Sci. **28**: 1987–1994.
45. JENKINS, J. S. & J. CONNOLLY. 1968. Adrenocortical response to ethanol in man. Br. Med. J. **2**: 804–805.
46. WRIGHT, J. 1983. Endocrine effects of alcohol. Clin. Endocrinol. Metab. **7**: 351–367.
47. SMALS, A. G. H., K. T. NJO, J. M. KNOBEN, C. M. RULAND & P. W. C. KLOPPENBORG. 1977. Alcohol-induced Cushingoid syndrome. J. R. Coll. Physicians Lond. **12**: 36–41.
48. REES, L. H., G. M. BESSER, W. J. JEFFCOATE, D. J. GOLDIE & V. MARKS. 1977. Alcohol-induced Pseudo-Cushing's syndrome. Lancet **4/2**: 726–728.
49. LAMBERTS, S. W. J., J. G. M. KLIJN, F. H. DE JONG & J. C. BIRKENHAGER. 1979. Hormone secretion in alcohol-induced Pseudo-Cushing's syndrome. J. Am. Med. Assoc. **242**: 1640–1643.
50. JENKINS, R. M. & M. McB. PAGE. 1981. Atypical case of alcohol-induced Cushingoid syndrome. Br. Med. J. **282**: 1117–1118.
51. FINK, R. S., F. SHORT, D. H. MARGOT & V. H. T. JAMES. 1981. Abnormal suppression of plasma cortisol during the intravenous infusion of dexamethasone to alcoholic patients. Clin. Endocrinol. **15**: 97–102.
52. SWARTZ, C. M. & F. J. DUNNER. 1982. Dexamethasone suppression testing of alcoholics. Arch. Gen. Psychiatry **39**: 1309–1312.
53. NEWSOM, G. & N. MURRAY. 1983. Reversal of dexamethasone suppression test nonsuppression in alcohol abusers. Am. J. Psychiatry **140**: 353–354.
54. KROLL, P., C. PALMER & J. F. GREDEN. 1983. The dexamethasone suppression test in patients with alcoholism. Biol. Psychiatry. **18**: 441–450.
55. ABOU-SALEH, M. T., J. MERRY & A. COPPEN. 1984. Dexamethasone suppression test in alcoholism. Acta Psychiatr. Scand. **69**: 112–116.
56. TARGUM, S. D., A. E. CAPODANNO, S. UNGER & M. ADVANI. 1984. Abnormal dexamethasone tests in withdrawing alcoholic patients. Biol. Psychiatry. **19**: 401–405.
57. DEL PORTO, J. A., M. G. MONTEIRO, R. R. LARANJEIRA, M. R. JORGE & J. MASUR. 1985. Reversal of abnormal dexamethasone suppression test in alcoholics abstinent for four weeks. Biol. Psychiatry. **20**: 1156–1160.

58. RIVIER, C., T. BRUHN & W. VALE. 1984. Effect of ethanol on the hypothalamic-pituitary-adrenal axis in the rat: Role of corticotropin-releasing factor (CRF). J. Pharmacol. Exp. Ther. **229**: 127–131.
59. EHLERS, C. L. & R. I. CHAPLIN. 1987. Chronic ethanol exposure potentiates the locomotor-activating effects of corticotropin-releasing factor (CRF) in rats. Regul. Pept. **19**: 345–353.
60. MENDELSON, J. H. & S. STEIN. 1966. Serum cortisol levels in alcoholic and nonalcoholic subjects during experimentally induced ethanol intoxication. Psychosom. Med. **28**: 616–626.
61. RIVIER, C., J. RIVIER & W. VALE. 1982. Inhibition of adrenocorticotrophic hormone secretion in the rat by immunoneutralization of corticotropin-releasing factor (CRF). Science **218**: 377–378.
62. DAVIDOFF, L. A. 1973. Alcohol and presynaptic inhibition in an isolated spinal cord preparation. Arch. Neurol. **28**: 60–63.
63. COTT, C. F., J. CARLSSON, J. A. ENGEL & M. LINDQVIST. 1976. Suppression of ethanol-induced locomotor stimulation by GABA-like drugs. Arch. Pharmacol. **295**: 203–209.
64. LILJEQUIST, S. & J. A. ENGEL. 1982. Effects of GABAergic agonist and antagonist on various ethanol-induced behavioral changes. Psychopharmacology **78**: 71–75.
65. NESTOROS, J. N. 1980. Ethanol specifically potentiates GABA-mediated neurotransmission in feline cerebral cortex. Science **209**: 708–710.
66. MANCILLAS, J. R., G. R. SIGGINS & F. E. BLOOM. 1986. Systemic ethanol: Selective enhancement of responses to acetylcholine and somatostatin in hippocampus. Science **231**: 161–163.
67. DAVIS, W. C. & M. K. TICKU. 1981. Ethanol enhances [^{3}H] diazepam binding at the benzodiazepine-GABA receptor-ionophore complex. Mol. Pharmacol. **20**: 287–294.
68. GREENBERG, D. A., E. C. COOPER, A. GORDON & I. DIAMOND. 1984. Ethanol and the γ-aminobutyric acid-benzodiazepine receptor complex. J. Neurochem. **42**: 1062–1068.
69. KOOB, G. F., R. E. STRECKER & F. BLOOM. 1980. Effects of naloxone on the anticonflict properties of alcohol and chlordiazepoxide. Subst. Alcohol Actions Misuse **1**: 447–457.
70. LILJEQUIST, S. & J. A. ENGEL. 1984. The effects of GABA and benzodiazepine receptor antagonists on the anti-conflict actions of diazepam or ethanol. Pharmacol. Biochem. Behav. **21**: 521–525.
71. BELLEVILLE, R. E. & H. F. FRASER. 1957. Tolerance to some effects of barbiturates. J. Pharmacol. Exp. Ther. **120**: 469–474.
72. GOLDSTEIN, D. B. 1973. Alcohol withdrawal reactions in mice: Effects of drugs that modify neurotransmission. J. Pharmacol. Exp. Ther. **186**: 1–9.
73. OLSEN, R. W. 1981. GABA-benzodiazepine-barbiturate receptor interactions. J. Neurochem. **37**: 1–13.
74. SKOLNICK, P. & S. M. PAUL. 1982. Benzodiazepine receptors in the central nervous system. Int. Rev. of Neurobiol. **23**: 103–140.
75. SUZDAK, P. D., R. D. SCHWARTZ, P. SKOLNICK & S. M. PAUL. 1988. Alcohol stimulates γ-aminobutyric acid receptor-mediated chloride uptake in brain vesicles: Correlation with intoxication potency. Brain Res. **444**: 340–345.
76. CALOGERO, A. E., W. T. GALLUCCI, G. P. CHROUSOS & P. W. GOLD. 1988. Interaction between GABAergic neurotransmission and rat hypothalamic corticotropin-releasing hormone secretion in vitro. Brain Res. **463**: 28–36.

Alterations in Biodistribution of 11C-Methamphetamine (MAP), 14C-MAP, and 123I-N-Isopropyl-Iodoamphetamine (IMP) in MAP- and Cocaine-sensitized Animals

YOHTARO NUMACHI, SUMIKO YOSHIDA,
TAKAO INOSAKA, AND MITSUMOTO SATO

Department of Psychiatry
Tohoku University School of Medicine
1-1 Seiryo-machi, Aoba-ku
Sendai Miyagi 980, Japan

MICHINAO MIZUGAKI, KATSUHIKO KIMURA,
AND TAKANORI HISHINUMA

Department of Pharmaceutical Sciences
Tohoku University Hospital
1-1 Seiryo-machi, Aoba-ku
Sendai Miyagi 980, Japan

INTRODUCTION

The behavioral sensitization induced by repeated administration of amphetamine (AMP), methamphetamine (MAP), and cocaine to experimental animals is widely used as an experimental model of stimulant-induced psychosis. Because AMP- and MAP-induced behavioral hypersensitivity is accompanied by an increased releasability of dopamine (DA) in the striatum and nucleus accumbens, enhanced synaptic transmission of DA neurons has been implicated in such behavioral sensitization, but the precise mechanism of this long-term increase in DA releasability is unknown.

In the present study, we investigate the alterations in biodistribution (especially in the brain) of 11C-MAP (Experiment 1), 14C-MAP (Experiment 2) and 123I-IMP (Experiment 3) in MAP- and cocaine-sensitized animals to study the mechanism involved in increased dopaminergic transmission and behavioral sensitization.

METHODS

Animals and Drug Schedule

In experiment 1, male ddY mice initially weighing 30–35 g were used. The experimental animals were housed under a 12-h light-dark cycle with free access to food and

153

water. The animals were injected intraperitoneally (i.p.) with 2 mg/kg of MAP hydrochloride (Dainippon Co., Japan) once daily for 7 consecutive days. The control animals
received an equal volume of saline for the same length of time. In experiment 2 and
3, male Sprague-Dawley rats (Clea Co., Japan) initially weighing 210–240 g were used.
The experimental animals were housed 4 to 5 per cage under a 12-h light-dark cycle
with free access to food and water. The animals in experiment 2 were injected with
4 mg/kg (i.p.) of MAP hydrochloride (Dainippon Co., Japan) once daily for 21 consecutive days. The animals in experiment 3 were injected with 4 mg/kg (i.p.) of MAP
hydrochloride and 20 mg/kg (i.p.) of cocaine hydrochloride (Takeda Co., Japan), respectively, once daily for 21 consecutive days. The control animals received an equal
volume of saline for the same length of time. On the 1st and the 21st days, the stereotyped behavior of the MAP- and the cocaine-treated rats was scored, using a stereotypy
rating scale of Creese and Iversen,[1] 30 min after the administration of the drug. The
statistical significance of the behavioral results was evaluated with the Mann-Whitney
U-test (two-tailed).

Synthesis of ^{11}C- and ^{14}C-MAP

^{11}C-MAP: For a simple and speedy method of observing the biodistribution, ^{11}C-
MAP was synthesized by the direct methylation of AMP using the ^{11}C-CO_2 devel-
oped by the Tohoku University Cyclotron Radioisotope Center. The synthesized ^{11}C-
MAP was then purified as a marker by high performance liquid chromatography
(HPLC). Then after its conversion to hydrochloride salt, it was used for experiment 1.
The radiochemical yield was 3 Ci/mmol at the end of the supply.

^{14}C-MAP: ^{14}C-MAP was synthesized by the N-(^{14}C-) methylation method using
trifluoroacetylamphetamine and purified by column chromatography and HPLC.
After its conversion to hydrochloride salt, it was used for experiment 2.

^{123}I-IMP: ^{123}I-IMP was purchased from Nihon Mediphysics Co. (Japan).

Brain Distribution of ^{11}C-MAP, ^{14}C-MAP and ^{123}I-IMP

Experiment 1

^{11}C-MAP (19.3 microCi/head) was applied to the MAP- and saline-treated mice 7
days after the last MAP or saline treatment. After a 15-min interval, the mice were
decapitated. The brains were dissected according to the method of Glowinski and
Iversen,[2] and radioactive distributions were determined.

Experiment 2

^{14}C-MAP (0.1 microCi/head) was applied to the MAP- and saline-pretreated rats
7 days after the last MAP or saline treatment. After a 30-min interval, the rats were
decapitated, and the striatum and limbic forebrain area (the nucleus accumbens plus
olfactory tubercle) were dissected according to an atlas of Pellegrino, Pellegrino and
Cushman.[3] The radioactivity of each brain region was counted with a liquid scintillation counter (LSC–1000, Aloka) and the differential absorption ratio (DAR) was
calculated.

Experiment 3

¹²³I-IMP (10 microCi/head) was applied to the cocaine-, MAP-, and saline-treated rats 7 days after the last treatment. In the cocaine-treated group, rats were decapitated after a 30-min interval. In the MAP-treated group, rats were decapitated after 30-min, 1-h and 2-h intervals. The striatum and limbic forebrain area (the nucleus accumbens plus olfactory tubercle) were dissected according to the above mentioned atlas. The radioactivity of each brain region was counted by a well-type gamma counter (ARC-501, Aloka) and the DAR was calculated.

The statistical significance of DAR was evaluated with the Student's *t*-test.

RESULTS

Behavioral Sensitization

In experiments 2 and 3, the stereotypy rating scores on the 21st days were significantly greater than scores on the 1st day for both MAP-pretreated animals and cocaine-pretreated animals ($p < 0.01$).

Brain Distribution of ¹¹C-MAP, ¹⁴C-MAP and ¹²³I-IMP

Experiment 1

DAR of ¹¹C-MAP in the striatum and hypothalamus of the MAP-pretreated mice was higher than that of saline-treated controls (FIG. 1).

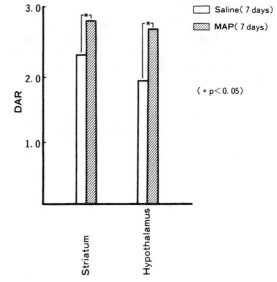

FIGURE 1. DAR of ¹¹C-MAP in the striatum and hypothalamus of the MAP-pretreated mice. DAR of ¹¹C-MAP in the striatum and hypothalamus of the MAP-pretreated mice was significantly higher than that of saline-pretreated controls (*: $p < 0.05$).

TABLE 1. DAR ^{14}C-MAP in Striatum and Limbic Forebrain Area

Brain Region	DAR	
	Saline-control	MAP-pretreatment
	*a	
Striatum	6.11 ± 1.56	22.68 ± 2.77
	(n = 7)	(n = 7)
	**	
Limbic forebrain	4.86 ± 1.18	31.69 ± 2.92
	(n = 8)	(n = 5)

^{a} *: $p < 0.05$ and **: $p < 0.01$.

Experiment 2

DAR increased significantly by 370% in the striatum ($p < 0.005$, n = 7) and by 650% in the limbic forebrain area ($p < 0.01$, n = 7) of the MAP-sensitized rats (TABLE 1).

Experiment 3

No difference was found in DAR between cocaine-sensitized rats and control rats 30 min after ^{123}I-IMP administration (TABLE 2). There was no difference in DAR between MAP-sensitized rats and controls rats 30 min, 1 h and 2 h after ^{123}I-IMP administration (TABLE 3).

DISCUSSION

We newly synthesized ^{11}C-MAP and ^{14}C-MAP and investigated their biodistribution in cocaine- and MAP-pretreated animals. The results of the present study first revealed the lasting and significant increase in both ^{11}C-MAP radioactivity in the striatum and hypothalamus of MAP-pretreated mice, and ^{14}C-MAP radioactivity in the striatum and limbic forebrain of MAP-sensitized rats. This finding is considered to be

TABLE 2. DAR of ^{123}I-IMP in the Cocaine-sensitized Rats and Controls

Brain Region	DAR	
	Saline-control	Cocaine-pretreatment
Striatum	4.02 ± 1.08	4.59 ± 0.98
	(n = 9)	(n = 10)
Limbic forebrain	3.37 ± 0.88	3.99 ± 0.81
	(n = 9)	(n = 10)
Cerebellum	3.12 ± 1.24	3.85 ± 0.96
	(n = 10)	(n = 10)

TABLE 3. DAR of ¹²³I-IMP in the MAP-sensitized Rats and Controls

Brain Region	Pretreatment	30 Minutes	DAR 1 Hour	2 Hours
Striatum	Saline	3.94 ± 0.14 (*n* = 5)	3.03 ± 0.57 (*n* = 3)	3.68 ± 0.26 (*n* = 4)
	MAP	3.60 ± 0.47 (*n* = 7)	3.36 ± 0.55 (*n* = 7)	3.58 ± 0.16 (*n* = 7)
Limbic forebrain	Saline	3.44 ± 0.13 (*n* = 5)	2.53 ± 0.32 (*n* = 3)	3.23 ± 0.12 (*n* = 4)
	MAP	3.17 ± 0.30 (*n* = 7)	2.93 ± 0.48 (*n* = 8)	3.73 ± 0.39 (*n* = 8)
Cerebellum	Saline	3.49 ± 0.11 (*n* = 6)	2.51 ± 0.51 (*n* = 3)	2.89 ± 0.11 (*n* = 4)
	MAP	3.37 ± 0.31 (*n* = 7)	2.79 ± 0.43 (*n* = 8)	2.55 ± 0.52 (*n* = 8)

important in discussing the mechanism involved in enhanced dopaminergic transmission, which has been implicated in behavioral sensitization. Kazahaya et al.[4] found that challenge injection of either cocaine or MAP after a 7-day interval free from chronic MAP treatment caused a marked increase in striatal DA efflux *in vivo* under behavioral sensitization in the MAP-sensitized rats. They concluded that the enhanced efflux of DA in the synaptic cleft may play a role in MAP-induced behavioral sensitization and cross-sensitization to cocaine. This finding is consistent with earlier findings by Robinson and Becker,[5] Kolta et al.[6] and Yamada et al.[7] that the AMP-stimulated release of DA increased in striatal slices of sensitized animals. In addition, Robinson et al.[8] found that AMP-induced long-term hypersensitivity was accompanied by a significantly elevated DA release in the nucleus accumbens of rats subjected to previous repeated AMP treatment. They also noted no change in the basal extracellular concentrations of DA, and concluded that the sensitization produced by chronic AMP use was due to the releasability of DA. Thus, MAP- and AMP-induced behavioral hypersensitivity appears, at least partially, to be due to an increased releasability of DA in the striatum and nucleus accumbens but the precise mechanism of this long-term increase in DA releasability is unknown. Reviewing previous reports, Robinson and Becker[9] pointed out two possibilities: i) the regulation of DA release by subsensitive autoreceptors which are located on the presynaptic terminals, and ii) presynaptic facilitation by hyperpolarization of the DA terminal via a presynaptic input or a shift in the distribution of DA terminal via a presynaptic input or a shift in the distribution of DA from a storage pool to a more releasable pool. As for ii), Paulson and Robinson[10] suggest that neural adaptations in DA terminal fields are sufficient for the expression of AMP sensitization, although an action on DA cell bodies may be required for the induction of AMP sensitization. In addition, Akiyama et al.[11] found that ouabain infusion into striatum of MAP-sensitized rats caused a significant increase in DA efflux, using *in vivo* dialysis. They suggest that subchronic MAP treatment causes some functional changes in DA transporting systems that are involved in DA release and uptake on presynaptic DA terminals.

A mechanism of exchange diffusion at the DA uptake carrier has been proposed as the method by which the releasing amines, such as MAP, stimulate the release of DA.[12] Exchange diffusion is a model in which the movement of releasing amines into synaptosomes stimulates the efflux of DA from the synaptosomes. The present finding of a lasting increase in [14]C- and ^{11}C-MAP radioactivity in the brain structures that include striatum and nucleus accumbens of MAP-sensitized animals and the previous findings of prominent cross-sensitivity to cocaine than to L-dopa and apomorphine in MAP-sensitized cats[13] suggest that subchronic MAP administration may result in a long-term change in the presynaptic cell membrane at the nerve terminal which may in turn cause an increase in both MAP and DA uptake accompanied by an increased release of DA at the synaptic cleft. For future clinical application of our finding of increased [11]C- and ^{14}C-MAP accumulation, we evaluated brain distribution of ^{123}I-IMP in MAP- or cocaine-sensitized rats, while no difference was found between sensitized animals and the control animals. This impaired membrane theory should be further examined using a tracer that reflects lasting changes in DA terminals.

SUMMARY

Alterations in brain distribution of ^{11}C-MAP, ^{14}C-MAP, and ^{123}I-IMP in MAP- and cocaine-sensitized animals were examined to investigate the mechanism involved in increased dopaminergic transmission and behavioral sensitization. First, a significant increase in ^{11}C-MAP radioactivity in the striatum and hypothalamus was found in the mice pretreated with MAP for 7 days. Secondly, in MAP-sensitized rats, marked increases in ^{14}C-MAP radioactivity were found in the striatum and limbic forebrain, respectively (370% and 650%). These findings may propose a new hypothesis that subchronic MAP administration may result in a long-term change in the presynaptic cell membrane at the nerve terminal which may in turn cause an increase in both MAP and DA uptake accompanied by an increased release of DA at the synaptic cleft.

REFERENCES

1. CREESE, I. & S. D. IVERSEN. 1973. Blockade of amphetamine induced motor stimulation and stereotypy in the adult rat following neonatal treatment with 6-hydroxydopamine. Brain Res. 55: 369–382.
2. GLOVINSKI, J. & L. L. IVERSEN. 1966. Regional studies of catecholamines in the rat brain-1: The disposition of [3H]norepinephrine, [3H]dopamine and [3H]dopa in various regions of the brain. J. Neurochem. 13: 655–669.
3. PELLEGRINO, L. J., A. S. PELLEGRINO & A. J. CUSHMAN. 1986. A Stereotaxic Atlas of the Rat Brain. 2nd edit. Plenum Press. New York.
4. KAZAHAYA, Y., K. AKIMOTO & S. OTSUKI. 1989. Subchronic methamphetamine treatment enhances methamphetamine- or cocaine-induced dopamine efflux in vivo. Biol. Psychiatry 25: 903–912.
5. ROBINSON, T. E. & J. B. BECKER. 1982. Behavioral sensitization is accompanied by enhancement in amphetamine-stimulated dopamine release from striatal tissue in vitro. Eur. J. Pharmacol. 85: 253–254.
6. KOLTA, M. G., P. SHREVE, V. DE SOUZA & N. J. URETSKY. 1985. Time course of the development of the enhanced behavioral and biochemical responses to amphetamine after pretreatment with amphetamine. Neuropharmacology 24: 823–829.
7. YAMADA, S., H. KOJIMA, H. YOKOO, K. TSUTSUMI, K. TAKAMUKI, S. ANRAKU, S. NISHI

& K. INANAGA. 1988. Enhancement of dopamine release from striatal slices of rats that were subchronically treated with methamphetamine. Biol. Psychiatry **24:** 399–408.

8. ROBINSON, T. E., P. A. JURSON, J. A. BENNETT & K. M. BENTGEN. 1988. Persistent sensitization of dopamine neurotransmission in ventral striatum (nucleus accumbens) produced by prior experience with (+)-amphetamine: A microdialysis study in freely moving rats. Brain Res. **462:** 211–222.

9. ROBINSON, T. E. & J. B. BECKER. 1986. Enduring changes in brain and behavior produced by chronic amphetamine administration: A review and evaluation of animal models of amphetamine psychosis. Brain Res. Rev. **11:** 157–198.

10. PAULSON, P. E. & T. E. ROBINSON. 1991. Sensitization to systemic amphetamine produces an enhanced locomotor response to a subsequent intra-accumbens amphetamine challenge in rats. Psychopharmacology **104:** 140–141.

11. KANZAKI, A., K. AKIYAMA, K. OKUMURA, H. UJIKE & S. OTSUKI. 1990. Effect of chronic methamphetamine on Na⁺, K⁺-ATPase in rats. Bull. Jpn. Neurochem. Soc. **29:** 142–143. (In Japanese.)

12. FISCHER, J. F. & A. K. CHO. 1979. Chemical release of dopamine from striatal homogenates: Evidence for an exchange diffusion model. J. Pharmacol. Exp. Ther. **208:** 203–209.

13. SATO, M. 1979. An experimental study of onset and relapsing mechanisms of chronic methamphetamine psychosis. Psychiat. Neurol. Jpn. **81:** 21–31. (In Japanese.)

A Lasting Vulnerability to Psychosis in Patients with Previous Methamphetamine Psychosis

MITSUMOTO SATO

Department of Psychiatry
Tohoku University School of Medicine
1-1 Seiryo-machi, Aoba-ku
Sendai Miyagi 980, Japan

INTRODUCTION

A number of cases of methamphetamine (MAP) psychosis were reported during the previous epidemic of MAP abuse (1945–1954) in Japan. Those reports indicated that the main cross-sectional clinical feature of this type of psychosis was a paranoid psychotic state with auditory or visual hallucination almost indistinguishable from schizophrenia. The duration of such episodes of paranoid psychosis was also reported to sometimes last quite long after excretion of MAP in the urine (see review in Sato and Kashihara,[1] 1986). Brain damage produced gradually during the period of chronic abuse of intravenous MAP (mostly 20–30 mg/shot) has been presumed to be the cause of MAP psychosis, its prolongation after excretion of MAP and the lasting susceptibility to relapse. However, the number of intensive studies to identify such brain damage decreased with the end of the first epidemic. Once again, an increasing number of patients with MAP psychosis, especially those with episodes of psychotic relapse (43%), has been reported in a second epidemic (1970–present). The brain damage produced secondarily during chronic abuse of MAP has called out attention to the need to investigate a possible lasting vulnerability to paranoid psychotic features in MAP psychosis.[2] Thus, the traditional Japanese concept of MAP psychosis, namely, that the psychotic episode develops on a base of MAP-induced brain damage appears essentially different from Connell's concept in which the psychotic episode is seen to be caused directly by the psychotogenic action of amphetamine (acute intoxication) and is never prolonged after excretion of amphetamine in the urine.[3] Clinical studies to examine this discrepancy often face difficulties due to the combined use of multiple drugs, a lack of urine test data for ethical reasons, and insufficient information on patterns of drug abuse, duration, and clinical features of the psychotic episodes. In Japan, MAP abuse is not usually accompanied by abuse of other controlled drugs such as cocaine, heroin, and marijuana. This situation in Japan provides an opportunity to investigate the long-term clinical course of MAP dependence in relation to evolution of MAP psychosis. The purpose of this study was to review previous studies on MAP-induced vulnerability of the brain to psychotic episodes with schizophrenic symptoms in light of the clinical studies reported mainly during the second epidemic of MAP abuse in Japan.

METHODS

To evaluate the nature of vulnerability to psychotic episodes in MAP psychosis, clinical studies after 1970 in Japan that reported recurrence of psychotic episodes in the second epidemic were selected mainly based on the following criteria: i) they included a detailed description of the clinical features and course, and ii) they contained reliable information on the status of intravenous MAP injections reported by a third person (usually a family member).

In addition, the findings of experimental studies using animals sensitized to MAP after repeated systemic administration of MAP for more than 2 weeks were selected to allow discussion of possible neuromechanisms of the vulnerability.

CLINICAL FEATURES OF MAP PSYCHOSIS

In the first epidemic of MAP abuse, Hayashi[4] (1955) and Tatetsu et al.[5] (1957) reported the incidence of the paranoid psychotic state with hallucinations to be 90% and 92%, respectively. Connell[3] also reported that the clinical picture of amphetamine psychosis was primarily that of paranoid psychosis with ideas of reference, delusions of persecution, and auditory and visual hallucinations, in a state of clear consciousness. He also indicated that the clinical picture may be indistinguishable from acute or chronic schizophrenia.

According to the studies reported in the second epidemic, a paranoid psychotic state with hallucinations appeared in more than 76.3% of the total cases (TABLE 1). When the studies that examined cross-sectional clinical features with questionnaire methods are excluded, the frequency of such psychotic features increases up to 90%, confirming the earlier findings of Hayashi and others. Based on these findings, the current concept of MAP psychosis in Japan has been defined as a paranoid psychotic state often accompanied by hallucinations, which develops in those with present or past MAP dependence. Sato et al.[7,14] reported that the symptoms of MAP psychosis included some symptoms also characteristic of the active phase of schizophrenia in DSM-III-R[15] or similar to Schneider's first rank symptoms.[16]

TABLE 1. Frequency of Paranoid Psychotic Features with Hallucinations in Methamphetamine Psychosis[a]

Authors	Subjects (n)	Frequency (%)
1st Epidemic (1945–1957)		
Hayashi, S.[4] (1955)	74	90
Tatetsu, M. et al.[5] (1957)	131	92
Aoki, Y.[17] (1958)	459	72.3*
2nd Epidemic (1970–present)		
Sato, M. et al.[7] (1982)	82	90
Konuma, S.[6] (1987)	192	80.2
Wada, K. & S. Fukui[18] (1991)	233	76.3**

[a] Multi-institutional examination with questionnaire at 6–12 months after discharge (*) or during administration in psychiatric wards.

TABLE 2. Comparison of Psychotic Relapses with the First Episode

	First Episodes (n = 21)		Relapsed Episodes (n = 16)	
Symptoms	n	%	n	%
Bizarre delusions[a]	5	23.8	6	37.5
Delusions with jealous or persecutory content	21	100	16	100
Auditory hallucinations	16	76.2	15	93.8
Visual hallucinations	8	38.1	7	43.8
Incoherence, loosening of associations	4	19	3	18.8

(Sato, M. et al.[14])

[a] Including delusions of being controlled, thought insertion, or thought broadcasting. No significant difference was found between the first and relapsed psychotic episodes (χ^2 test).

COMPARISON OF EPISODES OF LATER PSYCHOTIC RELAPSES WITH THE FIRST PSYCHOTIC EPISODE

The paranoid psychotic feature with hallucinations appears in both the first episode and subsequent episodes of relapses in MAP psychosis. In the second epidemic, cases with relapses of MAP psychosis admitted into psychiatric wards accounted for 43–49% of the total number of inpatients with MAP psychosis.[7,11] Cases characterized by frequent readmission due to episodes of psychotic relapses, i.e., more than 10 readmissions were also reported.[7,13] In those cases, clinical features of the episodes of psychotic relapses were compared with those of the first psychotic episodes (TABLE 2). Clinical features in both types of psychotic episodes were almost identical, and included symptoms such as bizarre delusions, delusions with jealous or persecutory content, auditory hallucinations, and incoherence or loosening of association. The frequency of hallucinations in the episodes of psychotic relapses was higher than that of the initial episodes.[14]

These results suggest that MAP abusers who had experienced the paranoid psychotic state with hallucinations acquired an established pattern of response to subsequent MAP with very similar psychotic episodes. In other words, long-term intravenous MAP abuse may produce a lasting vulnerability to psychotic episodes with schizophrenic symptoms.

DURATION OF MAP ABUSE REQUIRED FOR THE FIRST AND SUBSEQUENT PSYCHOTIC EPISODES

Results of the available reports are summarized in TABLE 3. In 75% of the patients admitted to the psychiatric wards at the time of the first psychotic episode, more than 3 months of MAP abuse was required for evolution of MAP psychosis, although there was a large variation among individuals. This variation may depend upon multiple factors other than disposition: e.g., the amount and quality of MAP, the routes of MAP intake, the combined use of alcohol or hypnotics, a previous history of solvent inha-

TABLE 3. Duration of MAP Abuse until the First and Subsequent Psychotic Episodes

Subjects and Duration	First Episode			Relapsed Episode 7 Reports[6,8-11]
	Tatetsu[5]	Konuma[6]	Sato[7]	
Number of subjects	100	136	35	73
Duration				
Within 1 week	–	8.8	0	100
1 week–1 month	6	4.4	0	0
1–3 months	19	9.6	8.6	0
3–6 months	23	8.1	8.6	0
6–12 months	27	16.1	2.8	0
More than 1 year	25	51.5	71.4	0
Undetermined	0	1.5	0	0

lation. Nevertheless, these findings indicate a gradual evolution of vulnerability to psychotic episodes with remarkable individual variation. Ellinwood et al.[19] divided the period of amphetamine abuse for evolving amphetamine psychosis into 3 stages: the early, intermediate and end stages. They noted curiosity with repetitive examining, searching, and sorting behaviors in the early stage; sustained suspiciousness in the intermediate stage; and ideas of reference, persecutory delusions, and hallucinations marked by a fearful, panic-stricken, agitated, overreactive state in the end stage. They also mentioned that the amphetamine psychosis develops over a period of time as the user gradually increases his or her intake of amphetamine to amounts ranging from 150 to 2,000 mg. However, MAP psychosis gradually developed even when the abusers injected a fixed amount of MAP ranging from 20 to 60 mg/day.[7]

Regarding 73 cases in 7 reports in TABLE 1 who were readmitted with episodes of psychotic relapses less than 1 week of MAP reabuse resulted in relapses, apparently less than the period of abuse leading up to the first episode. The decrease in the length of MAP abuse resulting in episodes of psychotic relapses indicates that a lasting sensitization to the psychotogenic action of MAP may have developed by the time of the first psychotic episode.

STATUS OF RELAPSE OF MAP PSYCHOSIS

Duration of MAP Abstinence and Amount of MAP Reuse

At least 27 cases with previous MAP psychosis were reported who again used MAP once or more after long-term abstinence from MAP (up to 5 years) and experienced acute exacerbation of a paranoid psychotic state almost identical to the initial psychotic episode (TABLE 4). Four of these cases relapsed following a single MAP reuse of an amount less than that initially used.[14] In the 8 patients, small doses of neuroleptics, e.g., 3 mg/day of haloperidol, prevented the acute recurrence of a psychotic state by MAP reuse. Subsequently, 3 of these 8 patients relapsed into a psychotic state following MAP reuse without concurrent haloperidol medication. These findings again indicate that vulnerability to paranoid psychotic episodes in cases with prior MAP psy-

TABLE 4. Relapse of MAP Psychosis with MAP Reuse

Authors	Duration of MAP Abstinence	Number of Cases
1) After reuse of lesser amount of MAP		
Sato, M.[8] (1978)	20 days–1 year	7
Sato, M. et al.[7] (1982)	1 month–5 years	16
Ebihara, H.[10] (1984)	more than 3 months	2
Takezaki, H.[12] (1984)	more than 3 years	1
Amagai, I.[21] (1987)	more than 3 months	1
2) Prevention of MAP-induced relapse by antipsychotics		
Sato, M. et al.[14] (1983)	1 month–5 years	8

chosis is the result of a long-term sensitization to the psychotogenic action of MAP, which endures long after MAP abstinence. The fact that small doses of haloperidol prevented relapse in cases of MAP reuse may suggest the possible involvement of central dopaminergic systems in such vulnerability.

Relapse after Alcohol Ingestion

Tohri and Fujimori[11] reported 5 patients with previous MAP psychosis whose episodes of psychotic relapses were due to ingestion of alcohol without MAP reuse (TABLE 5). These 5 cases had a long history of MAP abuse ranging from 3 to 24 years, and experienced relapses shortly after being discharged from the hospital or jail where they had discontinued abuse of MAP for 1 to 16 months. Four other reports include 22 cases with previous MAP psychosis who experienced relapses due to alcohol ingestion after long abstinence from MAP.[13,21-23] These observations may suggest that MAP-induced vulnerability can be activated not only by MAP reuse but also by alcohol ingestion. However, no information is available as to whether the acute pharmacological action of alcohol or the withdrawal from alcohol may precipitate such relapses.

Relapse without Substance Use

Twelve cases with previous MAP psychosis were reported in which a paranoid psychotic state similar to a MAP-induced psychotic episode with hallucinations recurred

TABLE 5. Relapse of MAP Psychosis after Alcohol Ingestion

Authors	Cases	Duration of MAP	Abstinence from MAP	Psychotic Features of Relapsed Episodes
Utena, H.[22] (1982)	1	more than 3 years	14 years	Paranoid hallucinatory
Suwaki, H.[23] (1985)	19	–	–	ditto
Amagai, I.[21] (1987)	1	more than 10 years	1 month	ditto
Nakatani, Y.[13] (1987)	1	more than 30 years	4 months	ditto
Tohri, K.[11] (1991)	5	more than 3 years	more than 1 month	ditto

TABLE 6. Relapse of MAP Psychosis without Substance Use

Case No.	Duration of MAP Abuse (years)	After Last Episode (months except as shown)	Life Events	Psychotic Features of Relapses
1[7]	4	2	divorce	Paranoid hallucinatory
2[6]	15	11	n.p.	ditto
3[6]	20	1	missing of wife & son	ditto
4[24]	10	1	discharge from jail	ditto
5[24]	13	2	n.p.	ditto
6[24]	12	3	n.p.	Paranoid state
7[24]	7	1	n.p.	Paranoid hallucinatory
8[24]	22	6	n.p.	ditto
9[11]	10	14	n.p.	ditto
10[11]	5	3	n.p.	ditto
11[12]	7	11 days	n.p.	ditto
12[12]	12	12 years	n.p.	ditto

despite the absence of substance use (TABLE 6). Whether the MAP-induced vulnerability of the brain may be activated by nonspecific factors including life events, such as in the case of schizophrenia, is an important question requiring investigation. For this reason, a representative case[9] is presented.

Case

A 42-year-old married male whose family history was unremarkable had been jailed for 1 year because of antisocial behavior at the age of 23. He had abused MAP intravenously since the age of 37 with 2 or 3 "runs" daily. In March 1977, the day after a MAP injection, he felt that someone was hiding in the ceiling and that people were walking beneath the floor. He felt panic, smelled foul odors in food, and was convinced he was under surveillance by "people in the background" using a strange machine. Frequently he heard a voice saying "he is escaping." He believed that his wife was being prostituted by the drug-seller. He had all her hair cut off and restricted her to the house until he went to the police asking for protection from someone trying to kill him. Under strict observation by relatives and a policeman, MAP abuse was discontinued and the above symptoms disappeared after several days. One month later, he reinjected one-third of the previous single amount (15 mg) of MAP. A second psychotic episode similar to the first recurred immediately. Again the symptoms were relieved by abstinence from MAP, under intensive observation by relatives. Thereafter, he remained in fair condition. On the night of April 19, 1979, he suddenly shouted, "I can't breath, no, no-, foul-," simultaneously becoming very violent. Members of his family denied that he had taken any stimulant prior to this third psychotic episode. He was admitted to Takaoka Hospital the next day where he received neuroleptics for 28 days. As he remained very suspicious and jealous when he was discharged, follow-up in the outpatient clinic continued for 9 months. Thereafter, the family did not notice any mental abnormality until a fourth episode occurred in January 1981. At that time, he was found standing at midnight, bowing toward the wall stereotypically. On re-admission to the hospital, paranoid delusions and auditory hallucinations were observed. Both he and his wife denied any MAP reuse, but his wife stated that he was agitated by the unexpected disclosure of his wife's original domicile, which had long been kept a secret from him.

NEUROMECHANISMS OF MAP-INDUCED VULNERABILITY TO PSYCHOTIC SYMPTOMS SIMILAR TO SCHIZOPHRENIA

Long-term Behavioral Sensitization

The characteristics in the course of MAP psychosis, namely, gradual evolution of the psychosis during chronic MAP abuse, prolongation of the psychotic episode after MAP excretion in the urine, episodes of psychotic relapses due to MAP reuse, alcohol ingestion and nonspecific factors other than substance abuse, and prevention of relapse with neuroleptics indicate a lasting vulnerability of the brain, presumably a lasting sensitization to the psychotogenic action of MAP with cross-sensitization to alcohol ingestion and psychological stressors. These characteristics may be reproduced in an animal model of MAP psychosis, which has been termed stimulant-induced lasting behavioral sensitization (LBS).

LBS characterized by stereotyped behavior or locomotor activities has been observed in many species of animals including primates. However, it is difficult to construct a behavioral index that reflects the psychotogenic action of the stimulants. In our previous study on cats, stereotypy not disrupted by loud noise was regarded arbitrarily as psychotic behavior because of the dissociation from the environment.[25] Such behavioral stereotypy developed 2 to 4 days after repeated administration of MAP at 4 to 6 mg/kg/day, and 13 to 18 days after 2 mg/kg/day of MAP. In these cats sensitized to MAP, stereotypy with dissociation was reproduced by an initially ineffective dose of MAP (1 or 2 mg/kg) 3 months after the end of repeated MAP administration. The cross-sensitization to a challenge dose of cocaine (5 mg/kg) was potent enough to reproduce the stereotypy with dissociation. The cross-sensitizations to 25 mg/kg of L-dopa and 0.4 mg/kg of apomorphine were positive, but not sensitive enough to reproduce the stereotypy with dissociation. These findings may suggest that the MAP and cocaine, rather than being direct or indirect dopamine agonists, may share common mechanisms for production of sensitized abnormal behavior.

Enhanced Increase of Dopamine Release in the Striatum and Nucleus Accumbens

Robinson and Becker,[26] Kolta et al.,[27] and Yamada et al.[28] reported that the amphetamine-induced release of dopamine was enhanced significantly in striatal slices of the rats with amphetamine-induced LBS. Moreover, in a microdialysis study, Robinson et al.[29] reported a marked hypersensitivity to the motor stimulating effects of an amphetamine challenge, which was accompanied by significant elevation of dopamine release in the nucleus accumbens of rats with amphetamine-induced LBS. They found no change in basal extracellular dopamine concentration. Kazahaya et al.[30] reported a significant enhancement of MAP- as well as a cocaine-induced increase in ex-

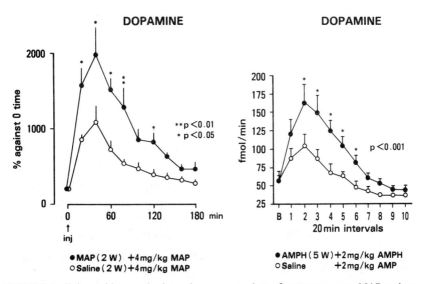

FIGURE 1. Enhanced increase in dopamine concentrations after reexposure to MAP and amphetamine in MAP- and amphetamine-sensitized rats. *Left*: Reexposure to MAP in MAP-sensitized rats. (striatum). (From Kazahaya *et al.*[30]) *Right*: Reexposure to amphetamine in amphetamine-sensitized rats. (nucleus accumbens). (From Robinson *et al.*[29])

tracellular dopamine concentration in the striatum of rats with MAP-induced LBS (FIG. 1).

Thus, stimulant-induced LBS to amphetamine and MAP are accompanied by a lasting enhancement of a stimulant-induced increase in dopamine release from nerve terminal fields of the striatum and nucleus accumbens, although no change was found in baseline dopamine concentration of extracellular dopamine in these structures.

A Possible Mechanism for Lasting Enhancement of MAP-induced Increase in Dopamine Release

Fischer and Cho[31] reported that dopamine and amphetamine share a common diffusion system for uptake into striatal homogenates, and constructed an exchange diffusion model with the exchange taking place at the binding site of the uptake carrier. In our recent studies (Numachi *et al.* in this volume), the uptake of intravenous ^{14}C-MAP increased by more than 5 times in both the striatum and nucleus accumbens of rats 7 days after MAP pretreatment for 3 weeks (FIG. 2). When the exchange diffusion model was applied to our evidence, a lasting increase in uptake of MAP into the synaptosomes accelerated the efflux of dopamine out of the synaptosomes. This hypothesis is consistent with recent findings of Paulson and Robinson[32] that an intra-accumbens amphetamine challenge enhanced the locomotor responses in rats sensitized with systemic amphetamine, and suggests a key role of the impaired uptake mechanisms of MAP and dopamine at terminal fields in both induction and expression of sensiti-

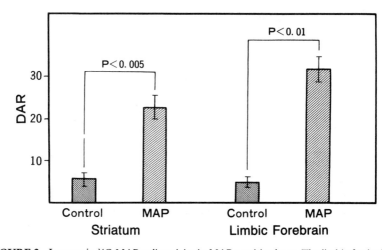

FIGURE 2. Increase in ¹⁴C-MAP radioactivity in MAP-sensitized rats. The limbic forebrain includes nucleus accumbens and olfactory tubercle.

zation. Butcher *et al.*[33] reported that ouabain, a specific Na^+, K^+-ATPase inhibitor known to affect the operation of the uptake carrier, facilitated the effect of amphetamine on the efflux of a newly synthesized pool of dopamine in the striatum. More recently, Kanzaki *et al.*[35] reported a significant enhancement of the ouabain-induced increase in dopamine efflux in the striatum of sensitized rats with repeated MAP. Further studies are needed to identify the change in stimulant-uptake mechanisms at neuronal membranes to understand the mechanisms for induction and the expression of the vulnerability to psychotic episodes in MAP psychosis.

SUMMARY

Chronic MAP abuse may produce a lasting vulnerability of the brain which leads to a paranoid delusional psychosis with hallucinations similar to schizophrenia. This view is based on the clinical observations that duration of the psychotic episodes could last quite long after excretion of MAP in the urine, and that reuse of MAP, alcohol ingestion and nonspecific psychological stressors lead to acute recurrence of psychotic episodes whose clinical features are almost identical to the initial episode in patients with prior MAP psychosis. The experimental studies indicate that a lasting change at the nerve terminal membranes, namely transporters of MAP and dopamine at the uptake sites, in the striatum and nucleus accumbens may be a cause for induction and expression of stimulant-induced sensitization, which may relate to vulnerability to schizophrenia-like psychotic episodes in MAP psychosis.

REFERENCES

1. SATO, M. & K. KASHIHARA. 1986. Methamphetamine Psychosis. Kongo-Syuppan. Tokyo. (In Japanese.)

2. SATO, M. 1986. Acute exacerbation of methamphetamine psychosis and lasting dopaminergic supersensitivity—A clinical survey. Psychopharmacol. Bull. **22**: 751–756.
3. CONNELL, P. H. 1958. Amphetamine Psychosis. Oxford University Press. London. Pp. 57–76.
4. HAYASHI, S. 1955. Wake-amine addiction. Sougo-Igaku **12**: 1–7. (In Japanese.)
5. TATETSU, S., A. GOTO & T. FUJIWARA. 1958. The Methamphetamine Psychosis. Igaku-Shoin. Tokyo. (In Japanese.)
6. KONUMA, K. 1984. Multiphasic clinical types of methamphetamine psychosis and its dependence. Psychiat. Neurol. Jpn. **86**: 315–339. (In Japanese.)
7. SATO, M., T. NAKASHIMA & S. OTSUKI. 1982. A clinical study of chronic methamphetamine psychoses. Clin. Psychiatry **24**(5): 481–489. (In Japanese.)
8. SATO, M. 1978. Acute reappearance of paranoid state by a small amount of methamphetamine injection in 7 cases of chronic methamphetamine psychoses. Clin. Psychiatry **20**: 643–648. (In Japanese.)
9. SATO, M., K. AKIYAMA, T. NAKASHIMA, S. OTSUKI, T. HARADA, M. FUNAKOSHI & T. NAGAO. 1982. Reverse tolerance phenomenon in the clinical course of chronic methamphetamine psychosis and prophylactic effects of antipsychotics on reuse of methamphetamine. Clin. Psychiatry **24**: 1333–1340. (In Japanese.)
10. EBIHARA, H. & F. SATO. 1984. Characteristics of the delusion of jealousy in methamphetamine abusers. Jpn. J. Clin. Psychiatry **86**: 315–339. (In Japanese.)
11. TOHRI, K. & H. FUJIMORI. 1991. Methamphetamine psychoses over the last 10 years examined from admitted cases to a psychiatric emergency ward. Clin. Psychiatry **33**: 101–108. (In Japanese.)
12. TAKEZAKI, H., T. INOUE, T. IKEDA & T. YASUOKA. 1984. A case of methamphetamine psychosis characterized by fancy delusions of grandeur. Psychiat. Neurol. Jpn. **86**: 621–630. (In Japanese.)
13. NAKATANI, Y., M. SAKAGUCHI & H. FUJIMORI. 1987. Revolving door patients of methamphetamine psychosis. Clin. Psychiatry **29**: 1327–1334. (In Japanese.)
14. SATO, M., C. C. CHEN, K. AKIYAMA & S. OTSUKI. 1983. Acute exacerbation of paranoid psychotic state after long-term abstinence in patients with previous methamphetamine psychosis. Biol. Psychiatry **18**: 429–440.
15. AMERICAN PSYCHIATRIC ASSOCIATION. 1987. Diagnostic and Statistical Manual of Mental Disorders (Third Edition-Revised), p. 195, Washington, D.C.
16. SCHNEIDER, K. 1967. Klinische Psychopathologie (8 Aufl). Thieme. Stuttgart.
17. AOKI, Y. 1958. On the treatment and prognosis of Benzedrinism. Psychiat. Neurol. Jpn. **60**: 341–351. (In Japanese.)
18. WADA, K. & S. FUKUI. 1990. Relationship between years of methamphetamine use and symptoms of methamphetamine psychosis. Jpn. J. Alcohol Drug Dependence **25**(3): 143–158. (In Japanese.)
19. ELLINWOOD, E. H., A. SUDILOVSKY & L. M. NELSON. 1973. Evolving behavior in the clinical and experimental amphetamine (model) psychosis. Am. J. Psychiatry **130**: 1088–1093.
20. EBIHARA, H. & F. SATO. 1984. Characteristics of symptomatology on the delusions of jealousy in methamphetamine abusers. Jpn. J. Clin. Psychiatry **13**: 101–108. (In Japanese.)
21. AMAGAI, I. 1987. Methamphetamine dependence and psychosis. Yokohama Med. J. **38**: 59–70. (In Japanese.)
22. UTENA, H. 1982. Recurrence of methamphetamine psychosis—Rireki phenomenon. Seisinka Mook **3**: 70–78. (In Japanese.)
23. SUWAKI, H., T. YOSHIDA & K. OHARA. 1985. A survey of methamphetamine abusers in prison, on probation and in mental hospitals in Kochi Prefecture. Jpn. J. Soc. Psychiatry **8**(2): 144–150. (In Japanese.)
24. HORIKOSHI, R., K. SATO, N. YAGINUMA, M. KANEKO & H. KUMASHIRO. 1988. Serum dopamine blocking activity in treatment of relapse of methamphetamine psychosis with antipsychotic drugs in prison. Acta Crim. Jpn. **54**(4): 169–174. (In Japanese.)
25. SATO, M. 1979. An experimental study of onset and relapsing mechanisms of chronic methamphetamine psychosis. Psychiatr. Neurol. Jpn. **81**: 21–32. (In Japanese.)
26. ROBINSON, T. E. & J. B. BECKER. 1982. Behavioral sensitization is accompanied by enhancement in amphetamine-stimulated dopamine release from striatal tissue *in vitro*. Eur. J. Pharmacol. **85**: 253–254.

27. KOLTA, M. G., P. SHREVE, V. DE SOUZA & N. J. URETSKY. 1985. Time course of the development of the enhanced behavioral and biochemical responses to amphetamine after pretreatment with amphetamine. Neuropharmacology 24: 823–829.
28. YAMADA, S., H. KOJIMA, H. TOKOO, K. TSUTSUMI, K. TAKAMUK, S. ANRAKU, S. NISHI & K. INANAGA. 1988. Enhancement of dopamine release from striatal slices of rats that were subchronically treated with methamphetamine. Biol. Psychiatry 24: 399–408.
29. ROBINSON, T. E., P. A. JURSON, J. A. BENNETT & K. M. BENTGEN. 1988. Persistent sensitization of dopamine neurotransmission in ventral striatum (nucleus accumbens) produced by prior experience with (+)-amphetamine: A microdialysis study in freely moving rats. Brain Res. 462: 211–222.
30. KAZAHAYA, Y., K. AKIMOTO & S. OTSUKI. 1989. Subchronic methamphetamine- or cocaine-induced dopamine efflux in vivo. Biol. Psychiatry 25: 903–912.
31. FISCHER, J. F. & A. K. CHO. 1979. Chemical release of dopamine from striatal homogenates: Evidence for an exchange diffusion model. J. Pharmacol. Exp. Ther. 208: 203–209.
32. PAULSON, P. E. & T. E. ROBINSON. 1991. Sensitization to systemic amphetamine produces an enhanced locomotor response to a subsequent intra-accumbens amphetamine challenge in rats. Psychopharmacology 104: 140–141.
33. BUTCHER, S. P., I. S. FAIRBROTHER, J. S. KELLY & G. W. ARBUTHNOTT. 1988. Amphetamine-induced dopamine release in the rat striatum: An in vivo microdialysis study. J. Neurochem. 50: 346–355.
34. KANZAKI, A., K. AKIYAMA, K. OKUMURA, H. UJIKE & S. OTSUKI. 1990. Effect of chronic methamphetamine on Na$^+$,K$^+$-ATPase in rats. Bull. Jpn. Neurochem. Soc. 29(1): 142–143. (In Japanese.)

Neural Mechanisms of Drug Reinforcement[a]

GEORGE F. KOOB

Department of Neuropharmacology
The Scripps Research Institute
10666 North Torrey Pines Road
La Jolla, California 92037

INTRODUCTION

Definitions of dependence and addiction emphasize two important phenomena: a compulsion to take the drug with a loss of control in limiting intake, and a characteristic withdrawal syndrome that results in physical signs as well as motivational signs of discomfort when the drug is removed. The search for neurobiological substrates for these phenomena has depended on the development of animal models, both for the acute reinforcing (or rewarding) effects of drugs, as well as for the withdrawal syndromes associated with the removal of the drug after chronic access or administration. The acute reinforcing properties of drug can be considered to be subsumed under the theoretical construct of the positive reinforcing action of the drug, while the motivational properties of drug withdrawal can be subsumed under the theoretical construct of the negative reinforcing actions of the drug.

Recent studies using animal models have brought the search for a neurobiological substrate for drug dependence to a focus on the medial forebrain and its connections with the region of the nucleus accumbens in the anterior part of the basal forebrain. The nucleus accumbens is well situated to integrate limbic function with the extrapyramidal motor system, and appears to play a critical role in mediating not only the acute reinforcing effects of drugs but also may be involved in the motivational aspects of drug withdrawal. The present manuscript will explore studies directed at elucidating the neural substrates for cocaine, opiate, and ethanol reinforcement.

NEURAL SUBSTRATES FOR THE ACUTE REINFORCING EFFECTS OF COCAINE

Animal models for the acute reinforcing effects of psychomotor stimulants have included measures of the effects of psychomotor stimulants on reward thresholds using intracranial self-stimulation, measures of preference for the environment paired with drug administration (place preference) and direct self-administration of the drug. In

[a] Preparation of this chapter was supported in part by NIAAA Specialized Center Grant AA 06420, NIAAA Grant AA 08459, NIDA Grant DA 04043, and NIDA Grant DA 04398.

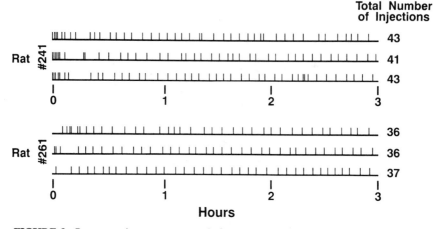

FIGURE 1. Representative response records for two rats self-administering cocaine. Test sessions were 3 h in duration. Each mark represents a response/infusion of intravenous drug (0.75 mg/kg/injection). (Taken with permission from Koob, 1991.[96])

studies involving direct self-administration of the drugs, rats with limited access to cocaine (3 h/day) will show a stable and regular drug intake over each daily session (FIG. 1). In addition, no obvious tolerance or dependence develops in these limited access (<6 h) situations. An important aspect of this model is that the rats regulate the amount of drug self-administered, such that lowering the dose from the training dose of 0.75 mg/kg per injection increases cocaine self-administration, whereas increasing the dose decreases cocaine self-administration.

Neuropharmacological studies of the acute reinforcing effects of cocaine have established an important role for dopamine. Low doses of dopamine receptor antagonists when injected systemically reliably increase cocaine self-administration[1-4] (FIG. 2). This has been interpreted as a partial blockade of the reinforcing actions of cocaine. Thus, the rats compensate for decreases in the magnitude of reinforcement with an increase in cocaine self-administration (or a decrease in the interinjection interval), similar to that observed by lowering the dose of cocaine in the self-administration session.

A role for dopamine in the reinforcing properties of cocaine was extended by the observation that 6-hydroxydopamine (6-OHDA) lesions of the nucleus accumbens produce extinction-like responding and a significant and long-lasting reduction in self-administration of cocaine over days.[5-7] This blockade of the reinforcing effects of cocaine has been replicated using a progressive ratio schedule.[8] Similar 6-OHDA lesions of the frontal cortex and caudate nucleus failed to significantly alter cocaine self-administration.[8,9]

Recent work using injections of selective dopamine receptor antagonists has shown that D-1 receptors may be particularly important for the reinforcing actions of cocaine. SCH 23390 significantly increases cocaine self-administration at doses as low as 5 μg/kg SC and appears to produce these anti-cocaine effects at doses that are not cataleptic[10] (FIG. 3). D-2 receptor antagonists are also effective but there is a narrow range between the anti-cocaine and motor impairing actions when they are injected systemically.[11]

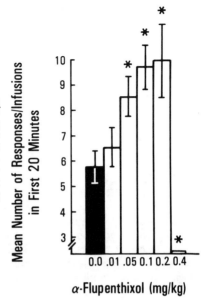

FIGURE 2. The effects of α-flupenthixol on the loading dose (infusions in the first 20 min of the 3-h test sessions) in cocaine-self-administering animals. *A posteriori* Newman-Keuls tests compared each treatment dose with the appropriate no-drug control. An asterisk in the base of histogram indicates that the treatment dose was reliably different from the no-drug saline condition ($p <$ 0.05). (Modified with permission from Ettenberg et al., 1982.[4])

In contrast, local intracerebral injections into the nucleus accumbens of both D-1 and D-2 antagonists produce significant increases in cocaine self-administration[12] (see this volume).

Previous work has established the substantia innominata-ventral pallidum as an important connection in the expression of behavioral stimulation produced by activation of the nucleus accumbens,[13] and there are established efferent connections between

FIGURE 3. Effects of subcutaneous injection of D1 dopamine receptor antagonist SCH 23390 (*left side*) and the D2 dopamine receptor antagonist spiperone (*right side*) on cocaine self-administration. Each point represents the average hourly intake of cocaine by injection ($n = 5$). Doses are in micrograms per kilogram. For SCH 23390, doses of 5, 10 and 20 μg/kg significantly increased cocaine self-administration ($p <$ 0.05 Newman-Keuls test following ANOVA). For spiperone, the dose of 10 μg/kg significantly increased cocaine self-administration ($p < 0.05$ paired t-test, overall ANOVA $p >$ 0.05). (Taken with permission from Koob et al., 1987a.[10])

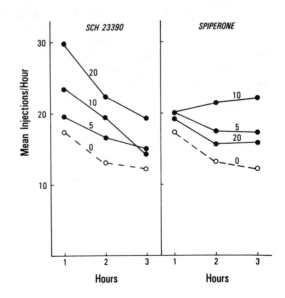

the nucleus accumbens and the substantia innominata-ventral pallidum. To test the hypothesis that the processing of the reinforcing properties of cocaine may also involve the substantia innominata-ventral pallidum, rats trained to intravenously self-administer cocaine received bilateral ibotenic acid lesions of the region of the substantia innominata-ventral pallidum.[14] The substantia innominata-ventral pallidum lesions significantly decreased baseline cocaine self-administration, and when the rats were subjected to a progressive ratio procedure, these lesions produced a significant decrease in the highest ratio obtained for cocaine.[14] These results suggest that the substantia innominata-ventral pallidum may be an important site for the processing of the reinforcing effects of cocaine.

NEURAL SUBSTRATES FOR THE NEGATIVE REINFORCING PROPERTIES OF COCAINE WITHDRAWAL

Following prolonged use of cocaine on a "binge," abstinence is characterized by severe depressive symptoms combined with irritability and anxiety.[15,16] These symptoms characterize the "crash" associated with the abstinence from cocaine in cocaine dependence and may last several hours to several days. Anhedonia is one of the more salient depressive symptoms and can be defined as the inability to derive pleasure from normally pleasurable stimuli.

A means of assessing anhedonia in animals has involved the use of measures of threshold for intracranial self-stimulation. Thresholds for intracranial self-stimulation have been hypothesized to reflect the hedonic state of an animal because animals will readily self-administer the stimulation to their own brains, and intracranial self-stimulation is thought to activate the same neural substrates that mediate the reinforcing effects of natural reinforcers (e.g., water, food).[17] Cocaine injected acutely, as well as other psychomotor stimulants, has been well documented to lower self-stimulation thresholds in rats.[18]

To explore the possibility that prolonged self-administration of cocaine may result in an increase in brain stimulation thresholds, animals were allowed to self-administer cocaine intravenously for long periods and reward thresholds were monitored during the course of cocaine withdrawal. Animals prepared with both chronic indwelling brain stimulation electrodes and chronic indwelling catheters were allowed to self-administer cocaine for various time periods and tested for brain stimulation thresholds during cocaine withdrawal.

During cocaine withdrawal brain stimulation reward thresholds were elevated compared to pre-drug baseline levels, and the magnitude and duration of the elevation in reward thresholds was proportional to the amount of cocaine self-administered (FIG. 4). This elevation in reward threshold may reflect an "anhedonic" state and as such it may be homologous to the anhedonia reported by human drug users following a cocaine binge.[19] In addition, these results suggest that cocaine can alter the function of the reward system(s) in the medial forebrain bundle during the course of a cocaine bout and withdrawal.

A likely neurochemical mechanism involved in this withdrawal state would be some hypoactivity of dopamine functioning.[20] There is some direct support for this hypothesis in studies of *in vivo* microdialysis during cocaine withdrawal (Weiss *et al.*,[72] 1992; this volume). However, there may also be separate neurochemical processes that op-

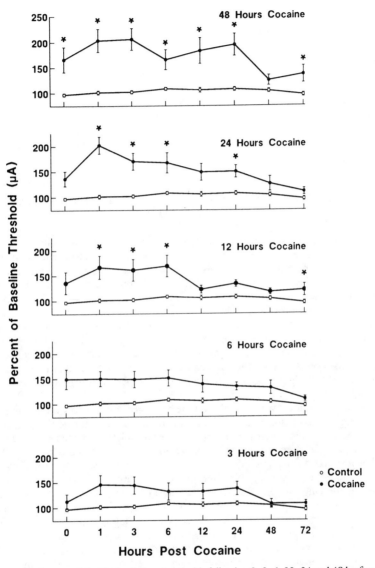

FIGURE 4. Intracranial self-stimulation thresholds following 0, 3, 6, 12, 24 and 48 h of cocaine self-administration at several time points postcocaine (0, 1, 3, 6, 12, 24, 48 and 72 h). The results are expressed as percent change from baseline threshold levels. The mean ± SEM baseline threshold for the experimental group was 37.4 ± 2.5 μA and for the control group 35.9 ± 3.1 μA. The asterisks indicate statistically significant differences ($p < 0.05$) between control and experimental groups with Dunnett's tests, following a significant group × hours interaction in an analysis of variance. (Taken with permission from Markou and Koob, 1991.[19])

pose the acute action of the drug, such as changes in a nucleus accumbens output system that may be overactive during cocaine withdrawal.

In summary, the acute reinforcing effects of cocaine appear to depend on the presynaptic release of dopamine within the region of the nucleus accumbens. Both D-1 and D-2 dopamine receptors may be important. Chronic access to cocaine produces a withdrawal state as reflected in increases in brain stimulation reward thresholds that appear to be opposite to the actions of the drug administered acutely. These effects are thought to reflect a change in the activity of neural elements in the medial forebrain bundle involved with the positive reinforcing effects of cocaine and thus may be responsible for the negative reinforcing state associated with the anhedonia of cocaine withdrawal.

NEURAL SUBSTRATES FOR THE ACUTE REINFORCING EFFECTS OF OPIATES

Opiate drugs such as heroin, if provided in limited access, are readily self-administered intravenously by rats much like cocaine (FIG. 5). Rats will maintain stable levels of drug intake on a daily basis without any major signs of physical dependence.[21] This behavior probably best reflects the human equivalent of "chipping,"[22] and has been used to study the neurobiologic basis of heroin reinforcement independent of the confounds of dependence.

As with cocaine, decreases in the dose of heroin available to the animal will change the pattern of self-administration such that the interinjection interval decreases and the number of injections increases.[8] Similar increases in the number of injections have been obtained by both systemic and central administration of competitive opiate antagonists,[4,21,23-25] suggesting that the animals attempt to compensate for the opiate antagonism by increasing the amount of drug injected.

A systematic series of studies exploring the opiate receptor subtype important for the reinforcing actions of opiates using selective opiate agonists and antagonists suggest that μ receptors play an important, if not critical, role in opiate reinforcement. Mu opioid agonists produce dose-dependent decreases in heroin self-administration and irreversible μ selective antagonists dose-dependently increase heroin self-administration.[26]

To explore the location of opioid receptors in the central nervous system important for the reinforcing properties of heroin, a series of studies was initiated using intracerebral injection of a quaternary derivative of naloxone, methylnaloxonium. Methylnaloxonium is charged and hydrophilic and does not readily spread from the sites in the brain at which it is injected.[27] Intracerebroventricular administration of methylnaloxonium dose-dependently increased heroin self-administration in non-dependent rats (FIG. 6). The region of the nucleus accumbens appeared to be particularly sensitive to the effects of methylnaloxonium on heroin self-administration[28] (FIG. 7). Injections of methylnaloxonium into the ventral tegmental area produced increases in heroin self-administration only at doses similar to those required by the intracerebroventricular route.

These results suggested that neural elements in the region of the nucleus accumbens are responsible for both the reinforcing properties of opiates and cocaine. Rats will also self-administer opioid peptides in the region of the nucleus accumbens.[29]

The exact neurochemical mechanisms mediating the reinforcing effect of opiates in the nucleus accumbens is unknown but some evidence exists to suggest that it is in-

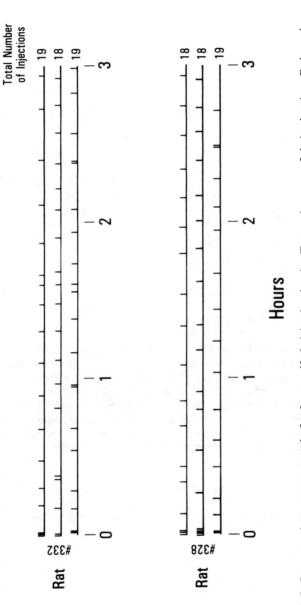

FIGURE 5. Representative response records for 2 rats self-administering heroin. Test sessions were 3 h in duration. Each mark represents a response/infusion of intravenous drug (0.06 mg/kg/injection). (Taken with permission from Koob, 1987.[8])

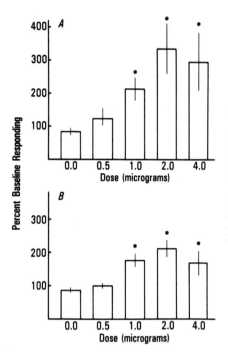

FIGURE 6. The effects of intracerebroventricular methylnaloxonium treatment on responding for heroin over the first hour (A) and over the total 3-h self-administration session (B). Response rates were expressed as the percentage of baseline responding. Asterisks indicate that the treatment dose was significantly different from the saline treatment, $p < 0.05$, Newman-Keuls test. Six rats were tested across all drug treatments. The day prior to ICV injections was used as the baseline day. (Taken with permission from Vaccarino et al., 1985.[25])

dependent of dopamine release. Rats trained to self-administer cocaine and heroin on alternate days and receiving 6-OHDA lesions of the nucleus accumbens showed a time-dependent decrease or extinction of cocaine self-administration, whereas heroin self-administration returned to near normal levels.[30] Similar results have been obtained using chronic dopamine receptor blockade and places preference for heroin and self-administration[31] (see this volume). However, opioids are self-administered directly into the source of the mesocorticolimbic dopamine system, the ventral tegmental area (VTA), and microinjections of opioids into the VTA lower brain stimulation reward thresholds and produce robust place preferences.[32,33] The place preferences produced by opioids appear to have a major dopaminergic component[31,32] (see both, this volume). Thus, the reinforcing actions of opiates may involve both a dopamine-dependent (VTA) and dopamine-independent (nucleus accumbens) mechanism.

There may be an interdependence of the neural substrates for the reinforcing stimuli of cocaine and heroin at the level of the nucleus accumbens post-synaptic to the dopamine innervation and at the level of the substantia innominata-ventral pallidum. Kainic acid lesions of the nucleus accumbens decrease both cocaine and heroin self-administration,[34] and ibotenic acid lesions of the substantia innominata-ventral pallidum also decrease heroin self-administration.[14] These results suggest that the substantia innominata-ventral pallidum may be an important part of the neural circuitry involved in the processing of the reinforcing effects of both cocaine and heroin (FIG. 8).

The processing of drug-reinforcing stimuli beyond the substantia innominata-ventral pallidum is unknown at this time. Evidence from locomotor activity studies

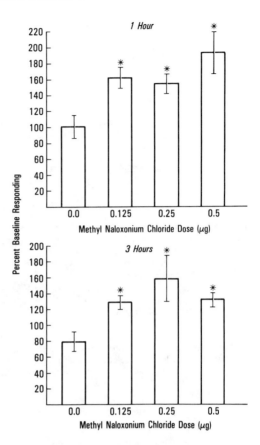

FIGURE 7. Percent baseline (predrug day) responding for IV heroin during the first hour (*top graph*) and for the total 3 hours (*bottom graph*) of the heroin self-administration session following methylnaloxonium injections into the nucleus accumbens. Asterisks indicate a significant difference ($p < 0.05$) from saline vehicle (0.0 dose), Duncan Multiple Range *a posteriori test*. (Taken with permission from Vaccarino *et al.*, 1985.[28])

suggests roles for both the dorsomedial thalamus and the pedunculopontine nucleus in psychomotor stimulant activation (FIG. 8). Limbic afferents to the nucleus accumbens include major projections from the frontal cortex, amygdala and hippocampus.[35] Thus, direct limbic information received by the nucleus accumbens may be directed to the appropriate motor groups to produce motivated behavior via the pallido-thalamic projections and perhaps thalamo-cortical projections (FIG. 8).

NEURAL SUBSTRATES FOR THE NEGATIVE REINFORCING PROPERTIES OF OPIATE WITHDRAWAL

Dependence on opiate drugs is defined by a characteristic withdrawal syndrome that appears with the abrupt termination of opiate administration or can be precipitated with administration of competitive opiate antagonists. Opiate withdrawal in humans is characterized by both physical and motivational symptoms such as nausea, gastrointestinal disturbances, chills, sympathetic reactions, and a painful flu-like dysphoric state.[36] In rats, opiate physical dependence has been characterized by an abstinence

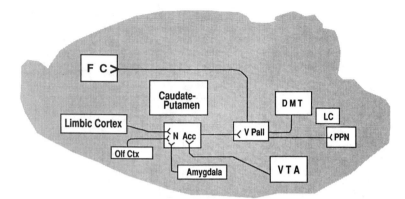

FIGURE 8. Schematic model of brain sites and circuitry that participate in the reinforcing and adaptive opposing actions of opiates and psychostimulants. The region of the nucleus accumbens (N Acc) is the target of a dopaminergic projection from the ventral tegmental area (VTA) and of afferents from olfactory cortex (Olf Ctx) and from limbic cortex. The nucleus accumbens projects, among other targets, to the ventral pallidum (V Pall), and also sends a reciprocal connection, believed to be GABA-mediated, back to the VTA. From the ventral pallidum, connections project to the pedunculopontine nucleus (PPN) and to the dorsal medial thalamus (DMT), which have been proposed as being functionally important in motor activation in the rat.[97] The ventral pallidum may also regulate responsiveness of neurons in the frontal cortex (FC), a site from which psychostimulant reinforcement has also been observed. Also illustrated as potentially important for the implementation of the adaptive opposing responses to the behavioral effects of these drugs, is the locus coeruleus (LC); although its connections are not shown, the LC projects to the amygdala and to olfactory, frontal, and limbic cortices. (Taken with permission from Koob and Bloom, 1988.[84])

syndrome that includes the appearance of ptosis, teeth chattering, wet dog shakes, and diarrhea,[37] and these symptoms can be dramatically precipitated in dependent animals by systemic injections of opiate antagonists.[37] More motivational measures have included the disruption of trained operant behavior for food reward or the development of place aversions following precipitated withdrawal with systemic opiate antagonist administration.[38]

Studies of the neural substrates of physical dependence on opiates have revealed multiple sites responsible for the classical opiate abstinence syndrome. Early studies implicated the periaqueductal gray[39,40] and dorsal thalamus.[41] More recent work using intracerebral microinjections of methylnaloxonium in rats dependent on morphine has revealed that the locus coeruleus is particularly important for the activating effects of opiate withdrawal.[42] Other physical signs appear to depend on a more widespread activation of opiate receptors.

The sites in the brain responsible for the negative reinforcing properties of opiate withdrawal appear to be more selective. The response-disruptive effects of local intracerebral administration of methylnaloxonium to rats physically dependent on morphine were explored by measuring performance on a fixed ratio-15 (FR-15) schedule during precipitated opiate withdrawal. Rats were implanted with cannulas aimed at the lateral ventricle periaqueductal gray, medial dorsal thalamus and nucleus accumbens,

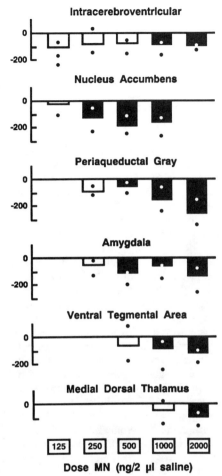

FIGURE 9. The effect of intracerebral methylnaloxonium paired with a particular environment on the amount of time spent in that environment during an injection-free test session. Values represent the median difference between the postconditioning score and the preconditioning score. Dots refer to the interquartile range of this distribution. Darkened bars represent those doses where the conditioning scores were significantly different from the preconditioning scores using the non-parametric Wilcoxon Matched Pairs Signed-Rank test. Significance was set at $p < 0.02$ to control for multiple comparisons. (Taken with permission from Stinus *et al.*, 1990.[45])

and were trained on an FR-15 schedule of reinforcement for food, and then made dependent on morphine using subcutaneous morphine pellets.

Very low doses of methylnaloxonium (4–64 ng) injected into the nucleus accumbens produced a disruption of food motivated operant responding, whereas injections of methylnaloxonium into the periaqueductal gray or dorsal thalamus produced a dose effect function similar to that following intracerebroventricular injection.[43] These results suggested that during the development of morphine dependence, neural elements in the region of the nucleus accumbens may have become sensitized to opiate antagonists and may be responsible for the negative stimulus effects of opiate withdrawal. Confirmation of a negative reinforcing effect for the withdrawal induced by intracerebral methylnaloxonium was shown using the place aversion procedure,[44] and the nucleus accumbens also proved to be the most sensitive site for intracerebral injections of methylnaloxonium to produce place aversions in dependent rats[45] (FIG. 9).

NEURAL SUBSTRATES FOR THE ACUTE REINFORCING
EFFECTS OF ETHANOL

Several brain neurotransmitter systems such as opioid peptides, serotonin, norepinephrine, dopamine, and GABA have been implicated in the reinforcing properties of ethanol based on pharmacological studies using either neurotransmitter agonists or antagonists. Direct intravenous self-administration of drugs has been an effective tool for the study of the neuropharmacology of the reinforcing actions of drugs such as cocaine and opiates (see above). However, intravenous self-administration of ethanol, and most sedative hypnotics, is not readily obtained in rats. The alternative model, oral ethanol self-administration in the rat, has been fraught with problems of taste, consummatory behavior confounds, and lack of reliable blood alcohol determinations, but several recent studies have provided reliable procedures for the initiation and maintenance of alcohol intake using taste adulteration procedures (sucrose or saccharine substitution). Reliable, sustained operant responding for 10% ethanol can be obtained in free-feeding and -drinking rats (non-deprived), even after complete removal of sweetener, provided that the sweetener is slowly withdrawn.[46-48]

The opiate antagonists naloxone and naltrexone have consistently been shown to decrease ethanol drinking,[49-53] and opiate agonists will enhance ethanol intake in limited access situations.[54-56] However, only relatively large opiate antagonist doses reduce ethanol drinking, in contrast to the small doses required for altering intravenous opiate self-administration.[50] Also, systemically administered naloxone and other opiate antagonists suppress food and water intake over a wide dose range,[57-59] and inhibitory effects of naloxone on ingestive behavior have been seen in non-deprived as well as deprived animals and extend to stimuli which are normally potent reinforcers (*e.g.*, sucrose and sweetened milk).[60,61] Thus, there is considerable evidence to suggest that opiate antagonists inhibit consummatory behavior in general.

Similar conclusions resulted from a recent study where non-motivationally constrained rats (Wistar and alcohol-preferring-P rats) were trained on a free-choice operant procedure to lever press for ethanol and were injected systemically with low doses of naloxone. Naloxone (0.125–0.5 mg/kg) produced dose-dependent reductions in responding for both ethanol and water, and consequently decreased the total amount of fluid intake.[48] However, ethanol preference was not altered in either strain of rats since the water-ethanol ratios remained constant across naloxone doses. The decreases in operant responding for both water and ethanol do not seem to support a selective role for opiate receptors in the reinforcing actions of ethanol, but appear more consistent with the well-documented inhibitory effects on consummatory behaviors of this opiate antagonist.

Neuropharmacological manipulation of serotonin systems has been shown to alter ethanol consumption in numerous studies. Treatments designed to increase the synaptic availability of serotonin such as a precursor loading (5-hydroxytryptophan), administration of serotonin re-uptake blockers, or central injection of serotonin itself reduce voluntary ethanol intake.[62-64] The results of neuropharmacological decreases in serotonin function on ethanol self-administration, however, are more difficult to interpret. Serotonin synthesis inhibitors, serotonin neurotoxins, and serotonin antagonists have been shown to decrease rather than increase voluntary ethanol drinking.[65-67]

Several studies have suggested that brain dopamine systems may be involved in the reinforcing properties of ethanol. Dopamine receptor antagonists have been shown to reduce lever-pressing for ethanol in non-deprived rats[68,69] and also reduce home cage ethanol drinking.[70] To test the hypothesis that dopamine receptors in the nucleus accumbens have a role in ethanol self-administration, non-motivationally constrained male Wistar rats were trained to orally self-administer ethanol in a two-lever, free-choice self-administration task. The animals were then prepared with chronic indwelling guide cannulas aimed above the nucleus accumbens. Fluphenazine decreased ethanol self-administration at doses of 2 and 4 μg; water self-administration was unaltered at 2 μg but slightly decreased at 4 μg.[71] These data, combined with observations of a release of dopamine as measured by *in vivo* microdialysis in the nucleus accumbens during ethanol self-administration[72] (see this volume), suggest that dopamine receptors in the region of the nucleus accumbens may be involved in ethanol reinforcement in the non-dependent rat.

GABA has long been hypothesized to have a role in the intoxicating effects of ethanol based on the ability of GABAergic antagonists to reverse many of the behavioral effects of ethanol, and GABAmimetic drugs can potentiate some of ethanol actions. For example, GABA antagonists decrease the ability of ethanol to produce ataxia, anesthesia and the release of punished responding (anti-conflict effects).[73–76] At a biochemical level, ethanol in the 10–50 mM range potentiates stimulation by GABA of Cl⁻ uptake in synaptosomes from the cerebral cortex[77] and cerebellum.[78] Further support for a role of brain GABA is the observation that the partial inverse benzodiazepine agonist, RO 15-4513, which has been shown to reverse some of the behavioral effects of ethanol,[79–81] produces a dose-dependent reduction of oral ethanol (10%) self-administration in non-deprived rats[81] and in an operant free-choice situation[82] (see this volume) (TABLE 1).

The neuropharmacological data reviewed above provide some evidence for the actions of four major neurotransmitter systems in ethanol reinforcement: opioid pep-

TABLE 1. Effects of Low Doses of Neurotransmitter Antagonists on Responding for 10% Ethanol and Water Using a Free-Choice Operant Task in Non-Deprived Rats[a]

Treatment	Ethanol Responding	Water Responding
Systemic		
• GABA complex-inverse agonist RO 15-4513	decrease	no change
• DA receptor antagonist	decrease	no change
• Calcium diacetyl homotaurine-glutamate antagonist	decrease	no change
• Isopropylbicyclophosphate-GABA/ picrotoxinin antagonist	decrease	no change
• Naloxone, opiate antagonist	decrease	decrease
• Methysergide, serotonin antagonist	no change	no change
Nucleus accumbens		
• Dopamine receptor antagonist	decrease	no change
• NMDA antagonist-APV	decrease	no change
Responding for 0.2% saccharin and water		
• GABA complex-inverse agonist RO 15-4513	no change	no change

[a] Results supporting these conclusions can be found in Weiss *et al.*, 1990[48] and Rassnick *et al.*, 1990[71] and 1992.[82]

tides, serotonin, dopamine and GABA. Other approaches involving biochemical measures, lesions and genetics also provide significant evidence for opioid peptides, serotonin, dopamine and GABA.[83] These neurotransmitters do form an intimate part of the brain circuitry hypothesized to be part of the systems involved in drug reinforcement in general (FIG. 8), but the exact site or sites for the reinforcing actions of ethanol will require further investigation.[84]

NEURAL SUBSTRATES FOR THE NEGATIVE REINFORCING PROPERTIES OF ETHANOL WITHDRAWAL

Ethanol withdrawal in humans is characterized in its early stages (first 1–2 days) by anxiety, anorexia, insomnia, tremor, some mild disorientation, and possibly hallucinations. This syndrome is accompanied by a major sympathetic hyperactivity including elevated blood pressure, heart rate and body temperature. Tonic-clonic seizures similar to those of grand mal epilepsy can be observed in the first 1–2 days. In later stages of severe withdrawal, a syndrome called delirium tremens may become manifest which is characterized by marked tremor, anxiety, insomnia, and autonomic hyperactivity. Subjects can become totally disoriented with respect to time and place, with vivid hallucinations and outbursts of irrational behavior. The pharmacological treatment for ethanol withdrawal has included barbiturates, phenothiazines, and antihistamines, but benzodiazepines are considered safer and more effective.

Ethanol withdrawal in animals is characterized by central nervous system hyperexcitability that results in both physical and motivational signs of dependence. Physical signs include tremor, lack of a ventromedial distal flexion, weight loss, and audiogenic or stress-induced seizures. More motivational measures have included disruption of operant behavior,[85] increased responsiveness in acoustic startle tests,[86] and increased sensitivity in the behavioral tests of anxiety such as the elevated plus maze test.[87]

Studies of the neurochemical bases for the physical signs of ethanol withdrawal have suggested a functional role for GABA. GABA agonists decrease the central nervous system hyperexcitability during ethanol withdrawal and ethanol withdrawal-induced convulsions.[88,89] GABA antagonists exacerbate many of the symptoms of ethanol withdrawal,[90] and the partial inverse benzodiazepine agonist RO 15-4513 has been shown to increase the incidence of seizures during ethanol withdrawal.[91]

GABA has also been implicated in more motivational measures of ethanol withdrawal. Using a drug discrimination procedure, ethanol withdrawal as a stimulus produces stimulus characteristics similar to injection of pentylenetetrazol (PTZ), an anxiogenic drug.[92] This PTZ-like interoceptive stimulus produced by ethanol withdrawal is potentiated by bicuculline and picrotoxin, suggesting that the anxiogenic-like response produced by ethanol withdrawal may be related to an ethanol-induced alteration in the function of the GABA-benzodiazepine ionophore complex.[93]

Another candidate possibly involved in the motivational aspects of ethanol withdrawal is the brain stress hormone, corticotropin-releasing factor (CRF). CRF is a neuropeptide widely distributed in the central nervous system and has been hypothesized to have a functional role in behavioral responses to stress. CRF itself has anxiogenic actions and a CRF antagonist, α-helical CRF can reverse some behavioral responses to stress.[94] Rats made dependent on ethanol and then subjected to abrupt withdrawal from chronic ethanol show an "anxiogenic-like" response in several "anxiety" tests, such as the elevated plus maze.[95] To explore the role of endogenous brain CRF sys-

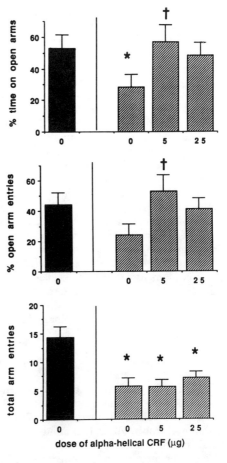

FIGURE 10. Effect of ICV administration of α-helical CRF to rats tested in the elevated plus-maze after ethanol withdrawal. The *left-hand bar* in each panel contains data from rats tested 8 h after withdrawal from control diet and 30 min after ICV vehicle administration ("controls"). The three *right-hand bars* in each panel contain data from rats tested 8 h after withdrawal from ethanol diet and 30 min after ICV α-helical CRF administration (0, 5 and 25 mg). The *top panel* shows mean (± SEM) % of time spent on the open arms. The *middle panel* shows the mean (± SEM) % number of entries onto the open arms. The *lower panel* shows the mean (± SEM) total number of arm entries. Difference from "controls": * $p < 0.05$ (ANOVA). Significantly different from group receiving ICV vehicle after ethanol withdrawal: † $p < 0.05$ (Newman-Keul's tests after ANOVA). (Taken with permission from Baldwin et al., 1991.[87])

tems in ethanol withdrawal, the effect of a CRF antagonist on the behavioral response of rats during withdrawal was examined. Rats chronically maintained (2–3 weeks) on a liquid diet showed a significant anxiogenic-like response in an elevated plus maze 8 hours into withdrawal. This anxiogenic-like response was reversed with intracerebroventricular administration of the CRF antagonist, α-helical CRF (FIG. 10).[87] These results suggest that CRF in the central nervous system may also be involved in some of the more motivational aspects of ethanol withdrawal.

SUMMARY AND CONCLUSIONS

The brain substrates involved in the effect of cocaine on brain stimulation reward, in the psychomotor activation associated with cocaine, and in cocaine self-administration appear to be focused on the medial forebrain bundle and its connections with the basal forebrain, notably the nucleus accumbens. Chronic access to cocaine produces a withdrawal state as reflected in increases in brain stimulation reward thresholds, and this change in reward threshold appears to be opposite to the actions of the drug administered acutely. These effects are thought to reflect a change in the activity of reward elements in the medial forebrain bundle and may be responsible for the negative reinforcing state associated with the anhedonia of cocaine withdrawal.

Opiate receptors particularly sensitive to the reinforcing effects of heroin also appear to be located in the region of the nucleus accumbens and the ventral tegmental area. There is good evidence for both dopamine-dependent and dopamine-independent opioid interactions in the ventral tegmental-nucleus accumbens connection. In addition, the opiate receptors in the region of the nucleus accumbens may become sensitized during the course of opiate withdrawal and thus become responsible for the aversive stimulus effects of opiate dependence.

Reliable measures of the acute reinforcing effects of ethanol have been established in rat models, and substantial evidence exists to show that non-deprived rats will orally self-administer pharmacologically relevant amounts of ethanol in lever-press choice situations. Neuropharmacological studies of ethanol reinforcement in non-dependent rats suggest important roles for serotonin, GABA and dopamine. A role for opioid peptides in ethanol reinforcement may reflect more general actions of opioid peptides in consummatory behavior. Studies of ethanol dependence have implicated brain GABAergic and CRF systems in the more motivational aspects of withdrawal. Future studies will need to focus on the common neurobiologic changes associated with all these drugs, particularly regarding their hedonic and motivational properties.

ACKNOWLEDGMENTS

Results discussed in this chapter are derived from studies with the following individuals: Stephen Negus, Patricia Robledo, Rafael Maldonado, Steve Heinrichs, Athina Markou, Stephanie Rassnick, Barak Caine, Helen Baldwin, Luigi Pulvirenti, Karen Britton, Friedbert Weiss, Luis Stinus and Floyd E. Bloom. I thank them for their help and collaboration. I thank Molecular and Experimental Medicine's Word Processing Center for their help in manuscript preparation.

REFERENCES

1. DAVIS, W. M. & S. G. SMITH. 1975. Effect of haloperidol on (+)-amphetamine self-administration. J. Pharm. Pharmacol. 27: 540–542.
2. YOKEL, R. A. & R. A. WISE. 1975. Increased lever pressing for amphetamine after pimozide in rats: Implications for a dopamine theory of reward. Science 187: 547–549.
3. YOKEL, R. A. & R. A. WISE. 1976. Attenuation of intravenous amphetamine reinforcement by central dopamine blockade in rats. Psychopharmacology 48: 311–318.
4. ETTENBERG, A., H. O. PETTIT, F. E. BLOOM & G. F. KOOB. 1982. Heroin and cocaine intravenous self-administration in rats: Mediation by separate neural systems. Psychopharmacology 78: 204–209.
5. ROBERTS, D. C. S., M. E. CORCORAN & H. C. FIBIGER. 1977. On the role of ascending catecholaminergic systems in intravenous self-administration of cocaine. Pharmacol. Biochem. Behav. 6: 615–620.
6. ROBERTS, D. C. S., G. F. KOOB, P. KLONOFF & H. C. FIBIGER. 1980. Extinction and re-

covery of cocaine self-administration following 6-hydroxydopamine lesions of the nucleus accumbens. Pharmacol. Biochem. Behav. **12:** 781–787.

7. LYNESS, W. H., N. M. FRIEDLE & K. E. MOORE. 1979. Destruction of dopaminergic nerve terminals in nucleus accumbens: Effect of d-amphetamine self-administration. Pharmacol. Biochem. Behav. **11:** 663–666.

8. KOOB, G. F., F. J. VACCARINO, M. AMALRIC & F. E. BLOOM. 1987. Positive reinforcement properties of drugs: Search for neural substrates. *In* Brain Reward Systems and Abuse. J. Engel & L. Oreland, Eds.: 35–50. Raven Press. New York.

9. MARTIN-IVERSON, M. T., C. SZOSTAK & H. C. FIBIGER. 1986. 6-Hydroxydopamine lesions of the medial prefrontal cortex fail to influence intravenous self-administration of cocaine. Psychopharmacology **88:** 310–314.

10. KOOB, G. F., H. T. LE & J. CREESE. 1987. D-1 and D-2 dopamine antagonists increase cocaine self-administration in the rat. Neurosci. Lett. **79:** 315–320.

11. CAINE, S. B., M. BERHOW, M. AMALRIC & G. F. KOOB. 1990. The D1 antagonist SCH 23390 and the D2 antagonist raclopride selectively decrease behavior maintained by cocaine or food in the rat. Soc. Neurosci. Abstr. **16:** 25a.

12. ROBLEDO, P., R. MALDONALDO-LOPEZ & G. F. KOOB. 1992. Role of dopamine receptors in the nucleus accumbens in the rewarding properties of cocaine. Ann. NY Acad. Sci. **654:** 509–512. This volume.

13. SWERDLOW, N. R., L. W. SWANSON & G. F. KOOB. 1984. Substantia innominata: Critical link in the behavioral expression of mesolimbic dopamine stimulation in the rat. Neurosci. Lett. **50:** 19–24.

14. HUBNER, C. B. & G. F. KOOB. 1990. The ventral pallidum plays a role in mediating cocaine and heroin self-administration in the rat. Brain Res. **508:** 20–29.

15. GAWIN, F. H. & H. D. KLEBER. 1986. Abstinence symptomatology and psychiatric diagnosis in cocaine abusers. Arch. Gen. Psychiatry **43:** 107–113.

16. ELLINWOOD, E. H. & W. M. PETRIE. 1977. Dependence on amphetamine, cocaine and other stimulants. *In* Drug Abuse: Clinical and Basic Aspects. S. N. Pradhan, Ed.: 248–262. Mosby. St. Louis.

17. STELLAR, J. R. & E. STELLAR. 1985. The Neurobiology of Reward and Motivation. Springer-Verlag. New York.

18. ESPOSITO, R. U., A. H. D. MOTOLA & C. KORNETSKY. 1978. Cocaine: Acute effects on reinforcement thresholds for self-stimulation behavior to the medial forebrain bundle. Pharmacol. Biochem. Behav. **8:** 437–439.

19. MARKOU, M. A. & G. F. KOOB. 1991. Postcocaine anhedonia: An animal model of cocaine withdrawal. Neuropsychopharmacology **4:** 17–26.

20. DACKIS, C. A. & M. S. GOLD. 1985. New concepts in cocaine addiction: The dopamine depletion hypothesis. Neurosci. Biobehav. Rev. **9:** 469–477.

21. KOOB, G. F., H. O. PETTIT, A. ETTENBERG & F. E. BLOOM. 1984. Effects of opiate antagonists and their quaternary derivatives on heroin self-administration in the rat. J. Pharmacol. Exp. Ther. **229:** 481–486.

22. ZINBERG, N. E. & R. C. JACOBSON. 1976. The natural history of "chipping." Am. J. Psychiatry **133:** 37–40.

23. GOLDBERG, S. R., J. H. WOODS & C. R. SCHUSTER. 1971. Nalorphine-induced changes in morphine self-administration rhesus monkeys. J. Pharmacol. Exp. Ther. **176:** 464–471.

24. WEEKS, J. R. & R. J. COLLINS. 1976. Changes in morphine self-administration in rats induced by prostaglandin E and naloxone. Prostaglandins **12:** 11–19.

25. VACCARINO, F. J., H. O. PETTIT, F. E. BLOOM & G. F. KOOB. 1985. Effects of intracerebroventricular administration of methylnaloxonium chloride on heroin self-administration in the rat. Pharmacol. Biochem. Behav. **23:** 495–498.

26. NEGUS, S. S., N. B. WEINGER, S. J. HENRICKSON & G. F. KOOB. 1991. Effect of mu, delta, and kappa opioid agonists on heroin maintained responding in the rat. Abstract Committee on Problems of Drug Dependence Meeting.

27. SCHROEDER, R. L., M. B. WEINGER, L. VAHASSIAN & G. F. KOOB. 1991. Methylnaloxonium diffuses out of the brain more slowly than naloxone after direct intracerebral injection. Neurosci. Lett. **12:** 173–177.

28. VACCARINO, F. J., F. E. BLOOM & G. F. KOOB. 1985. Blockade of nucleus accumbens opiate receptors attenuates intravenous heroin reward in the rat. Psychopharmacology (Berlin) **85:** 37–42.
29. GOEDERS, N. E., J. D. LANE & J. E. SMITH. 1984. Self-administration of methionine enkephalin into the nucleus accumbens. Pharmacol. Biochem. Behav. **20:** 451–455.
30. PETTIT, H. O., A. ETTENBERG, F. E. BLOOM & G. F. KOOB. 1984. Destruction of dopamine in the nucleus accumbens selectively attenuates cocaine but not heroin self-administration in rats. Psychopharmacology **84:** 167–173.
31. STINUS, L., M. CADOR & M. LE MOAL. 1992. Interaction between endogenous opioids and dopamine within the nucleus accumbens. Ann. N.Y. Acad. Sci. **654:** 254–273. This volume.
32. SHIPPENBERG, T. S., R. SPANAGEL & A. HERZ. 1992. Conditioning of opioid reinforcement: Neurochemical and neuroanatomical substrates. Ann. N.Y. Acad. Sci. **654:** 347–356. This volume.
33. WISE, R. A. 1992. Self-stimulation and drug reward mechanisms. Ann. N.Y. Acad. Sci. **654:** 192–198. This volume.
34. DE WIED, D. & B. BOHUS. 1979. Modulation of memory processes by neuropeptides of hypothalamic-neurohypophyseal origin. *In* Brain Mechanisms in Memory and Learning: From the Single Neuron to Man. M. A. B. Brazier, Ed.: 139–149. Raven Press. New York.
35. KELLEY, A. E. & L. STINUS. 1984. The distribution of the projection from the parataenial nucleus of the thalamus to the nucleus accumbens in the rat: An autoradiographic study. Exp. Brain Res. **54:** 499–512.
36. JAFFE, J. H. 1987. Drug addiction and drug abuse. *In* Goodman and Gilman's The Pharmacological Basis of Therapeutics. A. G. Gilman, L. S. Goodman & T. W. Rall, Eds. 7th Edit.: 532–580. MacMillan Publishing Co. New York.
37. WAY, E. L., H. H. LOH & F. H. SHEN. 1969. Simultaneous quantitative assessment of morphine tolerance and physical dependence. J. Pharmacol. Exp. Ther. **167:** 1–8.
38. GELLERT, V. F. & S. B. SPARBER. 1977. A comparison of the effects of naloxone upon body weight loss and suppression of fixed-ratio operant behavior in morphine-dependent rats. J. Pharmacol. Exp. Ther. **201:** 44–54.
39. WEI, E., H. H. LOH & E. L. WAY. 1972. Neuroanatomical correlates of morphine dependence. Science **177:** 616–617.
40. WEI, E., H. H. LOH & E. L. WAY. 1973. Brain sites of precipitated abstinence in morphine-dependent rats. J. Pharmacol. Exp. Ther. **185:** 108–115.
41. BOZARTH, M. A. & R. A. WISE. 1984. Anatomically distinct opiate receptor fields mediate reward and physical dependence. Science **224:** 516–517.
42. MALDONALDO, R., L. GOLD, L. STINUS & G. F. KOOB. 1992. Morphine withdrawal syndrome after local administration of methylnaloxonium in several brain structure. J. Pharmacol. Exp. Ther. In press.
43. KOOB, G. F., T. L. WALL & F. E. BLOOM. 1989. Nucleus accumbens as a substrate for the aversive stimulus effects of opiate withdrawal. Psychopharmacology (Berlin) **98:** 530–534.
44. HAND, T. H., G. F. KOOB, L. STINUS & M. LE MOAL. 1988. Aversive properties of opiate receptor blockade are centrally mediated and are potentiated by previous exposure to opiates. Brain Res. **474:** 364–368.
45. STINUS, L., M. LE MOAL & G. F. KOOB. 1990. The nucleus accumbens and amygdala as possible substrates for the aversive stimulus effects of opiate withdrawal. Neuroscience **37:** 767–773.
46. SAMSON, H. S. 1986. Initiation of ethanol reinforcement using a sucrose-substitution procedure in food- and water-sated rats. Alcoholism: Clinical and Experimental Research **10:** 436–442.
47. GRANT, K. A. & H. H. SAMSON. 1985. Induction and maintenance of ethanol self-administration without food deprivation in the rat. Psychopharmacology **86:** 475–479.
48. WEISS, F., M. MITCHINER, F. E. BLOOM & G. F. KOOB. 1990. Free-choice responding for ethanol versus water in Alcohol-Preferring (P) and unselected Wistar rats is differentially

altered by naloxone, bromocriptine and methysergide. Psychopharmacology **101:** 178–186.

49. PULVIRENTI, L. & A. J. KASTIN. 1988. Naloxone, but not Tyr-MIF-1, reduces volitional ethanol drinking in rats: Correlation with degree of spontaneous preferences. Pharmacol. Biochem. Behav. **31:** 129–134.

50. REID, L. D. & G. A. HUNTER. 1984. Morphine and naloxone modulate intake of ethanol. Alcohol **1:** 33–37.

51. SANDI, C., J. BORELL & C. GUZAZ. 1988. Naloxone decreases ethanol consumption within a free choice paradigm in rats. Pharmacol. Biochem. Behav. **29:** 39–43.

52. VOLPICELLI, R., M. A. DAVIS & J. E. OLGIN. 1986. Naltrexone blocks the post-shock increase of ethanol consumption. Life Sci. **38:** 841–847.

53. MARFAING-JALLAT, P., D. MICELI & J. LEMAGNEN. 1983. Decrease in ethanol consumption by naloxone in naive and dependent rats. Pharmacol. Biochem. Behav. **18:** 5355–5395.

54. HUNTER, G. A., C. M. BEAMAN, L. L. DUNN & L. D. REID. 1984. Selected opioids, ethanol and intake of alcohol. Alcohol **1:** 43–46.

55. HUBBELL, C. L., S. A. CZIRR & L. D. REID. 1987. Persistence and specificity of small doses of morphine on intake of alcoholic beverages. Alcohol **4:** 149–156.

56. REID, L. D., S. A. CZIRR, C. C. BENSINGER, C. L. HUBBELL & A. J. VOLANTH. 1987. Morphine and diprenorphine together potentiate intake of alcoholic beverages. Alcohol **4:** 161–168.

57. BROWN, D. R. & S. G. HOLTZMAN. 1979. Suppression of deprivation-induced food and water intake in rats and mice by naloxone. Pharmacol. Biochem. Behav. **11:** 567–573.

58. HOLTZMAN, S. G. 1979. Suppression of appetitive behavior in the rat by naloxone: Lack of effect of prior morphine dependence. Life Sci. **24:** 219–226.

59. HYNES, M. A., M. GALLAGHER & K. V. YACOS. 1981. Systemic and intraventricular naloxone administration: Effects on food and water intake. Behav. Neural Biol. **32:** 334–342.

60. COOPER, S. J. 1980. Naloxone: Effects on food and water consumption in the non-deprived and deprived rat. Psychopharmacology **71**(1): 1–6.

61. STAPLETON, J. M., N. L. OSTROWSKI, V. J. MERRIMAN, M. D. LIND & L. D. REID. 1979. Naloxone reduces fluid consumption in deprived and nondeprived rats. Bull. Psychon. Soc. **13:** 237–239.

62. AMIT, S., E. A. SUTHERLAND, K. BILL & S. O. OGREN. 1984. Zimelidine: A review of its effects on ethanol consumption. Neurosci. Biobehav. Rev. **8:** 35–54.

63. GELLER, I. 1973. Effects of para-chlorophenylalanine and 5-hydroxytryptophane on alcohol intake in rats. Pharmacol. Biochem. Behav. **1:** 361–365.

64. LAWRIN, M. O., C. A. NARANJO & E. M. SELLERS. 1986. Identification of new drugs for modulating alcohol consumption. Psychopharmacol. Bull. **22:** 1020–1025.

65. FREY, H-H., M. P. MAGNUSSEN & C. KAERGAARD NIELSEN. 1970. The effect of p-chloroamphetamine on the consumption of ethanol by rats. Arch. Int. Pharmacodyn. Ther. **183:** 165–172.

66. MYERS, R. D. & W. L. VEALE. 1968. Alcohol preference in the rats: Reduction following depletion of brain serotonin. Science **160:** 1469–1471.

67. VEALE, W. L. & R. D. MYERS. 1970. Decrease in ethanol intake in rats following administration of p-chlorophenylalanine. Neuropharmacology **9:** 317–326.

68. PFEFFER, A. O. & H. H. SAMSON. 1988. Haloperidol and apomorphine effects on ethanol reinforcement in free-feeding rats. Pharmacol. Biochem. Behav. **29:** 343–350.

69. PFEFFER, A. O. & H. H. SAMSON. 1985. Oral ethanol reinforcements: Interactive effects of amphetamine, pimozide and food restriction. Alcohol Drug Res. **6:** 37–48.

70. PFEFFER, A. O. & H. H. SAMSON. 1986. Effect of pimozide on home cage ethanol drinking in the rat: Dependence on drinking session length. Drug Alcohol Depend. **17:** 47–55.

71. RASSNICK, S., L. PULVIRENTI & G. F. KOOB. 1990. Modulation of ethanol self-administration by dopamine and GABA mechanisms within the nucleus accumbens. Abstract Research Society on Alcoholism, Toronto.

72. WEISS, F., Y. L. HURD, U. UNGERSTEDT, A. MARKOU, P. M. PLOTSKY & G. F. KOOB.

1992. Neurochemical correlates of cocaine and ethanol self-administration. Ann. N.Y. Acad. Sci. **654:** 220–241. This volume.

73. LILJEQUIST, S. & J. A. ENGEL. 1984. The effects of GABA and benzodiazepine receptor antagonists on the anti-conflict actions of diazepam or ethanol. Pharmacol. Biochem. Behav. **21:** 521–525.

74. KOOB, G. F., W. B. MENDELSON, J. SCHAFER, T. L. WALL, K. THATCHER-BRITTON & F. E. BLOOM. 1988. Picrotoxin receptor ligand blocks anti-punishment effects of alcohol. Alcohol **5:** 437–443.

75. FRYE, G. D. & G. R. BRESE. 1982. GABAergic modulation of ethanol-induced motor impairment. J. Pharmacol. Exp. Ther. **223:** 750–756.

76. LILJEQUIST, S. & J. ENGEL. 1982. Effects of GABAergic agonists and antagonists on various ethanol-induced behavioral changes. Psychopharmacology **78:** 7! 75.

77. SUZDAK, P. D., R. D. SCHWARTZ, P. SKOLNICK & S. M. PAUL. 1986. Ethanol stimulates gamma-aminobutyric acid receptor-mediated chloride transport in rat brain synaptoneurosome. Proc. Natl. Acad. Sci. USA **83:** 4071–4075.

78. ALLAN, A. M. & R. A. HARRIS. 1987. Acute and chronic ethanol treatments alter GABA receptor-operated chloride channels. Pharmacol. Biochem. Behav. **27:** 665–670.

79. SUZDAK, P. D., J. R. GLOWA, J. N. CRAWLEY, R. D. SCHWARTZ, P. SKOLNICK & S. M. PAUL. 1986. A selective imidazobenzodiazepine antagonist of ethanol in the rat. Science **236:** 1243–1247.

80. BRITTON, K. T., C. L. EHLERS & G. F. KOOB. 1988. Is ethanol antagonist RO 15-4513 selective for ethanol. Science **239:** 648–650.

81. SAMSON, H. H., G. A. TOLLIVER, A. O. PFEFFER, K. G. SADEGHI & F. G. MILLS. 1987. Oral ethanol reinforcement in the rat: Effect of the partial inverse benzodiazepine agonist RO15-4513. Pharmacol. Biochem. Behav. **27:** 517–519.

82. RASSNICK, S., L. D'AMICO, E. RILEY, L. PULVIRENTI, W. ZIEGLGÄNSBERGER & G. F. KOOB. 1992. GABA and nucleus accumbens glutamate neurotransmission modulate ethanol self-administration in rats. Ann. N.Y. Acad. Sci. **654:** 502–505. This volume.

83. DEITRICH, R. A., T. V. DUNWIDDIE, R. A. HARRIS & V. G. ERWIN. 1989. Mechanism of action of ethanol: Initial central nervous system actions. Pharmacol. Rev. **41:** 489–537.

84. KOOB, G. F. & F. E. BLOOM. 1988. Cellular and molecular mechanisms of drug dependence. Science **242:** 715–723.

85. DENOBLE, U. & H. BEGLEITER. 1976. Response suppression on a mixed schedule of reinforcement during alcohol withdrawal. Pharmacol. Biochem. Behav. **5:** 227–229.

86. RASSNICK, S., G. F. KOOB & M. A. GEYER. 1992. Responding to acoustic startle during chronic ethanol intoxication and withdrawal. Psychopharmacology **106:** 351–358.

87. BALDWIN, H. A., S. RASSNICK, J. RIVIER, G. F. KOOB & K. T. BRITTON. 1991. CRF antagonist reverses the "anxiogenic" response to ethanol withdrawal in the rat. Psychopharmacology **103:** 227–232.

88. COOPER, B. R., K. VIIK, R. M. FERRIS & H. L. WHITE. 1979. Antagonism of the enhanced susceptibility to audiogenic seizures during alcohol withdrawal in the rat by gamma-aminobutyric acid (GABA) and GABA-mimetics. J. Pharmacol. Exp. Ther. **209:** 396–408.

89. FRYE, G. D., T. J. MCCOWN & G. R. BREESE. 1983. Differential sensitivity of ethanol withdrawal signs in the rat to gamma-aminobutyric acid (GABA) mimetics: Blockade of audiogenic seizures but not forelimb tremors. JPET **226:** 720–723.

90. GOLDSTEIN, D. B. 1973. Alcohol withdrawal reaction in mice: Effects of drugs that modify neurotransmission. J. Pharmacol. Exp. Ther. **186:** 1–9.

91. LISTER, R. G. & J. W. KARANIAN. 1987. RO 15-4513 induces seizures in DBA/2 mice undergoing alcohol withdrawal. Alcohol 4(5): 409–411.

92. LAL, H., C. M. HARRIS, D. BENJAMIN, A. C. SPRINGFIELD, S. BLADRA & M. EMMETT-OGLESBY. 1988. Characterization of a pentylenetetrazol-like interoceptive stimulus produced by ethanol withdrawal. J. Pharmacol. Exp. Ther. **247:** 508–518.

93. INDEMUDIA, S. O., S. BLADRA & H. LAL. 1989. The pentylenetetrazol-like interoceptive stimulus produced by ethanol withdrawal is potentiated by bicuculline and picrotoxin. Neuropsychopharmacology **2:** 115–122.

94. BALDWIN, H. A., K. T. BRITTON & G. F. KOOB. 1990. Behavioral effects of CRF. *In* Behavioral Aspects of Neuroendocrinology. D. W. Pfaff & D. Ganten, Eds.: 1–14. Springer Verlag.
95. FILE, S. E., H. A. BALDWIN & P. K. HITCHCOTT. 1989. Flumazenil but not nitrendipine reverses the increased anxiety during ethanol withdrawal in the rat. Psychopharmacology **98:** 252–264.
96. KOOB, G. F. 1991. Neurobiological mechanisms in cocaine and opiate dependence. *In* Advances in Understanding the Addictive State. Raven Press. New York.
97. KOOB, G. F. & N. R. SWERDLOW. 1988. Functional output of the mesolimbic dopamine system. Ann. N.Y. Acad. Sci. **537:** 216–227.

Self-Stimulation and Drug Reward Mechanisms

ROY A. WISE, PASQUALINO BAUCO,
AND WILLIAM A. CARLEZON, JR.

Center for Studies in Behavioral Neurobiology
Concordia University
Montréal, Québec, Canada H3G 1M8

WERONIKA TROJNIAR

Department of Physiology
University of Gdansk
Gdansk, Poland

Important advances in our understanding of the habit-forming effects of drugs have come from an appreciation of the ability of drugs to serve as operant reinforcers. An operant reinforcer is a stimulus event which, when made contingent upon some act of an animal, increases the probability of recurrence of that act. Intravenous injections of habit-forming drugs establish and maintain such arbitrary habits as lever-pressing, and drug self-administration by lever-pressing has provided us with animal models of intravenous drug-seeking in humans.

Habit-forming drugs do more than merely serve as operant reinforcers, however. Animals learn to approach the portions of the environment where they have received drugs in the past,[1-3] and they do so through Pavlovian rather than operant conditioning.[4] Habit-forming drugs also reinstate or "prime" operant responding after periods of non-reward or temporarily disrupted responding.[5,6] Finally, they sometimes potentiate the effectiveness of other rewards: cannabis,[7-9] amphetamine,[10,11] and opiates[12,13] facilitate feeding; opiates facilitate sexual behavior[14] in animals; and cannabis is reported to enhance the rewarding effects of food, music, and sexual interaction in humans.

The ability of habit-forming drugs to potentiate the rewarding effects of medial forebrain bundle brain stimulation reward[15-17] offers a particularly useful model in which to quantify such interactions. Most classes of abused drugs have been shown to increase lever-pressing for brain stimulation reward; this is true of amphetamine,[18] cocaine,[19] nicotine,[20,21] opiates,[22] cannabis,[23] phencyclidine,[24] ethanol,[25] barbiturates,[26] and benzodiazepines.[27] In several cases it is clear that the drugs enhance the rewarding impact of the brain stimulation and do not merely enhance the response capacity of the animal.

The primary evidence that a drug enhances the rewarding effects of brain stimulation is that the drug reduces the amount of stimulation needed to motivate normal responding.[15] Rewarding stimulation is given in the form of brief trains of pulsed current, and the potency of each rewarding stimulation train is traditionally controlled by varying either the intensity or the frequency of stimulation. Typically, when one stimulation parameter is varied, the other stimulation parameters are held constant. Variations in the stimulation intensity alter the effective radius of current spread from the electrode tip, increasing or decreasing the size of the population of directly activated medial forebrain bundle fibers. Variations in the stimulation frequency alter the number of times per stimulation that action potentials are triggered in a fixed population of directly activated fibers. The minimum stimulation intensity or stimulation frequency required to sustain lever-pressing is defined as the intensity threshold or the frequency threshold; such thresholds vary with electrode characteristics, stimulation site, and with a variety of factors such as response requirements and drug treatments. Brain stimulation reward thresholds have been found to be lowered by amphetamine, cocaine, nicotine, phencyclidine, ethanol, and cannabis.[15-17]

Thresholds represent single points on the function relating rate or strength of responding to the intensity or frequency of stimulation. Rate-intensity or rate-frequency functions essentially represent brain stimulation reward "dose-effect" functions, where the rewarding "dose" of stimulation is inferred from the stimulation frequency or intensity.[28] These dose-response functions take the same general shape and behave in the same general manner as traditional pharmacological dose-effect curves. That is, the behavioral effect is nil if the dose of stimulation is too low, the behavioral effect is maximal if the dose of stimulation is beyond some upper limit, and the rate of stimulation increases relatively linearly with stimulation values between these extremes.[29]

Self-stimulation threshold can be defined in relation to a variety of arbitrary response criteria. Some workers demand a minimal absolute rate of responding (*e.g.*, 5 or 10 responses per minute) while others demand a minimal relative rate (5% or 50% of the maximal response rate for a given animal and a given electrode). In cases where the test drug causes a parallel shift of the rate-frequency function, the choice of response criterion is irrelevant; the effectiveness of the drug is the same regardless of what response criterion is used (FIG. 1).

Low and moderate doses of dopamine antagonists cause parallel rightward shifts of the rate-intensity[30] or rate-frequency[18]; higher doses can cause independent downward as well as rightward shifts.[31] The rightward shifts reflect what would be interpreted as competitive antagonism in a dose-response analysis; dopamine antagonists reduce the rewarding effectiveness of the stimulation. Amphetamine, an indirect dopamine agonist, causes parallel leftward shifts of the rate-frequency function and can reverse the effects of a dopamine antagonist.[18] Thus the effects of amphetamine synergize with the synaptic events triggered by the rewarding stimulation. It is generally assumed that it is amphetamine's ability to cause synaptic dopamine release that synergizes with the rewarding effects of stimulation and antagonizes the effects of dopamine blockers.

Parallel leftward shifts in the rate-frequency functions of animals lever-pressing for lateral hypothalamic or midline mesencephalic brain stimulation reward are typical not only of amphetamine but also of morphine,[31] cocaine (FIG. 1), nicotine (FIG. 2),[21] and phencyclidine (FIG. 3).[24] Each of these drugs, like amphetamine, can be considered an indirect dopamine agonist; each, like amphetamine, causes increases in synaptic dopamine levels.[32,33] In the case of morphine, sedative side-effects can obscure the reward-facilitating effects of the drug; however, if the drug is given centrally, in the ventral tegmental area, its ability to cause leftward shifts in the rate frequency function and its ability to reverse the effects of low doses of dopamine antagonists is readily demonstrated.[31] (Note that morphine and dopamine antagonists can synergize at

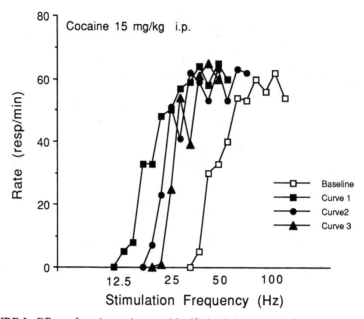

FIGURE 1. Effects of cocaine on intracranial self-stimulation rate as a function of stimulation frequency. Successive rate-frequency curves were taken at 30-min intervals. Cocaine caused large parallel leftward shifts in the rate-frequency functions.

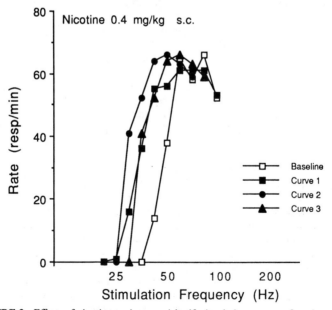

FIGURE 2. Effects of nicotine on intracranial self-stimulation rate as a function of stimulation frequency. Successive rate-frequency curves were taken at 15-min intervals. Nicotine caused moderate parallel leftward shifts in the rate-frequency functions.

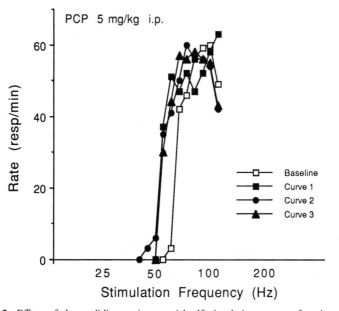

FIGURE 3. Effects of phencyclidine on intracranial self-stimulation rate as a function of stimulation frequency. Successive rate-frequency curves were taken at 18-min intervals. PCP caused minor parallel leftward shifts in the rate-frequency functions.

higher doses.[34]) Our current working hypothesis is that the rewarding effects of these drugs summate with the rewarding effects of stimulation, increasing the rewarding consequences of self-stimulation by increasing the synaptic levels of nucleus accumbens dopamine that are known to be caused by each treatment by itself.[4,35]

The case of ethanol is not so clear-cut, at least in our hands to date. We (Trojniar & Wise, in preparation) have attempted to assess the effects of ethanol in the "curve-shift" paradigm; we have dealt with the fact that ethanol has a half-life shorter than our typical testing periods by giving ethanol by intravenous drip. We see leftward shifts in some animals and rightward shifts in an approximately equal number of others; when we consider the effects of ethanol on our animals as a group, most animals show little or no effect of sub-intoxicating doses of ethanol and those animals that do seem to be affected are as likely to have their thresholds increased as to have them decreased. We have seen interesting differences between groups involving animals of different strains or different previous experience with ethanol, but these differences must be replicated before they are taken as more than chance differences. The one statistically reliable finding from this work is that ethanol increases the variability of our animals' behavior; it appears to do so by an order of magnitude. However, neither increases nor decreases in threshold appear to reflect parallel shifts of our rate-frequency functions. In each case, the thresholds shift without a corresponding shift in the behavior maintained by higher "doses" of stimulation. Without further study we can suggest no reasonable explanation of these findings.

Our current hypothesis is that the reward-facilitating effects of amphetamine, cocaine, morphine, phencyclidine, and nicotine each depends on the same brain mechanism of the direct rewarding effects of these substances.[4,35] In the case of morphine and amphetamine, we know that the brain sites where the drugs facilitate brain stimulation reward are brain sites where the drugs have rewarding actions in their own right. In the case of morphine, there are two such sites: the ventral tegmental area[36-38] and the nucleus accumbens.[39,40] In the case of amphetamine the reward-facilitating[41,42] and rewarding[43,44] actions are associated with nucleus accumbens. The site at which cocaine facilitates brain stimulation reward has not been determined; cocaine has local anesthetic properties that make it a poor choice for central injection studies. In the case of nicotine, the ventral tegmental area seems a likely site and is under current investigation.

Whether the reported reward-facilitating and rewarding effects of ethanol and cannabis depend on their known ability to increase synaptic dopamine concentrations remains to be confirmed; in neither case is the site of the rewarding or the reward-facilitating action known. Two drug classes that have abuse liability in humans and that are self-administered in lower animals but that do not increase—rather they decrease[45]—synaptic dopamine concentrations are barbiturates and benzodiazepines. These agents may act by reward mechanisms that are independent of the mesolimbic dopamine system, or they may simply act efferent to the dopaminergic link in the reward circuitry that seems common to the drugs discussed above.

REFERENCES

1. Spragg, S. D. S. 1940. Morphine addiction in chimpanzees. Comp. Psychol. Monogr. 15: 1-132.
2. Beach, H. D. 1957. Morphine addiction in rats. Can. J. Psychol. 11: 104-112.
3. Rossi, N. A. & L. D. Reid. 1976. Affective states associated with morphine injections. Physiol. Psychol. 4: 269-274.
4. Wise, R. A. 1989. The brain and reward. In The Neuropharmacological Basis of Reward. J. M. Liebman & S. J. Cooper, Eds.: 377-424. Oxford University Press. Oxford.
5. Gerber, G. J. & R. Stretch. 1975. Drug-induced reinstatement of extinguished self-administration behavior in monkeys. Pharmacol. Biochem. Behav. 3: 1055-1061.
6. Stewart, J. & H. de Wit. 1987. Reinstatement of drug-taking behavior as a method of assessing incentive motivational properties of drugs. In Methods of Assessing the Reinforcing Properties of Abused Drugs. M. A. Bozarth, Ed.: 211-227. Springer-Verlag. New York.
7. Glick, S. D. & S. Milloy. 1972. Increased and decreased eating following THC administration. Psychonom. Sci. 29: 6.
8. Hollister, L. E. 1971. Hunger and appetite after single doses of marijuana, alcohol and dextroamphetamine. Pharmacol. Ther. 12: 44-49.
9. Trojniar, W. & R. A. Wise. 1989. Facilitory effect of Δ⁹-tetrahydrocannabinol on hypothalamically induced feeding. Psychopharmacology 103: 172-176.
10. Blundell, J. E. & C. J. Latham. 1980. Characterization of adjustments to the structure of feeding behavior following pharmacological treatment: Effects of amphetamine and fenfluramine and the antagonism produced by pimozide and methergoline. Pharmacol. Biochem. Behav. 12: 717-722.
11. Colle, L. M. & R. A. Wise. 1988. Concurrent facilitory and inhibitory effects of amphetamine on stimulation-induced eating. Brain Res. 459: 356-360.
12. Jenck, F., A. Gratton & R. A. Wise. 1986. Opposite effects of ventral tegmental and periaqueductal gray morphine injections on lateral hypothalamic stimulation-induced feeding. Brain Res. 399: 24-32.

13. LIEBOWITZ, S. F. & L. HOR. 1982. Endorphinergic and α-noradrenergic systems in the paraventricular nucleus: Effects on eating behaviour. Peptides 3: 421–428.
14. MITCHELL, J. B. & J. STEWART. 1990. Facilitation of sexual behavior in the male rat associated with intra-VTA injections of opiates. Pharmacol. Biochem. Behav. 12: 717–722.
15. KORNETSKY, C., R. U. ESPOSITO, S. MCLEAN & J. D. JACOBSON. 1979. Intracranial self-stimulation thresholds: A model for the hedonic effects of drugs of abuse. Arch. Gen. Psychiat. 36: 289–292.
16. GARDNER, E. L. 1992. Brain reward systems and drug addiction. *In* Advances in Psychopharmacology and Behavioral Neurobiology. R. J. Birnbaum, J. F. Rosenbaum & M. Fava, Eds. Raven Press. New York. In press.
17. WISE, R. A. 1980. Action of drugs of abuse on brain reward systems. Pharmacol. Biochem. Behav. 13: 213–223.
18. GALLISTEL, C. R. & D. KARRAS. 1984. Pimozide and amphetamine have opposing effects on the reward summation function. Pharmacol. Biochem. Behav. 20: 73–77.
19. CROW, T. J. 1970. Enhancement by cocaine of intra-cranial self-stimulation in the rat. Life Sci. 9: 375–381.
20. CLARKE, P. B. S. & R. KUMAR. 1984. Effects of nicotine and *d*-amphetamine on intracranial self-stimulation in a shuttle box test in rats. Psychopharmacology 84: 109–114.
21. BAUCO, P. & R. A. WISE. 1990. Effect of repeated nicotine administration on dorsal raphe brain stimulation reward. Soc. Neurosci. Abstr. 16: 593.
22. BUSH, H. D., M. A. BUSH, M. A. MILLER & L. D. REID. 1976. Addictive agents and intracranial self-stimulation: Daily morphine and lateral hypothalamic self-stimulation. Physiol. Psychol. 4: 79–85.
23. GARDNER, E. L., W. PAREDES, D. SMITH, A. DONNER, C. MILLING, D. COHEN & D. MORRISON. 1988. Facilitation of brain stimulation reward by Δ⁹-tetrahydrocannabinol. Psychopharmacology 96: 142–144.
24. CARLEZON, W. A., JR. & R. A. WISE. 1991. The effects of repeated phencyclidine (PCP) on lateral hypothalamic brain stimulation reward (BSR) and locomotion in rats. Soc. Neurosci. Abstr. 17: 1237.
25. KORNETSKY, C., G. T. BAIN, E. M. UNTERWALD & M. J. LEWIS. 1988. Brain stimulation reward: Effects of ethanol. Alcoholism: Clin. Exp. Res. 12: 609–616.
26. REID, L. D., W. E. GIBSON, S. M. GLEDHILL & P. B. PORTER. 1964. Anticonvulsant drugs and self-stimulation behavior. J. Comp. Physiol. Psychol. 7: 353–356.
27. OLDS, J. 1966. Facilitatory action of diazepam and chlordiazepoxide on hypothalamic reward behavior. J. Comp. Physiol. Psychol. 62: 136–140.
28. LIEBMAN, J. M. 1983. Discriminating between reward and performance: A critical review of intracranial self-stimulation methodology. Neurosci. Biobehav. Rev. 7: 45–72.
29. MILIARESSIS, E., P.-P. ROMPRÉ, L. P. LAVIOLETTE, L. PHILIPPE & D. COULOMBE. 1986. The curve-shift paradigm in self-stimulation. Physiol. Behav. 37: 85–91.
30. LYNCH, M. R. & R. A. WISE. 1985. Relative effectiveness of pimozide, haloperidol and trifluoperazine on self-stimulation rate-intensity functions. Pharmacol. Biochem. Behav. 23: 777–780.
31. ROMPRÉ, P.-P. & R. A. WISE. 1989. Opioid-neuroleptic interaction in brainstem self-stimulation. Brain Res. 477: 144–151.
32. DI CHIARA, G. & A. IMPERATO. 1988. Drugs of abuse preferentially stimulate dopamine release in the mesolimbic system of freely moving rats. Proc. Natl. Acad. Sci. (USA) 85: 5274–5278.
33. NG CHEONG TON, J. M., G. A. GERHARDT, M. FRIEDEMANN, A. ETGEN, G. M. ROSE, N. S. SHARPLESS & E. L. GARDNER. 1988. The effects of Δ⁹-tetrahydrocannabinol on potassium-evoked release of dopamine in the rat caudate nucleus: An in vivo electrochemical and in vivo microdialysis study. Brain Res. 451: 59–68.
34. ROMPRÉ, P.-P. & R. A. WISE. 1989. Behavioral evidence for midbrain dopamine depolarization inactivation. Brain Res. 477: 152–156.
35. WISE, R. A. & M. A. BOZARTH. 1987. A psychomotor stimulant theory of addiction. Psychol. Rev. 94: 469–492.
36. BROEKKAMP, C. L. E., J. H. VAN DEN BOGAARD, H. J. HEIJNEN, R. H. ROPS, A. R. COOLS & J. M. VAN ROSSUM. 1976. Separation of inhibiting and stimulating effects of mor-

phine on self-stimulation behavior by intracerebral microinjections. Eur. J. Pharmacol. **36:** 443–446.

37. JENCK, F., A. GRATTON & R. A. WISE. 1987. Opioid receptor subtypes associated with ventral tegmental facilitation of lateral hypothalamic brain stimulation reward. Brain Res. **423:** 34–38.

38. BOZARTH, M. A. & R. A. WISE. 1981. Intracranial self-administration of morphine into the ventral tegmental area of rats. Life Sci. **28:** 551–555.

39. WEST, T. E. G. & R. A. WISE. 1988. Nucleus accumbens opioids facilitate brain stimulation reward. Soc. Neurosci. Abstr. **14:** 1102.

40. OLDS, M. E. 1982. Reinforcing effects of morphine in the nucleus accumbens. Brain Res. **237:** 429–440.

41. BROEKKAMP, C. L. E., A. J. J. PIJNENBURG, A. R. COOLS & J. M. VAN ROSSUM. 1975. The effect of microinjections of amphetamine into the neostriatum and the nucleus accumbens on self-stimulation behavior. Psychopharmacologia **42:** 179–183.

42. COLLE, L. M. & R. A. WISE. 1988. Effects of nucleus accumbens amphetamine on lateral hypothalamic brain stimulation reward. Brain Res. **459:** 361–368.

43. HOEBEL, B. G., A. P. MONACO, L. HERNANDEZ, E. F. AULISI, B. G. STANLEY & L. LENARD. 1983. Self-injection of amphetamine directly into the brain. Psychopharmacology **81:** 158–163.

44. CARR, G. D. & N. M. WHITE. 1983. Conditioned place preference from intra-accumbens but not intra-caudate amphetamine injections. Life Sci. **33:** 2551–2557.

45. WOOD, P. L. 1982. Actions of GABAergic agents on dopamine metabolism in the nigrostriatal pathway of the rat. J. Pharmacol. Exp. Ther. **222:** 674–679.

Self-Stimulation of the Ventral Tegmental Area Enhances Dopamine Release in the Nucleus Accumbens: A Microdialysis Study[a]

A. G. PHILLIPS,[b,c] A. COURY,[b] D. FIORINO,[b]
F. G. LePIANE,[b] E. BROWN,[d] AND H. C. FIBIGER[d]

[b]Department of Psychology and
[d]Division of Neurological Sciences
Department of Psychiatry
University of British Columbia
Vancouver, B.C., Canada V6T 1Z4

INTRODUCTION

Several groups[1-4] maintain that substances of abuse such as cocaine achieve their rewarding properties by the activation of a specific reward system in the brain that also will support intracranial self-stimulation (ICSS). There are a number of advantages in the use of the ICSS procedure to study the rewarding effects of drugs, including its methodological simplicity and the high concordance between the pharmacological facilitation of ICSS and human addiction liability data.[1] Most researchers who study the effects of drugs on ICSS are well aware of the possible confounds that can arise from unconditioned motor effects of the drugs and from fatigue. Accordingly, procedures have been developed to measure current thresholds required to maintain ICSS. Employing this procedure, Esposito *et al.*[5] showed that cocaine lowered the threshold for rewarding brain-stimulation, thereby extending Crow's[6] initial report of an increase in ICSS rate by cocaine.

A distinct advantage of using the ICSS procedure to study drug-reward is the information provided about neuronal circuits that may subserve the rewarding properties of drugs of abuse. A large body of data derived from pharmacological, neurotoxic lesion and postmortem neurochemical studies support the role of mesotelencephalic dopaminergic neurons in ICSS at sites in the ventral tegmental area (VTA) and parts of the medial forebrain bundle (MFB) (cf. refs. 2, 4, 7). Until recently however, critical *in vivo* evidence in support of this hypothesis was lacking. Two new techniques for mea-

[a] This research was supported by a Program Grant (PG-23) from the Medical Research Council of Canada.

[c] Address correspondence to: A. G. Phillips, Department of Psychology, The University of British Columbia, Vancouver, B.C., Canada V6T 1Z4; Tel.: (604) 822-4624; Fax: (604) 822-6923.

suring changes in extracellular concentrations of dopamine *in vivo* have been used to address this shortcoming. The first approach used the electrochemical technique of chronoamperometry to measure current resulting from the oxidation of dopamine in terminal regions of the mesotelencephalic dopamine systems, including the nucleus accumbens. An initial experiment with anesthetized rats previously trained to deliver stimulation to either the VTA or MFB, reported that electrical stimulation at reward-relevant sites produced transient releases of an electroactive species resembling dopamine in the nucleus accumbens, medial prefrontal cortex and striatum.[8] More prolonged stimulation of the MFB at rates comparable to normal ICSS rates produced a more sustained increase in an electrochemical signal thought to represent 3,4-dihydroxyphenylacetic acid (DOPAC). Subsequent studies with unanesthetized freely-moving rats showed conclusively that chronoamperometric signals in the nucleus accumbens could be increased in a current intensity-dependent manner coincidentally with increasing rates of ICSS.[9,10] These data were obtained with a stearate-modified carbon paste electrode that can measure the oxidation of dopamine unconfounded by DOPAC or ascorbic acid.[11] Furthermore, both the chronoamperometric signal and the ICSS rate were facilitated by dopamine uptake blockers including nomifensine, cocaine and GBR 12909, thereby providing independent confirmation that the signal reflected dopamine levels in the nucleus accumbens.

Very similar experiments have been conducted with a second *in vivo* technique, microdialysis, with high performance liquid chromatography and electrochemical detection (HPLC-EC). This procedure has the advantage of unequivocally measuring changes in several neurochemical species including dopamine, DOPAC, homovanillic acid (HVA) and 5-hydroxyindoleacetic acid (5-HIAA). The sampling rate of microdialysis is much slower than chronoamperometry, and care must be taken to ensure that sufficient time has elapsed between insertion of the probe into brain and sampling of the extracellular fluid. This is necessary to minimize non-physiological levels of dopamine and its metabolites arising from damaged neurons. It is now recommended that this period be at least 18 h.[12] Using a microdialysis system designed for chronic experiments, Nakahara *et al.*[13] reported that extracellular concentrations of DOPAC and HVA were increased in dialysate samples from the nucleus accumbens during spontaneous ICSS of the MFB in rats. Surprisingly, only a small increase in dopamine levels was observed and this failed to reach statistical significance. In a subsequent experiment this group[14] reported a significant increase in dopamine levels in the nucleus accumbens during MFB-ICSS by rats pretreated with nomifensine (1 mg/kg). The fact that similar changes were observed with experimenter-administered MFB stimulation suggested that the effects on dopamine levels were due to the rewarding effects of the brain-stimulation and not to the motor activity of bar-pressing.

Collectively, both chronoamperometry and microdialysis studies support a role for the mesotelencephalic dopamine system in brain-stimulation reward. However, the discrepancies in the results obtained to date cannot be overlooked, in particular the failure of microdialysis to detect an increase in dopamine levels in the nucleus accumbens during ICSS by rats untreated with a dopamine uptake blocker. Two factors may have militated against the predicted increase in dopamine, including the placement of stimulating electrodes in the MFB instead of the VTA, and sampling from the microdialysis probes just three hours after insertion into brain. The present experiment sought to re-examine the usefulness of microdialysis in monitoring changes in dopamine and its metabolites during ICSS; first by using electrode placements in the VTA and secondly by implanting a microdialysis probe into the nucleus accumbens via a chronic cannula guide, 18–24 h prior to the HPLC-EC analysis of dialysate samples during and after an ICSS session. Success in measuring increases in extracellular dopamine during ICSS would set the stage for a subsequent study of the effects of drugs of abuse such as cocaine on both ICSS behavior and the stimulated release of dopamine.

METHODS

Intracranial Self-Stimulation

Male Long-Evans rats (340–530 g) (Charles River Canada, Inc., St. Constance, Québec) were anesthetized with sodium pentobarbital (60 mg/kg) prior to stereotaxic implantation of a bipolar stimulating electrode (Plastic Products Co.) into the VTA (AP + 3.4 L ± 0.5 D/V + 1.8 from ear bars) and a 19 ga stainless steel guide cannulae dorsal to the nucleus accumbens (AP + 1.8, L ± 1 mm from Bregma and 1 mm below dura). Following a 5–7 day post-operative period, each rat was screened for ICSS behavior. Stimulation current parameters were 60 Hz sine wave, 200 msec trains, intensity 16–26 μA. Rats ($n = 4$) that maintained stable rates of ICSS (>750 presses/15 min) were selected for the microdialysis phase of the experiment. The test day consisted of four separate phases: 1) baseline measures of neurotransmitter and metabolites, in which the animal was connected to the stimulating lead and to a dual electrical/liquid swivel (modified Instech 375D) with the stimulator disconnected (60 min); 2) first ICSS period (15 min) where each animal engaged in bar pressing for VTA stimulation (current = 18–22 μA); 3) post-ICSS recovery with no brain-stimulation available for 90 min; and 4) second ICSS period initiated with identical stimulation parameters to the first ICSS session.

Microdialysis

The day before the experiment (18–24 h), the animals were briefly anesthetized with halothane to facilitate manual insertion of the microdialysis probe into the guide cannula to a depth of 7.8 mm below dura. Dialysis occurred across a 2 mm vertical portion of exposed membrane at the end of the probe. This post-insertion period greatly reduces the contribution of dopamine from damaged cells. We have also verified in these conditions that the levels of dopamine are Ca^{++}, TTX, and K^+ dependent. The animal was then placed into a test chamber and connected to the swivel. The probe was flushed overnight at 1.5 μl/min in a physiological perfusate made of 0.01 M sodium phosphate buffer (pH 7.4 with 1.3 mM Ca^{++}). On the day of the experiment, 15-min dialysis samples were collected and injected manually through an HPLC-EC system.

Characteristics of the Microdialysis Probe

The dialysis probe is of concentric design consisting of a semi permeable hollow fiber (OD 340 μ, 65,000 M.W. cut-off, Filtral 12, Hospal), a PE 50 inlet tubing, a fused silica outlet tubing (175 μ ID × 150 μ OD) and 24 ga stainless steel cannula. Epoxy (Devcon 2-Ton) was used to seal the joints and plug the dialysis fiber. The inlet tubing

13

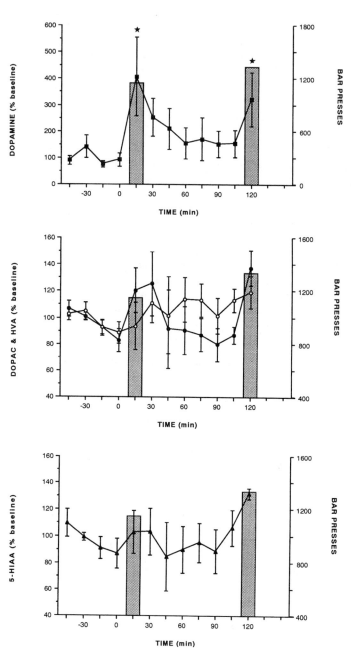

FIGURE 1. **Upper panel:** Changes in extracellular levels of dopamine in the nucleus accumbens during and between two 15 min sessions of VTA-ICSS. ICSS bar-press rates are indicated
by the two histograms at time 0 and 120 min. Data for dopamine levels are presented as % of
baseline values measured in four 15 min samples prior to ICSS. Basal values for dopamine were

was connected to a syringe pump (Harvard model 22). Typical *in vitro* recovery at 21°C and 1.5 μl/min is 15% for dopamine and 11% for the metabolites.

HPLC-EC

The compounds were separated by microbore reverse chromatography, Beckman column (ODS 5 μm, 15 cm, 2 mm i.d.) using 0.083 M sodium acetate buffer pH 3.5 with 4.2% methanol. The glassy carbon working electrode was set at +0.65 V. The apparatus consisted of a Spectra Physics 8810 HPLC pump, Rheodyne (7125) injector, electrochemical detector EEG400, and Shimadzu CR3A integrator.

RESULTS

VTA-ICSS

The four animals in this study averaged 1147 (range 977–1495) responses for rewarding VTA stimulation during the first 15 min ICSS session and the mean increased slightly to 1335 (range 827–1770) responses in the second ICSS session, 90 min later.

Dopamine Levels in the Nucleus Accumbens

As shown in the upper panel of FIGURE 1, basal levels of dopamine prior to the ICSS sessions averaged 0.763 ± 0.085 nM. Dopamine levels in the dialysate sampled during the first ICSS session increased significantly to 406 ± 148% ($p < 0.05$). Dopamine levels remained elevated but not significantly for 30 min after sessation of VTA stimulation. Dopamine levels were again increased significantly to 322 ± 102% ($p < 0.05$) during the second period of ICSS. A 1-way repeated measures ANOVA, $F = 4.29$, confirmed significant increases in dopamine levels during the 120 min period that included both ICSS sessions.

DOPAC and HVA Levels

Changes in the levels of the dopamine metabolites DOPAC and HVA are shown in the middle panel of FIGURE 1, and basal levels prior to VTA stimulation were $\overline{X}$ = 0.141 ± 0.024 μM and $\overline{X}$ = 0.104 ± 0.013 μM, respectively. DOPAC levels increased during the first ICSS session to 120% of baseline values. The levels of DOPAC

$\overline{X}$ = 0.763 ± 0.085 nM. * $p < 0.05$. **Middle panel:** Changes in extracellular levels of DOPAC (*closed circles*) and HVA (*open circles*) in the nucleus accumbens during and between two 15 min sessions of VTA-ICSS (*histograms*). Data for DOPAC and HVA levels are presented as % of baseline values. Basal values for DOPAC were $\overline{X}$ = 0.141 ± 0.024 μM, and for HVA, $\overline{X}$ = 0.104 ± 0.013 μM. **Lower panel:** Changes in extracellular levels of 5-HIAA in the nucleus accumbens during and between two 15 min sessions of VTA-ICSS (*histograms*). Data for 5-HIAA levels are presented as % of baseline values. Basal values were $\overline{X}$ = 0.046 ± 0.006 μM.

remained higher than baseline during the first 15 min post ICSS and had returned to baseline by 30 min. DOPAC levels were again increased to 137% of baseline during the second ICSS session. Changes in DOPAC levels were not statistically significant. The 1-way ANOVA failed to detect significant changes in HVA levels in the nucleus accumbens during or between the ICSS sessions.

5-HIAA Levels

5-HIAA levels in the nucleus accumbens were $\bar{X} = 0.046 \pm 0.006$ μM, prior to ICSS. A 1-way ANOVA failed to detect significant changes in 5-HIAA during or between the ICSS levels.

Histology

Histological analyses confirmed that the bipolar stimulating electrodes were located in the anterior region of the VTA. The exposed 2 mm sections of the microdialysis probes were also located accurately in the nucleus accumbens.

DISCUSSION

The present results provide clear evidence of increased release of dopamine in the nucleus accumbens during ICSS at electrode sites in the VTA. A 15-min ICSS session at near maximum current intensities was accompanied by a >300% increase in dopamine. The dopamine metabolites DOPAC and HVA were also elevated, to a much lesser degree (25% and 13%, respectively). It is important to note that dopamine levels remained elevated for 15–30 min after stimulation had terminated. These data are in general agreement with the conclusions drawn from the previous microdialysis studies of dopamine and its metabolites by Nakahara et al.,[13,14] but they differ in several respects. Employing stimulation sites in the MFB, this group failed to observe an increase in dopamine levels in the nucleus accumbens during ICSS, although significant increases in the dopamine metabolites DOPAC and HVA were reported. The fact that increased release of dopamine could be observed during ICSS when the rats were pretreated with the dopamine uptake blocker nomifensine,[14] led to the suggestion that MFB stimulation alone may have caused an increase in the uptake of dopamine into dopaminergic nerve terminals in the nucleus accumbens. A similar mechanism does not appear to be activated by VTA stimulation, as increased dopamine release was measured clearly in the present study in the absence of a dopamine uptake blocker. The success of the present procedure could reflect the site of stimulation or the longer period for equilibration of brain tissue following implantation of the microdialysis probe. It is also possible that the use of a more physiological level of $CaCl_2$ (1.3 mM versus 2.3 mM) may have contributed to our ability to detect the stimulated release of dopamine.

In all important respects, the pattern of results in the present study closely parallels the results obtained with chronoamperometry,[9,10] indicating that dopamine was the electroactive species monitored in those experiments. The electrochemical measures revealed an immediate increase in extracellular dopamine levels within the first min of the ICSS session. The elevated levels were sustained throughout the test session. In 10 min stimulation sessions with lower current intensities, the chronoamperometric measures had returned to baseline within 10 min post stimulation. The trend towards an extended duration of the post-stimulation increase in dopamine levels observed in the present dialysis study may reflect both the higher current intensities and longer duration of the ICSS sessions (15 min). Together these findings add to the support for the dopaminergic hypothesis of brain-stimulation reward at sites in the VTA.[2] Additional *in vivo* evidence includes 1) the increased activation of tyrosine hydroxylase as measured by DOPA accumulation following VTA-ICSS[15]; 2) the close relationship between the threshold current for VTA-ICSS and the threshold for evoked changes in chronoamperometric measures of dopamine in the nucleus accumbens[9]; and 3) the facilitation of both electrochemical measures of dopamine and concurrent ICSS rates by the dopamine uptake blockers nomifensine, cocaine, and GBR 12909.[9,10]

It is interesting to note that sustained increases in dopamine levels also have been observed in dialysates collected from the nucleus accumbens of male rats following a 30 min session of copulation.[16] Dopamine returned to precopulation levels within 20–30 min following removal of the receptive female from the test chamber. Further important parallels in the dynamic changes in extracellular dopamine levels in the nucleus accumbens during copulation and ICSS may be seen in the magnitude of change which averaged nearly 200% of baseline during mating behavior and 300% during ICSS. On the basis of these similarities it is tempting to speculate that the dopamine-mediated brain-stimulation reward accompanying VTA stimulation may be related phenomenologically to the reward accompanying copulation by male rats. This in turn may have important implications for the nature of reward produced by self-administration of psychomotor stimulants including amphetamine and cocaine. There is now an ample body of evidence indicating a critical role for increased dopamine release in the nucleus accumbens in mediating the rewarding effects of these drugs of abuse.[2] Accordingly, the subjective effects of amphetamine and cocaine self-administration may also mimic sexual pleasure in certain respects.

ACKNOWLEDGMENT

Thanks are extended to E. McCririck for her excellent assistance in typing the manuscript.

REFERENCES

1. BOZARTH, M. A. 1987. An overview of assessing drug reinforcement. *In* Methods of Assessing the Reinforcing Properties of Abused Drugs. M. A. Bozarth, Ed.: 635–658. Springer-Verlag. New York.
2. FIBIGER, H. C. & A. G. PHILLIPS. 1987. On the role of catecholamine neurotransmitters in brain reward systems: Implications for the neurobiology of affect. *In* Brain Reward Systems and Abuse. L. Oreland & J. Engel, Eds.: 61–74. Raven Press. New York.
3. KORNETSKY, C. & G. BAIN. 1987. Neuronal bases for hedonic effects of cocaine and opiates. *In* Cocaine: Clinical and Biobehavioral Aspects. S. Fisher, A. Raskin & E. H. Uhlenhuth, Eds.: 66–79. Oxford University Press. New York.
4. PHILLIPS, A. G. & H. C. FIBIGER. 1989. Neuroanatomical bases of intracranial self-stimulation: Untangling the Gordian knot. *In* The Neuropharmacological Basis of Reward. J. M. Liebman & S. J. Cooper, Eds.: 66–105. Oxford University Press. Oxford.

5. ESPOSITO, R. U., A. H. D. MOTOLA & C. KORNETSKY. 1978. Cocaine: Acute effects on reinforcement thresholds for self-stimulation behavior to the medial forebrain bundle. Pharmacol. Biochem. Behav. **8:** 437–439.
6. CROW, T. J. 1970. Enhancement by cocaine of intracranial self-stimulation in the rat. Life Sci. **9:** 375–381.
7. PHILLIPS, A. G. 1984. Brain reward circuitry: A case for separate systems. Brain Res. Bull. **12:** 195–201.
8. GRATTON, A., B. J. HOFFER & G. A. GERHARDT. 1989. Effects of electrical stimulation of brain reward sites on release of dopamine in rat: An in vivo electrochemical study. Brain Res. Bull. **21:** 319–324.
9. PHILLIPS, A. G., C. D. BLAHA & H. C. FIBIGER. 1989. Neurochemical correlates of brain-stimulation reward measured by ex vivo and in vivo analyses. Neurosci. Biobehav. Rev. **13:** 99–104.
10. BLAHA, C. D. & A. G. PHILLIPS. 1990. Application of in vivo electrochemistry to the measurement of changes in dopamine release during intracranial self-stimulation. J. Neurosci. Meth. **34:** 125–133.
11. BLAHA, C. D. & M. E. JUNG. 1991. Electrochemical evaluation of stearate-modified graphite paste electrodes: Selective detection of dopamine is maintained after exposure to brain tissue. J. Electroanal. Chem. **310:** 317–334.
12. WESTERINK, B. H. C., G. DAMSMA, H. ROLLEMA, J. B. DE VRIES & A. S. HORN. 1987. Scope and limitations of in vivo brain dialysis: A comparison of its applications to various neurotransmitter systems. Life Sci. **41:** 1763–1776.
13. NAKAHARA, D., N. OZAKI, Y. MIURA & T. NAGUTSU. 1989. Increased dopamine and serotonin metabolism in rat nucleus accumbens produced by intracranial self-stimulation of medial forebrain bundle as measured by in vivo microdialysis. Brain Res. **495:** 178–181.
14. NAKAHARA, D., N. OZAKI, N. KAPOOR & T. NAGUTSU. 1989. The effect of dopamine uptake inhibition on dopamine release from the nucleus accumbens during self- or forced stimulation of the medial forebrain bundle: A microdialysis study. Neurosci. Lett. **104:** 136–140.
15. PHILLIPS, A. G., A. JAKUBOVIC & H. C. FIBIGER. 1987. Increased in vivo tyrosine hydroxylase activity in the rat telencephalon produced by self-stimulation of the ventral tegmental area. Brain Res. **402:** 109–116.
16. PFAUS, J. G., G. DAMSMA, G. G. NOMIKOS, D. WENKSTERN, C. D. BLAHA, A. G. PHILLIPS & H. C. FIBIGER. 1990. Sexual behavior enhances central dopamine transmission in the male rat. Brain Res. **430:** 345–348.

Drug Motivation and Abuse: A Neurobiological Perspective

GAETANO DI CHIARA, ELIO ACQUAS,
AND EZIO CARBONI

Department of Toxicology
University of Cagliari
Viale Diaz, 182
09100 Cagliari, Italy

Stimuli are operationally defined by their ability to produce biological responses. Stimuli essential for survival of the self or of the species are provided with intrinsic motivational (goal-directed) properties which make them capable of producing specific motor responses directed to approach and prolong the stimulus (appetitive stimuli or primary incentives) or to terminate and avoid it (aversive stimuli or punishers). Repeated temporal association (pairing) of a neutral stimulus with a motivational (unconditioned) stimulus is known to result in transfer (conditioning) to the neutral stimulus of the response-eliciting properties of the unconditioned stimulus (incentive learning).

Many centrally acting drugs have motivational properties. Thus, in appropriate experimental conditions, narcotic analgesics, psychostimulants, nicotine, ethanol, benzodiazepines, and barbiturates can be shown to act as positive reinforcers. On the other hand, drugs like naloxone, picrotoxin, phencyclidine, lithium and k-opiate agonists show aversive properties.[1,2]

DOPAMINE AND DRUG-MOTIVATION

Dopamine (DA) is involved in the motivational properties of centrally acting drugs. Thus, psychostimulants such as amphetamine and cocaine stimulate DA transmission by releasing the transmitter and, respectively, by blocking its reuptake; the experimental evidence that DA is essential for the rewarding properties of these drugs is overwhelming. The role of DA in the motivational effects of most other drugs, however, has been uncertain and debated for at least two reasons: lack of studies on the effect of these drugs on *in vivo* dopaminergic transmission; lack of unequivocal experimental evidence in a variety of behavioral paradigms after manipulation of DA transmission.

With regard to the first issue, the advent of brain dialysis[3] (FIG. 1) has enabled the monitoring of DA release in specific brain areas of the freely moving rat and the correlation of DA release with behavior.

Mesolimbic Dopamine and Drugs of Abuse

In a series of studies from our laboratory,[4] it was shown that many drugs which

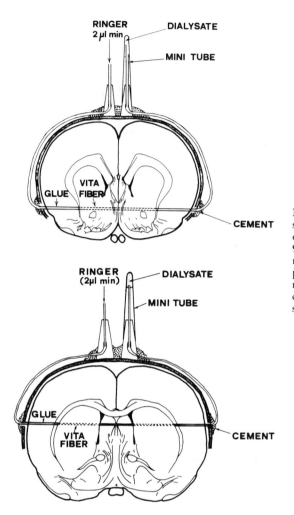

FIGURE 1. Diagram of dialysis tubes implanted at the level of the nucleus accumbens (A 9.6) and of the dorsal caudate nucleus (A 7.4). The stippled portion of the dialysis tube corresponds to the part that is not covered by glue and where dialysis takes place.

possess rewarding properties, such as morphine (FIG. 2) and narcotic analgesics (methadone and fentanyl),[5] ethanol (FIG. 3),[6] nicotine,[7] phencyclidine,[8] and nomifensine,[8] increase the extracellular concentration of DA preferentially in the nucleus accumbens as compared to the dorsal striatum. This effect is shared by classic psychostimulants such as amphetamine and cocaine (FIG. 4).[8]

Electrophysiological studies support a preferentially limbic effect of drugs of abuse. Thus, systemic morphine,[9] ethanol,[10] and nicotine[11] preferentially stimulate the firing activity of A10 as compared to A9 dopaminergic neurons. Since the nucleus accumbens is innervated mainly by mesolimbic A10 neurons arising from the ventral tegmental area and the dorsal caudate by A9 nigro-striatal neurons arising from the substantia nigra pars compacta, these results suggest that the differential effects on

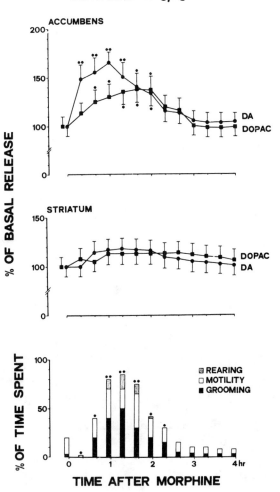

MORPHINE 1 mg/kg s.c.

FIGURE 2. Effect of morphine on dopamine and metabolite output from the accumbens and from the caudate. Results are expressed as percent of basal output (mean ± SEM of values obtained from at least four animals). $p < 0.05$ (*) is with respect to basal values.

morphine, ethanol and nicotine on DA release *in vivo* are directly related to a differential sensitivity to their stimulant effect of mesolimbic as compared to mesostriatal DA neurons.

Dopamine and Motivation: Active Role

Although brain dialysis in freely moving rats suggests the existence of a relationship between stimulation of DA transmission in the mesolimbic system and drug-induced behavioral activation, it might be argued that activation of behavior is the cause rather than the result of stimulation of DA release in the nucleus accumbens; in fact, arousing

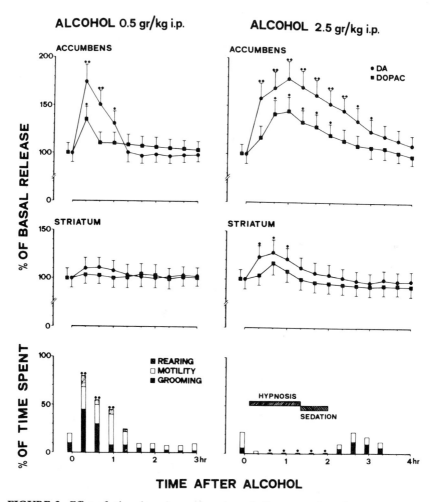

FIGURE 3. Effect of ethanol on dopamine and metabolite output from the accumbens and from the caudate. Results are percent of basal release (mean ± SEM of values obtained from at least four rats). $p < 0.05$ (*) with respect to basal values.

and stressful stimuli do activate DA release in the mesolimbic system.[12] However, pharmacological and lesion studies show that various stimuli (including stress and drugs) which activate behavior depend on DA for their behavioral stimulant properties. Thus, studies on the effects of narcotic analgesics, ethanol, nicotine, amphetamine, and cocaine on unlearned as well as on learned behavior (place preference and drug self-administration), show that the motor stimulant as well as the positive motivational properties of these drugs is severely disrupted by blockade of DA transmission, particularly at D_1 receptors.[13–16]

On the basis of these results, we have hypothesized[17] that motivation is related to

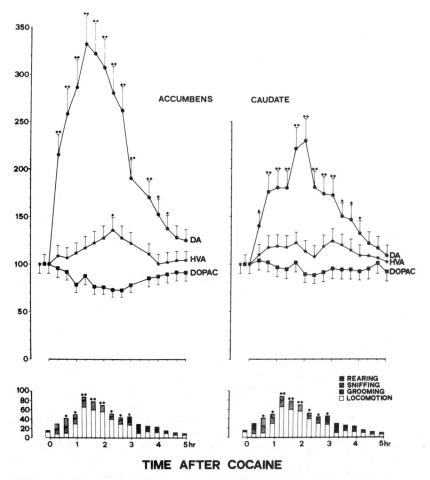

FIGURE 4. Effect of cocaine (5.0 mg/kg s.c.) on the output of dopamine (DA), dihydroxy-phenylacetic acid (DOPAC) and of homovanillic acid (HVA) from the accumbens and from the caudate. Results are expressed as percent of basal output (mean ± SEM of values obtained from four rats). $p < 0.05$ (*) and $p < 0.001$ (**) are with respect to basal values.

an active change of DA transmission in the mesolimbic system with reward or aversion depending on the sign of this change. Accordingly, stimulation of DA transmission would be rewarding while its inhibition would be aversive.

Stress, which is likely to be aversive, stimulates DA release in the mesolimbic system[12] rather than reducing it, as our hypothesis would predict. However, stimulation of DA release by stress could be a homeostatic reaction which tends to withdraw the animal from the stressful stimulus by promoting motor activity and to attenuate the aversive impact of stress by providing a pleasurable interoceptive cue.

Dopamine and Motivation: Permissive Role

Blockade of D_1 receptors by SCH 23390 prevents not only place preference elicited by drugs which stimulate DA release, *e.g.*, morphine, nicotine and amphetamine, but also the place aversion induced by drugs like naloxone, lithium, picrotoxin, phencyclidine[16] (Acquas *et al.*, 1989) and k-opioid agonists[18] which do not have consistent effects on DA transmission. Naloxone, for example, fails to affect DA transmission as estimated by brain dialysis in all the areas tested (nucleus accumbens, prefrontal cortex, hippocampus, and dorsal caudate). Phencyclidine stimulates DA release in all the areas investigated, but nonetheless elicits aversion[16]; k-agonists reduce DA release[5] and elicit place aversion which, as in the case of naloxone and phencyclidine, is blocked by SCH 23390.[18] These results are not compatible with a simple active role of DA in reward and aversion.

A way out of this is to postulate that DA plays not only an active role which relates to the ability of the stimulus (drug or other) to stimulate or to inhibit DA transmission and determines its intrinsic motivational properties (rewarding or aversive) but also a permissive role, related to a more general influence of DA on incentive learning.[17]

Dual Role of Dopamine in Motivation

According to our hypothesis, the affective state of the individual depends on the activity of DA transmission; increased DA transmission in mesolimbic areas would result in a positive mood state which is expressed as euphoria in man and forward locomotion in animals; reduced DA-transmission would result in dysphoria in man and reduced locomotion in animals; association of these neurochemical changes with environmental stimuli would confer to them positive or negative incentive properties depending on the sign of the change of DA transmission (incentive learning).

However, not all stimuli exert their primary incentive properties through an active change in DA transmission; naloxone, for example, probably elicits a negative mood state (aversion) by reducing transmission along an endogenous opioid reward system[19]; diazepam, on the other hand, might be rewarding independently from DA,[17] by potentiating GABA-ergic transmission. No matter which neurochemical change carries the motivational stimulus (DA or other neurotransmitters systems), the presence of DA appears essential for the ability of the active neurochemical change carrying the motivational stimulus to confer incentive properties to neutral stimuli paired with it (incentive learning); this associative process takes place also in the presence of a reduction of dopaminergic transmission but not in its complete absence. Thus, strong blockade of DA transmission (*e.g.*, by SCH 23390) impairs, not only positive but also negative incentive learning even by drugs such as k-agonist, which reduce DA transmission.[16,17]

DRUG ABUSE: A BIOLOGICAL PERSPECTIVE

The evidence showing that stimulation of DA transmission in the mesolimbic system relates to the rewarding properties of drugs of abuse brings one to ask what is the significance of the drug-induced changes in DA transmission.

In answering to this question one should consider that drugs act on biological organisms to the extent that they are able to activate biological processes which are operative independently from the drug itself; indeed, drugs do not invent anything new but just mimic or interfere with what is preformed. This principle also applies to drugs of abuse; thus, drugs owe their abuse liability to the fact that they activate certain neural pathways which carry natural rewarding stimuli.

Drugs of Abuse as Surrogates of Natural Rewards

Feeding, drinking, sexual, and maternal behavior are directed towards goals essential for survival of the self and of the species; natural selection, in order to ensure the accomplishment of these behaviors, has provided their goals with powerful rewarding properties. Thus, at least in higher phyla, natural stimuli such as food, water, sex, and mother are rewarding. Two aspects can be distinguished in natural rewards, an incentive or preparatory aspect and a consummatory one[20]; the incentive aspect of natural reward stimuli is provided by their distinctive sensory properties (smell, color, shape, taste, temperature, *etc.*) which readily identify them; on the other hand the consummatory aspect of natural rewards mainly involves the physiological and metabolic consequences of the contact, interaction, and eventual consumption of the rewarding stimulus itself. Each one of these aspects is pleasurable (*i.e.*, elicits a positive affective state) but both are necessary for natural reward to be fully reinforcing. Thus, for example, foods devoid of caloric (consummatory) properties are less rewarding than others provided with the same incentive properties (*e.g.*, sweetness). Vice versa, foods with the same caloric properties but differing in taste (incentive) can have opposite motivational properties. The incentive aspect of reward stimuli involves ergotropic changes such as arousal, activation of motor behavior, and of the sympathetic nervous system and catabolism while the consummatory aspect involves trophotropic changes such as rest, sedation, anabolism and activation of the parasympathetic nervous system (FIG. 5).

The incentive properties are essential for learning of a behavioral response directed to approach the reward stimulus itself; dopamine might play an important role in this process.[21]

In fact, the distinctive sensory properties of natural rewards have the ability of stimulating mesolimbic DA transmission; this effect has at least three consequences: one is that of eliciting arousal and forward locomotion which directly promotes approach to the stimulus; the second is that of conferring approach-eliciting properties and therefore positive incentive properties to otherwise neutral stimuli (secondary incentives) present in the environment and repeatedly associated with the natural reward (incentive learning)—by this mechanism the probability of the individual's coming into contact with the primary reward stimulus will be increased; the third property is that of activating the incentive properties of other environmental stimuli related to the same or to other rewards[22]—in this way reward-related stimuli can reacquire their incentive properties which had been reduced following extinction. While the ability of stimulating DA transmission in mesolimbic areas accounts for most of the properties of the incentive aspect of natural rewards, this may not be the case for the consummatory aspect, which might involve the activation of non-DA mechanisms such as, for example, the central opioid reward system.

Drugs of abuse can be regarded as surrogates of natural rewards (FIG. 5). In fact all drugs of abuse act as positive reinforcers and are provided with rewarding and appetitive properties. Moreover, most drugs of abuse share with natural rewards a fun-

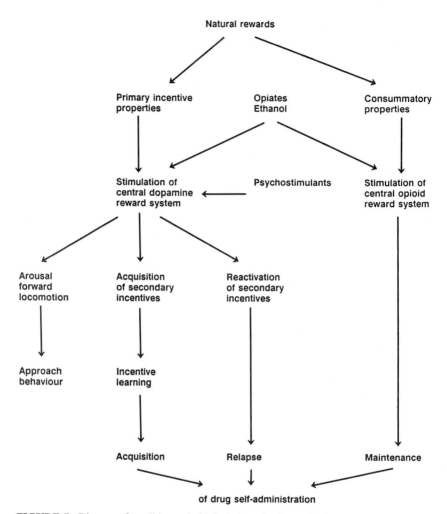

FIGURE 5. Diagram of possible psychobiological mechanisms of drug self-administration.

damental aspect of their incentive properties, namely the ability of stimulating DA transmission.[4]

It is important to note however, that, while in the case of natural rewards DA transmission is stimulated in response to the distinctive sensory properties of these stimuli, this happens to a lesser extent for drugs which are abused as chemicals and, as such, do not possess as salient sensory properties as natural rewards. For this reason, drug reward depends, more than natural reward, from incentive learning, that is, from the ability of drugs, related essentially to their intrinsic DA stimulant properties,[4] to promote the acquisition of secondary incentives.[23] Ethanol and opiates might best mimic the incentive and the consummatory aspects of natural reinforcers; given their ability to stimulate DA transmission[4] as well as the endogenous opioid reward system (opiates and ethanol). This system has been related to the sedative, anabolic, and reduced-drive state typical of the consummatory aspect of natural reward and accounts for the sedative, narcotic, and analgesic properties of opiates.[29] Ethanol in addition is provided with caloric properties which are typical of the consummatory aspect of natural rewards. Other drugs of abuse, like psychostimulants (cocaine and amphetamine) mimic only the incentive aspect of natural reward. Failure to mimic the consummatory aspect of natural reward might be the reason for the escalating tendency of psychostimulant abuse, which can result in exhaustion of the individual or acute toxicity and death (FIG. 5).

ROLE OF DOPAMINE IN DRUG-DEPENDENCE AND CRAVING

Repeated exposure to drugs of abuse results in profound biological changes which modify the function of the exposed organism. These properties are reflected in the ability of certain drugs like opiates, ethanol, and sedative-hypnotics to induce a state of physical dependence, expressed in the physical signs of the withdrawal syndrome.

Classic theories of addiction have assumed that withdrawal is a physical expression of distress and that drug-addiction results, at least in part, from the need to reduce such distress. Accordingly, craving would be a negatively reinforced behavior related to avoidance of withdrawal distress.

This hypothesis has been challenged on both experimental and clinical grounds; thus, some among the most abused drugs, like cocaine and psychostimulants, hardly induce physical dependence; moreover it has been shown that the degree of physical dependence for those drugs which induce this state (*e.g.*, opiates) does not predict the intensity of craving; moreover, detoxification and recovery from physical dependence on opiates does not prevent relapse into opiate-addiction.

This however does not exclude the possibility that motivational changes unrelated to the classical withdrawal symptoms, but nonetheless occurring following withdrawal, play a role in the maintenance of opiate-addiction.

In fact, spontaneous withdrawal from heroin in addicts is characterized by a syndrome of depressed mood and dysphoria, which can be considered as a reflection of psychological dependence. In animals, withdrawal from opiates results in place and taste aversion which appears unrelated to the pattern and intensity of the physical symptoms of withdrawal.[24] Withdrawal from chronic opiates and psychostimulants is also associated to impairment of responding for intracranial self-stimulation (reduction in rate and increase in current threshold).[25,26]

In rats made dependent by repeated non-contingent administration of morphine, spontaneous withdrawal results in a profound and long-lasting (at least 7 days) reduction of DA release in the nucleus accumbens indicative of a dependence state of mesolimbic DA neurons (FIG. 6).

Reduction of basal DA release in the nucleus accumbens has been observed also following withdrawal from repeated cocaine.[27,28]

These results are therefore consistent with the hypothesis that a common characteristic of withdrawal from different drugs of abuse might be a depression of DA transmission resulting in impairment of the central reward system which is reflected in a reduction of ICSS and in dysphoria. Since the abused drug effectively counteracts both withdrawal dysphoria and the reduction of DA transmission, it is proposed that

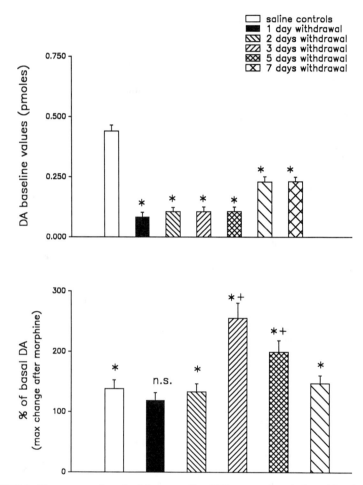

FIGURE 6. Time course of maximal decrease of basal DA output (pmoles/sample) and of maximal increase of DA output after morphine challenge (5.0 mg/kg s.c.) in dependent rats at various days of withdrawal from morphine. Results are means ± SEM of at least 5 animals per group. * $p < 0.05$ as compared to basal values; + $p < 0.05$ as compared to saline controls.

these changes contribute, by a negatively reinforcing mechanism, to maintain drug-addiction.[28]

Withdrawal from morphine is also associated with changes in the activity of morphine-induced stimulation of DA release in the nucleus accumbens. Thus, tolerance to morphine on day 1 of withdrawal is followed by a normal response on day 2 and by an increased response on day 3 and 5 with recovery to a normal response on day 7 (FIG. 6); these changes have been interpreted as the result of tolerance (day 1) and of supersensitivity (days 3 and 5) to the opiate as a result of withdrawal from the tonic influence of exogenous opiate. Such an increased sensitivity to the DA-stimulant properties of the abused drug might provide the substrate for a parallel magnification of its DA-dependent incentive properties. Therefore, a condition of dependence not only will induce a negative reinforcing mechanism in drug-directed behavior but will also potentiate the positive reinforcing properties of the drug by increasing its incentive aspects.[28]

CONCLUSIONS

We will now try to provide an interpretative framework of the psychobiological mechanisms of addiction to opiates and of craving for psychostimulants. As far as regards opiates, a DA theory of opiate reward[29] has been opposed to a non-DA theory[30]; moreover, a positive reinforcement mechanism of opiate-addiction[31] has been opposed to a negative reinforcement one.[32] These controversies might simply reflect the fact that more than one mechanism is involved in certain critical aspects of opiate-addiction. An integrative hypothesis will be proposed here.

Our interpretation starts from the view that opiate-reward mimics to a certain extent natural reward and that it possesses incentive as well as consummatory properties. DA seems involved in the incentive aspects of opiate reward and therefore in the mechanism of acquisition and reacquisition (relapse) of opiate self-administration.[4,31,33] Once acquired, maintenance of opiate self-administration relates not only to the incentive but also and particularly to the consummatory properties of the opiate stimulus which might be DA-independent.[30]

Opiate addiction, on the other hand, as distinguished from opiate self-administration, is a chronic condition in which maintenance of self-administration is associated with dependence. In this case the behavior is maintained both by the positively reinforcing (rewarding) properties of the opiate and by the negatively reinforcing (aversive) properties of dependence.

Again, DA could be involved in this aspect as from a reduction of its transmission in the mesolimbic system might derive the aversive effects of withdrawal.[28]

Therefore, at least two systems, a DA-ergic and a non-DA-ergic (endogenous opiate reward system?) might contribute to opiate self-administration and two mechanisms, a positively and a negatively reinforcing one, might play a role in opiate-addiction.

As far as regards abuse of psychostimulants such as cocaine amphetamine and phencyclidine, a differential feature with opiate abuse is given by the absence of a true biological consummatory aspect in the reward they elicit; thus, paradoxically, while actual consumption of the drug should coincide with a consummatory phase, its effects are purely incentive in nature. As already pointed out, this might be the reason for the escalating and compulsive character (craving) of psychostimulant abuse.

REFERENCES

1. CARR, A., H. C. FIBIGER & A. G. PHILLIPS. 1989. Conditioned place preference as a measure of drug rewards. *In* The Neuropharmacological Basis of Rewards. J. M. Liebman & S. J. Cooper, Eds.: 264–319. Oxford University Press. Oxford.
2. LIEBMAN, J. M. & S. J. COOPER, Eds. 1989. The Neuropharmacological Basis of Reward. Oxford. Oxford University Press.
3. DI CHIARA, G. 1990. In-vivo brain dialysis of neurotransmitters. TIPS 11: 116–121.
4. DI CHIARA, G. & A. IMPERATO. 1988. Drugs abused by humans preferentially increase syn-

aptic dopamine concentrations in the mesolimbic system of freely moving rats. Proc. Natl. Acad. Sci. USA **85**: 5274–5278.

5. DI CHIARA, G. & A. IMPERATO. 1988. Opposite effects of μ and k-opiate agonists on dopamine-release in the nucleus accumbens and in the dorsal caudate of freely moving rats. J. Pharmacol. Exp. Ther. **244**: 1067–1080.

6. IMPERATO, A. & G. DI CHIARA. 1986. Preferential stimulation of dopamine-release in the accumbens of freely moving rats by ethanol. J. Pharmacol. Exp. Ther. **239**: 219–228.

7. IMPERATO, A., A. MULAS & G. DI CHIARA. 1986. Nicotine preferentially stimulates dopamine release in the limbic system of freely moving rats. Eur. J. Pharmacol. **132**: 337–338.

8. CARBONI, E., A. IMPERATO, L. PEREZZANI & G. DI CHIARA. 1989. Amphetamine, cocaine, phencyclidine and nomifensine increase extracellular dopamine concentrations preferentially in the nucleus accumbens of freely moving rats. Neuroscience **28**: 653–661.

9. MATTHEWS, G. P. & D. C. GERMAN. 1984. Electrophysiological evidence for excitation of rat ventral tegmental area dopamine neurons by morphine. Neuroscience **11**: 617–625.

10. GESSA, G. L., F. MUNTONI, M. COLLU, L. VARGIU & G. P. MEREU. 1985. Low doses of ethanol activate dopaminergic neurons in the ventral tegmental area. Brain. Res. **348**: 201–203.

11. MEREU, G. P., P. WOOM, V. BOI, G. L. GESSA, L. NAESA & T. C. WESTERFALL. 1987. Preferential stimulation of ventral tegmental area dopaminergic neurons by nicotine. Eur. J. Pharmacol. **141**: 393–395.

12. ABERCROMBIE, E. D., K. A. KEEFE, D. S. DIFRISCHIA & M. J. ZIGMOND. 1989. Differential effect of stress on in vivo dopamine release in striatum, nucleus accumbens, and medial frontal cortex. J. Neurochem. **52**: 1655–1658.

13. LEONE, P. & G. DI CHIARA. 1987. Blockade of D-1 receptors by SCH 23390 antagonized morphine- and amphetamine-induced place preference conditioning. Eur. J. Pharmacol. **135**: 251–254.

14. LONGONI, R., L. SPINA & G. DI CHIARA. 1987. Dopaminergic D-1 receptors: Essential role in morphine-induced hypermotility. Psychopharmacology **93**: 401–402.

15. KOOB, G. F., H. T. LE & I. CREESE. 1987. The D_1 dopamine receptor antagonist SCH 23390 increases cocaine self-administration in the rat. Neuroscience Lett. **79**: 315–320.

16. ACQUAS, E., E. CARBONI, P. LEONE & G. DI CHIARA. 1989. SCH 23390 blocks drug-conditioned place-preference and place-aversion: Anhedonia (lack of reward) or apathy (lack of motivation) after dopamine-receptor blockade? Psychopharmacology **99**: 151–155.

17. DI CHIARA, G., E. ACQUAS & E. CARBONI. 1991. Role of mesolimbic dopamine in the motivational effects of drugs: Brain dialysis and place preference studies. *In* The Mesolimbic Dopamine System: From Motivation to Action. P. Willner & J. Scheel-Krüger, Eds.: 367–384. John Wiley & Sons Ltd. Chichester, UK.

18. SHIPPENBERG, T. S. & A. HERZ. 1987. Place preference conditioning reveals the involvement of D_1-dopamine receptors in the motivational properties of μ- and k-opioid agonists. Brain Res. **436**: 169–172.

19. BELLUZZI, J. D. & L. STEIN. 1977. Enkephalin may mediate euphoria and drive-reduction. Nature **266**: 556–558.

20. KONORSKI, J. 1967. Integrative Activity of the Brain. University of Chicago Press. Chicago.

21. PHILLIPS, A. G., J. G. PFAUS & C. D. BLAHA. 1991. Dopamine and motivated behavior: Insights provided by in vivo analyses. *In* The Mesolimbic Dopamine System: From Motivation to Action. P. Willner & J. Scheel-Krüger, Eds. John Wiley & Sons, Ltd. Chichester, UK.

22. TAYLOR, J. R. & T. W. ROBBINS. 1984. Enhanced behavioral control by conditioned reinforcers following microinjections of d-amphetamine into the nucleus accumbens. Psychopharmacology **84**: 405–412.

23. BENINGER, R. J. 1983. The role of dopamine in locomotor activity and learning. Brain Res. Rev. **6**: 173–196.

24. MUCHA, R. F. 1987. Is the motivational effect of opiate withdrawal reflected by common somatic indices of precipitated withdrawal? A place conditioning study in the rat. Brain Res. **418**: 21–220.

25. SHAEFER, G. J. & R. P. MICHAEL. 1986. Changes in response rates and reinforcement

thresholds for intracranial self-administration during morphine withdrawal. Pharmacol. Biochem. Behav. **25:** 1263–1269.

26. MARCOU, A. & G. F. KOOB. 1991. Post cocaine anhedonia: An animal model of cocaine withdrawal. Neuropsychopharmacology **4:** 17–26.

27. ACQUAS, E., E. CARBONI & G. DI CHIARA. 1991. Profound depression of mesolimbic dopamine release after withdrawal in dependent rats. Eur. J. Pharmacol. **193:** 133–134.

28. ACQUAS, E. & G. DI CHIARA. 1992. Depression of mesolimbic dopamine-transmission and sensitization to morphine during opiate abstinence. J. Neurochem. In press.

29. BOZARTH, M. A. & R. A. WISE. 1981. Heroin reward is dependent on a dopaminergic substrate. Life Sci. **29:** 1881–1886.

30. ETTENBERG, A., H. O. PETTIT, F. E. BLOOM & G. F. KOOB. 1982. Heroin and cocaine intravenous self-administration in rats: Mediation by separate neural systems. Psychopharmacology **78:** 204–209.

31. STEWART, J., H. DE WIT & R. EIKELBOOM. 1984. Role of unconditioned and conditioned drug effects in the self-administration of opiates and stimulants. Psychol. Rev. **91:** 251–268.

32. WIKLER, A. & F. T. PESCOR. 1967. Classical conditioning of a morphine abstinence phenomenon reinforcement of opioid-drinking behavior and relapse in morphine addicted rats. Psychopharmacologia **10:** 255–284.

33. WISE, R. A. & M. A. BOZARTH. 1987. A psychomotor stimulant theory of addiction. Psychol. Rev. **94:** 469–492.

Neurochemical Correlates of Cocaine and Ethanol Self-Administration[a]

FRIEDBERT WEISS,[b,e] YASMIN L. HURD,[c]
URBAN UNGERSTEDT,[c] ATHINA MARKOU,[b]
PAUL M. PLOTSKY,[d] AND GEORGE F. KOOB[b]

[b] Department of Neuropharmacology
The Scripps Research Institute
10666 North Torrey Pines Road
La Jolla, California 92037

[c] Department of Pharmacology
Karolinska Institute
S-104 01 Stockholm, Sweden

[d] The Clayton Foundation Laboratories for Peptide Biology
Salk Institute
La Jolla, California 92186

Self-administration procedures have been an effective tool to study the neuropharmacology of psychostimulant and opiate reward.[1-4] On the basis of this work, biological theories of drug reinforcement have emerged that center around the assumption that drugs of abuse directly or indirectly activate central "reward substrates" that mediate motivated behavior and reinforcement.[5-9] In particular, self-administration studies have established an important role for dopamine in the acute reinforcing effects of psychostimulant drugs including cocaine and d-amphetamine.[10-13] Relative to the advances in identifying critical circuitries for psychostimulant reward, little is known about the neuropharmacological bases of ethanol reward. Progress toward the identification of neurobiological substrates of ethanol reward has been impeded, in part, by the difficulty in establishing orally presented ethanol as a reinforcer in the absence of food or fluid restrictions, or the addition of sweeteners (for review see refs. 14–16). However, novel procedures for the initiation of ethanol self-administration have recently been developed in which oral ethanol intake is maintained more clearly by pharmacological motivation rather than nutritional appetite or thirst.[15,17] These models may allow a systematic exploration of the physiological systems involved in ethanol preference and reward. A number of neuropharmacological investigations using these procedures have since suggested a role for dopamine neurotransmission in low-dose ethanol reinforcement[18,19] (Samson *et al.*, this volume). The present series of experiments sought to extend previous work on the role of dopamine in cocaine and ethanol

[a] This work was supported in part by NIDA grants DA 05843 and DA 04398, NIAAA grant DA 07348, NIAAA Specialized Center Grant AA 06420, and a grant from the Swedish Medical Research Council B88-14X-03574-17B.

[e] Address correspondence to: Friedbert Weiss, Ph.D. Tel.: (619) 554-7068; Fax: (619) 554-6480.

reward by examining the significance of dopamine release in the region of the nucleus accumbens in the acute, reinforcing actions of these drugs as well as in cocaine dependence and withdrawal.

COCAINE SELF-ADMINISTRATION

A substantial body of evidence implicates the mesocorticolimbic dopamine system in the mediation of the acute reinforcing effects of intravenous cocaine self-administration.[11-13] For example, selective 6-hydroxydopamine (6-OHDA) lesions of A10 dopamine cell bodies in the ventral tegmental area, or of dopamine terminals in the nucleus accumbens abolish cocaine self-administration.[12,13] In contrast, 6-OHDA lesions of the caudate nucleus or frontal cortex do not alter cocaine self-administration.[9,11,13] A specific involvement of dopaminergic transmission in the nucleus accumbens in cocaine reward is further suggested by the observation that intra-accumbens administration of selective D_1 and D_2 antagonist drugs attenuates the reinforcing efficacy of cocaine (Robledo *et al.*, this volume).

When access to cocaine is limited to only few hours per day, cocaine self-administering rats develop a highly consistent and reproducible pattern of responding.[9,12,13] This behavior is characterized by an initial "loading phase" followed by the development of dose-titration. During this stage the duration of interresponse intervals is almost identical and the response density (*i.e.*, the number of injections per unit time) is inversely related to the dose of cocaine.[20,21] The titration to a given dose as well as the compensatory changes in response rates after a change in dose suggest that self-administering animals regulate their drug intake in a manner that maintains not only stable plasma concentrations,[22] but sustained and stable neurochemical activation of a specific—presumably dopaminergic—reward substrate. Given the evidence that the reinforcing actions of cocaine depend on its property to increase dopamine accumulation in the nucleus accumbens, cocaine self-administration patterns may serve to increase and maintain stable synaptic dopamine levels in this brain region. This hypothesis was explored in the first series of experiments using *in vivo* microdialysis procedures in awake, cocaine self-administering rats.

Effects of Limited-Access Cocaine Self-Administration on Extracellular Dopamine Levels in the Nucleus Accumbens

To examine the relationship between accumulation of dopamine and responding for cocaine (0.75 mg/kg/injection), extracellular dopamine levels were determined from microdialysate fractions collected from the nucleus accumbens of cocaine self-administering rats during 3-hour limited-access sessions. The animals had been trained to self-administer cocaine in 8–15 limited-access training sessions and developed dose-titrated response patterns prior to the test.

In all animals a close correspondence between response patterns and accumbens dopamine levels was observed. Extracellular dopamine concentrations typically increased during the loading phase early during self-administration until the onset of dose-titrated responding (FIGS. 1 and 2B). During this period neurotransmitter levels oscillated around a stable mean value until access to cocaine was discontinued. After substitution of cocaine by saline, dopamine concentration began to decrease toward

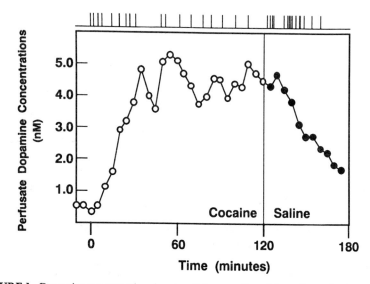

FIGURE 1. Dopamine concentrations in microdialysates collected from the nucleus accumbens of a trained, dose-titrated rat during cocaine self-administration and after substitution of cocaine by saline (0.1 ml/injection). Event recorder tracing on top of the figure indicates response rate. Each lever-press produced one intravenous injection of cocaine (0.75 mg/kg/injection) or saline (0.1 ml/injection) infused over 4 seconds.

basal levels. Behaviorally, the decline in dopamine accumulation was accompanied by a transient increase in responding ("frustration bursts") and eventual extinction (FIG. 1). No change in extracellular dopamine levels was seen in rats that received intravenous injections of saline (FIG. 2, Panel C). A clear relationship between dopamine overflow and responding was also evident in drug-naive rats during the acquisition of cocaine self-administration (FIG. 2, Panel A).

Mean extracellular dopamine levels and response rates across a group of self-administering rats are shown in FIGURE 3. Like the individual records, the grouped data illustrate that extracellular accumbens dopamine concentrations increase after initiation of self-administration and remain stable within a specific range throughout the entire session. While dopamine levels were significantly and consistently elevated over basal levels, the mean increase of 165% ± 12.75 (percent of basal: Mean ± SEM of all observation points after the 10 minute loading phase) was surprisingly low. This is in sharp contrast to the substantial mean (± SEM) increase of 435% ± 232 (percent of basal) observed in earlier work with drug-naive rats[23] that received intravenous cocaine injections at comparable doses by means of a yoking procedure (FIG. 4).

COCAINE WITHDRAWAL

While limited-access self-administration procedures provide a useful tool to examine the acute reinforcing actions of cocaine, investigations of the neuropharma-

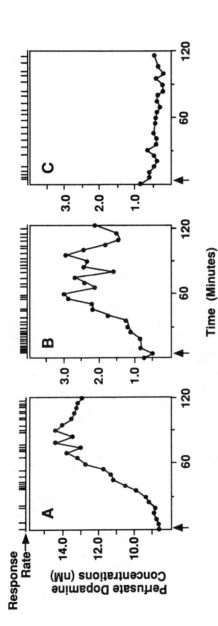
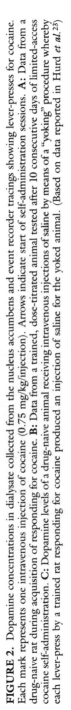

FIGURE 2. Dopamine concentrations in dialysate collected from the nucleus accumbens and event recorder tracings showing lever-presses for cocaine. Each mark represents one intravenous injection of cocaine (0.75 mg/kg/injection). Arrows indicate start of self-administration sessions. **A:** Data from a drug-naive rat during acquisition of responding for cocaine. **B:** Data from a trained, dose-titrated animal tested after 10 consecutive days of limited-access cocaine self-administration. **C:** Dopamine levels of a drug-naive animal receiving intravenous injections of saline by means of a "yoking" procedure whereby each lever-press by a trained rat responding for cocaine produced an injection of saline for the yoked animal. (Based on data reported in Hurd *et al.*[23])

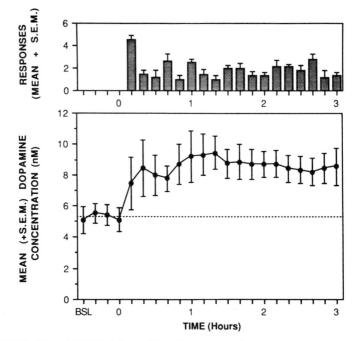

FIGURE 3. Mean (±SEM) dialysate dopamine concentrations and response rates at 10-min intervals over a 3-hour cocaine self-administration session. All rats ($n = 6$) had been trained to self-administer cocaine in 8–15 self-administration sessions and had developed stable, dose-titrated baselines of responding prior to testing. The increase in dopamine overflow over the 3-h session was significantly increased over basal levels [$F(14,70) = 5.07$; $p < 0.001$]. Dotted line indicates mean pre-cocaine basal dopamine concentration.

cology of cocaine dependence and withdrawal require episodes of unlimited access. When given unlimited access to cocaine, animals and humans will self-administer cocaine in repetitive episodes or "binges" which last for many hours or even days.[24–26] In humans the end of such binges is associated with a withdrawal syndrome resembling an episode of major depression.[27] In rats a similar syndrome of "post-cocaine anhedonia" has been observed following extended periods of unlimited-access cocaine self-administration.[26,28] In this work[26] the reward thresholds for lateral hypothalamic intracranial self-stimulation were significantly elevated over baseline levels when assessed after 6 to 48 hours of continuous access to cocaine. The reduced reinforcing efficacy of electrical brain stimulation during cocaine withdrawal presumably reflects a condition of anhedonia or diminished ability to experience rewarding stimulation, a condition that may be comparable to the dysphoria experienced by humans during cocaine withdrawal[26,27] (Koob, this volume). In view of the evidence implicating dopamine neurotransmission in the nucleus accumbens in the mediation of the acute reinforcing effects of cocaine it is possible that the same system is also involved in the dysphoric

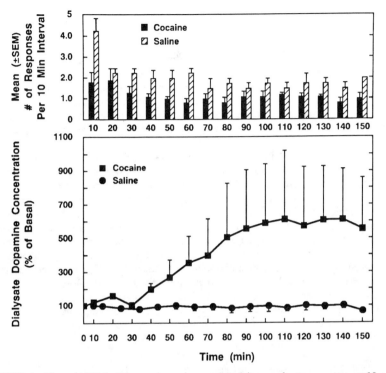

FIGURE 4. Mean (±SEM) dialysate dopamine concentrations and response rates at 10-min intervals in drug-naive rats receiving intravenous injections of cocaine (0.75 mg/kg/injection) or saline (0.1 ml/injection) by means of a "yoking" procedure. Cocaine produced significant increases in dopamine overflow [$F_{(16,96)}$ = 1.176; $p < 0.05$ (interaction, mixed-factorial ANOVA)]. Saline injections did not alter basal dopamine levels. (Modified from Hurd *et al.*[23])

aspects of the cocaine withdrawal syndrome. Although there is, to date, little direct evidence in favor of this position, the withdrawal-associated attenuation of brain stimulation reward offers some support for this hypothesis. The rewarding effects of lateral hypothalamic brain stimulation are thought to depend, at least in part, on dopamine neurotransmission in the nucleus accumbens (see ref. 29 for review). Thus, the reductions in brain stimulation reward during cocaine withdrawal may reflect a specific impairment in dopaminergic neurotransmission in the accumbens. Consistent with this possibility, a deficiency in releasable dopamine following chronic cocaine abuse has also been implicated as a possible physiological basis of the cocaine withdrawal syndrome by the dopamine depletion hypothesis.[30] The purpose of the following experiment was, therefore, to study dopamine release in the nucleus accumbens during withdrawal from cocaine following unlimited-access self-administration, and to determine whether the attenuation of brain stimulation reward observed in earlier work[26] is paralleled by a specific impairment in mesolimbic dopamine function.

Effects of Cocaine Withdrawal after Unlimited-Access Self-Administration on
Dopamine Release

Rats were trained to intravenously self-administer cocaine (0.75 mg/kg/injection) in daily 3-hour limited-access sessions. Testing began 3 to 5 days after dose-titration and stable baselines of limited-access responding were obtained. On the test day rats were given unlimited-access to cocaine until they ceased responding for a minimum of 3 hours. Dialysate was collected from the nucleus accumbens at 20 minute intervals during cocaine self-administration, and for an additional 12 hours during cocaine withdrawal.

The duration of self-administration among individual rats varied from 9.5 to 21.75 hours (Mean ± SEM: 14.13 ± 2.13). As with limited-access conditions dopamine levels were significantly increased by cocaine and remained elevated at a stable mean level (212.89 ± 22.64 percent of basal) throughout most of the session. In some animals dopamine levels began to decrease shortly before cessation of self-administration in spite of continued cocaine intake. Cocaine withdrawal was associated with marked reductions in basal dopamine release below levels recorded prior to the start of the cocaine binge. The magnitude of this inhibition increased as a function of the length of the preceding self-administration episode ($r = 0.96$; $p < 0.003$). The largest decreases in basal release occurred 4–6 hours after onset of withdrawal. Dopamine release returned to pre-cocaine levels between 7 and 12 hours post-cocaine. No deviations from basal concentrations were seen in drug-naive control animals placed in the self-administration environment for 30 hours without access to cocaine. These data are summarized in FIGURE 5.

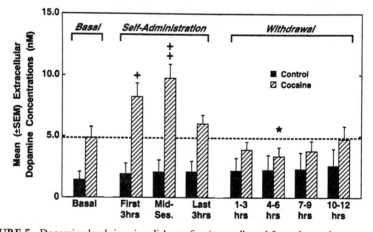

FIGURE 5. Dopamine levels in microdialysate fractions collected from the nucleus accumbens of rats ($n = 5$) during unlimited-access cocaine self-administration (0.75 mg/kg/injection) and cocaine withdrawal. Control rats ($n = 3$) were drug-naive animals placed into the self-administration chambers for 30 hours without access to cocaine. Dopamine release was significantly suppressed below basal levels between 4–6 hours post-cocaine. Note also that pre-cocaine basal dopamine levels in trained, self-administering rats were significantly higher than in drug-naive control rats (see text). $^+$ $p < 0.05$, significant increases over basal; $^{++}$ $p < 0.01$, significant increases over basal; * $p < 0.05$, significant decreases below basal (Newman-Keuls after ANOVAs).

Effects of Repeated Exposure to Cocaine on Dopamine Levels in the Nucleus Accumbens

The cocaine withdrawal experiments revealed a large difference in basal dopamine levels between trained, cocaine-acclimated and control animals: $F(1,3) = 15.44$; $p < 0.005$ (over 4 consecutive 10-min basal fractions). Pre-cocaine basal dopamine levels were close to 4-fold higher in rats that had been previously exposed to cocaine in 10–15 limited-access self-administration training sessions than in drug-naive control rats (FIG. 5). The effects of repeated cocaine exposure on basal dopamine activity were, therefore, examined more systematically in rats pretreated with one daily injection of cocaine (30 mg/kg; IP) or saline (1 ml/kg) over 10 consecutive days. Basal extracellular dopamine concentrations in the nucleus accumbens were then determined by *in vivo* microdialysis under halothane anesthesia on Day 1 (24 hrs), Day 3, and Day 7 after the final chronic cocaine injection in separate groups of rats. In addition, accumulation of extracellular dopamine in response to a cocaine challenge injection (30 mg/kg; IP) was examined at the same time points.

Ten days of repeated cocaine administration resulted in a substantial increase in basal dialysate dopamine concentrations (FIG. 6A) similar to that observed in self-administering animals (FIG. 5). This effect was most pronounced on Day 1 (Mean +

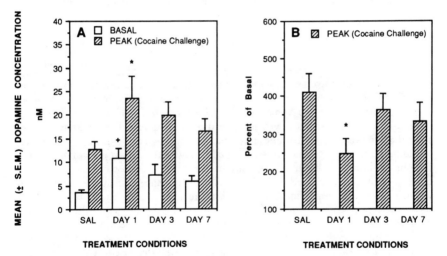

FIGURE 6. Effect of daily intraperitoneal injections of cocaine (30 mg/kg) or saline (Sal) on basal dopamine release (Basal) and peak dopamine accumulation (Peak) after cocaine challenge injections (10 mg/kg; IP). Dopamine concentrations were determined in separate groups of hal-othane anesthetized rats 1, 3 and 7 days following the end of chronic treatments. Data in **A** represent absolute (nanomolar) dialysate dopamine concentrations. **B** shows the same data with peak dopamine concentrations expressed as percent of basal levels. Compared to chronic saline (Sal), chronic cocaine pretreatment produced elevations in basal dopamine levels on Day 1 ($p < 0.05$; Newman-Keuls after ANOVA) and increased absolute extracellular dopamine concentrations in response to cocaine challenge injections on Days 1 and 3 ($p < 0.05$) (**A**). Although absolute dopamine levels after cocaine challenge injections were higher in chronic cocaine than in chronic saline-treated animals, the relative, percent of basal increase in dopamine overflow was, in fact, reduced by chronic cocaine treatment (**B**). This reduction was significant on Day 1 ($p < 0.05$).

SEM chronic saline: 3.58 ± 0.57 nM vs. Mean + SEM chronic cocaine: 10.79 ± 2.19 nM) and decreased progressively with time. Moderate increases were still evident on Posttreatment Days 3 and 7 but did not differ statistically from chronic saline-treated control rats (FIG. 6A).

Cocaine challenge injections produced significant increases in dopamine accumulation in chronic saline and chronic cocaine-treated rats at all 3 posttreatment intervals. However, there were marked, statistically reliable differences in the magnitude of cocaine effects depending on pretreatment conditions and interval length between chronic and challenge treatments. Extracellular dopamine concentrations reached higher absolute peak levels after challenge injections in chronic cocaine than in chronic saline-treated rats (FIG. 6A). Like the increases in basal concentrations this effect was strongest on Day 1 (Mean $\pm$ SEM chronic saline: $12.61 + 1.76$ nM vs. chronic cocaine: $23.6 + 4.63$ nM) and decreased over time in the Day 3 and Day 7 challenge groups. To compensate for the systematic differences in basal DA overflow among treatment groups, changes in perfusate dopamine concentrations were also examined in relation to their corresponding basal values. When expressed in terms of percent of basal concentrations the cocaine challenge-induced increases in extracellular dopamine were, in fact, smaller after repeated cocaine as opposed to saline pretreatments (FIG. 6B). In particular, on Challenge Day 1 cocaine produced a mean maximal increase to 412 ($\pm$49) percent of basal dopamine levels in the chronic saline group. In contrast, the corresponding peak increase in chronic cocaine-treated rats was only 252 ($\pm$39) percent.

Discussion

Consistent with its dopamine reuptake blocking properties, cocaine produced a gradual increase in dopamine levels in the nucleus accumbens in a manner well correlated with the self-administration response patterns. Regardless of the length of access, all animals appeared to regulate their cocaine intake so as to maintain stable dopamine concentrations within a specific range above basal levels. The failure to observe additional increases in dopamine accumulation during the "titrated" stage of responding cannot be attributed to a ceiling effect since extracellular dopamine concentrations can increase substantially beyond this level when the dose or frequency of cocaine injections are increased.[31,32] These results, then, suggest that the range within which extracellular dopamine concentrations are regulated by the dose-titrated response pattern of cocaine self-administering rats corresponds to a "window" of dopaminergic activity at which some optimal hedonic state is achieved. As a consequence, when dopamine levels are near or below the lower limit of this range animals respond for additional cocaine injections. When dopamine levels decrease further, responding is no longer supported as indicated by the behavioral extinction following substitution of cocaine with saline. Conversely, dopamine levels exceeding the upper boundary of this range may be aversive and intake is controlled accordingly. Evidence for the reinitiation of responding when dopamine levels approach the lower limit of this range has been provided by pharmacokinetic calculations.[32] Together, these findings provide further evidence for the existence of a dopaminergic "reward threshold" in the reinforcing effects of psychostimulant drugs as suggested by others.[22,33,34] The evidence for an upper threshold beyond which dopaminergic activation may become aversive is more controversial. The present data as well as related work[32] appear to support the existence of an upper "reward limit." This possibility seems to be supported also by the finding that animals compensate for an increase in cocaine dose by a proportional decrease in cocaine intake.[20] However, this response adjustment is not sufficient to maintain accumbens dopamine at the level induced by lower cocaine doses. Instead, dopamine levels in the accumbens increase with increasing cocaine doses in spite of compensatory decreases in cocaine intake.[21] This finding is difficult to reconcile with the hypothesis that cocaine intake is limited by the aversive effects of dopaminergic activation exceeding a certain level unless some tolerance to the reinforcing actions of cocaine develops. While these issues remain for further research, the limited-access self-administration data confirm and extend previous behavioral work with selective dopaminergic lesions that have demonstrated a critical role of mesolimbic dopamine in the reinforcing effects of intravenous cocaine self-administration.[9,11,12,13]

As pointed out above, the neuropharmacological bases of the cocaine withdrawal syndrome have remained largely unclear. Data from animal models of cocaine withdrawal suggest that some functional impairment in dopamine neurotransmission may underlie the behavioral manifestations of the post-cocaine "anhedonia" demonstrated in brain stimulation work[26] (Koob, this volume). The present results confirm this hypothesis by demonstrating that self-administration of cocaine under conditions of unlimited access is followed by a strong "rebound" inhibition of basal dopamine release. Like the elevation in reward thresholds, the inhibition of basal dopamine release increased as a function of the length of the preceding cocaine "binge." Similarly, maximal attenuation of dopamine release and brain stimulation reward were both observed between one and six hours post-cocaine. Given this close correspondence it would seem that the depression in basal dopamine release after extended periods of cocaine self-administration may be an important neurochemical correlate of the cocaine withdrawal syndrome as measured by intracranial self-stimulation thresholds. These observations suggest that the behavioral manifestations of dysphoria and anhedonia during cocaine withdrawal may reflect a cellular adaptation or overadaptation of mesolimbic dopamine neurons to the effects of sustained exposure to cocaine. Thus, the cocaine withdrawal syndrome may, at least in part, be the result of a within-systems adaptation[35] whereby the same neuronal system that mediates the reinforcing/euphorigenic actions of cocaine produces dysphoric effects after withdrawal of the drug due to physiological changes that serve to oppose or neutralize the cellular actions of the drug.

Reduced dopaminergic activity has also been implicated in cocaine craving and withdrawal by the dopamine depletion hypothesis.[30] The present data confirm that cocaine withdrawal is associated with some impairment in mesolimbic dopamine release. However, the physiological changes responsible for this condition remain to be elucidated. It is unclear for example whether this finding can be attributed to a depletion of intraneuronal dopamine pools as postulated by the dopamine depletion hypothesis. In earlier work no differences were found in accumbens tissue dopamine levels of rats before and after ten consecutive days of limited-access cocaine self-administration.[23] Alternatively, factors such as increased sensitivity of presynaptic, release-regulating receptors[36,37] (but see ref. 38), enhanced dopamine uptake,[43,44] or reduced dopamine synthesis[39,40] may account for the observed reductions in basal dopamine levels during cocaine withdrawal. However, the latter observations have all been made with repeated single or twice-daily bolus injection regimens. Future work should, therefore, be directed at identifying the precise changes in dopamine synaptic function that occur during withdrawal after periods of unlimited access to cocaine.

Repeated cocaine exposure increased basal release and significantly altered the effects of cocaine challenge injections on dopamine accumulation in the nucleus accumbens. In spite of the depression in dopamine release observed in trained, self-administering rats during cocaine withdrawal, basal dopamine concentrations in these animals were considerably higher than in drug-naive control rats (FIG. 5). A comparable increase in basal dopamine release was also observed following ten days of daily intraperitoneal cocaine injections. The same chronic cocaine pretreatment produced significantly greater elevations in extracellular dopamine concentrations after cocaine challenge than in chronic-saline controls. Repeated cocaine administration has been shown to induce a subsensitivity of somatodendritic, impulse-regulating, dopamine autoreceptors[41,42] (White et al., this volume). These changes were associated with increases in both firing rate and the number of spontaneously active A10 dopamine neurons. Interestingly, the autoreceptor subsensitivity reported in electrophysiological work persisted for four, but not eight days after repeated cocaine treatment[41] and thus, follows the same time course as the changes in basal release in the present work. The enhanced basal dopamine release after repeated cocaine administration, therefore, appears to reflect the changes in somatodendritic dopamine autoreceptor sensitivity. By extension, attenuated feedback inhibition due to autoreceptor subsensitivity in these animals may account for the significantly higher peak dopamine levels in response to cocaine challenge injections in the chronic-cocaine group. It is important to note, however, that while cocaine challenge-induced dopamine concentrations were increased by chronic cocaine pretreatment (FIG. 6A), the relative increase over basal levels was considerably reduced (FIG. 6B). It is unclear, at present, whether this relative reduction in the degree of dopaminergic activation over basal levels is the result of the development of supersensitivity in release-regulating, dopamine terminal autoreceptors in the nucleus accumbens,[36,37] increased dopamine uptake,[43,44] or a "ceiling effect."

Reduced dopamine accumulation in cocaine-experienced, self-administering animals compared to drug-naive controls was also evident in earlier work[23] (see also FIG. 3 vs. FIG. 4). In this situation both peak absolute dopamine concentrations and relative increases over basal levels were diminished. These results may suggest that self-administering animals develop some tolerance to the drug during the training period. These "acute-chronic" differences are, however, difficult to interpret because of possible stress effects associated with the first exposure to intravenous cocaine. Thus, the greater mean increase in dopamine levels in drug-naive over cocaine-experienced animals, may reflect some additive effect of the pharmacological action of cocaine and factors related to stress.

The changes in dopamine function observed after repeated exposure to cocaine may have important implications with regard to the neuropharmacology of cocaine reward, behavioral activation, and the pathological side effects associated with chronic abuse. First, repeated cocaine administration is accompanied by the emergence of reverse tolerance or sensitization to the motor stimulant actions of the drug (see ref. 45 for review; Post et al.; Kalivas et al., this volume). The strong augmentation of absolute dopamine concentrations in chronically pretreated rats after cocaine challenge is consistent with other reports showing that the increased motoric response in sensitized animals is paralleled by increased extracellular dopamine levels in the nucleus accumbens[46,47] (Kalivas et al., this volume). The cocaine challenge data suggest, however, that this apparent neurochemical "sensitization" is the result of a sustained overall augmentation of dopamine activity–reflected by decreased somatodendritic dopamine autoreceptor sensitivity[41,42] and increased basal dopamine release–rather than a sensitization to the pharmacological actions of cocaine. Second, in contrast to its motor stimulant effects, the reinforcing properties of cocaine appear to be subject to tolerance in both rats and humans[48,49] (Emmett-Oglesby, this volume). Also, cocaine self-administering animals increase their cocaine intake over a 10 day acquisition period by more than 100%, a finding which may suggest that these animals are compensating for developing tolerance (Weiss & Koob, unpublished observations). In the present work, repeated cocaine pretreatment produced a considerable reduction in the potency of cocaine to increase extracellular dopamine when expressed in terms of percent of basal levels. This effect may, in part, account for the apparent tolerance to the reinforcing effects of cocaine. However, this interpretation rests on the assumption that behavioral activation (sensitization) increases with increased absolute extracellular dopamine concentrations while the reinforcing effects of cocaine depend on the relative change in dopamine levels.

Clearly, additional research to elucidate the changes in dopamine function responsible for tolerance to the rewarding effects of cocaine is necessary. Finally, the increase in tonic, basal dopamine release after repeated cocaine treatments may play a role in post-cocaine psychopathology. Dopaminergic hyperactivity has long been implicated in the pathophysiology of (paranoid) schizophrenia and amphetamine psychosis.[51-53] By extension, it is possible that enhanced basal dopamine activity may play a role in the psychotic-like symptoms associated with chronic use and abuse of cocaine.[50]

ETHANOL SELF-ADMINISTRATION

Considerable evidence suggests that the reinforcing effects of a great variety of stimuli, and in particular many drugs of abuse, are dopamine-dependent (*e.g.*, refs. 5, 54, 55). Although there is convincing evidence for a dopaminergic involvement in psychostimulant reward, it remains to be established whether this also applies to ethanol.

A possible role for dopamine in the acute reinforcing actions of ethanol is suggested by several independent findings. Systemic administration of low doses of ethanol stimulates locomotor activity and produces marked increases in extracellular dopamine levels particularly in the nucleus accumbens where neurotransmitter release is closely time-locked to the behavioral activation.[56] Data from genetic models of ethanol preference indicate that ethanol-induced dopamine release as estimated from dopamine metabolite levels is greater in a line of rats outbred for ethanol preference (*s*P-rats) than in rats selected for non-preference (*s*NP-rats).[57] Additionally, low doses of ethanol were shown to stimulate spontaneous locomotor activity in Alcohol-Preferring (P-) and Maudsley Reactive (MR/N) rats, but not in Alcohol-Nonpreferring (NP-) and Maudsley Nonreactive (MNR/N) rats.[58] These findings are of particular importance in view of evidence suggesting that the rewarding as well as the locomotor stimulatory effects of psychostimulant drugs depend on increased dopamine activity in the nucleus accumbens.[3] Therefore, it is possible that the locomotor enhancing effects of ethanol reflect the reinforcing properties of this drug, and that both the locomotor and acute reinforcing actions of low doses of ethanol are the result of its ability to stimulate dopamine release in the nucleus accumbens. In support of this account recent reports indicate that alcohol self-administration and preference are modified by pharmacological manipulations of dopamine neurotransmission in a direction consistent with a role of dopamine in ethanol reward.[18,19,59-61]

The following experiments were designed to directly test the hypothesis that stimulation of dopamine release is involved in the acute reinforcing actions of ethanol using *in vivo* microdialysis procedures in rats operantly trained to self-administer ethanol. In

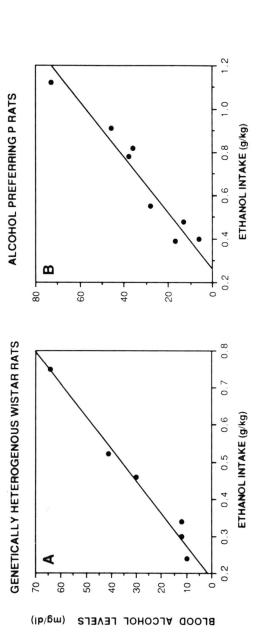

FIGURE 7. Relationship between ethanol intake (g/kg) and Blood Alcohol Levels (mg%) in genetically heterogeneous Wistar ($r = 0.98$; $p < 0.002$) and Alcohol-Preferring (P) rats ($r = 0.96$; $p < 0.001$).

addition, it was of interest to examine the possibility that alterations in dopamine function may be associated with the ethanol preference of Alcohol Preferring (P-) rats.

Effects of Voluntary Alcohol Self-Administration on Dopamine Release in the Nucleus Accumbens

Rats were trained to respond for ethanol or water in a two-lever, free-choice operant task (for details of the training procedures see refs. 16, 18). During daily 30 minute sessions responses at the appropriate lever produced delivery of 0.1 ml ethanol solution (10% w/v) or water on a concurrent schedule of continuous reinforcement. All training and testing occurred in the absence of food or fluid restrictions. To control for nonspecific changes in dopamine release related to factors such as "arousal" (as a result of moving animals from home to operant cage), or the "expectancy" of ethanol (due to the predictive nature of the operant environment for impending ethanol availability), a 15-minute waiting period was introduced before ethanol (and water) was made available by extension of the levers.

Rats of both strains showed a marked preference for ethanol over water at the end of the initiation procedures. Mean (±SEM) ethanol intake on the test day was 0.68 (±0.09) g/kg in P-rats and 0.44 (±0.08) g/kg in the Wistar group. Ethanol intake was sufficient to produce pharmacologically relevant mean blood alcohol levels (BALs) which ranged from 6.0 to 73.0 mg% (mean ± SEM: 32.13 ± 7.57 mg%) in P-rats

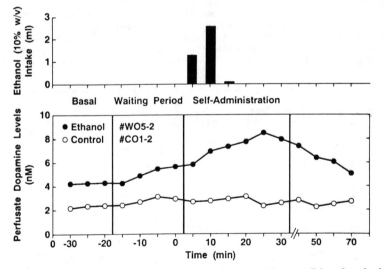

FIGURE 8. Individual records of an ethanol self-administering Wistar rat (Ethanol) and a drug-naive Wistar control rat trained to respond for water (Control). Dopamine overflow in the accumbens before, during and after the 30-minute self-administration session is shown in the lower panel. Amounts of 10% ethanol ingested per 5-minute interval are represented in the upper panel. Note that dopamine overflow increased already during the presession waiting period in the ethanol-expecting animal prior to ethanol availability. Dopamine overflow increased further during ethanol self-administration and reached peak 15 min after peak intake.

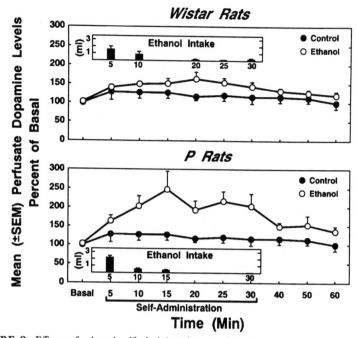

FIGURE 9. Effects of ethanol self-administration on dopamine release in the nucleus accumbens in genetically heterogeneous Wistar ($n = 5$) and Alcohol Preferring (P) rats ($n = 7$). Data of both strains of rats are contrasted against the same control group ($n = 4$) consisting of ethanol-naive Wistar and P-rats trained to respond for water. Ethanol produced significant increases in dopamine release in both strains of rats [Wistar: $F(1,9) = 5.3$; $p < 0.05$; P-rats: $F(1,11) = 11.4$; $p < 0.01$]. Insets show mean ($\pm$SEM) ethanol intake per 5-minute intervals.

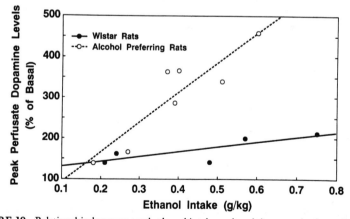

FIGURE 10. Relationship between total ethanol intake and peak increases in dopamine release in genetically heterogeneous Wistar and P-rats. A clear dose-response relationship was evident in both strains of rats (Wistar: $r = 0.79$; $0.1 > p > 0.05$; P-rats: $r = 0.91$; $p < 0.0005$). However, the slope of the dose-response function was significantly steeper in P-rats ($p < 0.001$). Thus, with increasing doses ethanol produced a progressively greater stimulation of dopamine release in P- than in Wistar rats.

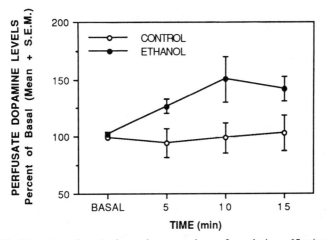

FIGURE 11. Dopamine release in the nucleus accumbens of rats during a 15-minute waiting period prior to onset of ethanol self-administration. Dialysate dopamine levels were significantly increased at the 10-minute ($p < 0.01$) and 15-minute ($p < 0.05$) intervals in rats ($n = 9$) expecting to receive access to ethanol (Ethanol), but not in rats ($n = 4$) anticipating water (Control) [simple effects after mixed-factorial ANOVAs (pooled data from both rat strains)].

and from 10.0 to 64.3 mg% (mean ± SEM: 28.22 ± 8.8 mg%) in genetically heterogeneous Wistar rats (FIG. 7). Self-administration of ethanol was associated with significant, dose-dependent increases in extracellular dopamine levels in the nucleus accumbens in both strains of rats (FIGS. 9 and 10). The stimulation of dopamine release by ethanol was also clearly time-locked to ethanol self-administration patterns such that peak dopamine levels occurred at 10–15 minutes following peak ethanol intake (FIGS. 8, 9 and 10).

As illustrated in FIGURES 8 and 11, extracellular dopamine levels were also significantly increased (Mean ± SEM: 150.21 ± 19.95 percent of basal levels) during the 15-minute waiting period prior to ethanol availability. No statistically reliable increases in dopamine overflow during the waiting period were noted in drug-naive control animals trained to self-administer water.

Strain Differences in Ethanol-induced Dopamine Release: Alcohol-Preferring (P) versus Genetically Heterogeneous Wistar Rats

To examine the possibility that strain differences in dopamine function may contribute to the differences in ethanol preference, basal and ethanol-induced dopamine release in genetically heterogeneous Wistar rats was compared to that of Alcohol Preferring (P-) rats.

The average ethanol intake and BALs in Alcohol-Preferring rats were only marginally higher than in genetically heterogeneous Wistar rats. However, the dose-effect functions of the relationship between ethanol intake (g/kg) and increases in dopamine release (percent of basal) revealed considerable strain differences (FIG. 10). In P-rats, ethanol produced a significantly greater enhancement of dopamine release at a given dose than in unselected Wistars. Over the near identical range of doses self-administered by rats of both strains, ethanol produced increases in dopamine overflow ranging from 120% to 460% (of basal levels) in Alcohol-Preferring, but only from 120% to 200% (of basal levels) in Wistar rats. There was also a tendency for P-rats to show lower (although not statistically different) mean (±SEM) levels of basal dopamine release than Wistar rats (P-rats: 1.14 ± 0.46 nM; Wistar: 2.17 ± 0.81 nM).

In order to differentiate the pharmacological effects of ethanol on dopamine release from the effects of responding for a reinforcer *per se*, one group of animals (P-rats) was tested during self-administration of a weak saccharine (0.05% w/v) solution one day after ethanol self-administration testing. In contrast to ethanol, self-administration of saccharine produced only a small increase in dopamine levels (data not shown). Saccharine not only failed to induce substantial enhancements of dopamine release, but these (marginal) effects also followed a different time course than the ethanol-induced changes in extracellular dopamine. Although there were no differences in the distribution of ethanol and saccharine intake over the 30 minute test sessions, peak dopamine levels during saccharine self-administration occurred in parallel with peak intake at the beginning of the sessions; in contrast peak dopamine levels were observed 10–15 minutes *after* peak ethanol intake.

Discussion

Consistent with previous reports showing that systemically administered ethanol stimulates dopamine release from terminal areas of the mesolimbic dopamine system,[56] these findings demonstrate that the self-administration of ethanol is followed by significant, dose-dependent increases in extracellular dopamine levels in the nucleus accumbens. An alternative reinforcer, saccharine failed to produce reliable changes in dopamine release. Although ethanol intake during the 30 minute self-administration sessions was not sufficient to produce gross behavioral signs of intoxication, ethanol intake and BALs in the observed range appear to be nonetheless relevant to the reinforcing actions of ethanol. First, while of shorter duration, the increases in dopamine release elicited by ethanol doses above 0.5 g/kg were comparable to those commonly associated with the self-administration of cocaine[23,32] (COCAINE SELF-ADMINISTRATION above). Second, doses of ethanol which produce BALs comparable to those in the present work have discriminative stimulus properties[62] and consequently, are "meaningful" to animals. Third, systemically administered ethanol at doses as low as 0.12 g/kg to 0.25 g/kg stimulate spontaneous locomotor activity in some strains of rats, a finding which has been interpreted as an expression of the positively reinforcing effects of ethanol.[55,56,58] Finally, BALs and amounts of ethanol ingested by rats of both strains corresponded well to those reported in other work where pharmacological manipulation of dopamine neurotransmission was shown to modify ethanol reward.[17-19,59-61]

The present results, then, further confirm a possibly important role for mesolimbic dopamine in low-dose ethanol reinforcement in non-dependent rats. In particular, the absence of a comparable effect of saccharine on dopamine overflow suggests that the enhancement of dopamine release by ethanol is a direct consequence of its pharmacological actions and cannot be explained solely on the basis of motivational processes associated with responding for a reinforcer *per se*. This account is also supported by the dose-dependency of ethanol effects as well as by the time-lag between ethanol intake and peak dopamine stimulation. The observed delays are consistent with the pharmacokinetic properties of ethanol and the time required to reach peak brain alcohol concentrations.[63,64] Moreover, the peak intake-to-effect delays correspond closely with other work in which peak locomotor stimulatory effects [58] and peak dopamine release in the nucleus accumbens[56] were reported to occur with similar delays following systemic administration of ethanol.

Although the failure to obtain dopamine stimulatory effects with saccharine strongly suggests that the augmentation of dopamine release by ethanol is the result of its pharmacological actions, a rise in extracellular dopamine levels was also observed in the absence of ethanol during the presession waiting period. Since comparable effects were not evident in ethanol-naive control animals one may speculate that dopamine release in this situation was triggered by the "expectancy" of access to alcohol. Similar results have recently been reported in work with *in vivo* dopamine binding techniques where self-administration and anticipation of ethanol produced identical amounts of dopaminergic activation.[65] It is likely that this anticipatory dopaminergic response depends on the presence of incentive motivational stimuli in the operant environment which are associated with the impending availability of the drug. Additional work to identify these stimuli, their relative contribution to the anticipatory stimulation of dopamine release, and the precise conditions under which they activate dopamine release in the accumbens will be needed in order to establish their significance in ethanol-related motivational processes and reinforcement.

The results revealed striking strain differences with regard to the magnitude of the dopaminergic stimulation induced by ethanol. Alcohol-Preferring rats have a number of neurochemical deficiencies including a 25% reduction in dopamine content in the nucleus accumbens, which has been suggested to be an important determinant of the ethanol preference in this line of rats.[66] Consistent with these reports, in the present study there was a tendency toward reduced basal dopamine release in P-rats. However, ethanol self-administration produced a considerably greater relative stimulation of dopamine release in this strain than in genetically heterogeneous Wistar rats. Enhanced dopaminergic activity in *s*P- compared to *s*NP-rats has also been reported following systemic ethanol administration.[57] It seems, therefore, that in spite of their deficiency in accumbens dopamine content, P-rats respond to ethanol with a greater relative enhancement in dopamine release. This "sensitization" with regard to the dopamine stimulatory effects of ethanol may be one of the neurobiological bases of the ethanol preference in this line of rats.

GENERAL CONCLUSIONS

Previous research has implicated a role for dopamine release in the nucleus accumbens in the reinforcing actions of many drugs of abuse. The present results provide additional support for this hypothesis with respect to cocaine and ethanol. Self-administration of both cocaine and ethanol was followed by an increase in extracellular dopamine levels in the nucleus accumbens. With both cocaine and ethanol, a consistent and reliable relationship was evident between dopamine release and the pattern or amount of the self-administered drug. Dopamine neurotransmission in the nucleus accumbens appears to play a critical role not only in the reinforcing actions of cocaine, but also in withdrawal. Marked rebound inhibition of basal dopamine release observed

after unlimited-access self-administration may be an important neurochemical correlate of the anhedonia and dysphoria associated with cocaine withdrawal.
    While it is well established that the increase in extracellular dopamine associated
with the self-administration of cocaine is a direct result of its pharmacological actions,
the present results suggest that this applies to ethanol as well. Moreover, stimulation
of dopamine release by ethanol was greater in a strain of rats selectively outbred for
ethanol preference (P-rats) than in genetically heterogeneous strain (Wistar) suggesting
that dopamine neurotransmission may be an important factor in ethanol preference.
Dopamine release in the case of ethanol can, however, also be stimulated independently of its pharmacological actions presumably by the presence of incentive stimuli
related to the motivational properties of this drug. Such neurochemical responses may
be of particular importance with regard to drug-seeking behaviors and craving elicited
by conditioned stimuli associated with drugs of abuse in general.

ACKNOWLEDGMENTS

    We wish to thank Marge T. Lorang, Robert Lintz, and Ilham Polis for their excel-
lent technical assistance.

REFERENCES

1. BOZARTH, M. A. 1982. Opiate reward mechanisms mapped by intracranial self-administra-
    tion. *In* Neurobiology of Opiate Reward. J. E. Smith & J. D. Lane, Eds. Raven Press.
    New York.
2. GOEDERS, N. E. & J. E. SMITH. 1987. Intracranial self-administration methodologies.
    Neurosci. Biobehav. Rev. 11: 319–329.
3. KOOB, G. F., F. J. VACCARINO, M. AMALRIC & F. E. BLOOM. 1987. Positive reinforcement
    properties of drugs: Search for neural substrates. *In* Brain Reward Systems and Abuse.
    J. Engel & L. Oreland, Eds.: 35–50. Raven Press. New York.
4. WISE, R. A. 1984. Neural mechanisms of the reinforcing actions of cocaine. *In* NIDA Research
    Monograph Cocaine: Pharmacology, Effects, and Treatment of Abuse. J. Grabowski,
    Ed.: 15–33. NIDA. Rockville, MD.
5. FIBIGER, H. C. 1978. Drugs and reinforcement mechanisms: A critical review of the cat-
    echolamine theory. Ann. Rev. Pharmacol. Toxicol. 18: 37–56.
6. KOOB, G. F. & N. E. GOEDERS. 1988. Neuroanatomical substrates of drug self-
    administration. *In* The Neuropharmacological Basis of Reward. J. Liebman & S. Cooper,
    Eds.: 216–263. Oxford University Press. Oxford.
7. WISE, R. A. 1980. Action of drugs of abuse on brain reward systems. Pharmacol. Biochem.
    Behav. 13(Suppl. 1): 213–232.
8. WISE, R. A. & M. A. BOZARTH. 1982. Action of drugs of abuse on brain reward systems:
    An update with specific attention to opiates. Pharmacol. Biochem. Behav. 17: 239–243.
9. KOOB, G. F., F. J. VACCARINO, M. AMALRIC & N. R. SWERDLOW. 1987. Neural substrates
    for cocaine and opiate reinforcement. *In* Cocaine: Clinical and Biobehavioral Aspects.
    S. Fischer, A. Raskin & E. H. Uhlenhuth, Eds.: 80–108. Oxford University Press. New
    York.
10. LYNESS, W. H., N. M. FRIEDLE & K. E. MOORE. 1979. Destruction of dopaminergic nerve
    terminals in nucleus accumbens: Effect of *d*-amphetamine self-administration. Phar-
    macol. Biochem. Behav. 11: 663–666.
11. ROBERTS, D. C. S., M. E. CORCORAN & H. C. FIBIGER. 1977. On the role of ascending
    catecholaminergic systems in intravenous self-administration of cocaine. Pharmacol. Bio-
    chem. Behav. 6: 615–620.

12. ROBERTS, D. C. S., G. F. KOOB, P. KLONOFF & H. C. FIBIGER. 1980. Extinction and recovery of cocaine self-administration following 6-hydroxydopamine lesions of the nucleus accumbens. Pharmacol. Biochem. Behav. 12: 781–787.
13. ROBERTS, D. C. S. & G. F. KOOB. 1982. Disruption of cocaine self-administration following 6-hydroxydopamine lesions of the ventral tegmental area in rats. Pharmacol. Biochem. Behav. 17: 901–904.
14. MEISCH, R. A. 1982. Animal studies of alcohol intake. J. Psychiatr. Res. 141: 113–120.
15. SAMSON, H. H. 1987. Initiation of ethanol-maintained behavior: A comparison of animal models and their implication to human drinking. *In* Neurobehavioral Pharmacology. T. Thompson, P. Dews & J. Barret, Eds. 6th Edit. Erlbaum Associates. New Jersey.
16. WEISS, F. & G. F. KOOB. 1991. The neuropharmacology of ethanol self-administration. *In* Neuropharmacology of Ethanol: New Approaches. R. E. Meyer, G. F. Koob, M. J. Lewis & S. M. Paul, Eds. Birkhauser. Boston.
17. GRANT, K. A. & H. H. SAMSON. 1985. Induction and maintenance of ethanol self-administration without food deprivation in the rat. Psychopharmacology 86: 475–479.
18. WEISS, F., M. MITCHINER, F. E. BLOOM & G. F. KOOB. 1990. Free-choice responding for ethanol versus water in Alcohol-Preferring (P) and unselected Wistar rats is differentially altered by naloxone, bromocriptine and methysergide. Psychopharmacology 101: 178–186.
19. PFEFFER, A. O. & H. H. SAMSON. 1988. Haloperidol and apomorphine effects on ethanol reinforcement in free-feeding rats. Pharmacol. Biochem. Behav. 29: 343–350.
20. KOOB, G. F. 1991. The reward system and abuse with cocaine. *In* The Biological Basis of Substance Abuse. S. G. Korenman & J. D. Barchas, Eds. Oxford University Press. New York.
21. PETTIT, H.-O. & J. B. JUSTICE, JR. 1991. Effect of dose on cocaine self-administration behavior and dopamine levels in the nucleus accumbens. Brain Res. 539: 94–102.
22. YOKEL, R. A. & R. PICKENS. 1974. Drug level of *d*- and *l*-amphetamine during intravenous self-administration. Psychopharmacology (Berlin) 34: 255–264.
23. HURD, Y. L., F. WEISS, G. F. KOOB, N.-E. ANDEN & U. UNGERSTEDT. 1989. Reinforcing effects of cocaine are dissociated from dopamine release in rat nucleus accumbens: An in vivo microdialysis study. Brain Res. 489: 199–203.
24. DENEAU, G. A., T. YANAGITA & M. H. SEEVERS. 1969. Self-administration of psychoactive substances by the monkeys. Psychopharmacologia 16: 30–48.
25. BOZARTH, M. A. & R. A. WISE. 1985. Toxicity associated with long-term intravenous heroin and cocaine self-administration in the rat. J. Am. Med. Assoc. 254: 81–83.
26. MARKOU, A. & G. F. KOOB. 1991. Post cocaine anhedonia. An animal model of cocaine withdrawal. Neuropharmacology 4: 17–26.
27. GAWIN, F. H. & H. D. KLEBER. 1986. Abstinence symptomatology and psychiatric diagnosis in cocaine abusers. Arch. Gen. Psychiatry 43: 107–113.
28. KOKKINIDIS, L. & B. D. MCCARTER. 1990. Postcocaine depression and sensitization of brain stimulation reward: Analysis of reinforcement and performance effects. Pharmacol. Biochem. Behav. 36: 463–471.
29. STELLAR, J. R. & M. B. RICE. 1989. Pharmacological basis of intracranial self-stimulation reward. *In* The Neuropharmacological Basis of Reward. J. M. Liebman & S. J. Cooper, Eds.: 14–65. Clarendon Press. Oxford.
30. DACKIS, C. A. & M. S. GOLD. 1985. New concepts in cocaine addiction: The dopamine depletion hypothesis. Neurosci. Biobehav. Rev. 9: 469–477.
31. HURD, Y. L. & U. UNGERSTEDT. 1989. Cocaine: An *in vivo* microdialysis evaluation of its acute actions on dopamine transmission in rat striatum. Synapse 3: 48–54.
32. PETTIT, H.-O. & J. B. JUSTICE, JR. 1989. Dopamine in the nucleus accumbens during cocaine self-administration as studied by *in vivo* microdialysis. Pharmacol. Biochem. Behav. 34: 899–904.
33. YOKEL, R. A. & R. A. WISE. 1973. Increased lever-pressing for amphetamine reinforcement after pimozide in rats: Implications for a dopamine theory of reward. Science 187: 547–549.
34. WISE, R. A. & M. A. BOZARTH. 1987. A psychomotor stimulant theory of addiction. Psychol. Rev. 94: 469–492.

35. KOOB, G. F. & F. E. BLOOM. 1988. Cellular and molecular mechanisms of drug dependence. Science 242: 715–723.
36. DWOSKIN, L. P., J. PERIS, R. P. YASUDA, K. PHILPOTT & N. R. ZAHNISER. 1988. Repeated cocaine administration results in supersensitivity of striatal D-2 dopamine autoreceptors to pergolide. Life Sci. 42: 255–262.
37. WEISS, F., Y. L. HURD, U. UNGERSTEDT & G. F. KOOB. 1989. Repeated cocaine administration potentiates the hypomotility effects of apomorphine. Soc. Neurosci. Abstr. 15: 250.
38. YI, S.-J. & K. J. JOHNSON. 1990. Chronic cocaine treatment impairs the regulation of synaptosomal ^{3}H-DA release by D_2 autoreceptors. Pharmacol. Biochem. Behav. 36: 457–461.
39. BROCK, J. W., J. P. NG & J. B. JUSTICE, JR. 1990. Effect of chronic cocaine on dopamine synthesis in the nucleus accumbens as determined by microdialysis perfusion with NSDO-1015. Neurosci. Lett. 117: 234–239.
40. TRULSON, M. E. & M. J. ULISSEY. 1987. Chronic cocaine administration decreases dopamine synthesis rate and increases [^{3}H] spiroperidol binding in rat brain. Brain Res. Bull. 19: 35–38.
41. ACKERMAN, J. M. & F. J. WHITE. 1990. A10 somatodendritic dopamine autoreceptor sensitivity following withdrawal from repeated cocaine treatment. Neurosci. Lett. 117: 181–187.
42. HENRY, D. J., M. A. GREENE & F. J. WHITE. 1989. Electrophysiological effects of cocaine in the mesoaccumbens dopamine system: Repeated administration. J. Pharmacol. Exp. Ther. 251: 833–839.
43. NG, J. P., G. W. HUBERT & J. B. JUSTICE, JR. 1991. Increased stimulated release and uptake of dopamine in the nucleus accumbens after repeated cocaine administration as measured by in vivo voltammetry. J. Neurochem. 56: 1485–1492.
44. YI, S.-J. & K. J. JOHNSON. 1991. Effects of acute and chronic administration of cocaine on striatal uptake, compartmentalization and release of [^{3}H]dopamine. Neuropharmacology 29: 475–486.
45. POST, R. M. & S. R. B. WEISS. 1988. Psychomotor stimulant vs. local anesthetic effects of cocaine: Role of behavioral sensitization and kindling. NIDA Res. Monogr. 88: 217–238.
46. KALIVAS, P. W. & P. DUFFY. 1990. The effect of acute and daily cocaine treatment on extracellular dopamine in the nucleus accumbens. Synapse 5: 48–58.
47. PETTIT, H.-O., H.-T. PAN, L. H. PARSONS & J. B. JUSTICE, JR. 1990. Extracellular concentrations of cocaine and dopamine are enhanced during chronic cocaine administration. J. Neurochem. 55: 798–804.
48. WOOD, D. M. & M. W. EMMET-OGLESBY. 1986. Characteristics of tolerance, recovery from tolerance and cross-tolerance for cocaine used as a discriminative stimulus. J. Pharmacol. Exp. Ther. 237: 120–125.
49. FISHMAN, M. W., C. R. SCHUSTER, J. JAVAID, Y. HATANO & J. DAVIS. 1985. Acute tolerance to the cardiovascular and subjective effects of cocaine. J. Pharmacol. Exp. Ther. 235: 677–682.
50. POST, R. M. & R. T. KOPANDA. 1976. Cocaine, kindling and psychosis. Am. J. Psychiatry 133: 627–634.
51. STEVENS, J. R. 1979. Schizophrenia and dopamine regulation in the mesolimbic system. Trends Neurosci. 2: 102–105.
52. SNYDER, S. H. 1973. Amphetamine psychosis: A model schizophrenia mediated by catecholamines. Am. J. Psychiatry 130: 61–67.
53. ROBINSON, T. E. & J. B. BECKER. 1986. Enduring changes in brain and behavior produced by chronic amphetamine administration: A review and evaluation of animal models of amphetamine psychosis. Brain Res. Rev. 11: 157–198.
54. WISE, R. A. 1978. Catecholamine theories of reward: A critical review. Brain Res. 152: 215–217.
55. DI CHIARA, G. & A. IMPERATO. 1988. Drugs abused by humans preferentially increase synaptic dopamine concentrations in the mesolimbic system of freely moving rats. Proc. Natl. Acad. Sci. USA 85: 5274–5278.
56. IMPERATO, A. & G. DICHIARA. 1986. Preferential stimulation of dopamine release in the

nucleus accumbens of freely moving rats by ethanol. J. Pharmacol. Exp. Ther. **239**: 219–239.

57. FADDA, F., E. MOSCA, G. COLOMBO & G. L. GESSA. 1989. Effects of spontaneous ingestion of ethanol on brain dopamine metabolism. Life Sci. **44**: 281–287.
58. WALLER, M. B., J. M. MURPHY, W. J. MCBRIDE, L. LUMENG & T.-K. LI. 1986. Effect of low-dose ethanol on spontaneous motor activity in alcohol-preferring and nonpreferring rats. Pharmacol. Biochem. Behav. **24**: 617–623.
59. PFEFFER, A. O. & H. H. SAMSON. 1986. Effect of pimozide on home cage ethanol drinking in the rat: Dependence on drinking session length. Drug Alcohol Depend. **17**: 47–55.
60. PFEFFER, A. O. & H. H. SAMSON. 1985. Oral ethanol reinforcements: Interactive effects of amphetamine, pimozide and food restriction. Alcohol Drug Res. **6**: 37–48.
61. RASSNICK, N., L. PULVIRENTI & G. F. KOOB. 1989. Effects of a novel dopamine agonist, Sandoz 205-152, on ethanol self-administration. Soc. Neurosci. Abstr.
62. YORK, J. L. 1978. A comparison of the discriminative stimulus properties of ethanol, barbital, and phenobarbital in rats. Psychopharmacology **60**: 19–23.
63. GOLDSTEIN, D. B. 1983. Pharmacology of Alcohol. Oxford University Press. New York.
64. LUMENG, L., M. B. WALLER, W. J. MCBRIDE & T.-K. LI. 1982. Different sensitivities to ethanol in alcohol-preferring and non-preferring rats. Pharmacol. Biochem. Behav. **16**: 125–130.
65. VAVROUSEK-JAKUBA, E., C. A. COHEN & W. J. SHOEMAKER. 1991. Ethanol effects on dopamine receptors: *In vivo* binding following voluntary ethanol (ETOH) intake in rats. *In* Novel Pharmacological Interventions for Alcoholism. C. E. Naranjo & E. M. Sellers, Eds. Springer Verlag. New York.
66. MURPHY, J. M., W. J. MCBRIDE, L. LUMENG & T-K LI. 1987. Contents of monoamines in forebrain regions of alcohol-preferring (P) and non-preferring (NP) lines of rats. Pharmacol. Biochem. Behav. **26**: 389–392.

Alcohol Self-Administration: Role of Mesolimbic Dopamine[a]

HERMAN H. SAMSON,[b] GERALD A. TOLLIVER,
MIKI HARAGUCHI, AND CLYDE W. HODGE

Alcohol and Drug Abuse Institute (NL-15)
University of Washington
3937 15th Avenue, N.E.
Seattle, Washington 98195

INTRODUCTION

The involvement of the mesocorticolimbic dopamine (DA) system has been implicated in reinforcement processes in general,[1-4] including the self-administration of drugs of abuse.[5-7] However, for oral ethanol self-administration, no direct evidence for its involvement has been demonstrated.

When ethanol is administered to rats, various techniques have indicated that the mesocorticolimbic DA system is activated. Several studies have found increased DA or DA metabolite levels in the ventral striatum following administration of ethanol at doses ranging from 1 to 3 g/kg.[8-10] Other investigators have demonstrated that low doses of ethanol, administered IV to rats, increased firing of DA cell bodies in the ventral tegmental area (VTA).[11] Also, low concentrations of alcohol perfused into the bathing medium of the VTA slice preparation increased DA cell body firing.[12] Using microdialysis, Imperato and Di Chiara found that administration of low doses of ethanol resulted in preferential release of DA from the nucleus accumbens compared to striatum.[13] Taken together, these studies indicate that investigator administered ethanol can result in the activation and release of DA from portions of the mesocorticolimbic DA system. However, in none of these studies did the animal self-administer (voluntarily drink) ethanol.

In studies in which rats are drinking ethanol, systemic injection of DA agonists and antagonists have resulted in mixed effects. In 24-hour home-cage ethanol-drinking studies, either decreases or no effects of a variety of DA agents have been reported.[14-18] When ethanol is available only during limited time periods each day in the home cage, decreases in ethanol intake have been reported for both agonists and antagonists.[17,18] However, decreases in water consumption also occurred in one study,[17] suggesting a non-specific effect.

When operant self-administration procedures are employed, systemic administra-

[a] This work was supported in part by grants from the National Institute on Alcohol Abuse and Alcoholism (AA06845 and AA07404 to HHS) and by the Alcohol and Drug Abuse Institute of the University of Washington.
[b] Author to whom correspondence should be addressed.

tion of agonists and antagonists[19-22] have been found to decrease ethanol-reinforced responding. However, the effect on response pattern is different between agonists and antagonists. Agonists were found to break up the regular high-rate momentary responding which generally occurs during the first 10 min of a 30-min session.[20,21] However, antagonists did not break up this high-rate responding, but instead resulted in an early termination of the normal response pattern.[20,21] Although both agonists and antagonists decrease total ethanol self-administration, it would appear that they do so by different mechanisms.

EFFECT OF MICROINJECTION IN N. ACCUMBENS ON ETHANOL SELF-ADMINISTRATION

While the data discussed above suggest that DA is related to ethanol self-administration, they do not provide direct evidence that the mesocorticolimbic DA reinforcement pathways are involved in ethanol reinforcement. In order to assess more directly the involvement of this pathway in ethanol reinforcement, the effects of microinjection of DA agonists and antagonists into the nucleus accumbens on ethanol self-administration were tested using an operant self-administration procedure.

Rats, initiated with the sucrose-substitution procedure,[23] to lever press using ethanol reinforcement (10%, v/v) were surgically implanted with guide cannulae located to permit microinjection into nucleus accumbens. All injections and sham control were performed 10 min prior to the daily 30-min operant session (for a complete description of the methods and procedures see ref. 24). To date, the effects of the mixed agonist *d*-amphetamine, the D_2 agonist quinpirole (LY171555), and the D_2 antagonist raclopride have been examined.

Effects of the Mixed Agonist, d-Amphetamine

Microinjection of *d*-amphetamine significantly increased total session responding at the 20 μg/brain dose, with 9 out of 12 rats having increased responding, 2 rats showing decreased responding and one rat in which no effect was observed (FIG. 1). This increased responding resulted in a significant increase in ethanol intake (Values are mean and SEM. All rats: sham = 0.46[0.05] g ethanol/kg body weight; 20 μg dose = 0.58 g/kg[0.08], t(11) = 2.39, $p < 0.05$; nine rats who increased responding: sham = 0.50 g/kg[0.05], 20 μg dose = 0.74 g/kg[0.05]). For some animals, increases were seen at the 4 μg and 10 μg/brain doses as well, but these doses were not effective in all animals tested.

Increased total responding usually resulted from a slowing of momentary response rate compared to sham or no injection control conditions, accompanied by a prolonged continuation of responding throughout the 30-min session (see response records in FIG. 1). This effect of slowing of response rate is somewhat similar to that seen when *d*-amphetamine is injected systemically,[20] but with systemic injections, a more marked disruption of response pattern consistently resulted in decreased rather than increased ethanol intake. Chronic systemic administration of *d*-amphetamine has been reported to increase ethanol intakes.[25-27] The relationship between acute systemic injection, acute nucleus accumbens microinjection, and chronic systemic administration is unclear. It is possible that some alteration in DA sensitivity after chronic systemic

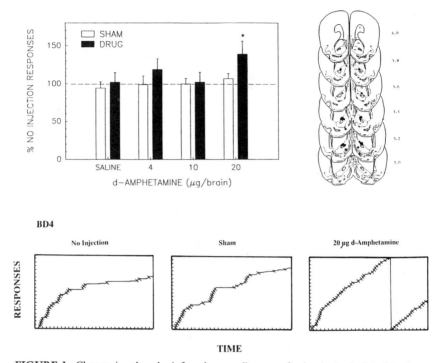

FIGURE 1. Changes in ethanol reinforced responding on a fixed ratio 4 schedule (FR 4) as a function of microinjection of *d*-amphetamine into the nucleus accumbens. The top left graph shows percent of sham/drug responding compared to non-injection control sessions (Mean and SEM; * = significant from control at $p < 0.05$, ** = significant from control at $p < 0.01$). The top right of the figure shows the localization of microinjection position for animals included in graph to the left. The bottom three records are representative cumulative response records from one animal (BD4) for each experimental condition. The scale for time on the X-axis represents one minute/division. The scale for responses on the Y-axis represents 8 responses/division. The cross-marks on each record indicate where ethanol dipper reinforcements were presented.

administration results in altered activation of nucleus accumbens DA, producing ethanol intakes similar to those noted in the present microinjection studies.

It should be noted that other investigators have found that microinjections of 20 μg/brain of *d*-amphetamine into the nucleus accumbens can cause increased motor activity, with some cases of mild stereotopy being observed.[28,29] In our studies, we have noticed on a few occasions that individual rats have failed to drink the ethanol when it was presented (*i.e.*, the change in fluid volume from the dipper reservoir following a session was less than that required by the number of dippers presented). Generally, however, the animals appear to drink the ethanol throughout the session. No excessive motor activation or stereotopy was observed. Additionally, no difficulty in handling the rats, nor signs of repetitive motor behaviors in the operant chamber were noted after the *d*-amphetamine injections.

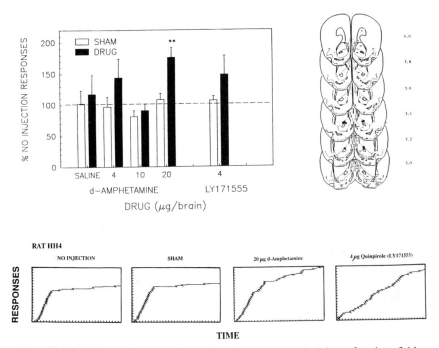

FIGURE 2. Changes in ethanol reinforced responding on a FR 4 schedule as a function of either *d*-amphetamine or quinpirole (LY171555) microinjected into the nucleus accumbens. See FIGURE 1 for a description of each portion of the figure.

Effects of the D₂ Agonist, Quinpirole (LY171555)

To date, we have only systematically tested a single dose of quinpirole (4 μg/brain), using 4 of the rats who were part of the *d*-amphetamine group described above. Comparison between the effects of amphetamine and quinpirole suggests that the increased and altered pattern of responding observed with amphetamine are at least in part a result of its action at the D_2 receptor site (FIG. 2). Although the limited data collected so far fail to reach statistical significance ($p < 0.19$), they are in the same direction as that of amphetamine (FIG. 2). In 3 of the 4 rats, the 4 μg/brain dose resulted in a similar effect to that of amphetamine (FIG. 2). In the remaining rat, this dose had no effect, but a 6 μg/brain dose resulted in an amphetamine-like effect.

The microinjection of 0.1 μg/brain quinpirole into the nucleus accumbens has been shown to slightly increase the number of cue-directed behaviors in a swimming test.[30] However, there were no effects on non cue-directed motor behaviors at this dose. Injection of 6 μg/brain of quinpirole in the nucleus accumbens slightly increased sniffing behavior, but had no other effects on other measures of locomotor activity.[31] A 10 μg/brain microinjection of quinpirole into the ventral striatum had no significant effect upon jaw movements.[32] From these data, it seems unlikely that the increased ethanol-reinforced responding reported above was due to a non-specific motor activa-

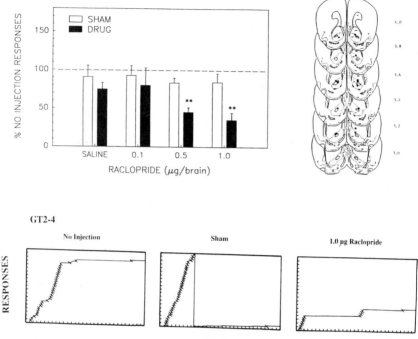

FIGURE 3. Changes in ethanol reinforced responding on a FR 4 schedule as a function of raclopride microinjected into the nucleus accumbens. See FIGURE 1 for a description of each portion of the figure.

tion effect of quinpirole. No gross behavioral changes in the animals' motor abilities or stereotypic behaviors in the operant chamber were noted. In all cases, the animals appeared to drink the ethanol presented.

Effects of the D_2 Antagonist, Raclopride

Unlike the DA agonists, raclopride decreased total responding and resulted in decreased ethanol intakes at doses of both 0.5 and 1.0 μg/brain (FIG. 3) (Mean [SEM] g ethanol/kg body weight values: sham = 0.51 g/kg (0.12); 0.5 μg/brain raclopride = 0.30 g/kg (0.07) [paired t(7) = 3.003, $p < 0.02$]; sham = 0.45 g/kg (0.06); 1.0 μg/brain raclopride = 0.27 g/kg [paired t(9) = 3.006, $p < 0.02$]). The effect upon response pattern (see response records of FIG. 3) was similar to that observed when the DA antagonists haloperidol and pimozide were administered systemically.[20,21] There was little effect on initial momentary response rates but responding termination after only a brief amount of time.

This result is opposite to that reported by Levy et al.[33] in which ethanol drinking was increased following microinjection of the D_2 antagonist sulpiride into the nucleus accumbens. In this study, a limited access home-cage ethanol drinking procedure was employed with rats from the genetically selected ethanol-preferring (P) line. There are several methodological differences between these studies which could account for this discrepancy. As well, the use of the selected P line rats, which are known to have decreased DA levels in nucleus accumbens,[34] could be an important difference which might determine the effects of DA antagonists. It should be noted that systemic administration of sulpiride has been shown to decrease drinking of other fluids,[35] which corresponds to our studies on systemic administration of other D_2 DA antagonists.[20,21] Thus, it is unlikely that the differences between the Levy *et al.* study[33] and our raclopride observations is because of a difference between raclopride and sulpiride.

Microinjection of 1.0 μg/brain of raclopride has been reported to result in a slight decrease in spontaneous motor activity[36] (this was an approximately 15% reduction in ambulation). Observation of our animals found no gross effects on motor behavior following the microinjection at any dose tested.

Implication of Microinjection Data

The above studies provide support for the hypothesis that DA in the nucleus accumbens is involved in oral ethanol reinforcement. While there are various interpretations as to what role the nucleus accumbens plays in reinforcement processes,[2,4] it appears that ethanol's reinforcing properties include the ability to access this part of the mesolimbic DA system. Given the data reviewed in the introduction related to the activation of this system by investigator administered ethanol, it would appear reasonable to hypothesize that oral ethanol self-administration results in similar activation. However, there is no direct evidence that this occurs and further experimentation is required to validate this hypothesis. It should be pointed out that investigator administered and self-administered drugs result in major differences in their effects, both on behavioral and neurological measures.[37,38] Thus, until direct evidence is provided that self-administered ethanol results in DA activation, caution should be used in assuming that the effects of the microinjection studies reported above are a result of specific ethanol DA activation in the nucleus accumbens.

THE MESOCORTICOLIMBIC DOPAMINE SYSTEM AND ORAL ETHANOL SELF-ADMINISTRATION CONTROL

A variety of complex factors interact to control ethanol self-administration. Genetics can clearly impact the amount of ethanol an animal self-administers.[39] It is of interest to note that in those animals genetically selected for ethanol preference, decreased levels of DA are found in several parts of the mesocorticolimbic DA system.[10,34] Behavioral initiation history has been shown to interact with these genetic predispositions to alter drinking behavior.[40,41] This would suggest that both genetic and environmental variables are important in regulating ethanol consumption. It remains unclear how these variables are related to the functioning of the mesocorticolimbic DA system or how alteration of this DA system may influence ethanol consumption.

When examining the effects of both genetic and environmental factors controlling

LH9

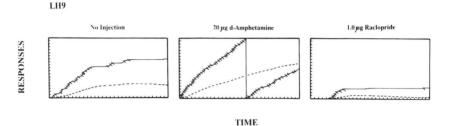

FIGURE 4. Representative ethanol reinforced cumulative response records for an animal who received both the dopamine agonist, *d*-amphetamine, and the dopamine antagonist, raclopride. The dashed lines are computer-generated estimated blood ethanol levels. See FIGURE 1 for the scale representations.

drinking, one main feature of interest is the process that controls individual drinking episodes. Our data suggest that control of these drinking bouts can be conceptualized as a regulatory process consisting of three phases: an initial *onset phase* in which the drinking behavior begins; a *maintenance phase* during which drinking continues at some fairly constant rate; and then a *termination phase* which ends a drinking episode. The following is a discussion of the microinjection data presented above in the context of these three phases.

Onset Phase

Clearly for oral ethanol self-administration, given the factors of adsorption and distribution, there can be no central DA effects produced until some time after drinking has started and blood/brain ethanol levels have reached some level. Using a modified computer blood ethanol estimation program,[42] we have found that predicted blood ethanol patterns are quite different depending upon the pattern of drinking (FIG. 4). As can be seen from the No Injection condition (FIG. 4), blood ethanol lags behind intake. Thus, the CNS processes related to the onset of drinking behavior and the drinking which follows immediately thereafter, may involve different subsets of actions upon the DA reinforcement system than the processes related to maintenance and termination. There is no evidence from the above microinjection studies that either DA agonists or antagonists have any marked effect upon the regulatory processes which control the onset of a drinking bout. Neither DA agonists nor antagonists appeared to systematically delay, or block drinking onset, although in some cases, the DA antagonist raclopride did appear to delay the onset of responding.

However, once begun, drinking which occurs prior to any direct ethanol actions upon the CNS can be affected by raclopride. It has been demonstrated that DA release in the nucleus accumbens occurs following the presentation of external stimuli.[2] It is a major assumption of this chapter, that DA release in nucleus accumbens by psychoactive drugs is involved in their reinforcing action.[5-7] Therefore, it is plausible that if initially neutral stimuli are paired with increased mesolimbic DA activity resultant from drug action, these stimuli could become conditioned so as to produce changes in DA activity. This process has been demonstrated in several different learning procedures.[43,44] These conditioned stimuli can then function as conditioned reinforcers and maintain a variety of behaviors.

We have postulated that one of the functions of ethanol initiation procedures is to associate the taste and smell of ethanol with the delayed onset of its pharmacological effects.[45] It could be hypothesized that these conditioned taste and smell stimuli can activate the DA reinforcement system and provide the reinforcing stimuli required to maintain the initial onset of drinking until such time that the direct effects of ethanol can access the system. It would appear, that the effects of raclopride injected into the nucleus accumbens interferes with this process, resulting in a rapid termination of drinking behavior. This rapid termination suggests that little to no blood ethanol is present based on estimated values for this drinking pattern (FIG. 4, raclopride figure). If this is the case, these low blood levels would reduce the probability that any direct effect of ethanol upon the DA system could even occur. It is difficult to state that the decreased responding produced by raclopride is equivalent to behavioral extinction phenomena, but the pattern is similar to that observed when either water or an empty dipper is presented to rats initiated with ethanol reinforcement.[46] It could be hypothesized that raclopride blocks any DA effect resultant from the presentation of the conditioned ethanol stimuli (*e.g.*, the smell and taste of ethanol), which are necessary to maintain responding during the early parts of the drinking bout by serving as conditioned reinforcers.

Maintenance Phase

Once a drinking episode (bout) has begun, in rats initiated to respond using ethanol reinforcement,[23,45] the sequence of lever responding and drinking from the dipper proceed at a fairly consistent rate, with only short pauses after the delivery of several reinforcers (No Injection and Sham conditions for all figures). While the rate of responding during this phase varies somewhat across animals, it remains a dominant feature of the initiated animals' drinking bout. As described above, the initial segments of this bout are probably maintained by conditioned reinforcement. However, as blood ethanol increases, direct pharmacological actions occur which could provide reinforcement (FIG. 4, No Injection condition). It would seem most consistent with the data that the transition from conditioned to pharmacological reinforcement occurs after approximately 30% to 50% of a drinking bout has transpired. However, there is no direct evidence as to when or if any DA release in nucleus accumbens occurs during oral ethanol self-administration, and thus this transition hypothesis remains speculative.

Termination Phase

Perhaps the most critical process in ethanol drinking regulation is the control of drinking termination. Understanding the variables controlling this phase of the process has important implications for alcohol abuse and alcoholism. From previous studies,[45] it appears that one major termination variable is blood ethanol level. While these levels range widely when measured at the end of a 30-min drinking session,[46,47] computer estimation at the time of drinking termination during a drinking bout appears to be more related to rising blood levels. Other investigators have also suggested that blood levels combined with the rate of development of acute tolerance could be central to termination processes.[48]

From the data presented above, dopamine agonists microinjected into the nucleus accumbens increased ethanol self-administration by prolonging drinking in most cases. This finding suggests that drinking termination processes were either blocked (FIGS. 1 and 4) or to some degree interferred with (FIG. 2) following the agonist injection. Examination of estimated blood ethanol found that with amphetamine, blood ethanol levels continued to rise during the session (FIG. 4), reaching levels greater than those estimated at drinking termination in the non-injection control condition. If blood levels are relevant to termination, this would suggest that the effect of the DA agonists was to interfere with the termination processes produced at these higher blood ethanol levels. There are several different hypotheses that could be proposed as to why this effect occurred, but one possible explanation is that the presence of increased DA activity in nucleus accumbens prolonged and perhaps enhanced the signals which are part of the maintenance phase. As such, the normal signals which would terminate drinking were ineffective or reduced in their efficacy. Where these termination processes act within the overall regulation of drinking cannot be determined from these studies, but it is clear that the termination processes can be negated to some extent with additional DA stimulation of the nucleus accumbens.

SUMMARY

It appears clear that ethanol reinforcement, like that of many abused drugs, utilizes the mesolimbic DA pathways. From the data presented on microinjection of DA agonists and antagonists, it would seem that only part of the regulatory process controlling ethanol drinking is directly involved with this pathway. Once drinking has begun, the DA antagonist raclopride results in a rapid termination of drinking. This appears to be a blocking effect of what may be conditioned reinforcement resulting from prior ethanol reinforcement initiation procedures. Microinjection of the DA agonists d-amphetamine and quinpirole prolonged drinking, with little signs of normal termination apparent in the 30-min session in many animals. This appeared to be the result of interference with normal termination processes. While it remains to be demonstrated that oral ethanol consumption results in the release of DA in the nucleus accumbens, evidence from prior work and the present studies support a role for the mesolimbic DA system in ethanol reinforcement.

ACKNOWLEDGMENTS

The authors wish to thank Ms. C. M. Andrews and Ms. P. A. Pang for their assistance with the research reported. Quinpirole was generously supplied by Lilly Research Laboratories and Raclopride by the Astra Research Centre, Sweden.

REFERENCES

1. FIBIGER, H. C. & A. G. PHILLIPS. 1986. Reward, motivation, cognition: Psychobiology of mesotelencephalic dopamine systems. In Handbook of Physiology. The Nervous

System. Intrinsic Regulatory System of the Brain. Vol. IV: 647–674. American Physiological Society. Bethesda, MD.

2. LE MOAL, M. & H. SIMON. 1991. Mesocorticolimbic dopamine network: Functional and regulatory roles. Physiol. Rev. 71: 155–234.

3. LIEBMAN, J. M. & S. J. COOPER, Eds. 1989. Topics in Experimental Psychopharmacology: The Neuropharmacological Basis of Reward. Vol. 1. Oxford University Press. Oxford.

4. WILLNER, P. & J. SCHEEL-KRUGER, Eds. 1991. The Mesolimbic Dopamine System: From Motivation to Action. John Wiley & Sons. New York.

5. DWORKIN, S. I. & J. E. SMITH. 1987. Neurobiological aspects of drug-seeking behaviors. In Advances in Behavioral Pharmacology: Neurobehavioral Pharmacology. T. Thompson, P. B. Dews & J. E. Barrett, Eds. Vol. 6: 1–44. Erlbaum Press. Hillsdale.

6. KOOB, G. F. & N. E. GOEDERS. 1989. Neuroanatomical substrates of drug self-administration. In Topics in Experimental Psychopharmacology: The Neuropharmacological Basis of Reward. J. M. Liebman & S. J. Cooper, Eds. Vol. 1: 214–263. Oxford University Press. Oxford.

7. WISE, R. A. & P.-P. ROMPRE. 1989. Brain dopamine and reward. Ann. Rev. Psychol. 40: 191–225.

8. BARBACCIA, M. L., A. BOSIO, P. F. SPANO & M. TRABUCCHI. 1982. Ethanol metabolism and striatal dopamine systems. Pharmacol. Biochem. Behav. 18(Suppl. 1): 169–177.

9. RUSSELL, V. A., M. C. L. LAMM & J. J. F. TALJAARD. 1988. Effect of ethanol on [³H]dopamine release in rat nucleus accumbens and striatal slices. Neurochem. Res. 13: 487–492.

10. FADDA, F., E. MOSCA, G. COLOMBO & G. L. GESSA. 1990. Alcohol-preferring rats: Genetic sensitivity to alcohol induced stimulation of dopamine metabolism. Physiol. Behav. 47: 727–729.

11. GESSA, G. L., F. MUNTONI, M. COLLU, L. VARGUI & G. MEREU. 1985. Low doses of ethanol activate dopaminergic neurons in the ventral tegmental area. Brain Res. 348: 201–203.

12. BRODIE, M. S., S. A. SHEFNER & T. V. DUNWIDDIE. 1990. Ethanol increases the firing rate of dopamine neurons in the rat ventral tegmental area in vitro. Brain Res. 508: 65–69.

13. IMPERATO, A. & G. DI CHIARA. 1986. Preferential stimulation of dopamine release in the nucleus accumbens of freely moving rats by ethanol. J. Pharmacol. Exp. Ther. 239: 219–228.

14. BROWN, Z. W., K. GILL, M. ABITBOL & Z. AMIT. 1982. Lack of effect of dopamine receptor blockade on voluntary ethanol consumption. Behav. Neural Biol. 36: 291–294.

15. DAOUST, M., N. MOORE, C. SALLIGAUT, J. P. LHUINTRE, P. CHRETIEN & F. BOISMARE. 1986. Striatal dopamine does not appear to be involved in the voluntary intake of ethanol by rats. Alcohol 3: 15–17.

16. FADDA, F., E. MOSCA, G. COLOMBO & G. L. GESSA. 1989. Effects of spontaneous ingestion of ethanol on brain dopamine metabolism. Life Sci. 44: 281–287.

17. LINSEMAN, M. A. 1990. Effects of dopaminergic agents on alcohol consumption by rats in a limited access paradigm. Psychopharmacology 100: 195–200.

18. PFEFFER, A. O. & H. H. SAMSON. 1986. Effect of pimozide on homecage ethanol drinking in the rat: Dependence on drinking session length. Drug Alcohol Depend. 17: 47–55.

19. PFEFFER, A. O. & H. H. SAMSON. 1985. Oral ethanol self-administration in the rat: Effects of acute amphetamine. Alcohol 2: 693–697.

20. PFEFFER, A. O. & H. H. SAMSON. 1985. Oral ethanol reinforcement: Interactive effects of amphetamine, pimozide and food restriction. Alcohol Drug Res. 6: 37–48.

21. PFEFFER, A. O. & H. H. SAMSON. 1988. Haloperidol and apomorphine effects on ethanol reinforcement in free-feeding rats. Pharmacol. Biochem. Behav. 29: 343–350.

22. SAMSON, H. H., G. A. TOLLIVER & K. SCHWARZ-STEVENS. 1990. Oral ethanol self-administration: A behavioral pharmacological approach to CNS control mechanisms. Alcohol 7: 187–191.

23. SAMSON, H. H. 1986. Initiation of ethanol reinforcement using a sucrose-substitution procedure in food- and water-sated rats. Alcoholism: Clin. Exp. Res. 10: 436–442.

24. SAMSON, H. H., G. A. TOLLIVER, M. HARAGUCHI & P. W. KALIVAS. 1991. Effects of d-amphetamine injected into the n. accumbens on ethanol reinforced behavior. Brain Res. Bull. 27: 267–271.

25. POTTHOFF, A. D. & G. ELLISON. 1982. Low-level continuous amphetamine administration selectively increases alcohol consumption. Psychopharmacology 77: 242–245.
26. POTTHOFF, A. D., G. ELLISON & L. NELSON. 1983. Ethanol intake increases during continuous administration of amphetamine and nicotine, but not by several other drugs. Pharmacol. Biochem. Behav. 18: 489–493.
27. LEVY, A. D. & G. ELLISON. 1985. Amphetamine-induced enhancement of ethanol consumption: Role of central catecholamines. Psychopharmacology 86: 233–236.
28. KELLEY, A. E., A. M. GAUTHIER & C. G. LANG. 1989. Amphetamine microinjections into distinct striatal subregions cause dissociable effects on motor and ingestive behaviors. Behav. Brain Res. 35: 27–39.
29. MAJ, J., K. WEDZONY & V. KLIMEK. 1987. Desipramine given repeatedly enhances behavioural effects of dopamine and d-amphetamine injected into the nucleus accumbens. Eur. J. Pharmacol. 140: 179–185.
30. VAN DEN BOS, R., G. A. C. ORTIZ, A. C. BERGMANS & A. R. COOLS. 1991. Evidence that dopamine in the nucleus accumbens is involved in the ability of rats to switch to cue-directed behaviours. Behav. Brain Res. 42: 107–114.
31. BREESE, G. R., G. E. DUNCAN, T. C. NAPIER, S. C. BONDY, L. C. IORIO & R. A. MUELLER. 1987. 6-Hydroxydopamine treatments enhance behavioral responses to intracerebral microinjection of D1- and D2-dopamine agonists into the nucleus accumbens and striatum without changing dopamine antagonist binding. J. Pharmacol. Exp. Ther. 240: 167–176.
32. KOSHIKAWA, N., F. KOSHIKAWA, K. TOMIYAMA, K. K. DE BELTRAN, F. KAMIIMURA & M. KOBAYASHI. 1990. Effects of dopamine D1 and D2 agonists and antagonists injected into the nucleus accumbens and globus pallidus on jaw movements of rats. Eur. J. Pharmacol. 182: 375–380.
33. LEVY, A. D., J. M. MURPHY, W. J. MCBRIDE, L. LUMENG & T.-K. LI. 1990. Microinjection of sulpiride into the nucleus accumbens increases drinking in alcohol-preferring (P) rats. Alcoholism: Clin. Exp. Res. 15: 145.
34. MCBRIDE, W. J., J. M. MURPHY, L. LUMENG & T.-K. LI. 1990. Serotonin, dopamine and GABA involvement in alcohol drinking of selectively bred rats. Alcohol 7: 199–205.
35. GILBERT, D. B. & S. J. COOPER. 1987. Effects of the dopamine D-1 antagonist SCH23390 and the D-2 antagonist sulpiride on saline acceptance-rejection in water-deprived rats. Pharmacol. Biochem. Behav. 26: 687–691.
36. VAN DEN BOS, R., A. R. COOLS & S.-O. OGREN. 1988. Differential effects of the selective D2-antagonist raclopride in the nucleus accumbens of the rat on spontaneous and d-amphetamine-induced activity. Psychopharmacol. 95: 447–451.
37. PORRINO, L. J., R. U. ESPOSITO, T. F. SEEGER, A. M. CRANE, A. PERT & L. SOKOLOFF. 1984. Metabolic mapping of the brain during rewarding self-stimulation. Science 224: 306–309.
38. SMITH, J. E. & S. I. DWORKIN. 1990. Behavioral contingencies determine changes in drug-induced neurotransmitter turnover. Drug Devel. Res. 20: 337–348.
39. MCCLEARN, G. E., R. A. DEITRICH & V. G. ERWIN, Eds. 1981. Development of animal models as pharmacogenetic tools. NIAAA Research Mono. No. 6, U. S. Govern. Printing Off. DHHS Pub. No. (ADM)81-1133. Washington, D.C.
40. SAMSON, H. H., G. A. TOLLIVER, L. LUMENG & T.-K. LI. 1988. Ethanol reinforcement in the alcohol nonpreferring (NP) rat: Initiation using behavioral techniques without food restriction. Alcoholism: Clin. Exp. Res. 13: 378–385.
41. SCHWARZ-STEVENS, K., H. H. SAMSON, G. A. TOLLIVER, L. L. LUMENG & T.-K. LI. 1991. The effects of ethanol initiation procedures on ethanol reinforced behaviors in the alcohol preferring (P) rat. Alcoholism: Clin. Exp. Res. 15: 277–285.
42. DOLE, V. P. & R. T. GENTRY. 1984. Towards an analogue of alcoholism in mice: Scale factors in the model. Proc. Natl. Acad. Sci. USA 81: 3543–3546.
43. BARRETT, J. E. & M. A. NADER. 1990. Neurochemical correlates of behavioral processes. Drug Devel. Res. 20: 313–335.
44. WHITE, N. M., M. G. PACKARD & N. HIROI. 1991. Place conditioning with dopamine D1 and D2 agonists injected peripherally or into nucleus accumbens. Psychopharmacology 103: 271–276.

45. SAMSON, H. H., A. O. PFEFFER & G. A. TOLLIVER. 1988. Oral ethanol self-administration in rats: Models of ethanol seeking behavior. Alcoholism: Clin. Exp. Res. **12:** 591–598.
46. GRANT, K. A. 1984. An experimental analysis of oral ethanol self-administration in the free feeding rat. Unpublished Doctoral Dissertation. University of Washington. Seattle.
47. GRANT, K. A. & H. H. SAMSON. 1985. Oral self-administration of ethanol in free feeding rats. Alcohol **2:** 317–322.
48. LI, T.-K., L. LUMENG, D. P. DOOLITTLE, W. J. MCBRIDE, J. M. MURPHY, J. C. FROEHLICH & S. MORZORATI. 1988. Behavioral and neurochemical associations of alcohol-seeking behavior. *In* Biomedical and Social Aspects of Alcohol and Alcoholism. K. Kuriyama, A. Takada & H. Ishii, Eds.: 435–438. Excerpta Medica International Series. Elsevier. Amsterdam.

Interaction between Endogenous Opioids and Dopamine within the Nucleus Accumbens[a]

L. STINUS, M. CADOR, AND M. LE MOAL

Laboratoire de Psychobiologie des Comportements Adaptatifs
INSERM U. 259
Université de Bordeaux II
Domaine de Carreire–Rue Camille Saint-Saëns
33077 Bordeaux Cedex, France

INTRODUCTION

A high density of enkephalin and opiate receptors has been observed in limbic and forebrain structures[1,2,34,48]; these regions have been implicated in the regulation of emotional and motivational states. There is a close association between the distribution of enkephalin-containing fibers and dopaminergic neurons,[38,39] and high concentrations of enkephalin, neutral endopeptidases, μ and δ receptors have been detected in the nucleus accumbens (N. Acc) and ventral tegmental area (VTA).[88]

In recent years, there has been much interest in identifying the neural bases for the reinforcing and locomotor-activating properties of psychostimulants, opiates and opioid peptides (see ref. 46 for review). The purpose of this chapter is to review evidence for potential opioid interactions in relation to reward. We will take into account not only the anatomy of mesolimbic DA neurons but also the varieties of opioid receptors and the distinction between D_1 and D_2 DA receptors. Although we will focus our attention mainly on N. Acc, this topic cannot be approached without first rapidly reviewing our knowledge concerning opioid-DA interaction within the VTA.

OPIOID-DOPAMINE INTERACTION WITHIN THE VENTRAL TEGMENTAL AREA

Bilateral injections of opiate peptides into the VTA induce behavioral activation characterized by increased locomotion, rearing, licking and sniffing which is reversed by either naloxone, systemic or intra-accumbens injection of DA antagonists or by specific lesions of DA-A10 neurons.[5,40,42,43,71,78] VTA infusion of opioid peptides increased DA turnover in DA-A10 terminal regions.[6,42,74] Moreover, morphine or DADLE VTA-iontophoretic application activates DA-A10 neurons (non–naloxone-

[a] Supported in part by the University of Bordeaux II, CNRS, INSERM, Regional Council of Aquitaine and Mission Interministerielle pour la Lutte contre la Toxicomanie (MILT).

reversible) and reduces the activity of non-DA neurons (naloxone-reversible).[30] Dilsts and Kalivas[21] showed that the activation of DA-A10 neurons by μ agonists could be triggered in part by inhibition of non-DA neurons of the VTA.

It is thus clear that VTA-opiate receptor stimulation activates DA-A10 neurons. However, VTA opiate microinfusion inhibits the evoked responses of spontaneously inactive cells in N. Acc elicited by stimulation of hippocampal afferents to the N. Acc. This inhibition is reversed by naloxone but not by α-flupenthixol, implying also a VTA-mediated non-DA mechanism.[31]

Laterner *et al.*[49] attempted to identify the opioid receptor type that mediated these effects. They showed that the specific μ receptor agonist DAGO was more potent than the δ receptor agonist DPDPE in stimulating locomotor activity and also in increasing DA metabolism in the terminal fields of DA-A10 neurons. However, more recent data indicate that behavioral effects induced by VTA-infusion of opiate agonists depend upon the anxiogenic degree of the experimental conditions.[8] VTA infusion of δ and μ agonists both induced behavioral activation in a familiar environment (photocell cages); however, when rats were introduced into a novel environment such as an open field or a hole-board, the δ agonists (BUBU, DTLET, and DSTBULET) increased exploratory behaviors which were reduced by NALTRINDOLE or ICI 174,864, specific δ antagonists. On the contrary, DAGO, a μ agonist, increased latency to move and decreased locomotion and hole visits. These effects were naloxone reversible. Moreover intra-accumbens 6-hydroxydopamine (lesion of DA-A10 neurons) prevented the effects induced by VTA infusion of δ agonists, while the effects of DAGO (μ agonist) were unchanged. In addition to the complexity of VTA interactions between DA and non-DA neurons, and the multiplicity of opioid receptors, these results indicate that the behavioral effects induced by the stimulation of a specific set of opioid receptors depend on the behavioral situations and the tasks that are used to explore the functional role of a particular neuronal mechanism (*e.g.*, the level of arousal, motivation, anxiety).

Neuronal mechanisms within the VTA are at least in part responsible for opioid-induced reward. Morphine is directly self-administered to the VTA.[3] Furthermore VTA infusion of an opioid antagonist resulted in a compensatory increase in the rate of intravenous heroin self-administration.[4] Moreover, infusion of morphine, DALA or the enkephalinase inhibitor thiorphan into the VTA could serve as a reinforcer in the conditioning of a place preference[27,61,62] and these effects were blocked either by haloperidol or by 6-OHDA lesions of ascending DA pathways.[63] Stimulation of either receptor subtypes (icv μ and δ agonists) is sufficient to produce a reward effect and these effects appear to be independent of each other.[73] However, considering the anxiogenic properties of VTA infusion of DAGO (μ agonist)[8] we suggest that opioid-induced reward in the VTA is mainly mediated by δ receptor stimulation.

NUCLEUS ACCUMBENS OPIOID/DOPAMINE INTERACTION

Intra-accumbens application of DA or opioid agonists has strikingly similar effects since both of them induce behavioral activation and rewarding effects. Opioids may interact with dopaminergic activity not only by their actions at receptors located in the VTA but also through their action at receptors located within the terminal fields. However, less than 30% of opioid receptors are located presynaptically in N. Acc DA terminals.[64] In the following paragraphs we will try to answer the following questions. Does opioid activity in the nucleus accumbens modulate or mediate DA functions or are there two separate neuronal systems and if so what is the interaction between them?

Nucleus Accumbens and Psychostimulant Drugs

Several groups have reported that injection of DA or DA agonists into the N. Acc induces a behavioral activation which could be reversed by DA antagonists or by the specific lesion of DA-A10 neurons (10 for review). These data are consistent with numerous studies suggesting that activation of forebrain DA mechanisms underlies the reinforcing effects of intracranial and intravenous administration of stimulants. Rats learn to self-administer DA[29] or d-amphetamine[33] into the N. Acc. 6-OHDA lesions of the N. Acc or VTA produces a long-lasting reduction in self-administration of cocaine and amphetamine.[52,66,68,69] Moreover a partial blockade of DA receptors[24] or a partial lesion of DA-A10 neurons by radiofrequency lesions of VTA[50] produced a compensatory increase of cocaine and amphetamine self-administration. Subsequent studies have shown that 6-OHDA lesions of the frontal cortex[54] and corpus striatum[47] do not produce this extinction-like responding. Finally, the increase of DA release in the N. Acc induced by cocaine and amphetamine[18] was prevented by specific lesions of DA-A10 neurons.[9,19] Furthermore, a directly acting DA receptor agonist apomorphine becomes a more effective reinforcer in rats with 6-OHDA lesions of the N. Acc due to the development of post-synaptic or receptor supersensitivity.[67] Altogether these results indicate that the N. Acc is the main neurobiological substrate for the rewarding effects of psychostimulants. Since the blockade of opioid receptors did not alter cocaine self-administration,[24] we can postulate that its rewarding effects are not opioid dependent.

Nucleus Accumbens, Opiates, and Opioid Peptides

Both the stimulation of opioid and DA receptors of N. Acc induce behavioral activation. However, Pert and Sivit[58] observed that administration of morphine or the long-acting enkephalin analogue DALA[57] into the N. Acc produced an increase of locomotor activity which was prevented by naloxone but not by a DA receptor antagonist. At a higher dose, intra-accumbens morphine injection induced a biphasic effect: first there was a behavioral depression which was followed by increased locomotor activity.[12,32] This apparent discrepancy has been explained by the use of specific opioid receptor agonists.[13] The intra-accumbens injection of DTLET a selective delta agonist or kelatorphan produced locomotor activation reversed by naloxone (high dose) and by ICI 174,864 a selective δ receptor antagonist. Thus, endogenous enkephalins acting at δ receptors in the N. Acc may be responsible of behavioral activation. In contrast, injection of a μ agonist DAGO produced initial suppression of activity. Thus, μ receptor stimulation appears to trigger the akinetic and cataleptic effects of opioids in the N. Acc. Moreover Dauge et al.[14] observed that thioproperazine, a DA receptor antagonist which reversed intra-caudate opiate-induced behavioral effects, was ineffective in blocking behavioral activation or inhibition produced respectively by intra-accumbens of δ and μ receptor agonists. Nevertheless, Longoni *et al.*[51] have reported that the behavioral stimulant effect induced by intra-accumbens infusion of ala-deltorphin, a δ selective agonist, could be blocked by SCH 23390, a selective D_1 antagonist. However, a chronic occupancy of DA receptors with SCH 23390 failed to reduce intra-accumbens kelatorphan-induced behavioral activation,[53] a δ-agonist-like effect.[13]

All together, these results indicate that behavioral effects induced by acute stimulation of opioid receptors in N. Acc are not reversed by the impairment of DA meso-limbic activity and that systemic effects of opiates in N. Acc activity can be mediated directly in the N. Acc. This assumption is in agreement with biochemical, electrophysiological and behavioral effects produced by systemic administration of opiates. Intra-accumbens infusion of DALA[42] or μ or δ receptor agonists[59] did not alter DA activity in the N. Acc. Electrophoretically applied morphine in N. Acc, inhibits spontaneously active N. Acc units, and this effect was blocked by simultaneous ejection of naloxone.[31] Moreover, behavioral activation induced by systemic heroin administration was completely abolished by intra-accumbens infusion of methylnaloxonium.[85] Intra-accumbens DA and opioid mechanisms appear then to be mainly independent.

Important interactions between these mechanisms could however exist. To evaluate these interactions we will analyze the effects of N. Acc opiate receptor stimulation after specific lesion of mesolimbic DA neurons originating in VTA and projecting to N. Acc.

Therefore, in the following paragraphs we will analyze the behavioral effects of the stimulation of the opioid receptor population which *is not* localized on DA terminals (70%), since the opioid receptors on the N. Acc DA terminals have degenerated.

Increased Locomotor Responsiveness to Intra-Accumbens Opiates by Mesolimbic DA Lesions

While lesions of mesolimbic DA neurons completely reversed the behavioral activation induced by VTA infusion of opioid peptides (FIG. 1),[43,77,78] the locomotor activity response to intra-accumbens injection of DALA or morphine was actually enhanced.[41,76,81] This behavioral potentiation was specific of DA lesions. As indicated in FIGURE 2 behavioral supersensitivity to intra-accumbens opioid peptides, measured in photocell activity cages, was induced by destruction of DA-A10 neurons produced by the infusion of the catecholaminergic neuron neurotoxin 6-OHDA either at the cell body site in the VTA, or in the N. Acc, a DA-A10 terminal field. On the contrary, the behavioral response was not changed after specific lesions of ascending norepinephrine pathways produced by local intracerebral infusion of 6-OHDA at the level of the superior cerebellar peduncles (6-OHDA-PCS).[77] This behavioral sensitization was a function of the extent of the DA-A10 lesion. Only in rats having a 68–100% depletion of N. Acc-DA did DALA produce a significant elevation in photocell counts compared with sham-operated rats, while the behavioral effects did not correlate with striatal-DA depletion.[41] Moreover, the threshold dose of DALA to produce significant behavioral hyperactivity in 6-OHDA-treated rats was 10–100 ng whereas, in sham-operated rats the threshold was 1000–3300 ng.[41] We have obtained similar results after chronic pharmacological blockade of DA receptors.[80,81]

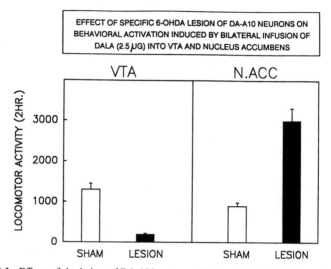

FIGURE 1. Effects of the lesion of DA-A10 neurons (N. Acc 6-OHDA infusion 8 μg by side) on behavioral activation induced by either injection of DALA (2.5 μg each side) in the ventral tegmental area (VTA, *left-panel*) or in the nucleus accumbens (N. Acc, *right panel*). Locomotor activity was recorded for 2 h in photocell activity cages, one month after the lesion.[77]

INCREASED LOCOMOTOR RESPONSIVENESS TO INTRA-ACCUMBENS OPIATES BY CHRONIC PHARMACOLOGICAL BLOCKADE OF DA ACTIVITY

We have shown that chronic treatment (one month) with six different neuroleptics (DA receptor antagonists) that are currently in human therapeutic use, induced a dramatic potentiation of locomotor response to intra-accumbens injection of DALA (FIG. 2). Rats were tested during permanent occupancy of DA receptors by neuroleptics. Behavioral activation was measured in photocell activity cages. Haloperidol and sulpiride were administered twice daily while long-acting neuroleptics were injected every 10 days for flupenthixol decanoate and a once a month for perphenazine enanthate and pipotiazine palmitate.[77,80,81] The amplitude and the time course of this behavioral sensitization was similar in DA-lesioned and neuroleptic-treated rats (FIG. 3). These effects were specific of central opioid receptor stimulation since they are reversed by systemic injection of naloxone but not of methylnaloxonium, an opioid receptor antagonist which does not cross the blood brain barrier.[77] Moreover, the behavioral effects induced by intra-accumbens injection of 1 μl of isotonic saline were similar in all rat groups. FIGURE 4 (*left panel*) indicates that rats injected with DALA into the N. Acc showed a dose-related increase in spontaneous motor activity. In both control and neuroleptic-treated (flupentixol decanoate) rats the peak response was at 2500 ng. However, the rats with permanent blockade of DA receptors (for one month) had a significantly greater response to DALA than control rats. Moreover, the threshold dose of DALA to produce significant behavioral hyperactivity in neuroleptic-treated rats was 64–160 ng and 1000–2500 ng in control rats (15.6 times reduction of the effective

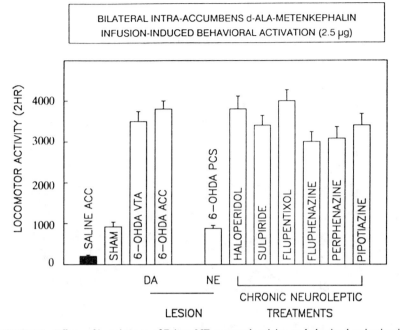

FIGURE 2. Effects of impairment of DA or NE neuronal activity on behavioral activation induced by intra-accumbens injection of DALA. The first bar on the left indicates the mean effect of N. Acc application of solvent (isotonic saline 1 μl). DA lesions were induced by intracerebral injection of 6-OHDA into the ventral tegmental area (6-OHDA VTA 4 μg) or into the nucleus accumbens (6-OHDA Acc 8 μg). NE lesions were induced by intracerebral injection of 6-OHDA at the level of superior cerebellar peduncles (6-OHDA PCS 6 μg). Rats were tested one month after the lesion. Chronic blockade of DA receptors was induced by long-term application (one month) of six different neuroleptics that are currently in human therapeutic use. Behavioral testing was performed during permanent occupancy of DA receptors by neuroleptics.[77]

dose). However, if investigatory behavior was evaluated in an automated eight-hole box, we observed that the increased locomotor activity recorded in photocell activity cages was not associated with an increase of hole visits. As indicated in FIGURE 4 (*right panel*) we observed a dose-related increase of the number of hole visits after intra-accumbens DALA injection. However, unlike the effects on locomotor activity, a significant increase in hole visits occurred for the same threshold dose 1000–2500 ng. Moreover, rats treated with lower doses of neuroleptics developed less investigatory behaviors than controls. Thus, it appears that locomotor hyperactivity induced by DALA-N. Acc injection consists of automatic locomotor activity disconnected from environmental cues. Interestingly, systemic or intra-accumbens injection of amphetamine increases investigatory behavior[44] and stimulus-reward association dose dependently.[7,26] Altogether, these results could indicate in part, separate neural mechanisms underlying behavioral activation induced by intra-accumbens opioid and DA agonists. The enhanced locomotor response developed progressively during the chronic neuroleptic treatment (FIG. 5) reaching a maximum at 2–3 weeks. It is evident

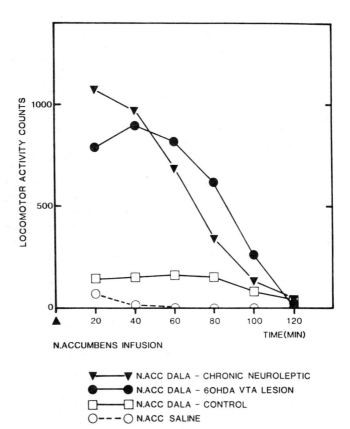

FIGURE 3. Time course of behavioral activation induced by bilateral intra-accumbens injection of DALA (2.5 μg by side) in sham, DA-A10 lesioned or chronic neuroleptic-treated rats ($n = 10$ for each group). DA-A10 lesions were produced by VTA injection of 6-OHDA (4 μg). Chronic neuroleptic treatment consisted of one injection every 10 days (for one month) of the long-acting neuroleptic fluanxol (flupentixol decanoate 12 mg/kg sc). Rats were tested under permanent neuroleptic impregnation.[81]

that the antipsychotic properties of neuroleptics are not all directly linked to blockade of DA receptors, as a delay of several weeks between the beginning of treatment and the appearance of the antipsychotic effect is generally observed ("therapeutic lag"). This phenomenon suggests that long-term neuronal changes that occur gradually underlie the development of the antipsychotic effect. The results reported suggest that a good candidate for such putative neuronal changes would be alterations in endogenous opioid systems or other peptidergic neurons.

From our results we could not have any clear evidence of D_1 or D_2 DA receptor blockade involvement in the potentiation of intra-accumbens opiate effects since, except for sulpiride which is a specific D_2 antagonist, all the other neuroleptics used (FIG. 2) inhibit both D_1 and D_2 DA receptor activity. However, it has been shown

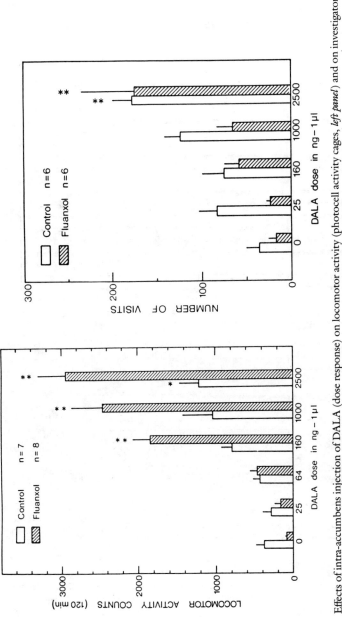

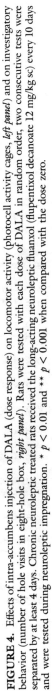

FIGURE 4. Effects of intra-accumbens injection of DALA (dose response) on locomotor activity (photocell activity cages, *left panel*) and on investigatory behavior (number of hole visits in eight-hole box, *right panel*). Rats were tested with each dose of DALA in random order, two consecutive tests were separated by at least 4 days. Chronic neuroleptic treated rats received the long-acting neuroleptic fluanxol (flupentixol decanoate 12 mg/kg sc) every 10 days and were tested during neuroleptic impregnation. * $p < 0.01$ and ** $p < 0.001$ when compared with the dose zero.

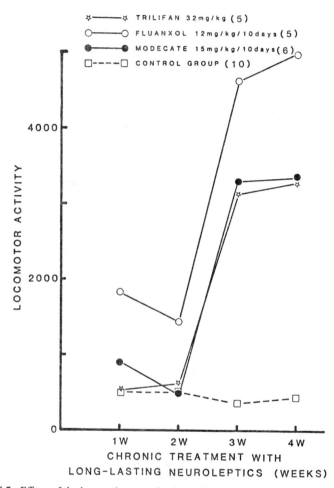

FIGURE 5. Effects of the long-acting neuroleptics Trilifan (perphenazine enanthate), Fluanxol (flupentixol decanoate), and Modecate (fluphenazine decanoate) on behavioral activation induced by D-Ala-Met-enkaphalin (2.5 μg-1 μl) infusion into the nucleus accumbens. *Abscissa,* duration of the neuroleptic treatment; *ordinate,* mean locomotor activity score recorded for 120 min following the intracerebral infusion of DALA. The number of animals in each group is shown in parentheses. Rats were tested during permanent neuroleptic impregnation.[80]

recently that chronic D_2 (sulpiride) but not D_1-dopamine receptor blockade (SCH 23390) facilitates behavioral responses to N. Acc opioid receptor stimulation.[53] Moreover, this sensitization exists not only in response to exogenous application of opiates or opioid peptides but also to N. Acc release of endogenous enkephalin since sulpiride potentiates the behavioral activation induced by intra-accumbens application of kelatorphan, an inhibitor of enkephalin degradating enzymes.[53] Both VTA and N. Acc play an essential role in mediating the reinforcing effects of opiates. However, we have

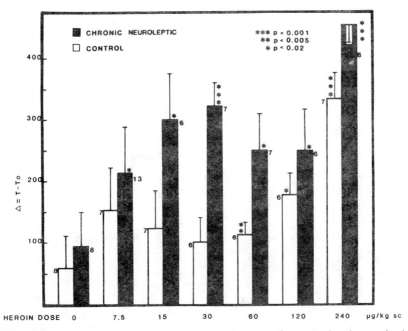

FIGURE 6. Dose-response curves for heroin-induced place preference in chronic neuroleptic-treated and control rats. Note that whereas 60 µg/kg heroin is required in controls, the lowest dose tested (7.5 µg/kg) was sufficient in the neuroleptic-treated rats. The y-axis depicts postconditioning minus preconditioning time spent in the compartment paired with heroin. Ranges are standard errors. Chronic neuroleptic treated rats received the long acting neuroleptic fluanxol (flupenthixol decanoate 12 mg/kg sc) every 10 days. Behavioral testing was conducted under permanent occupancy of DA receptors by the neuroleptic.[79]

shown that whereas both intra-VTA and intra-N. Acc application of opioid peptides induced behavioral activation, the chronic blockade of mesolimbic DA activity produced either by DA-A10 lesions or by chronic application of neuroleptics reverses the first effect while potentiating the second.[77] What, then, will be the consequence of the chronic blockade of DA activity upon the reinforcing effects of systemic administration of heroin or morphine?

Potentiation of the Reinforcing Properties of Systemic Opiates after Chronic Impairment of DA Mesolimbic Activity

To address the previous question, we have tested the effects of chronic blockade of mesolimbic DA receptors by long-term application of the long-acting neuroleptic flupenthixol decanoate (12 mg/kg sc every 10 days) on morphine-induced eating, heroin-induced place preference, and intravenous self-administration of heroin. In other words, we asked the behaving animal to tell us what the modifications of the hedonic value of systemic application of opiate drugs are during chronic impairment of DA-A10 activity.

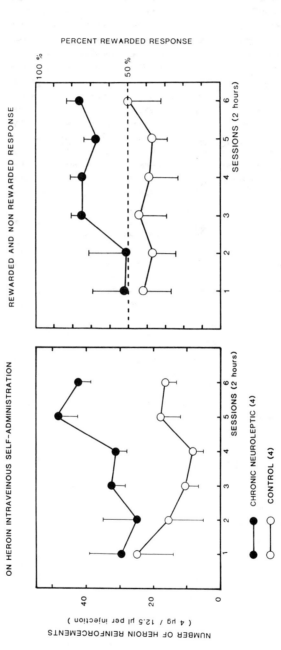

FIGURE 7. Effect of chronic neuroleptic treatment on heroin intravenous self-administration (IVSA). Each nose poke in the rewarded hole delivered a very low dose of heroin (4 μg), a sub-threshold drug dose unable to induce IVSA in control rats. *Left panel*: number of heroin reinforcements obtained during six sessions of 2 h (one daily session). *Right panel*: the percent of rewarded responses (rewarded responses/rewarded plus non-rewarded responses × 100), 50% represents the random level. Chronic neuroleptic-treated rats received the long-acting neuroleptic fluanxol (flupenthixol decanoate 12 mg/kg sc) every 10 days. Behavioral testing was conducted under permanent occupancy of DA receptors by the neuroleptic.[79]

Morphine-induced Eating

It has been recently shown that opiate signals influence feeding by acting on reward-relevant sites to increase the rewarding properties of food or eating.[25] We decided to inject rats every week, after the beginning of the neuroleptic treatment, with a sub-threshold dose of morphine (0.5 mg/kg sc). The threshold dose for morphine-induced feeding being 1 mg/kg sc. Food intake was measured for two hours following the drug injection in food-satiated animals. After one month of permanent occupancy of DA receptors by the neuroleptic, morphine-induced eating was significantly enhanced (sham + saline: 3.6 ± 0.5 g, sham + morphine: 4.0 ± 0.4, chronic neuroleptic + saline: 2.6 ± 1.0 and chronic neuroleptic + morphine: 5.8 ± 0.5 g, $p < 0.05$).[55] Interestingly this effect was statistically significant as early as the third week of neuroleptic treatment.[86] It should be noted that the evolution of this morphine-induced eating paralleled the increased behavioral activation reported in FIGURE 5.

Heroin-induced Place Preference

We determined the dose-response curve of the effects of systemic heroin (sc) administration on place-preference conditioning in control rats and in rats that had undergone the chronic neuroleptic regimen described above.[79] Place-preference conditioning was conducted in rectangular chambers, each containing two compartments. They were differentiated by two sets of sensory cues, the color of the walls (black or white) and the texture of the floor (rough or semi-rough).

A preconditioning test day, during which the rats' preference was measured, was followed by a 6-day conditioning phase during which rats were confined in one of the compartments after injection of solvent, and in the other after injection of heroin (3 pairings of each). The animals were then tested for changes in preference, one, two and eight days after the final conditioning trial. The difference in time spent in the heroin-paired compartment after minus before pairing was calculated. A positive difference indicated a preference for heroin. As shown in FIGURE 6, heroin induced a dose-related place preference. The threshold dose of peripheral heroin required to induce place preference in control rats was 60 μg. While, for chronic neuroleptic-treated rats the lowest dose tested (7.5 μg/kg) was still found to be effective. Our data show that chronic DA receptor blockade markedly reduces (at least 8 times less) the dose of systemically administered heroin required to act as a reinforcing and discriminative stimulus.[79]

Heroin-induced Intravenous Self-Administration

This experiment was designed to test whether or not chronic neuroleptic treatment could enhance the addictive properties of self-administered intravenous heroin. For this purpose, a sub-threshold dose of heroin in control rats was used (4 μg by intravenous injection). Rats were introduced into a cylindrical operant chamber equipped with two holes. Nose pokes activated infra-red photocells situated outside the chamber. The interruption of one of the photocell beams activated a syringe pump that delivered heroin (rewarded response), nose pokes in the other hole were recorded but had no scheduled consequences (non-rewarded response). Rats underwent a 2-h session each day for 6 days. As shown in FIGURE 7 (*left panel*) rewarded responses did not increase in control rats during the six 2-h sessions although they did so in the neuroleptic-treated subjects ($p = 0.04$). Furthermore, while control rats did not discriminate between rewarded and non-rewarded responses, treated rats did so from the 3rd session, since 77% of the responses were heroin rewarded ($p = 0.03$).[79]

DISCUSSION

It is essential to keep in mind that in the experiments describing intra-accumbens opioid injections, opioid receptor stimulation was solely applied to those which were not localized on mesolimbic DA terminals since, the opioid receptors on the DA terminals were either destroyed by the lesions of DA-A10 neurons or their physiological role inhibited by the DA receptor blockade.

Overall our results indicate that the chronic inhibition of mesolimbic DA activity induced by either lesions (6-OHDA VTA or 6-OHDA N. Acc) or by permanent occupancy of DA D_2 receptors (chronic neuroleptic treatment) produced a behavioral supersensitivity to opiate infusion into the N. Acc. In contrast, the behavioral effects induced by VTA infusion of opiates were completely abolished by the same treatments. Nevertheless, using the same animal model (chronic neuroleptic treatment), we have directly demonstrated by three different and complementary approaches that the reinforcing properties of systemic administration of opiates is increased. This indicates first, that non-opioid-dependent intra-accumbens mechanisms can trigger rewarding effects, second, that not only is the N. Acc sufficient to maintain positive opioid effects but it has a pre-eminent role when compared to the VTA opiate effects and third, when DA related reward mechanisms are impaired, opioid-related reward mechanisms are increased in a somehow homeostatic manner.

In Nucleus Accumbens, Opioid-mediated Reward Mechanisms Are Not DA-Dependent

Along with VTA, N. Acc is a critical structure mediating opiate reward since rats learn to self-administer morphine[56] and met-enkephalin[28] directly into the N. Acc. Consistent with these results are conditioned place-preference findings showing that microinjections of morphine into N. Acc will produce a conditioned place preference.[87] In this chapter we have shown that behavioral activation induced by intra-accumbens opiate injection and the reinforcing properties of systemic opiates were actually enhanced by the blockade of DA-A10 neuronal activity. These results indicate that N. Acc opioid-mediated reward mechanisms are DA-independent. Since systemic heroin reward is enhanced after DA activity blockade, while intra-VTA opiate-induced effects are reversed, we can postulate a pre-eminence of the N. Acc non-DA-dependent opioid reward upon the VTA DA-dependent opioid reward mechanisms. Interestingly, VTA and N. Acc intracerebral injection of an opiate receptor antagonist, which had no effect on cocaine intravenous self-administration, increased heroin self-administration because rats compensate for a lower effect of the drug at receptor sites; however, N. Acc injections were significantly more effective.[11,46,84]

While a non-cataleptic dose of α-flupenthixol, a DA antagonist, produced changes in cocaine self-administration heroin intake was unchanged.[24] Selective lesion of the presynaptic DA input to the N. Acc can significantly attenuate cocaine self-administration, without influencing heroin responding.[22,60] Furthermore, the behavioral characteristics of the locomotor activation induced by intra-accumbens injections of psychostimulants or opiates are completely different since in the first case the behavior is intimately related to the environment while in the second it is not. Thus, N. Acc DA-related and opioid-related reinforcing mechanisms appear to be different. However, ibotenic acid lesions of the ventral pallidum, which is one of the main outputs of N. Acc and critical to behavioral activation produced by stimulants, produced significant decreases of both cocaine and heroin self-administration. Neuronal elements which project from N. Acc to the ventral pallidum may be a common pathway mediating the expression of both stimulant and opiate reinforcement.[37]

Homeostatic Regulation of Opioid and DA-Dependent Reward Mechanisms

Several studies have reported increased met-enkephalin mRNA levels in the rat nucleus accumbens and striatum after chronic treatment with dopamine receptor blockers or 6-OHDA-induced lesions.[15,16,35,36,70,72,82,83] These data are confirmed by clinical observations since increased concentrations of met-enkephalin has been de-

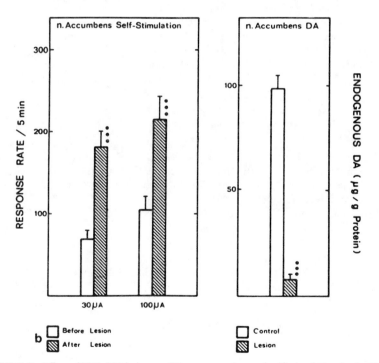

FIGURE 8. Effect of VTA-A10 lesion on DA concentration and self-stimulation in the N. accumbens. Note that a dramatic loss of DA does not alter the self-stimulation rate from medial prefrontal cortex ($n = 6$) but produced a significant increase of this behavior in the N. accumbens ($n = 10$). *** $p < .001$ compared prelesion value.[75]

tected in CSF of patients treated chronically by neuroleptics.[45] In contrast, chronic treatment with a DA agonist decreases the behavioral effects induced by DALA intra-accumbens injection (Stinus et al., in preparation). Taken together, these findings suggest that the chronic blockade of DA activity results in an enhancement of the synaptic biodisponibility of endogenous met-enkephalin within the nucleus accumbens. The above hypothesis is in agreement with the potentiation of intra-accumbens kelatorphan-induced behavioral activation observed after chronic impairment of DA activity.[53]

Except for one result indicating an increase of δ receptors seven days after 6-OHDA-N. Acc lesion,[23] all the other data obtained 3 to 4 weeks post-lesion indicate a decrease of about 20 to 30% of the number of μ (DAGO-binding) and δ (DSTLE-binding) opioid receptors in nucleus accumbens and dorsal striatum.[64,65,77] Moreover, chronic haloperidol or pipotiazine palmitate treatment failed to alter the number and the sensitivity of opioid receptors in DA terminal fields.[17,77]

Thus, the potentiation of intra-accumbens opioid-induced behavioral activation and the enhancement of the reinforcing effects of systemically applied opiates cannot be explained by a modification of opioid receptors. Instead it implicates the development, in the N. Acc or forward, of post-synaptic neuronal circuits hypersensitive to the effects triggered by opioid receptor stimulation within the N. Acc. This hypothesis is in agreement with our previous results on N. Acc intracranial self-stimulation (ICSS) published in 1979,[75] which we could not clearly explain at the time. FIGURE 8 shows the evolution of N. Acc ICSS after complete destruction of DA-A10 neurons by radio-frequency VTA lesions (remaining N. Acc DA: 8%). Both at low and medium current intensity N. Acc ICSS responses were increased after lesion (30 μA: 314 ± 42%, 100 μA: 202 ± 21% responses expressed in % of prelesion scores). The ICSS potentiation induced by DA-A10 lesion was observed in each of the rats tested (n = 10).

CONCLUSION

The reinforcing effects of opiates are believed to result from activation of central opioid primarily in the VTA and in the N. Acc. In VTA, opiate effects are mediated through the activation of mesolimbic DA-A10 neurons while in N. Acc, the main effects of opiates are not DA-dependent.

Permanent inhibition of DA-A10 activity completely inhibits VTA opiate-mediated effects while N. Acc effects are potentiated. Since in this situation, the reinforcing effects of systemic heroin are enhanced, the N. Acc non-DA-dependent effects are clearly pre-eminent.

Finally, as pointed out for the first time by Kalivas and Bronson (1985)[41] the increase in enkephalin tone following chronic DA blockade and the increase in post-synaptic responsiveness to N. Acc opioid receptor stimulation can be considered as a homeostatic response to maintain a steady state of neuronal tone for behavioral activation, incentive-motivation, and response initiation.

REFERENCES

1. ATWEH, S. F. & M. J. KUHAR. 1977. Autoradiographic localization of opiate receptors in rat brain. II. The brain stem. Brain Res. 129: 1–12.

2. ATWEH, S. F. & M. J. KUHAR. 1977. Autoradiographic localization of opiate receptors in rat brain. III. The telencephalon. Brain Res. **143:** 393–450.

3. BOZARTH, M. A. & R. A. WISE. 1981. Intracranial self-administration on morphine into the ventral tegmental area in rats. Life Sci. **28:** 551–555.

4. BRITT, M. F. & R. A. WISE. 1983. Ventral tegmental site of opiate reward: Antagonism by a hydrophilic opiate receptor blocker. Brain Res. **258:** 105–108.

5. BROEKKAMP, C. L. E., A. G. PHILLIPS & A. R. COLLS. 1979. Stimulant effects of enkephalin microinjection into the dopaminergic A10 area. Nature Lond. **278:** 560–562.

6. CADOR, M., J. M. RIVET, A. E. KELLEY, M. LE MOAL & L. STINUS. 1989. Substance P, neurotensin and enkephalin injections into the ventral tegmental area: Comparative study on dopamine turnover in several forebrain structures. Brain Res. **486:** 357–363.

7. CADOR, M., T. W. ROBBINS & B. J. EVERITT. 1989. Involvement of the amygdala in stimulus-reward associations: Interaction with the ventral striatum. Neuroscience **30:** 77–86.

8. CALENKO-CHOUKROUM, G., V. DAUGE, G. GACEL, J. FEGER & B. P. ROQUES. 1989. Opioid delta agonist and endogenous enkephalin induced different emotional reactivity than mu agonist after injection in the rat ventral tegmental area. Psychopharmacology **103:** 493–502.

9. CARBONI, E., A. IMPERATO, L. PEREZZANI & G. DI CHIARA. 1989. Amphetamine, cocaine, phencyclidine and nomifensine increase extracellular dopamine concentrations preferentially in the nucleus accumbens of freely moving rats. Neuroscience **28:** 653–661.

10. COOPER, J. 1991. Interactions between endogenous opioids and dopamine: Implications for reward and aversion. *In* The Mesolimbic Dopamine System: From Motivation to Action. P. Willner & J. Scheel-Kruger, Eds.: 331–366. Wiley & Sons. New York.

11. CORRIGAL, W. A. & F. J. VACCARINO. 1988. Antagonist treatment in nucleus accumbens or periacqueducal grey affects heroin self-administration. Pharmacol. Biochem. Behav. **30:** 443–450.

12. COSTALL, B., D. H. FORTUNE & R. J. NAYLOR. 1978. The induction of catalepsy and hyperactivity by morphine administered directly into the nucleus accumbens of rats. Eur. J. Pharmacol. **49:** 49–64.

13. DAUGE, V., P. ROSSIGNOL & B. P. ROQUES. 1988. Comparison of the behavioral effects induced by administration in rat nucleus accumbens or nucleus caudatus of selective mu and delta opioid peptides or kelatorphan, an inhibitor of enkephalin-metabolism. Psychopharmacology **96:** 343–352.

14. DAUGE, V., P. ROSSIGNOL & B. P. ROQUES. 1989. Blockade of dopamine receptors reverses the behavioral effects of endogenous enkephalins in the nucleus caudatus but not in the nucleus accumbens: Involvement of delta and mu opioid receptors. Psychopharmacology **99:** 168–175.

15. DE CEBALLOS, M. L., S. BOYCE, P. JENNER & C. D. MARSDEN. 1986. Alterations in [Met[5]]- and [Leu[5]]enkephalin and neurotensin content in basal ganglia induced by the long-term administration of dopamine agonist and antagonist drugs to rats. Eur. J. Pharmacol. **130:** 305–309.

16. DE CEBALLOS, M. L., P. JENNER & C. D. MARSDEN. 1986. Acute and repeated administration of sulpiride alters met- and leu-enkephalin content of rat brain. Neurosci. Lett. **68:** 322–326.

17. DELAY-GOYET, P., J. M. ZAJAC & B. P. ROQUES. 1989. Effects of repeated treatment with haloperidol on rat striatal neutral endopeptidase and on mu and delta-opioid binding sites: Comparison with chronic morphine and chronic kelatorphan. Neurosci. Lett. **103:** 197–202.

18. DI CHIARA, G. & A. IMPERATO. 1986. Preferential stimulation of dopamine release in the nucleus accumbens by opiates, alcohol and barbiturates: Studies with transcerebral dialysis in freely moving rats. Ann. NY Acad. Sci. **473:** 367–381.

19. DI CHIARA, G. & A. IMPERATO. 1988. Drugs abused by humans preferentially increase synaptic dopamine concentrations in the mesolimbic system of freely moving rats. Proc. Natl. Acad. Sci. USA **85:** 5274–5278.

20. DI CHIARA, G. J. & A. IMPERATO. 1988. Opposite effects of mu and kappa opiate agonists on dopamine release in the nucleus accumbens and in the dorsal of freely moving rats. J. Pharmacol. Exp. Ther. **244:** 1067–1080.

21. DILTS, R. P. & P. W. KALIVAS. 1988. Localization of mu opioid and neurotensin receptors within the A10 region of the rat. Annals NY Acad. Sci. **537:** 472–474.
22. DWORKIN, S. I., G. F. GUERIN, N. E. GOEDERS & I. E. SMITH. 1988. Lack of an effect of 6-hydroxydopamine lesions of the nucleus accumbens on intravenous morphine self-administration. Pharmacol. Biochem. Behav. **30:** 1051–1057.
23. ESPOSITO, E., L. CERVO, P. PETRILLO, M. SBACCHI, A. TAVANI & R. SAMANIN. 1987. Dopamine denervation of the nucleus accumbens induces a selective increase in the number of opioid binding sites. Brain Res. **436:** 25–29.
24. ETTENBERG, A., H. O. PETTIT, F. E. BLOOM & G. F. KOOB. 1982. Heroin and cocaine intravenous self-administration in rats: Mediation by separate neural systems. Psychopharmacology **78:** 204–209.
25. EVANS, K. R. & F. J. VACCARINO. 1990. Amphetamine and morphine-induced feeding: Evidence for involvement of reward mechanisms. Neurosci. Biobehav. Rev. **14:** 9–12.
26. EVERITT, B. J., M. CADOR & T. W. ROBBINS. 1989. Interactions between the amygdala and ventral striatum in stimulus-reward associations: Studies using a second-order schedule of sexual reinforcement. Neuroscience **30:** 63–75.
27. GLIMCHER, P. W., A. A. GIOVINO, D. H. MARGOLIN & B. G. HOEBEL. 1984. Endogenous opiate reward induced by an enkephalinase inhibitor, thiorphan, injected into the ventral midbrain. Behav. Neurosci. **98:** 262–268.
28. GOEDERS, N. E., J. D. LANE & J. E. SMITH. 1984. Self-administration of methionine enkephalin into the nucleus accumbens. Pharmacology Biochem. Behav. **20:** 441–455.
29. GUERIN, B., N. E. GOEDERS, S. I. DWORKIN & J. E. SMITH. 1984. Intracranial self-administration of dopamine into the nucleus accumbens. Soc. Neurosci. Abstr. **10:** 1072.
30. GYSLING, K. & R. Y. WANG. 1983. Morphine-induced activation of A10 dopamine neurons in the rat. Brian Res. **277:** 119–127.
31. HAKAN, R. L. & S. J. HENRIKSEN. 1989. Opiate influences on nucleus accumbens neuronal electrophysiology: Dopamine and non-dopamine mechanisms. J. Neurosci. **10:** 3538–3546.
32. HAVEMANN, U. & K. KUSCHINSKY. 1985. Locomotor activity of rats after injection of various opioids into the nucleus accumbens and the septum mediale. Naunyn-Schmiedebergs Arch. Pharmacol. **331:** 175–180.
33. HOEBEL, B. G., A. P. MONACO, L. HERNANDEZ, E. F. AULISI, B. G. STANLEY & L. LENARD. 1983. Self-injection of amphetamine directly into the brain. Psychopharmacology **81:** 158–163.
34. HONG, J. S., H. Y. T. YANG, W. FRATTA & E. COSTA. 1977. Determination of methionine enkephalin in discrete regions of rat brain. Brain Res. **134:** 383–386.
35. HONG, J. S., H. Y. T. YANG, W. FRATTA & E. COSTA. 1978. Rat striatal methionine-enkephalin content after chronic treatment with cataleptogenic and non cataleptogenic antischizophrenic drugs. J. Pharmacol. Exp. Ther. **205:** 141–147.
36. HONG, J. S., H. Y. T. YANG, J. C. GILLIN, A. M. DIGIULIO, W. FRATTA & E. COSTA. 1979. Chronic treatment with haloperidol accelerates biosynthesis of enkephalin in rat striatum. Brain Res. **160:** 192–195.
37. HUBNER, C. B. & G. F. KOOB. 1990. The ventral pallidum plays a role in mediating cocaïne and heroin self-administration in the rat. Brain Res. **508:** 20–29.
38. IWATSUBO, K. & D. H. CLOUET. 1977. Effects of morphine and haloperidol on the electrical activity of rat nigrostriatal neurons. J. Pharmacol. Exp. Ther. **202:** 429–436.
39. JOHNSON, R. P., M. SAR & W. E. STUMP. 1981. A topographic localization of enkephalin on the dopamine neurons of the rat substantia nigra and ventral tegmental area demonstrated by combined histofluorescence-immunohistochemistry. Brain Res. **194:** 566–571.
40. JOYCE, E. M. & S. D. IVERSEN. 1979. The effect of morphine applied locally to mesencephalic dopamine cell bodies on spontaneous motor activity in the rat. Neurosci. Lett. **14:** 207–212.
41. KALIVAS, P. W. & M. BRONSON. 1985. Mesolimbic dopamine lesions produce an augmented behavioral response to enkephalin. Neuropharmacology **24:** 931–936.
42. KALIVAS, P. W., E. WIDERLÖV, D. STANLEY, G. BREESE & A. J. PRANGE, JR. 1983. Enkephalin action on the mesolimbic system: A dopamine-dependent and a dopamine-independent increase in locomotor activity. J. Pharm. Exp. Ther. **227:** 229–237.

43. KELLEY, A. E., L. STINUS & S. D. IVERSEN. 1980. Interaction between d-ala-met-enkephalin, A10 dopaminergic neurons, and spontaneous behavior in the rat. Behav. Brain Res. 1: 3–24.
44. KELLEY, A. E., M. WINNOCK & L. STINUS. 1986. Amphetamine, apomorphine and investigatory behavior in the rat: Analysis of the structure and pattern of responses. Psychopharmacology 88: 66–74.
45. KLEINE, T. O., K. KLEMPEL & E. W. FÜNFGELD. 1986. Leucine (Leu)-enkephalin and methionine (Met)-enkephalin in cerebrospinal fluid (CSF) of chronic schizophrenics correlation with psychopathological states. In Biological Psychiatry, 1985, Developments in Psychiatry. C. Shagass, R. C. Josiassen, W. H. Bridger, K. J. Weiss, D. Stoff & G. M. Simpson, Eds. 7: 296–298. Elsevier Science Publishing Co. New York.
46. KOOB, G. F. & N. GOEDERS. 1989. Neuroanatomical substrates of drug self-administration. In Neuropharmacological Basis of Reward. J. M. Liebman & S. J. Cooper, Eds.: 214–263. Oxford University Press. Oxford.
47. KOOB, G. F., F. J. VACCARINO, M. ALMARIC & F. E. BLOOM. 1987. Positive reinforcement properties of drugs: Search for neural substrates. In Brain Reward Systems and Abuse. J. Engel & L. Oreland, Eds.: 35–50. Raven-Press. New York.
48. LA MOTTE, C. C., A. SNOWMAN, C. C. PERT & S. H. SNYDER. 1978. Opiate receptor binding in rhesus monkey brain: Association with limbic structures. Brain Res. 155: 374–379.
49. LATIMER, L. F., P. DUFFY & P. W. KALIVAS. 1987. Mu opioid receptor involvement in enkephalin activation of dopamine neurons in the ventral tegmental area. J. Pharmacol. Exp. Ther. 241: 328–337.
50. LE MOAL, M., L. STINUS & H. SIMON. 1979. Increased sensitivity to (+)-amphetamine self-administrated by rats following mesocorticolimbic dopamine neurone destruction. Nature 280: 156–158.
51. LONGONI, R., A. MULAS, L. SPINA, P. MELCHIORRI & G. DI CHIARA. 1989. Stimulation of delta opioid receptors in the accumbens elicits D-1 dependent stimulation of motor activity and stereotypes. Behav. Pharmacol. 1(Suppl. 1): 38.
52. LYNESS, W. H., N. M. FRIEDLE & K. E. MOORE. 1979. Destruction of dopaminergic nerve terminals in nucleus accumbens: Effect of d-amphetamine self-administration. Pharmacol. Biochem. Behav. 11: 553–556.
53. MALDONADO, R., V. DAUGE & B. P. ROQUES. 1990. Chronic D2 but not D1-dopamine receptor blockade facilitates behavioural responses to endogenous enkephalins protected by kelatorphan intraaccumbens administration in rats. Neuropharmacology 29: 215–223.
54. MARTIN-IVERSON, M. T., C. SZOSTAK & H. C. FIBIGER. 1986. 6-hydroxydopamine lesions of the medial prefrontal cortex fail to influence intravenous self-administration of cocaïne. Psychopharmacology 88: 310–314.
55. MOGIL, J. S., F. J. VACCARINO & L. STINUS. 1989. Chronic neuroleptic treatment induces a supersensitive feeding response to morphine. Soc. Neurosci. Abstract. 15(1): 248.
56. OLDS, M. E. 1982. Reinforcing effects of morphine in the nucleus accumbens. Brain Res. 237: 429–440.
57. PERT, B. C. & A. PERT. 1976. [D-ALA2]-Met-enkephalinamide: A potent, long-lasting synthetic pentapeptide analgesic. Science 194: 330–332.
58. PERT, C. B. & C. SIVIT. 1977. Neuroanatomical focus for morphine and enkephalin induced hypermobility. Nature 265: 645–664.
59. PETIT, F., M. HAMON, M. C. FOURNIE-ZALUSKI, B. P. ROQUES & J. GLOWINSKI. 1986. Further evidence for a role of delta-opiate receptors in the presynaptic regulation of newly synthetized dopamine release. Eur. J. Pharmacol. 126: 1–9.
60. PETTIT, H. O., A. ETTENBERG, F. E. BLOOM & G. F. KOOB. 1984. Destruction of dopamine in the nucleus accumbens attenuates cocaine but not heroin self-administration in rat. Psychopharmacology 84: 167–173.
61. PHILLIPS, A. G. & F. G. LE PIANE. 1980. Reinforcing effects of morphine microinjection into the ventral tegmental area. Pharmacol. Biochem. Behav. 12: 965–968.
62. PHILLIPS, A. G. & F. G. LE PIANE. 1982. Reward produced by microinjection of [D-Ala2], Met5-enkephalinamide into the ventral tegmental area. Behav. Brain Res. 5: 225–229.

63. PHILLIPS, A. G., F. G. LE PIANE & H. C. FIBIGER. 1983. Dopaminergic mediation of reward produced by direct injection of enkephalin into the ventral tegmental area of the rat. Life Sci. **33:** 2505–2511.
64. POLLARD, H., C. LLORENS-CORTES, J. J. BONNET, J. CONSTENTIN & J. C. SCHWARTZ. 1977. Opiate receptors on mesolimbic dopaminergic neurons. Neurosci. Lett. **7:** 295–299.
65. POLLARD, H., C. LLORENS-CORTES & J. C. SCHWARTZ. 1977. Enkephalin receptors on dopaminergic neurons in rat striatum. Nature **268:** 745–747.
66. ROBERTS, D. C. S. & G. F. KOOB. 1982. Disruption of cocaine self-administration following 6-hydroxydopamine lesions of the ventral tegmental area in rats. Pharmacol. Biochem. Behav. **17:** 901–904.
67. ROBERTS, D. C. S. 1989. Breaking points on a progressive ratio schedule reinforced by intravenous apomorphine increase daily following 6-hydroxydopamine lesions of the nucleus accumbens. Pharmacol. Biochem. Behav. **32:** 43–47.
68. ROBERTS, D. C. S., M. E. CORCORAN & H. C. FIBIGER. 1977. On the role of ascending catecholaminergic systems in intravenous self-administration of cocaine. Pharmacol. Biochem. Behav. **6:** 615–620.
69. ROBERTS, D. C. S., G. F. KOOB, P. KLONOFF & H. C. FIBIGER. 1980. Extinction & recovery of cocaine self-administration following 6-hydroxydopamine lesions of the nucleus accumbens. Pharmacol. Biochem. Behav. **12:** 781–787.
70. SABOL, S. L., K. YOSHIKAMA & J. S. HONG. 1983. Regulation of methionine-enkephalin precursor messenger RNA in rat striatum by haloperidol and lithium. Biochem. Biophys. Res. Commun. **113:** 391–399.
71. SCHEEL-KRÜGER, J., K. GOLEMBIOWSKA & E. MOGILNICKA. 1977. Evidence for increased apomorphine-sensitive dopaminergic effects after acute treatment with morphine. Psychopharmacology **53:** 55–63.
72. SCOTT YOUNG III, W., T. I. BONNER & M. R. BRANN. 1986. Mesencephalic dopamine neurons regulate the expression of neuropeptide mRNAs in the rat forebrain. Proc. Natl. Acad. Sci. USA **83:** 9827–9831.
73. SHIPPENBERG, T. S., R. BALS-KUBIK & A. HERTZ. 1987. Motivational properties of opioids: Evidence that an activation of delta-receptors mediates reinforcing processes. Brain Res. **436:** 234–239.
74. SHIPPENBERG, T. S., R. BALS-KUBIK, R. SPANAGEL & A. HERTZ. 1989. Reinforcing and aversive effects of opioid agonists involvement of the mesolimbic dopamine system. Behav. Pharmaco. **1**(Suppl. 1): 18.
75. SIMON, H., L. STINUS, J. P. TASSIN, S. LAVIELLE, G. BLANC, A. M. THIERRY, J. GLOWINSKI & M. LE MOAL. 1979. Is the dopaminergic mesocorticolimbic system necessary for intracranial self-stimulation? Biochemical and behavioral studies from A10 cell bodies and terminals. Behav. Neural. Biol. **27:** 125–145.
76. STINUS, L. 1982. Interaction entre systèmes peptidergiques opioïdes et neurones dopaminergiques mésolimbiques: Analyse comportementale. *In* Actualités de Chimie Thérapeutique, 2ème série, Technique et documentation. :275–284. Lavoisier. Paris.
77. STINUS, L., F. CESSELIN, J. M. DEMINIERE, S. BOURGOUIN, M. HAMON & M. LE MOAL. 1989. Effets toxicophiliques des morphinominétiques. Interactions dopamine-enképhaline dans l'aire tegmentale ventrale et dans le noyau accumbens. L'encéphale. **XV:** 95–104.
78. STINUS, L., G. F. KOOB, N. LING, F. E. BLOOM & M. LE MOAL. 1980. Locomotor activation induced by infusion of endorphins into the ventral tegmental area: Evidence for opiate-dopamine interactions. Proc. Nat. Acad. Sci. USA **77:** 2323–2327.
79. STINUS, L., D. NADAUD, J. M. DEMINIERE, J. JAUREGUI, T. H. HAND & M. LE MOAL. 1989. Chronic flupentixol treatment potentiates the reinforcing properties of peripheral heroïn administration. Biol. Psychiat. **26:** 363–371.
80. STINUS, L., D. NADAUD, J. JAUREGUI & A. E. KELLEY. 1986. Chronic treatment with five different neuroleptics elicits behavioral supersensitivity to opiate infusion into the nucleus accumbens. Biol. Psychiatry **21:** 34–48.

81. STINUS, L., M. WINNOCK & A. E. KELLEY. 1985. Chronic neuroleptic treatment and meso-limbic dopamine denervation induce behavioural hypersensitivity to opiates. Psychopharmacology **85**: 323–328.

82. TANG, F., E. COSTA & J. P. SCHWARTZ. 1983. Increase of proenkephalin mRNA and enkephalin content of rat striatum after daily injection of haloperidol for 2 to 3 weeks. Proc. Natl. Acad. Sci. USA **80**: 3841–3844.

83. THAL, L. J., N. S. SHARPLESS, I. D. HIRSCHORN, S. G. HOROWITZ & M. H. MAKMAN. 1983. Striatal met-enkephalin concentration increases following nigrostriatal denervation. Biochem. Pharmacol. **32**: 3297–3301.

84. VACCARINO, F. J., F. E. BLOOM & G. F. KOOB. 1985. Blockade of nucleus accumbens opiate receptors attenuates intravenous heroin reward in the rat. Psychopharmacology **86**: 37–42.

85. VACCARINO, F. J. & W. A. CORRIGAL. 1987. Effects of opiate antagonist treatment into either the periacqueducal grey or nucleus accumbens on heroin-induced locomotor activation. Brain Res. Bull. **19**: 545–549.

86. VACCARINO, F. J., J. MOGIL & L. STINUS. 1992. Chronic DA blockade and opiate-induced feeding. Psychopharmacology. Submitted.

87. VAN DER KOY, D., R. F. MUCHA, M. O'SHAUGHNESSY & P. BUCENIEKS. 1982. Reinforcing effects of brain microinjections of morphine revealed by conditioned place preference. Brain Res. **243**: 107–117.

88. WAKSMAN, G., E. HAMEL, P. DELAY-GOYET & B. P. ROQUES. 1986. Autoradiographic comparison of the distribution of the neutral endopeptidase "enkephalinase" and of mu and delta opioid receptors in rat brain. Proc. Natl. Acad. Sci. USA **83**: 1523–1527.

Cortical Regulation of Self-Administration[a]

STEVEN I. DWORKIN AND JAMES E. SMITH

Department of Physiology and Pharmacology
Bowman Gray School of Medicine
Wake Forest University
Winston–Salem, North Carolina 27157

The potential role of the cerebral cortex in the brain processes that underlie reinforcement has not been extensively studied. The concentration on the dopamine hypotheses of reward has minimized the contributions of the neocortex since dopaminergic innervations are sparse in most cortical regions. This chapter reviews research on the involvement of the cerebral cortex in positive reinforcement with special emphasis on drug self-administration. This includes discussions of cortical sites of electrical self-stimulation and those activated by such stimulation, cortical regions affected by intravenous self-administration, and cortical regions supporting direct drug self-administration into the brain.

CORTICAL SITES SUPPORTING INTRACRANIAL SELF-STIMULATION

The involvement of cortical regions in brain processes mediating positive reinforcement was first indicated by studies showing electrical stimulation of cortical areas maintained responding. Cortical regions that support intracranial self-stimulation (ICSS) include the prefrontal cortex,[1] medial prefrontal cortex,[2] sulcal prefrontal cortex,[3] pyriform cortex,[4] entorhinal cortex,[5] and medial entorhinal cortex[6] (TABLE 1). Although the rates of responding maintained by cortical stimulation are generally lower than that observed with ventral tegmental region or medial forebrain bundle stimulation, the data indicate that stimulation of these regions does initiate neuronal activity that has reinforcing consequences. Such stimulation has been thought to directly activate the neuronal circuits and networks that underlie positive reinforcement.

Several studies have attempted to define the type of neurons involved in cortical ICSS by utilizing pharmacological manipulations. Systemic administration of pimozide or spiroperidol decreased the rates of self-stimulation of the medial prefrontal cortex while sulpiride had no effect.[2] These data may indirectly support a role for dopaminergic D_1 receptors in these processes since sulpiride is a more specific D_2 antagonist than the other two drugs. Opioid receptors also have been implicated in self-

[a] Research for this paper was supported in part by USPHS Research Grants DA-01999, DA-03628, DA-03832, DA-06634, and DAKO5 00114 and by NIDA Contract 271-87-8118.

274

TABLE 1. Cortical Sites Supporting ICSS

Region	Reference
Prefrontal cortex	Routtenberg & Sloan, 1972
Medial prefrontal cortex	Ferrer et al., 1983
Sulcal prefrontal cortex	Clavier & Gerfen, 1979
Pyriform cortex	Prado-Alcala et al., 1984
Entorhinal cortex	Ott et al., 1980
Medial entorhinal cortex	Reymann et al., 1986

stimulation of the medial entorhinal cortex since systemic naloxone decreased rates of stimulation.[6] Two investigations[2,6] evaluated the effects of these opiate and dopamine antagonists on ICSS rates of responding. Data on response rates, however, are often difficult to interpret since drugs have both rate-dependent and unconditioned effects that can result in decreased response rates independent of effects on reinforcing efficacy. Another study utilized central administration of pimozide and spiroperidol directly into the site of stimulation in the medial prefrontal cortex[7] and found effects on rates that were similar to those seen with systemic administration.[2] Since central administration is less likely to produce the unconditioned effects that may be present with systemic administration, these data suggest that the effects on ICSS observed after systemic administration[2] may be a more specific result of modulating the reinforcing efficacy of the stimulation. Pharmacological manipulations using intracranial administration of neurotoxins also have been used to define the neuronal systems involved in cortical ICSS. Lesions of neurons of origin at the site of self-stimulation in the medial prefrontal cortex with ibotenate[8] or kainate[9] or in the sulcal prefrontal cortex with kainate[10] decreased rates of self-stimulation. 6-Hydroxydopamine lesions of the substantia nigra had mixed effects on medial prefrontal cortex self-stimulation, with half the animals showing decreases in rates of ICSS both contralateral and ipsilateral to the lesion while the other half showed no effects.[11] These lesion studies suffer from the same interpretation problems as mentioned above since rates of responding were assessed. In spite of these limitations, these data generally support a role for dopamine, opioid and neurons of origin in the medial prefrontal and medial entorhinal cortex in the processes maintaining ICSS at these sites.

CORTICAL GLUCOSE UTILIZATION DURING SELF-STIMULATION

Another series of studies has sought to identify the brain regions involved in ICSS using 2-deoxyglucose autoradiography for assessment of glucose utilization.[12-14] The distribution of 2-deoxyglucose has been evaluated in brain regions of rats receiving either response dependent or response independent brain stimulation of the substantia nigra.[12] Rats receiving contingent stimulation showed significant increases in glucose utilization bilaterally in the prefrontal and anterior cingulate cortices compared to response independently stimulated controls. This same laboratory has also investigated brain glucose utilization in rats receiving contingent and noncontingent stimulation of the ventral tegmental area[13] and medial forebrain bundle.[14] Rats receiving response contingent stimulation of these two regions showed increases in activity ipsilaterally to the stimulating electrode in the medial prefrontal cortex. The medial prefrontal cortex was the only cortical region that showed increases after stimulation of all three brain regions, which demonstrates the importance of this region in reinforcement produced by brain electrical stimulation.

A recent investigation which has concurrently measured glucose utilization and biogenic amine turnover rates in animals self-stimulating the ventral tegmental area found increases in dopamine turnover in the contralateral prefrontal cortex compared to response independently stimulated controls.[15] These same animals showed decreases in dopamine turnover from the elevated level in the response independently stimulated controls on the ipsilateral side which was still significantly above that seen in non-stimulated controls. These data indicate that the medial prefrontal cortex is important to ICSS of several brain sites and that dopamine is also involved in these processes.

CORTICAL LESIONS AND INTRAVENOUS DRUG SELF-ADMINISTRATION

Several studies have attempted to identify brain regions involved in intravenous drug self-administration by assessing the effects of cortical lesions on drug intake. Electrolytic lesions of the anterior cingulate cortex[16] and the frontal cortex[17] increased the intravenous self-administration of morphine. The dose intake relationship was shifted to the right suggesting a decrease in reinforcing efficacy after the frontal cortex lesions.[17] While these lesions are somewhat nonspecific, the data suggests that neuronal pathways either passing through or originating in these areas could be involved in the processes responsible for self-administration.

Neurotoxin-induced lesions have also been used to identify more specifically the neuronal systems important to self-administration. Bilateral 6-OHDA lesions of the medial prefrontal cortex either did not alter[18] or increased[19] the reinforcing efficacy of intravenous cocaine. These lesions in the latter study resulted in significant increases in the intake of low doses of cocaine while intake of higher doses was not altered.[19] Doses that were too low to maintain responding in the sham-lesioned rats would maintain significant levels of self-administration in the lesioned animals. The study that reported no effect of this lesion[19] evaluated only a single relatively high dose of cocaine which may have obscured the detection of potential low dose effects. These data collectively suggest the involvement of frontal cortical regions and dopamine innervations of the prefrontal cortex in the processes maintaining intravenous opiate and cocaine self-administration.

CORTICAL NEUROTRANSMITTERS AND SELF-ADMINISTRATION

Several studies have attempted to identify the neuronal systems involved in opiate self-administration by assessing the turnover rates and receptor densities for several neurotransmitters in self-administering animals (SA) in a number of brain regions and comparing these to yoked drug (YD) and yoked saline (YS) infused controls. One study assessed the turnover rates of dopamine, norepinephrine, serotonin, aspartate, glutamate and gamma-aminobutyric acid[20] while another addressed the turnover rates of acetylcholine and densities of muscarinic cholinergic receptors[21,22] intravenous mor-

TABLE 2. Percent Changes of the Significant Differences in the Turnover Rates of Dopamine, Aspartate, Glutamate and GABA in Cortical Regions between Intravenous Morphine Self-Administering Rats and Yoked Morphine-infused Controls

Brain Region	Neurotransmitter			
	DA	Asp	Glu	GABA
Frontal-pyriform cortex	270	58	106	42
Motor-somatosensory cortex	–	70	101	90

TABLE 3. Percent Changes of the Significant Differences in the Turnover Rates of Acetylcholine and Muscarinic Cholinergic Receptor Binding in Cortical Regions between Intravenous Morphine Self-Administering Rats and Yoked Morphine-infused Controls

Brain Region	ACh	QNB
Frontal cortex	44	−29
Pyriform cortex	−46	–
Entorhinal-subicular cortex	–	−19

phine self-administering animals. Several cortical regions showed significant changes in turnover rates and receptor densities between the self-administering and yoked-morphine infused controls (TABLES 2 and 3). These changes may be related to the differences between response-contingent (reinforcing effects) and response-independent presentation (pharmacologic actions). The differences that were observed comparing the SA to the YC subjects included increased turnover rates of acetylcholine, dopamine, aspartate, glutamate and gamma-aminobutyric acid in the frontal cortex and motor-somatosensory cortex and decreased acetylcholine turnover in the entorhinal-subicular cortex. These data implicate the mesocortical dopamine and basal forebrain cholinergic innervations of the frontal cortex in the neuronal processes involved in intravenous morphine self-administration. The amino acid turnover increases in the frontal cortex are more difficult to interpret, but may represent increases in activity of cortical association fibers in the self-administering animals. The increases in amino acid turnover in the motor-somatosensory cortex may be related to the directed drug seeking responses and not differences in activity between the yoked infused and self-administering animals. It also appears that cholinergic innervations of the pyriform cortex and entorhinal-subicular cortex may be involved in these processes.

CORTICAL AREAS SUPPORTING INTRACRANIAL
DRUG SELF-ADMINISTRATION

The neuronal circuits that mediate ICSS may also mediate drug reinforcement. The sites in the brain at which drugs initiate such activity have been investigated with intracranial self-administration techniques. These self-administration techniques suggest stimulants to initiate reinforcing neuronal activity from sites in the orbitofrontal[23] and medial prefrontal cortex.[24,25] Amphetamine was self-administered at nmol doses into the orbitofrontal cortex of monkeys[23] while cocaine[24] and ethylcocaine[25] were self-administered into the medial prefrontal cortex of rats at pmole doses. The self-administration of cocaine was dose dependent, receptor specific and site specific. The dose intake functions were inverted U shape functions with maximal rates of intake obtained with 90–120 pmole doses. The self-administration was blocked by concurrent infusion of sulpiride suggesting dopamine D_2 receptors to be necessary. Dopamine innervations are also necessary since 6-OHDA lesions of the medial prefrontal cortex self-administration site attenuate intake.[26] However, activation of postsynaptic dopamine receptors were shown to be still capable of initiative reinforcing neuronal activity since those lesioned animals would self-administer 300 pmole doses of dopamine into the medial prefrontal site that previously supported cocaine self-administration.[26] Ethylcocaine self-administration into this same brain region was shown to maintain responding on a lever that resulted in drug presentation but not on a second lever that did not.[25] Self-administration of ethylcocaine was also in the same dose range as cocaine (50 pmol). These data collectively suggest that the medial prefrontal cortex in rats and the orbitofrontal cortex in monkeys are sites at which stimulants may directly initiate neuronal activity in circuits that mediate reinforcement.

CORTICAL REGIONS INVOLVED IN WITHDRAWAL FROM SELF-ADMINISTERED DRUGS

A study recently completed in our laboratories attempted to identify the neuronal systems involved in cocaine withdrawal. The turnover rates for several neurotransmitters in a number of brain regions following 24-h withdrawal period from self-

TABLE 4A. Percent Changes of Significant Differences in Neuro-transmitter Turnover Rates in Cortical Regions between Chronic Intravenous Cocaine Self-administering and Yoked Cocaine-infused Controls 24 hours after a Self-Administration Session

Region	Neurotransmitter	
	5-HT	GABA
Pyriform cortex	144	
Motor somatosensory cortex	−41	84%

B. Percent Changes of Significant Differences in Neurotransmitter Turnover Rates in Cortical Regions between Chronic Yoked Cocaine-infused and Yoked Vehicle-infused Controls 24 hours after a Session

Region	Neurotransmitter			
	DA	NE	5-HT	Glu
Frontal cortex			−43	
Cingulate cortex	−70	−44		
Pyriform cortex		203		94
Motor-somatosensory cortex	−40			
Visual cortex	−89			

administering cocaine (SA) was compared to those found in subjects previously receiving yoked drug (YD) and yoked saline (YS) infusions (TABLE 4). The withdrawal from cocaine self-administration compared to withdrawal from yoked response-independent infusions resulted in three significant differences in cortical regions. These differences shown in TABLE 4 (top) included significant increases in serotonin and GABA turnover in the pyriform cortex and motor somatosensory cortex, respectively. Significant decreases in serotonin turnover in the motor somatosensory cortex in SA animals were also observed. Withdrawal from response-independent infusions of cocaine compared to yoked vehicle-infused subjects also indicated that a number of cortical regions are altered by withdrawal from the pharmacologic actions of the drug (see TABLE 4, bottom). It remains to be determined if cortical regions differentially activated by the self-administration of a drug are also directly involved in withdrawal from the drug.

CONCLUSION

The search for the physical substrates of reinforcement began shortly after the initial demonstration that animals would emit a response that had previously resulted in the delivery of an electrical stimulus to a discrete brain region.[27] This intracranial electrical self-stimulation was assumed to result in the activation of neuronal pathways responsible for the processes underlying reinforcement elicited by natural products. Considerable information has been obtained concerning the nature of these processes with several theories proposed suggesting one or two neuronal systems to be responsible for reward phenomena. The evidence for the involvement of cortical regions in these processes as reviewed here is significant. The medial prefrontal cortex has a central role in the circuits proposed to mediate opiate reinforcement[21] and in the limbic-motor reinforcement circuit recently outlined.[28] These two hypothesis propose complex circuits to mediate these processes.

There are advantages for considering the neurons that mediate reinforcement to be neuronal systems or networks over attributing such complex processes to one or two pathways or neurotransmitter releasing neuronal systems. A concentration on neuronal systems will encourage the potential integration of behavioral, neurochemical, neuroanatomical and molecular and cellular aspects of reinforcement. A systems approach will also allow for the inclusion of potential differences related to behavioral variables (i.e. the contingent and noncontingent administration of the drug and the organism's behavioral and drug history) and pharmacologic variables including drug class, dose, and route of administration. The utility of a neuronal systems approach is exemplified by the data indicating that different systems are activated by opiates and stimulants. Moreover, the observation that different neuronal systems are activated by the contingent and noncontingent administration of morphine and cocaine suggests that a systems approach can lead to the identification of the neuronal processes directly related to drug abuse differentiated from those neurobiological changes only indirectly involved. The systems approach is more consistent with what is known about complex brain function, since it is unlikely that a neuronal system in the CNS is independent of influences from other neurons or that intricate behavioral processes can be mediated by one or two neuronal pathways. Furthermore, it is likely that a single neuronal pathway or neurotransmitter releasing system has multiple functions that could not be understood in the absence of a model of specific systems and pathways.

Reinforcers are not immutable or constant. The state of the organism (deprivation, satiation) modulates the saliency of a putative reinforcer. Many reinforcers do not have inherent response strengthening properties but develop reinforcing efficacy through manipulations of behavioral and drug histories, and other aspects of conditioning. All of these factors are important to the processes that comprise reinforcement. It is not likely that one or two neuronal pathways control and integrate these complex phenomena. Neuronal circuits or networks involving a number of pathways and neurotransmitters are necessary for such complex actions.

Discrete and perhaps dedicated neuronal networks likely mediate reinforcement and perhaps drug withdrawal. These neuronal networks may be artificially activated by direct electrical stimulation or by chemical stimulation with drugs. Drugs may initiate or modulate activity in these circuits by interacting with receptors on component neurons of neuronal circuits dedicated to these functions or on neurons that modulate these circuits. A neuronal systems approach can provide the integration of behavioral and neurobiologic data that will be necessary to understand the intricate aspects of substance abuse.

REFERENCES

1. ROUTTENBERG, A. & M. SLOAN. 1972. Self-stimulation of the frontal cortex in Rattus Norvegicus. Behav. Biol. 7: 567–572.
2. FERRER, J. M. R., A. M. SANGUINETTI, F. VIVES & F. MORA. 1983. Effects of agonists and antagonists of D_1 and D_2 dopamine receptors on self-stimulation of the medial prefrontal cortex in the rat. Pharmacol. Biochem. Behav. 19: 211–217.
3. CLAVIER, R. M. & C. R. GERFEN. 1979. Self-stimulation of the sulcal prefrontal cortex in the rat: direct evidence for ascending dopaminergic mediation. Neurosci. Lett. 12: 183–187.
4. PRADO-ALCALA, R., A. STREATHER & R. A. WISE. 1984. Brain stimulation reward and dopamine terminal fields. II. Septal and cortical projections. Brain Res. 301: 209–219.
5. OTT, T., C. DESTRADE & H. RÜTHRICH. 1980. Introduction of self-stimulation behavior derived from a brain region lacking in dopaminergic innervation. Behav. Neurol. Biol. 28: 512–516.
6. REYMANN, K. G., S. MULCKO, T. OTT & H. MATTHIES. 1986. Opioid-receptor blockade reduces nose-poke self-stimulation derived from medial entorhinal cortex. Pharmacol. Biochem. Behav. 24: 439–443.
7. ROBERTSON, A. & G. J. MOGENSON. 1978. Evidence for a role for dopamine in self-stimulation of the nucleus accumbens of the rat. Can. J. Psychol. 32: 67–76.
8. NASSIF, S., B. CARDO, F. LIBERSAT & L. VELLEY. 1985. Comparison of deficits in electrical self-stimulation after ibotenic acid lesions of the lateral hypothalamus and the medial prefrontal cortex. Brain Res. 332: 247–257.
9. FERRER, J. M. R., R. D. MYERS & F. MORA. 1985. Suppression of self-stimulation of the medial prefrontal cortex after local microinjection of kainic acid in the rat. Brain Res. Bull. 15: 225–228.
10. GERFEN, C. R. & R. M. CLAVIER. 1981. Intracranial self-stimulation from the sulcal prefrontal cortex in the rat: The effect of 6-OHDA or kainic acid lesions at the site of stimulation. Brain Res. 224: 291–304.
11. CAREY, R. J. 1982. Unilateral 6-hydroxydopamine lesions of dopamine neurons produce bilateral self-stimulation deficits. Behav. Brain Res. 6: 101–114.
12. PORRINO, L. J. 1987. Cerebral metabolic changes associated with activation of reward systems. In Brain Reward Systems. J. Engel & L. Oreland, Eds.: 51–60. Raven Press. New York.
13. PORRINO, L. J., R. U. ESPOSITO, T. F. SEEGER, A. M. CRANE, A. PERT & L. SOKOLOFF.

1984. Metabolic mapping of brain during rewarding self-stimulation. Science 224: 306–309.

14. PORRINO, L. J., D. HUSTON-LYONS, G. BAIN, L. SOKOLOFF & C. KORNETSKY. 1990. The distribution of changes in local cerebral energy metabolism associated with brain stimulation reward to the MFB in the rat. Brain Res. 511: 1–6.

15. SMITH, J. E., S. I. DWORKIN, C. Co & L. J. PORRINO. 1990. Concurrent brain glucose utilization and biogenic monoamine turnover rates with VTA brain stimulation reinforcement. Neurosci. Abstr. 16: 753.

16. TRAFTON, C. I. & P. R. MARQUES. 1971. Effects of septal area and cingulate cortex lesions on opiate addiction behavior in rats. J. Comp. Physiol. Psychol. 75: 277–285.

17. GLICK, S. D. & R. D. COX. 1978. Changes in morphine self-administration after teldiencephalic lesions in rats. Psychopharmacologia (Berlin) 57: 283–288.

18. MARTIN-IVERSON, M. T., C. SZOSTAK & H. C. FIBIGER. 1986. 6-Hydroxydopamine lesions of the medial prefrontal cortex fail to influence intravenous self-administration of cocaine. Psychopharmacology 88: 310–314.

19. SCHENK, S., B. A. HORGER, R. PELTIER & K. SHELTON. 1991. Supersensitivity to the reinforcing effects of cocaine following 6-hydroxydopamine lesions to the medial prefrontal cortex in rats. Brain Res. 543: 227–235.

20. SMITH, J. E., C. Co, M. E. FREEMAN & J. D. LANE. 1982. Brain neurotransmitter turnover correlated with morphine-seeking behavior in rats. Pharmacol. Biochem. Behav. 16: 509–519.

21. SMITH, J. E., C. Co & J. D. LANE. 1984. Limbic acetylcholine turnover rates correlated with rat morphine-seeking behaviors. Pharmacol. Biochem. Behav. 20: 429–441.

22. SMITH, J. E., C. Co & J. D. LANE. 1984. Limbic muscarinic cholinergic and benzodiazepine receptor changes with chronic intravenous morphine and self-administration. Pharmacol. Biochem. Behav. 20: 443–450.

23. PHILLIPS, A. G. & E. T. ROLLS. 1981. Intracerebral self-administration of amphetamine by rhesus monkeys. Neurosci. Lett. 24: 81–86.

24. GOEDERS, N. E., S. I. DWORKIN & J. E. SMITH. 1986. Neuropharmacological assessment of cocaine self-administration into the medial prefrontal cortex. Pharmacol. Biochem. Behav. 24: 1429–1440.

25. MURPHY, J. M., G. J. GATTO, R. A. DEAN & W. F. BOSRON. 1991. Intracranial self-administration (ICSA) of ethylcholine (EC), an active metabolite of ethanol and cocaine, to the prefrontal cortex in rats. Alcoholism: Clin. Exp. Res. 15: 315 (Abstr.).

26. GOEDERS, N. E. & J. E. SMITH. 1986. Reinforcing properties of cocaine in the medial prefrontal cortex: Primary action on presynaptic dopaminergic terminals. Pharmacol. Biochem. Behav. 25: 191–199.

27. OLDS, J. & P. MILNER. 1954. Positive reinforcement produced by electrical stimulation of septal area and other regions of rat brain. J. Comp. Physiol. Psychol. 47: 419–427.

28. WATSON, S. J., K. A. TRUJILLO, J. P. HERMAN & H. AKIL. 1989. Neuroanatomical and neurochemical substrates of drug-seeking behavior: Overview and future directions. In Molecular and Cellular Aspects of the Drug Addictions. A. Goldstein, Ed.: 29–91. Springer-Verlag. New York.

High Potency Cocaine Analogs: Neurochemical, Imaging, and Behavioral Studies

J. W. BOJA,[a] E. J. CLINE,[a] F. I. CARROLL,[b]
A. H. LEWIN,[b] A. PHILIP,[b] R. DANNALS,[c]
D. WONG,[c] U. SCHEFFEL,[c] AND M. J. KUHAR[a]

[a] Neuroscience Branch, National Institute on Drug Abuse
Addiction Research Center
P.O. Box 5180
Baltimore, Maryland 21224

[b] Chemistry and Life Sciences
Research Triangle Institute
P.O. Box 12194
Research Triangle Park, North Carolina 27709

[c] Division of Nuclear Medicine
and Radiation Health Sciences
Johns Hopkins Medical Institute
Baltimore, Maryland 21205

INTRODUCTION

Recent evidence suggests the behavioral properties of cocaine are related to its ability to inhibit dopamine (DA) reuptake.[1,2] Specific binding sites for cocaine have been identified with a host of ligands, including [³H]cocaine.[3-5] However, the use of [³H]cocaine as a ligand presents many problems, including its low affinity and rapid dissociation rate. While other non-cocaine-like ligands such as GBR 12935, mazindol, and nomifensine overcome the problems of low affinity and rapid dissociation, they present problems of their own. These ligands bind to a single high affinity site, while cocaine binds to both a high and low affinity site. Furthermore, Madras et al.[6] reported that [³H]cocaine was not fully displaced by these non-cocaine-like drugs. Thus it appears that in order to correctly identify the molecular structural requirements for cocaine binding one must utilize cocaine or cocaine analogs.

It was reported by Clarke et al.[7] that removal of the ester linkage between the phenyl ring and tropane ring of cocaine (FIG. 1) results in the compound designated WIN 35,065-2. This compound demonstrated a higher affinity for the dopamine transporter than cocaine itself. Addition of fluorine to the para-position of the phenyl ring (WIN 35,428, also designated CFT) further enhanced potency. Both WIN 35,065-2 and WIN 35,428 have been radioactively labeled and have proven to be superior ligands for in vitro binding studies when compared to cocaine.[6,8]

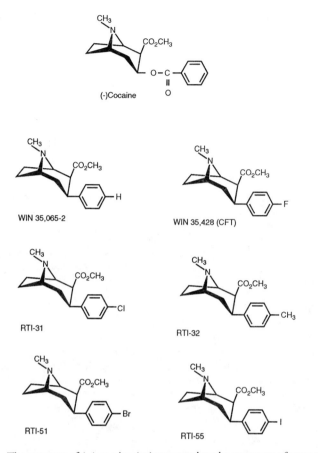

FIGURE 1. The structure of (−) cocaine (*top*) compared to the structures of some various cocaine analogs: WIN 35,065-2 (3β-(4-phenyl)tropan-2β-carboxylic acid methyl ester); WIN 35,428 (3β-(4-fluorophenyl) tropan-2β-carboxylic acid methyl ester); RTI-31 (3β-(4-chlorophenyl) tropan-2β-carboxylic acid methyl ester); RTI-32 3β-(4-methylphenyl) tropan-2β-carboxylic acid methyl ester); RTI-51 (3β-(4-bromophenyl) tropan-2β-carboxylic acid methyl ester); RTI-55 (3β-(4-iodophenyl) tropan-2β-carboxylic acid methyl ester).

In an ongoing structure-activity study,[9–12] the affinities for the dopamine transporter have been determined for several novel highly potent cocaine analogs. Some of the compounds (FIG. 1) include the chloro- and methylphenyl analogs of cocaine, designated RTI-31, RTI-32,[13] and the bromo- and iodophenyl analogs of cocaine, designated RTI-51 and RTI-55.[14] This paper will provide an overview of the *in vitro* receptor binding, dopamine (DA) reuptake inhibition, *in vivo* receptor binding, potential use as imaging agents, and behavioral effects of these compounds.

IN VITRO BINDING STUDIES AND [³H]DOPAMINE
REUPTAKE INHIBITION

The ability of several of the novel cocaine analogs to displace the binding of 0.5 nM [³H]WIN 35,428 to rat striatal membranes is shown in TABLE 1. As previously stated, the elimination of the ester linkage between the tropane ring and the phenyl ring (WIN 35,065-2) increased potency approximately 5-fold over (−)cocaine. Addition of a fluorine (WIN 35,428) to the *para* position of the phenyl ring further increased potency over the non-halogenated compound. Substitution of the fluorine with either a bromine (RTI-51), iodine (RTI-55), chlorine (RTI-31) or methyl (RTI-32) group further enhanced potency. In addition to binding to the DA transporter in striatal tissue, cocaine binds to other transporters as well, including the norepinephrine (NE) and serotonin (5-HT) transporters.[15] In the current studies, as shown in TABLE 1, increases in potency at the DA transporter were generally followed by increased potency at the other binding sites.[14] However, some exceptions exist; WIN 35,065-2 demonstrated increased potency at the DA transporter, but decreased potency at the NE transporter. Likewise, WIN 35,428 demonstrated increased potency at both the DA and 5-HT transporter, but decreased potency at the NE transporter.

In addition to competing with [³H]WIN 35,428 for the cocaine binding site, these compounds are also potent inhibitors of [³H]DA uptake in striatal synaptosomes.[16] The overall rank order of inhibition of [³H]DA is consistent with those observed for inhibition of [³H]WIN 35,428 binding, and the IC$_{50}$ values of these compounds to inhibit [³H]WIN 35,428 binding correlate significantly with the IC$_{50}$ values for the inhibition of [³H]DA uptake as shown in FIGURE 2.

A number of these compounds have been radiolabeled and tested for their suitability as ligands. The various affinities of these ligands for binding to striatal membranes are shown in TABLE 2. As expected, the affinities follow the same rank order as determined by their potencies for displacing [³H]WIN 35,428 binding.

The use of these ligands as a substitute for cocaine depends upon a pharmacology that is identical to cocaine. The pharmacology of [³H]WIN 35,056-2,[8] [³H]WIN

TABLE 1. Affinities of Cocaine and Various Cocaine Analogs for the DA,* NE,** and 5-HT*** Transporters[a]

Compound	[³H]WIN 35,428* IC$_{50}$ (nM)	[³H]Mazindol** K$_i$ (nM)	[³H]Paroxetine*** K$_i$ (nM)
(−)Cocaine	89.0	1866.1	43.9
WIN 35,065-2	23.0	949.4	66.6
WIN 35,428	15.7	563.5	25.3
RTI-51	1.8	22.1	0.9
RTI-32	1.7	22.4	22.2
RTI-55	1.3	16.4	0.4
RTI-31	1.2	19.7	4.3

[a] Data from Boja *et al.*[14] The IC$_{50}$ values for the various drugs at the DA transporter were obtained following the displacement of 0.5 nM [³H]WIN 35,428. K$_i$ values for the various drugs at the NE and 5-HT transporters were obtained by the displacement of 0.5 nM [³H]mazindol and 0.2 nM [³H]paroxetine respectively.[14] All values were determined using the EBDA software package (BIOSOFT).

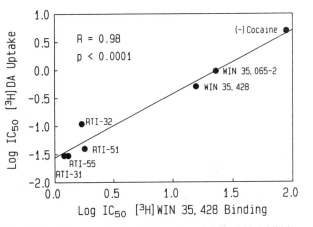

FIGURE 2. Correlation between the log IC_{50} values for binding inhibition of 0.5 nM [³H]WIN 35,428 to rat striatal membranes and the IC_{50} values for the inhibition of the uptake of 1 μM [³H]DA into rat synaptosomes. (Data from Boja *et al.*[14])

35,428,[6] and [¹²⁵I]RTI-55[13] matches that of [³H]cocaine[4,5,17] in the striatum, which contains a vast number of DA transporters. However, one may ask what the binding profile of these compounds outside the striatum looks like since these other areas do not contain the vast numbers of DA transporters relative to other binding sites.

Owing to its very high affinity, high specific to non-specific binding ratio and very high specific activity, [¹²⁵I]RTI-55 was used to examine the binding profiles of areas other than the striatum. As previously mentioned the binding profile of [¹²⁵I]RTI-55 in the striatum is that of the DA transporter. Additionally, in the striatum [¹²⁵I]RTI-55 binds to both a high ($K_d = 0.15$ nM) and a low ($K_d = 5.79$ nM) affinity site. However, in the cerebral cortex the binding profile demonstrated is consistent with that of the 5-HT transporter.[18] Furthermore, in the cerebral cortex [¹²⁵I]RTI-55 binds to only a single high affinity site ($K_d = 0.17$ nm). In other areas, such as the hypothalamus and brain stem, the displacement curves of [¹²⁵I]RTI-55 generated using selec-

TABLE 2. High and Low Affinity Constants for Cocaine and its Various Analogs

Ligand	$K_{d_{high}}$ (nM)	$K_{d_{low}}$ (nM)	Reference
[³H]Cocaine	530	25900	17
	16.0	660	4
	19.2	1120	5
[³H]WIN 35,065-2	5.6	160	8
[³H]WIN 35,428	4.7	60–66	6
	7.1	77.9	36
[¹²⁵I]RTI-55	0.15	5.79	18
[³H]RTI-31	0.12[a]		Boja unpublished

[a] One site only.

tive uptake inhibitors are biphasic and difficult to interpret indicating several possible binding sites (Boja, unpublished data). Further work will be necessary to resolve this observation.

IN VIVO BINDING AND IMAGING STUDIES

In addition to pharmacological evaluation using in vitro binding and uptake procedures, WIN 35,065-2, WIN 35,428, RTI-55 and the other para-substituted 3β-phenyltropane cocaine analogs described above have been examined as DA transporter ligands for both in vivo binding and imaging procedures. Development of these compounds as imaging agents will not only allow for the study of the effects of cocaine, but may permit accurate clinical diagnostic evaluation of DA transporters in pathological states such as Parkinson's disease, for example.[19]

In binding studies aimed at establishing an animal model for labeling the cocaine binding site in vivo, time course and regional binding of [³H]WIN 35,065-2 and [³H]WIN 35,428 was carried out following i.v. injection in mice.[20] In these initial studies, regional accumulation of these ligands peaked at approximately 60 minutes, and demonstrated a pharmacological profile consistent with binding to striatal DA transporters, in that binding was inhibited by the DA uptake inhibitors GBR 12909, nomifensine, and (−)cocaine, but not by 5-HT or NE uptake inhibitors such as paroxetine or desipramine. WIN 35,065-2 and especially WIN 35,428 produced higher ratios of specific to non-specific binding than cocaine, and in later studies[21] this binding was shown to be saturable at increasing doses and as before displayed the appropriate pharmacology. The ED_{50} values for the in vivo inhibition of mouse striatal [³H]WIN 35,428 binding by various DA uptake inhibitors correlated well with the in vitro IC_{50} values for inhibition of striatal membrane [³H]WIN 35,428 binding by these same compounds.[16]

More recently, some of the novel para-substituted cocaine analogs described earlier have also been tested in vivo following i.v. injection in the mouse.[22] The potencies of RTI-31, -32, -51 and -55 were slightly higher than that of WIN 35,428 and significantly greater than that of (−)cocaine in inhibiting the binding of [³H]WIN 35,428 in brain regions with high concentrations of the DA transporter. Following injection of ^{125}I-radiolabeled RTI-55 in mice, autoradiograms demonstrated binding primarily to DA transporters with slightly less binding to 5-HT transporters.[22] Cline et al.,[22] and Scheffel et al.[23] demonstrated that the in vivo binding to the serotonin transporter was inhibited by the 5-HT uptake inhibitor paroxetine, but not the DA uptake inhibitor GBR 12909.

Three studies have imaged both dopamine and serotonin transporters with [¹²³I]RTI-55 using single photon emission computed tomography (SPECT). Three hours following i.v. injection of [¹²³I]RTI-55 into a baboon, binding was apparent in the striatum and cerebral cortex. However, after 21 hours only striatal binding was observed.[24] If the baboon was unilaterally injected with the neurotoxin 1-methyl-4-phenyl-1,2,3,6-tetrahydropyridine (MPTP) [¹²³I]RTI-55 binding was absent in the pretreated striatum.[25] Innis et al.[26] also used [¹²³I]RTI-55 to image dopamine and serotonin transporters in the baboon. The apparent half-life of [¹²³I]RTI-55 in the striatum was approximately 27 hours. High [¹²³I]RTI-55 binding levels were observed in the striatum with slightly less binding in the hypothalamus and cerebral cortex. Both (−)cocaine and WIN 35,428 caused a rapid dose-dependent displacement of both striatal and hypothalamic binding. In contrast, the selective serotonin uptake inhibitor citalopram only displaced hypothalamic binding.[26] Thus, [^{123}I]RTI-55 binds *in vivo* to both dopamine and serotonin transporters.

BEHAVIORAL STUDIES

As an important adjunct to evaluation using *in vitro* and *in vivo* binding and uptake, the cocaine analogs discussed above have also been examined in various behavioral procedures. While it is difficult to extrapolate directly from either the *in vitro* or *in vivo* binding studies to the behavioral studies, the high potency of these analogs has been paralleled by the results of the behavioral studies to date.

Initial studies by Clarke *et al.*[7] included assessment of the locomotor activity effects produced by WIN 35,065-2 and WIN 35,428. They demonstrated that WIN 35,065-2 and WIN 35,428 were approximately 16 and 64 times more potent than cocaine, respectively, in inducing locomotor activity in mice. Subsequent studies by Heikkila *et al.*[27] demonstrated that WIN 35,428 was more potent than (−)cocaine in producing ipsilateral rotations in rats with unilateral 6-hydroxydopamine lesions of the substantia nigra.

In a variation on classical structure-activity studies, Reith *et al.*[28] compared the structural requirements necessary for various cocaine congeners including WIN 35,065-2 and WIN 35,428, to inhibit Na$^+$ dependent [^{3}H]cocaine binding in the

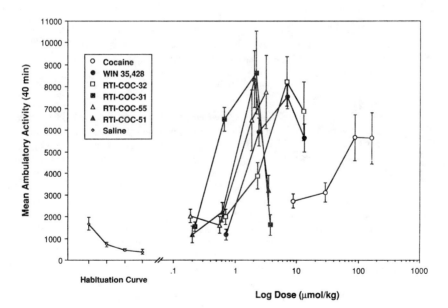

FIGURE 3. Dose-effect relationships for locomotor activity produced by cocaine and various analogs of cocaine (data from Cline *et al.*[32]). Curves represent mean ambulatory activity (± SEM) for a 40-min test period. Drugs were administered cumulatively, i.p.; *n* = 6 for each drug curve and *n* = 12 for the saline habituation curve.

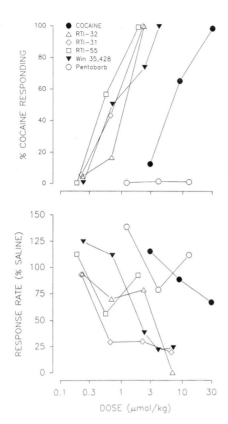

FIGURE 4. Effects of cocaine, sodium pentobarbital, and the 4-substituted phenyl tropane analogs in rats trained to discriminate cocaine from saline injections (data are from Cline et al.[33]). **Ordinate,** *top panel*: percentage of responses on the cocaine appropriate lever. **Ordinate,** *bottom panel*: response rates as percentage of control responding. **Abscissa:** drug dose in μmol/kg. Each point represents the mean of 3 to 5 rats.

striatum with the potency of these same congeners to induce stereotyped sniffing following intraventricular infusion in mice. They reported a significant correlation ($r = 0.84$, $p < 0.002$) for binding inhibition and sniffing stimulation threshold. These data are in agreement with the hypothesis that the DA transporter is involved in elements of cocaine-induced stereotypic behavior.

The cocaine analogs WIN 35,065-2 and WIN 35,428 have also been evaluated in studies of schedule controlled operant behavior. Spealman et al.[29] reported that WIN 35,065-2 and WIN 35,428 were 3 to 10 times more potent than cocaine at altering schedule controlled responding for food or shock termination. This study also demonstrated that these analogs had a slower onset of action and longer duration of action. D'Mello et al.[30] examined the effects of WIN 35,428 and cocaine on the rate of responding under a FR-30 schedule of food reinforcement and found the WIN 35,428 was approximately 34 times more potent than cocaine at decreasing response rates under this schedule. More recently, Spealman et al.[31] have reported WIN 35,428 to be 6 times more potent than cocaine in producing self-administration in primates.

As discussed previously, methyl or halogen substitutions to the phenyl ring of WIN 35,065-2 produce further increases in binding potency. Observations from our laboratory indicate that these increases in binding potency are paralleled by increased be-

TABLE 3. Average Effective Doses and Inhibitory Concentrations of Cocaine and Various Analogs[a]

Compound	In Vitro IC$_{50}$ (nM)	In Vivo ED$_{50}$ (μmol/kg)	Behavioral ED$_{50}$ (μmol/kg)
(−)Cocaine	89.0	40.93	45.52
WIN 35,428	15.7	0.46	1.55
RTI-31	1.2	0.18	0.46
RTI-32	1.7	0.31	2.18
RTI-51	1.8	0.31	0.68
RTI-55	1.3	0.26	1.01

[a] From Cline et al.[32] The IC$_{50}$ values for the various drugs at the DA transporter were obtained following the displacement of 0.5 nM [^{3}H]WIN 35,428.[14] In vivo ED$_{50}$ values were obtained following the i.v. injection of 2 μCi [^{3}H]WIN 35,428 in 0.2 ml saline in mice. Behavioral ED$_{50}$ values were calculated based on mean ambulatory activity for a 40-min test period following an i.p. cumulative dosing procedure.

havioral potency over cocaine, both in producing locomotor activity in mice[32] (FIG. 3) and in substituting for a cocaine discriminative stimulus in rats (FIG. 4).[33] Comparisons were made between the average effective doses (ED$_{50}$ values) for behavioral dose-effect curves, the ED$_{50}$ values for inhibition of [^{3}H]WIN 35,428 binding in vivo, and the IC$_{50}$ values for inhibition of [^{3}H]WIN 35,428 binding in vitro. These values are shown in TABLE 3.[32] In addition, the locomotor activity observed following adminis-

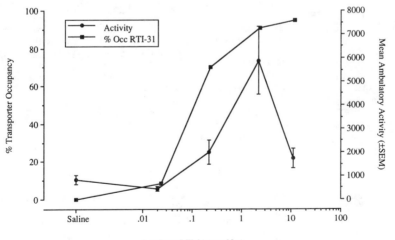

FIGURE 5. Comparison between dose-effect relationship for locomotor activity produced by RTI-31 after i.v. administration and in vivo displacement of [^{3}H]WIN 35,428 by RTI-31 given i.v. *Left ordinate* expressed as % occupancy by RTI-31, based on striatal specific to non-specific binding ratios. *Right ordinate* data again representing mean ambulatory activity (± SEM) for 40-min test, n = 6 mice per point. Maximal locomotor effects correspond to 91% occupancy at 2–3 μmol/kg, while higher doses produced stereotypy. (Data adapted from Cline et al.[32])

tration of the various analogs can be related to receptor occupancy. Comparison of the activity and binding data following i.v. administration of RTI-31 demonstrated that maximal ambulatory activity occurred when there was approximately maximal (91%) receptor occupancy (FIG. 5).[32] Additional receptor occupancy resulted in stereotypic behavior. These behavioral results expand upon the results from previous structure activity studies and the *in vivo* binding studies to emphasize the relationship between increased binding potency of these cocaine analogs at monoamine transporters and their potency in different relevant behavioral procedures.

CONCLUSION

The results of these studies demonstrate the profound effect phenyl substitution has upon the affinity of various cocaine analogs. It is hoped that continued structure-activity studies will allow for the modeling of the cocaine-binding site, thought to be located on the dopamine transporter.[34] Data obtained using CoMFA analysis have allowed for a preliminary pharmacophore of the binding site to be constructed.[12] According to this model there exist hydrogen binding sites and a hydrophobic pocket.[35] Further modifications of this model and the subsequent cloning of the DA transporter will perhaps allow for the development of a possible pharmacological intervention in the treatment of cocaine abuse.

REFERENCES

1. RITZ, M. C., R. J. LAMB & S. R. GOLDBERG. 1987. Science **237:** 1219–1223.
2. BERGMAN, J., B. K. MADRAS, S. E. JOHNSON & R. D. SPEALMAN. 1989. J. Pharmacol. Exp. Ther. **219:** 150–155.
3. REITH, M. E. A., H. SHERSHEN & A. LAJTHA. 1980. Life Sci. **27:** 1055–1062.
4. CALLIGARO, D. O. & M. E. ELDEFRAWI. 1987. J. Pharmacol. Exp. Ther. **243:** 61–67.
5. MADRAS, B. K., M. A. FAHEY, J. BERGMAN, D. R. CANFIELD & R. D. SPEALMAN. 1989. J. Pharmacol. Exp. Ther. **251:** 131–141.
6. MADRAS, B. K., R. D. SPEALMAN, M. A. FAHEY, J. L. NEUMEYER, J. K. SAHA & R. A. MILIUS. 1989. Mol. Pharmacol. **36:** 518–524.
7. CLARKE, R. L., S. J. DAUM, A. J. GAMBINO, M. D. ACETO, J. PEARL, M. LEVITT, W. R. CUMISKEY & E. F. BOGADO. 1973. J. Med. Chem. **16:** 1260–1267.
8. RITZ, M. C., J. W. BOJA, D. GRIGORIADIS, R. ZACZEK, F. I. CARROLL, A. H. LEWIN & M. J. KUHAR. 1990. J. Neurochem. **55:** 1556–1562.
9. CARROLL, F. I., A. H. LEWIN, A. PHILIP, K. PARHAM, J. W. BOJA & M. J. KUHAR. 1991. J. Med. Chem. **34:** 883–886.
10. LEWIN, A. H., Y. GAO, P. ABRAHAM, J. W. BOJA, M. J. KUHAR & F. I. CARROLL. 1992. J. Med. Chem. **35:** 135–140.
11. ABRAHAM, P., J. B. PITNER, LEWIN, A. H., J. W. BOJA, M. J. KUHAR & F. I. CARROLL. 1992. J. Med. Chem. **35:** 140–144.
12. CARROLL, F. I., Y. GAO, M. A. RAHMAN, A. PHILIP, K. PARHAM, A. H. LEWIN, J. W. BOJA & M. J. KUHAR. 1991. J. Med. Chem. **34:** 2719–2725.
13. BOJA, J. W., F. I. CARROLL, M. A. RAHMAN, A. PHILIP, A. H. LEWIN & M. J. KUHAR. 1990. Eur. J. Pharmacol. **184:** 329–332.
14. BOJA, J. W., F. I. CARROLL, M. A. RAHMAN, A. PHILIP, A. H. LEWIN & M. J. KUHAR. 1991. The Pharmacologist **33:** 161.
15. HYTTEL, J. 1982. Prog. Neuro-Psychopharmacol. & Biol. Psychiatr. **6:** 277–295.
16. BOJA, J. W., A. PATEL, F. I. CARROLL, M. A. RAHMAN, A. H. LEWIN, T. A. KOPAJTIC & M. J. KUHAR. 1990. Society for Neurosci. **16:** 428 (Abstract).

17. SHOEMAKER, H., C. PIMOULE, S. ARBILLA, B. SCATTOM, F. JAVOY-AGID & S. Z. LANGER. 1985. Naunyn Schmiedebergs Arch. Pharmacol. **329**: 227–235.
18. BOJA, J. W., W. M. MITCHELL, A. PATEL, T. A. KOPAJTIC, F. I. CARROLL, A. H. LEWIN, P. ABRAHAM & M. J. KUHAR. 1992. Synapse. In press.
19. CANFIELD, D. R., R. D. SPEALMAN, M. J. KAUFMAN & B. K. MADRAS. 1990. Synapse **6**: 189–195.
20. SCHEFFEL, U., J. W. BOJA & M. J. KUHAR. 1989. Synapse **4**: 390–394.
21. SCHEFFEL, U., P. POGUN, M. STATHIS, J. W. BOJA & M. J. KUHAR. 1991. J. Pharmacol. Exp. Ther. **257**: 954–958.
22. CLINE, E. J., U. SCHEFFEL, J. W. BOJA, W. M. MITCHELL, F. I. CARROLL, P. ABRAHAM, A. H. LEWIN & M. J. KUHAR. 1992. Synapse. In press.
23. SCHEFFEL, U., R. F. DANNALS, E. J. CLINE, G. A. RICAURTE, F. I. CARROLL, P. ABRAHAM, A. H. LEWIN & M. J. KUHAR. 1992. Synapse **10**: 169–172.
24. CARROLL, F. I., M. A. RAHMAN, P. ABRAHAM, K. PARHAM, A. H. LEWIN, R. F. DANNALS, E. SHAYA, U. SCHEFFEL, D. F. WONG, J. W. BOJA & M. J. KUHAR. 1991. Med. Chem. Res. **1**: 289–294.
25. SHAYA, E. U., SCHEFFEL, R. F. DANNALS, G. A. RICAURTE, F. I. CARROLL, H. N. WAGNER, JR., M. J. KUHAR & D. F. WONG. 1992. Synapse **10**: 169–172.
26. INNIS, R., R. BALDWIN, E. SYBIRSKA, Y. ZEA, M. LARUELLE, M. AL-TIKRITI, D. CHARNEY, S. ZOGHBI, E. SMITH, G. WISNIEWSKI, P. HOFFER, S. WANG, R. MILIUS & J. NEUMEYER. 1991. Eur. J. Pharmacol. **200**: 369–370.
27. HEIKKILA, R. E., F. S. CABBAT, L. MANZINO & R. C. DUVOISIN. 1979. J. Pharmacol. Exp. Ther. **211**: 189–194.
28. REITH, M. E. A., B. E. MEISLER, H. SERSHEN & A. LAJTHA. 1986. Biochem. Pharmacol. **35**: 1123–1129.
29. SPEALMAN, R. D., S. R. GOLDBERG, R. T. KELLEHER, D. GOLDBERG & J. P. CHARLTON. 1977. J. Pharmacol. Exp. Ther. **202**: 500–509.
30. D'MELLO, G. D., D. M. GOLDBERG, S. R. GOLDBERG & I. P. STOLERMAN. 1981. J. Pharmacol. Exp. Ther. **219**: 60–68.
31. SPEALMAN, R. D., J. BERGMAN & B. K. MADRAS. 1991. Pharmacol. Biochem. Behav. **39**: 1011–1013.
32. CLINE, E. J., U. SCHEFFEL, J. W. BOJA, F. I. CARROLL, J. L. KATZ & M. J. KUHAR. 1992. J. Pharmacol. Exp. Ther. **260**: 1174–1179.
33. CLINE, E. J., P. TERRY, F. I. CARROLL, M. J. KUHAR & J. L. KATZ. 1992. Behav. Pharmacol. **3**:.
34. KUHAR, M. J., M. C. RITZ & J. W. BOJA. 1991. TINS **14**: 299–302.
35. CARROLL, F. I., A. H. LEWIN, J. W. BOJA & M. J. KUHAR. 1992. J. Med. Chem. In press.
36. BOJA, J. W., M. A. RAHMAN, A. PHILIP, A. H. LEWIN, F. I. CARROLL & M. J. KUHAR. 1991. Mol. Pharmacol. **39**: 339–345.

Methamphetamine-induced Neurotoxicity: Structure Activity Relationships

MARK S. KLEVEN AND LEWIS S. SEIDEN

Department of Pharmacological and Physiological Sciences
Department of Psychiatry
The University of Chicago
Chicago, Illinois 60637

INTRODUCTION

It is well established that amphetamine (phenylisopropylamine; PIA) and a number of closely related analogs have toxic effects upon dopaminergic and/or serotonergic neurons.[1] In this paper we discuss structural similarities among amphetamine analogs which have been demonstrated to have effects consistent with neurotoxic activity, as well as some common neuropharmacological actions which might be related to drug-induced neurotoxic effects. Ring-, side chain-, or N-terminal-substituted amphetamines have been tested for neurotoxic activity, and certain compounds from each of these classes have been demonstrated to have neurotoxic activity. Of the various analogs which have been investigated, the long-term effects of the N-methyl derivative, methamphetamine (MA) have been well characterized. In addition, sufficient evidence is available to conclude that several ring-substituted analogs including *para*-chloroamphetamine, fenfluramine (*m*-trifluoromethyl, N-ethyl-phenylisopropylamine), 3,4-methylenedioxyamphetamine (MDA), and 3,4-methylenedioxy-methylamphetamine (MDMA) are toxic to serotonin (5-hydroxytryptamine; 5-HT) and/or dopamine (DA) containing neurons.[1] Many N-and ring-substituted compounds have been shown to cause long-lasting depletions of DA and/or 5-HT, reductions in the number of high affinity monoamine uptake sites, and decreased activity of synthetic enzymes.[1] MA, MDA, MDMA, and fenfluramine, in addition to causing prolonged depletions of biogenic amine transmitters, the intraneuronal enzymes required for their synthesis, as well as monoamine uptake sites, also cause alterations in neuronal morphology indicative of neuronal degeneration. These three factors taken together strongly suggest that these drugs exert neurotoxic effects. For some of the compounds we will discuss in this article, these three criteria have been demonstrated, whereas for others, generally only one or two of the criteria have been demonstrated since morphological evidence of the neurotoxic effect has been the most difficult to obtain.

Several species including rats, mice, cats and rhesus monkeys have been examined for drug-induced neurotoxicity and for some drugs, toxicity has been demonstrated at varying doses to DA- and 5-HT-containing nerve terminals. In general, the effects do not differ from species to species but the dose and frequency of administration may reveal important differences.[2] Some compounds have been shown to be neurotoxic in several species; for example MA has been shown to have effects on the DA and 5-HT system in rats, guinea pigs, mice, cats, and rhesus monkeys. In the face of this species generalization one can confidently conclude that a high dose exposure to humans would cause similar damage. At the same time, although there is considerable data on these drugs regarding their neurotoxicity, the differences between species, doses, and patterns of drug administration make inferences about structure-activity relationships difficult.

Several other factors limit drawing firm structure activity relationships for amphetamine-induced neurotoxicity are that not enough analogs have been tested and the endpoints are not always consistent between studies. Relatively few structurally similar analogs of amphetamine, other than the series of ring-halogenated analogs, have been extensively examined, and few of these compounds have met the strictest criteria of cytotoxicity. On the other hand, many more compounds have been demonstrated to have long-lasting neurochemical effects which highly suggest that they possess neurotoxic activity. This paucity of material limits generalizations regarding structure activity relationships (SAR). Therefore, strict quantitative analysis of the relative potencies of related drugs must remain a future task and in this review we necessarily make qualitative judgements about the ability of substituted amphetamines to cause neurotoxicity.

BEHAVIORAL PHARMACOLOGY OF AMPHETAMINE ANALOGS

A large number of amphetamine analogs have been investigated for their psychopharmacological effects in man,[3-5] and many of these derivatives have potent hallucinogenic or stimulant effects which contribute to their abuse potential. In addition, amphetamine suppresses food intake, interferes with sleep, and in large repeated doses induces stereotypic behaviors and even episodes of paranoid psychosis resembling that seen in schizophrenia. Some members of this class of drugs are useful in the treatment of obesity, narcolepsy, and attention deficit disorder with hyperkinesis. Amphetamine enhances release and blocks reuptake of DA, 5-HT, and norepinephrine (NE), and is also a monoamine oxidase inhibitor.[6-8] As a result of these effects, amphetamine and many of its derivatives are potent indirect agonists at monoaminergic receptors, however, depending upon the site and degree of substitution, amphetamine derivatives may also have direct receptor agonist activity.[9]

For amphetamines without ring substitutions, pharmacologically active compounds tend to be psychomotor stimulants, possessing sympathomimetic, antifatique, and reinforcing effects in humans. Derivatives of amphetamine with side chain substitutions tend to be mainly psychomotor stimulants or anorectics; derivatives with terminal amine substitutions have psychomotor stimulant effects at low doses and hallucinogenic activity at higher doses. Comparisons of the compounds tested for neurotoxic activity makes it clear that, as with stimulant effects, side-chain substitution can yield varying degrees of neurotoxic activity. In fact, compounds with single substitutions in any of the possible side-chain positions—α-carbon, β-carbon, or terminal nitrogen—have exhibited neurotoxic potential.

Amphetamine derivatives with aromatic ring substitutions are usually weak stimulants, but some possess hallucinogenic activity and therefore also generally have abuse potential.[9] Certain alkyloxy amphetamine derivatives have been examined for their ability to produce hallucinations in humans.[5] Compounds such as 2,5-dimethoxy-phenylisopropylamine (DMA), 2,5-dimethoxy-4-methylphenylisopropylamine (DOM), 3,4,5-trimethoxyamphetamine all tend to exhibit a profile of sensory, behavioral and physiological effects that are similar to lysergic acid LSD.[5,9,10] Amphetamine derivatives with methylenedioxy substitutions on the phenyl ring such as MDA or MDMA have both hallucinogenic and stimulant actions at relatively low doses[11] and may represent a novel class of hallucinogen. With the exception of the methylenedioxy and ring-halogenated amphetamine derivatives which are potent 5-HT neurotoxins, long-lasting effects of ring-substituted amphetamines have not been extensively investigated.

NEUROTOXICITY OF AMPHETAMINE ANALOGS

Side Chain–substituted Analogs

MA and amphetamine are toxic to certain monoamine-containing fibers in the central nervous system. MA is toxic to both DA- and 5-HT-containing nerve terminals in several regions of the brain where these terminal fields are located. MA reduces DA for eight weeks and longer in the olfactory tubercle, the frontal cortex, the septum, the striatum and the accumbens; DA in the brainstem and the hypothalamus is not affected by toxic dosing regimes of amphetamine. MA is toxic to 5-HT-containing cells in the olfactory tubercles, the cerebral cortex, striatum, hippocampus, accumbens, and hypothalamus. Levels of serotonin in the brain stem are not reduced by MA. MA-induced toxicity is dependent on both the size of the dose and the length of time over which it is administered. A single injection of 100 mg/kg can produce neurotoxicity and continuous infusion of as little as 2 mg/kg for 3 days can also produce neurotoxicity. With regard to magnitude or extent of neurotoxicity, amphetamine has not been as extensively studied as MA, but, it is generally observed that the extent of DA toxicity caused by amphetamine is greater than 5-HT toxicity. This relationship is reversed for most if not all of the other compounds which have been tested.

A number of N-alkyl amphetamine derivatives have been reported to possess neurotoxic activity, primarily to 5-HT neurons (see TABLES 1 and 2 for structures): MA, N-N-dimethylamphetamine (N,N-DMA),[12] benzphetamine,[13] MDA, MDMA,[14,15] and N-ethyl-MDA (MDE).[16] Considering potency differences between either amphetamine, N,N-DMA and MA, or between MDA, MDMA, and MDE, it appears that N-substitutions larger than a single methyl group generally reduce neurotoxic activity. Corresponding differences in psychomotor stimulant activity among N-alkylated amphetamine derivatives have been noted previously.[3,17,18] An apparent exception to this relationship is benzphetamine (N-benzyl, N-methyl amphetamine) which causes long-term depletions of DA and 5-HT,[13] but is approximately 10-fold less potent than amphetamine as a locomotor stimulant.[17] In this case, however, it is possible that neurotoxic effects are due to N-dealkylation, yielding amphetamine or methamphetamine. It must be considered that N-dealkylation could play an important role in neurotoxic effects, particularly since high dosage regimens are often required to demonstrate long-lasting effects.

The α-methyl group is another possible substitution point. One such substituted amphetamine available clinically is the anorectic phentermine (α,α, dimethyl-phenyl-ethylamine) and some recent data indicate that it may be neurotoxic.[13] Following repeated administration, phentermine was shown to produce long-lasting depletions of both DA and 5-HT in brain regions previously shown to be sensitive to the neurotoxic

TABLE 1. Side Chain Derivatives of Amphetamine

Drug	β	α	R₁	R₂
AMPH	–	–	–	–
MA	–	–	–	CH_3
N,N-DMA	–	–	CH_3	CH_3
Benzphetamine	–	–	C_6H_5	CH_3
PPA	OH	–	–	–
Cathinone	=O	–	–	–
Diethylpropion	=O	–	CH_2CH_3	CH_2CH_3
Phentermine	–	CH_3	–	–

effects of MA and a variety of congeners.[19] The finding that doses of phentermine as low as 5-fold higher than behaviorally active doses caused long-term decreases of DA and 5-HT suggests that this compound may possess significant neurotoxic liability. The ability of phentermine to cause long-lasting depletions of DA and 5-HT is consistent with several previous observations. Firstly, it has been suggested previously that the 4-chloro analog, chlorphentermine, is neurotoxic.[20] Since ring-halogenated compounds exhibit much greater potency relative to amphetamine,[21] it is not unexpected

TABLE 2. Alkyl and Alkyloxy Derivatives of Methylenedioxyamphetamine

Drug	R₁	R₂	α	N
MDA	–	–	–	–
MDMA	–	–	–	CH_3
MDE	–	–	–	CH_2CH_3
MBDB	–	–	CH_2CH_3	–
MMDA	OCH_3	–	–	–
MMDA-2	–	OCH_3	–	–

that phentermine itself would possess some degree of neurotoxic activity. Secondly, other α-substituted PIA homologs such as the α-ethyl analogs of MDMA[22] (MBDB) and *para*-chloroamphetamine (*p*-CA)[23] have recently been demonstrated to have long-lasting effects on DA and/or 5-HT neurons in the rat. Thus a number of studies confirm the idea that relatively simple side-chain substituted amphetamine analogs are likely to retain neurotoxic activity.

Several β-substituted amphetamines-phenylpropanolamine (PPA), cathinone, and diethylpropion-have been tested for possible neurotoxic effects. In a previous study conducted in this laboratory, phenylpropanolamine showed no toxic effects on DA or 5-HT in any of the doses tested, but at the higher doses caused a 20% depletion of NE in the cerebral cortex of rats,[24] whereas cathinone was demonstrated to cause long-term decreases in DA levels and *in vitro* DA reuptake.[25] We have recently tested diethylpropion, the N,N-diethyl derivative of cathinone, and found that it also causes long-term depletions of 5-HT (Kleven *et al.*, unpublished data), a finding also consistent with N-substitutions discussed above.

Lastly in terms of side-chain modifications, phenethylamine derivatives in which the aminoalkyl side chain is cyclized retain significant stimulant and/or anorectic activity.[3] We have recently reported that two phenylmorpholine derivatives of amphetamine, phenmetrazine and phendimetrazine (FIG. 1) apparently lack neurotoxic activity.[13] Cyclization of the side chain may not entirely explain the lack of toxicity since the oxazoline homolog, 4-methyl-aminorex has been reported to possess neurotoxic activity.[26] On the other hand, several other cyclized amphetamine derivatives such as methylphenidate (α-phenyl-2-piperidineacetic acid) and pemoline (2-amino-5-phenyl-4(5H)-oxazolone) also do not appear to have neurotoxic activity.[27-29] Unlike both of these latter compounds, phenmetrazine and 4-methyl-aminorex can be considered conformationally restricted N-monoalkyl PIAs,[30] whereas phendimetrazine is a N-dialkyl PIA derivative. As noted above, a number of N-monoalkyl derivatives tested thus far show some toxic effects, although compounds with larger alkyl

phenmetrazine   **pemoline**

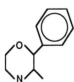

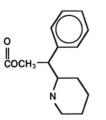

methylphenidate   **α -methyl aminorex**

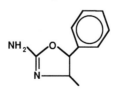

FIGURE 1. Structures of cyclized amphetamine derivatives.

groups or dialkyl derivatives such as N,N-DMA are generally less effective than amphetamine. On the basis of these observations, one might expect that phenmetrazine would also be neurotoxic, yet may not be as potent as amphetamine.

It is interesting that the β-keto amphetamine derivative, cathinone possesses neurotoxic activity whereas the β-hydroxy derivative, PPA apparently does not.[24,25] Although this is only a single substitution, it can result in substantial alteration of conformation and interactions *in vivo*. Among a number of possibilities, neurotoxic actions could be retained due to stabilization of the β-carbon due to side chain oxidation in cathinone. Alternatively, the β-hydroxy group of PPA may facilitate hydrogen bonding or increase polarity, therefore reducing interactions at monoamine high affinity reuptake sites. Although only a handful of compounds have been screened for neurotoxic activity it is already apparent that much can be gained in terms of SAR by further testing more amphetamine analogs. Nonetheless, it is clear from the various compounds tested so far that minimal changes of the side-chain can substantially alter neurotoxic activity.

Ring-substituted Analogs

Early work conducted by Sanders-Bush *et al.*[31,32] and Fuller *et al.*[21,33] demonstrated that 4-chloroamphetamine (*p*-CA) is a potent and selective 5-HT neurotoxin. A large series of ring-halogenated analogs has been examined for the ability to cause long-term depletions of 5-HT and the SAR among these compounds is discussed in an excellent review by Fuller.[34] The remaining mono-chloro substituted amphetamines, *ortho*- and *meta*-chloroamphetamine, are relatively less toxic,[21] a finding attributed in the rat to rapid *para*-hydroxylation.[34] However, when metabolism is reduced by cotreatment with iprindole or desmethylimipramine, *meta*- but not *ortho*-chloroamphetamine depletes 5-HT,[34] suggesting that substitution in the *ortho* position reduces neurotoxicity. At least one *meta*-substituted amphetamine, norfenfluramine (*m*-trifluoromethyl-phenylisopropylamine) and its N-ethyl analog, fenfluramine have been demonstrated to have long-term effects consistent with neurotoxic activity.[35–37] It can be inferred from these findings that the presence of electron withdrawing substituents such as halogens positioned away from the side chain yields substantial 5-HT neurotoxic activity.

It was reported in 1985 that the 3,4-methylenedioxyamphetamine (MDA) was neurotoxic.[38] It was subsequently discovered that both the N-methyl and N-ethyl derivatives of MDA are also neurotoxic,[14,15,39,40] consistent with the effects of N-alkyl substitutions discussed previously. We recently compared the long-lasting effects of two ring monomethoxy derivatives of 3,4-MDA, MMDA and MMDA-2, which differ only in the position of the methoxy group. MMDA has a methoxy group in the *meta* position, whereas MMDA-2 has the group in the *ortho* position. It was shown that MMDA, but not MMDA-2, caused long-lasting depletions of 5-HT similar to those caused by MDA.[41] These results have several implications. Firstly, it is clear that ring methoxy groups do not interfere with neurotoxicity, a finding also supported by recent data showing that the monomethoxy amphetamine derivative, PMA may possess 5-HT neurotoxic actions.[42] Secondly, taken together with a variety of other findings for other amphetamine analogs, these results are consistent with the idea that *ortho* substituents may abolish neurotoxic activity.

We recently examined several dimethoxy amphetamine analogs: 2,5-dimethoxy-

TABLE 3. Alkyl and Alkyloxy Derivatives of Amphetamine

Drug	R_1	R_2	R_3
PMA	–	4-OCH_3	–
DMA	OCH	–	OCH_3
DOM	OCH_3	CH_3	OCH_3
DOET	OCH_3	CH_2CH_3	OCH_3

substituted amphetamine (2,5-DMA) and the 4-methyl and 4-ethyl (DOM and DOET, respectively, TABLE 3) for their ability to cause long-lasting depletions of CNS monoamines.[42] In contrast to that seen with MMDA and PMA, none of the 2,5-dimethoxy analogs had long-lasting effects on DA or 5-HT levels in rat brain. Since all of these compounds have an *ortho* methoxy group, it is possible that this is the reason for the lack of neurotoxic activity. Although more comparisons, particularly of the mono-methoxy-amphetamine series (PMA, MMA, and OMA) should be made before this hypothesis can be supported, the findings with MMDA and MMDA-2, as well as the SAR reported previously for mono-chloroamphetamine derivatives,[34] suggest that *ortho* substituents interfere with neurotoxic activity. In the case of methoxy substitutions, it is possible either that ionic bonding or steric hindrance between the *ortho* methoxy group and the amine side chain introduces conformational restriction. It has been noted previously regarding hallucinogenic amphetamine analogs that such stabilization of the side chain by ring formation with an *ortho* methoxy group confers structural similarity to LSD.[43] The observation that rigid analogs of *p*-chloroamphetamine (6-chloro-2-aminotetralin)[44] and MDA (5,6-methylenedioxy-2-aminoindan)[45] do not have long-lasting effects on monoamines further suggests that free rotation about the side chain carbon-carbon bond is a requirement for neurotoxic activity.

BEHAVIORAL PHARMACOLOGY OF AMPHETAMINE ANALOGS: RELATIONSHIPS AMONG NEUROTOXIC ANALOGS

Up to this point we have been discussing structural features which may be related to the ability of amphetamine analogs to exert neurotoxic actions. It will now be considered that common behavioral or neurochemical effects can also be related to these same structural features. It is well known that amphetamine and methamphetamine are potent, efficacious psychomotor stimulants and comprehensive reviews of SAR among the behavioral effects of related psychoactive amphetamine analogs have been presented previously.[3,5,9,46] For the purposes of this paper, we will consider only those compounds which have been tested for neurotoxic activity. This level of analysis may be of some value in predicting such activity in amphetamine analogs with a similar profile of behavioral actions.

Many of the compounds which have demonstrated neurotoxic effects – with the important exceptions of fenfluramine and p-CA – are more or less effective locomotor stimulants (see ref. 3). On the other hand, not all stimulants possess neurotoxic actions, since many of the cyclized phenethylamine derivatives which have been tested for neurotoxicity-pemoline, methylphenidate, phenmetrazine, phendimetrazine, and 4-methyl-aminorex[47] are psychomotor stimulants, but only 4-methyl-aminorex has been demonstrated to have neurotoxic effects. Nonetheless, there are potency differences between analogs consistent with observed neurotoxic effects. It has been noted previously that, although β-keto derivatives such as cathinone show reduced potency as stimulants relative to amphetamine, β-hydroxy derivatives such as PPA are extremely weak stimulants.[17] Among the ring-monomethoxy derivatives, PMA has predominantly amphetamine-like activity, demonstrated using drug discrimination[9] and physiological measures,[48] whereas MMA and OMA are relatively less potent in comparison to PMA.[9,17]

Racemic 3,4-MDA and 3,4-MDMA substitute for the amphetamine discriminative stimulus in both rats and monkeys[9,49,50] indicating that they could have CNS mechanisms in common with amphetamine. Comparisons of the methoxy derivatives of MDA and the 2,5 DMA analogs also reveal a distinct behavioral profile associated with neurotoxicity. MMDA has also been reported to be amphetamine-like.[10,48] However, MMDA-2 substitutes completely for the DOM discriminative stimulus, indicating that it has hallucinogenic activity,[9] although it was not tested for amphetamine substitution. The hallucinogen 2,5-DMA produces only partial generalization to the discriminative stimulus effects of amphetamine in rats,[9] whereas it has been shown that 2-5-DMA is a direct agonist of 5-HT receptors.[51]

Taken together, the data indicate that amphetamine derivatives which possess a high degree of stimulant activity (e.g., PMA and MMDA) are likely to also have neurotoxic actions, whereas drugs which are primarily hallucinogens are not likely to have amphetamine-like neurotoxic effects. It must be noted, however, that stimulant activity is necessary but not sufficient to predict neurotoxicity since several compounds with this behavioral profile such as phenmetrazine and methylphenidate are apparently not toxic to CNS monoamine neurons.

NEUROPHARMACOLOGICAL EFFECTS OF AMPHETAMINE ANALOGS: RELATIONSHIP TO NEUROTOXICITY

There is a reasonable correspondence between neurotoxicity and the ability of amphetamine analogs to cause monoamine release. Similar to effects of MA, its neurotoxic analogs, PMA, MDMA, MDA have all been shown to be potent releasers of both DA and 5-HT.[40,52,53] PMA is comparatively more potent than amphetamine as a 5-HT releasing agent in vivo,[51] consistent with its MA-like, rather than amphetamine-like neurotoxic effects. In contrast, the non-neurotoxic amphetamine analog 2,5-DMA is a comparatively weak DA- or 5-HT-releasing agent.[54-56] Therefore, the ability of ring-substituted amphetamines to cause long-lasting depletions of monoamines is consistent with release of monoamines.

In summary, the available data show that compounds with ring methoxy substitutions are generally less potent neurotoxins in comparison to amphetamine itself. That this may be reflected in other pharmacological measures has implications for the screening of potential amphetamine-like neurotoxins. The current data suggest further that the ability of such compounds to cause release of DA and/or 5-HT is directly correlated with subsequent stimulant activity as well as neurotoxic activity. Ring substituted analogs such as the 2,5-dimethoxy-substituted amphetamines have a substantially reduced potential to cause long-lasting monoamine depletions. The results also suggest that conformational restriction due to substitution in the *ortho* position may abolish neurotoxic activity. Finally, since many amphetamine derivatives may be readily metabolized, the neurotoxic potential of primary metabolites must also be considered. Although studies to date have provided limited information, particularly with regard to α and β-carbon and ring substitutions, much remains to be understood about structure activity relationships and long-lasting neurochemical effects.

REFERENCES

1. SEIDEN, L. S. & G. A. RICAURTE. 1987. *In* Psychopharmacology: The Third Generation of Progress. H. Y. Meltzer, Ed.: 359–366. Raven Press. New York.
2. STONE, D. M., G. R. HANSON & J. W. GIBB. 1987. Neuropharmacology **26**: 1657–1661.
3. BIEL, J. H. & B. A. BOPP. 1978. *In* Stimulants. L. L. Iversen, S. D. Iversen & S. H. Snyder, Eds.: 1–39. Plenum Press. New York.
4. ANGRIST, B. & A. SUDILOVSKY. 1978. *In* Stimulants. L. L. Iversen, S. D. Iversen & S. H. Snyder, Eds.: 99–165. Plenum Press. New York.
5. SHULGIN, A. T. 1978. *In* Handbook of Psychopharmacology. L. L. Iversen, S. D. Iversen & S. H. Snyder, Eds.: 243–333. Plenum Press. New York.
6. LEWANDER, T. 1978. *In* Central Mechanisms of Anorectic Drugs. S. Garattini & R. Samanin, Eds. 343–356. Raven Press. New York.
7. LEWANDER, T. 1977. *In* Drug Addiction II. W. R. Martin, Eds.: 33. Springer Verlag. New York.
8. MOORE, K. E. 1978. *In* Handbook of Psychopharmacology: Stimulants. I. L. L. Iversen, S. D. Iversen & S. H. Snyder, Eds.: 41–98. Plenum Press. New York.
9. GLENNON, R. A. 1986. Drug Alcohol Depend. **17**: 119–134.
10. MARTIN, W. R., D. B. VAUPEL, M. NOZAKI & L. D. BRIGHT. 1978. Drug Alcohol Depend. **3**: 113–123.
11. CLIMKO, R. P., H. ROEHRICH, D. R. SWEENEY & J. AL-RAZI. 1986. Int. J. Psychiatry Med. **16**: 359–372.
12. RICAURTE, G. A., L. E. DELANNEY, I. IRWIN, J. M. WITKIN, J. L. KATZ & J. W. LANGSTON. 1989. Brain Res. **490**: 301–306.
13. KLEVEN, M. S., W. L. WOOLVERTON & L. S. SEIDEN. 1991. Soc. Neurosci. Abs. **17**: 1488.
14. COMMINS, D. L., G. VOSMER, R. M. VIRUS, W. L. WOOLVERTON, C. R. SCHUSTER & L. S. SEIDEN. 1987. J. Pharmacol. Exp. Ther. **241**: 338–345.
15. STONE, D. M., D. C. STAHL, G. R. HANSON & J. W. GIBB. 1986. Eur. J. Pharmacol. **128**: 41–48.
16. STONE, D. M., M. JOHNSON, G. R. HANSON & J. W. GIBB. 1987. Eur. J. Pharmacol. **134**: 245–248.
17. VAN DER SCHOOT, J. B., E. J. ARIENS, J. M. VAN ROSSUM & J. A. HURKMANS. 1961. Arzneim-Forschung **9**: 902–907.
18. WOOLVERTON, W. L., G. SHYBUT & C. E. JOHANSON. 1980. Pharmacol. Biochem. Behav. **13**: 869–876.
19. SEIDEN, L. S., D. L. COMMINS, G. VOSMER, K. AXT & G. MAREK. 1988. *In* The Mesocorticolimbic Dopamine System. P. W. Kalivas & C. B. Nemeroff, Eds. Ann. NY Acad. Sci. **537**: 161–172.
20. ADACHI, M., L. SCHNECK & B. W. VOLK. 1977. *In* Neurotoxicology. L. Roizin, S. Hiraki & N. Grcevic, Eds.: 497–501. Raven Press. New York.
21. HARVEY, J. A., S. E. MCMASTER & R. W. FULLER. 1977. J. Pharmacol. Exp. Ther. **202**: 581–589.

22. JOHNSON, M. P. & D. E. NICHOLS. 1989. Pharmacol. Biochem. Behav. **33:** 105–108.
23. JOHNSON, M. P., X. HUANG, R. OBERLENDER, J. F. NASH & D. E. NICHOLS. 1990. Eur. J. Pharmacol. **191:** 1–10.
24. WOOLVERTON, W. L., C. E. JOHANSON, D.-G. R., S. ELLIS, L. S. SEIDEN & C. R. SCHUSTER. 1986. J. Pharmacol. Exp. Ther. **237:** 926–930.
25. WAGNER, G. C., K. PRESTON, G. A. RICAURTE, C. R. SCHUSTER & L. S. SEIDEN. 1982. Drug Alcohol Depend. **9:** 279–284.
26. BUNKER, C. F., M. JOHNSON, J. W. GIBB, L. G. BUSH & G. R. HANSON. 1990. Eur. J. Pharmacol. **180:** 103–111.
27. WAGNER, G. C., G. A. RICAURTE, C. E. JOHANSON, C. R. SCHUSTER & L. S. SEIDEN. 1980. Neurology **20:** 547–550.
28. ZACZEK, R., G. BATTAGLIA, J. F. CONTRERA, S. CULP & E. B. DESOUZA. 1989. Tox. Appl. Pharmacol. **100:** 227–233.
29. MOLINA, V. A. & O. A. ORSINGHER. 1981. Arch. Int. Pharmacodyn. Ther. **251:** 66.
30. GLENNON, R. A., M. YOUSIF, N. NAIMAN & P. KALIX. 1987. Pharmacol. Biochem. Behav. **26:** 547–551.
31. SANDERS-BUSH, E., J. A. BUSHING & F. SULSER. 1975. J. Pharmacol. Exp. Ther. **192:** 33–41.
32. SANDERS-BUSH, E., J. BUSHING & F. SULSER. 1972. Eur. J. Pharmacol. **20:** 385–388.
33. FULLER, R. W., C. W. HINES & K. W. PERRY. 1974. Brain Res. **82:** 383–385.
34. FULLER, R. W. 1978. *In* Serotonin Neurotoxins. J. H. Jacoby & L. D. Lytle, Eds. Ann. NY Acad. Sci. **305:** 147–159.
35. STERANKA, L. R. & E. SANDERS-BUSH. 1979. Neuropharmacology **18:** 895–903.
36. SCHUSTER, C. R., M. LEWIS & L. S. SEIDEN. 1986. Psychopharmacol. Bull. **22:** 148–151.
37. JOHNSON, M. P. & D. E. NICHOLS. 1990. Pharmacol. Biochem. Behav. **36:** 105–109.
38. RICAURTE, G. A., G. BRYAN, L. STRAUSS, L. S. SEIDEN & C. R. SCHUSTER. 1985. Science **229:** 986–988.
39. RICAURTE, G. A., K. F. FINNEGAN, D. E. NICHOLS, L. E. DELANNEY, I. IRWIN & J. W. LANGSTON. 1987. Eur. J. Pharmacol. **137:** 265–268.
40. JOHNSON, M. P., A. J. HOFFMAN & D. E. NICHOLS. 1986. Eur. J. Pharmacol. **132:** 269–276.
41. FARFEL, G. M., M. S. KLEVEN, W. L. WOOLVERTON & L. S. SEIDEN. 1989. Fed. Am. Soc. Exp. Biol. J. A1036.
42. KLEVEN, M. S., G. M. FARFEL, W. L. WOOLVERTON & L. S. SEIDEN. 1990. Soc. Neurosci. Abs. **16:** 13.
43. SNYDER, S. H. & E. RICHELSON. 1968. *In* Psychopharmacology: A Review of Progress 1957–1967. D. H. Efron, Ed.: 1199–1210. U.S. Government Printing Office. Washington, D.C.
44. FULLER, R. W., K. W. PERRY, J. C. BAKER & B. B. MOLLOY. 1974. Arch. Int. Pharmacodyn. **212:** 141–153.
45. NICHOLS, D. E., W. K. BREWSTER, M. P. JOHNSON, R. OBERLENDER & R. M. RIGGS. 1990. J. Med. Chem. **33:** 703–710.
46. GLENNON, R. A. 1987. *In* Psychopharmacology: The Third Generation of Progress. H. Y. Meltzer, Ed.: 1627–1634. Raven Press. New York.
47. GLENNON, R. A. & B. MISENHEIMER. 1990. Pharmacol. Biochem. Behav. **35:** 517–521.
48. NOZAKI, M., D. B. VAUPEL, L. D. BRIGHT & W. R. MARTIN. 1978. Drug Alcohol Depend. **3:** 153–163.
49. OBERLENDER, R. & D. E. NICHOLS. 1988. Psychopharmacology **95:** 71–76.
50. KAMIEN, J. B., C. E. JOHANSON, C. R. SCHUSTER & W. L. WOOLVERTON. 1986. Drug Alcohol Depend. **18:** 139–147.
51. TSENG, L., K. M. MENON & H. H. LOH. 1976. J. Pharmacol. Exp. Ther. **197:** 263–271.
52. NICHOLS, D. E., D. H. LLODY, A. J. HOFFMAN, M. B. NICHOLS & G. K. W. YIM. 1982. J. Med. Chem. **25:** 530–535.
53. SCHMIDT, C. J., J. A. LEVIN & W. LOVENBERG. 1987. Biochem. Pharmacol. **36:** 747–755.
54. VRBANAC, J. J., H. A. TILSON, K. E. MOORE & R. H. RECH. 1975. Pharmacol. Biochem. Behav. **3:** 57–64.
55. ANDÉN, N.-E., H. CORRODI, K. FUXI & J. L. MEEK. 1974. Eur. J. Pharmacol. **25:** 176–184.
56. TSENG, L.-F. 1978. Naunyn-Schmiedeberg's Arch. Pharmacol. **304:** 101–105.

Genetic Determinants of Ethanol Reinforcement[a]

JOHN C. CRABBE,[b,c,d,e] TAMARA J. PHILLIPS,[b,c]
CHRIS L. CUNNINGHAM,[c]
AND JOHN K. BELKNAP[b,c]

[b]Research Service (151 W)
Department of Veterans Affairs Medical Center
3710 S.W. U.S. Veterans Hospital Road
Portland, Oregon 97201

[c]Department of Medical Psychology (L-470)
[d]Department of Pharmacology
Oregon Health Sciences University
3181 S.W. Sam Jackson Park Road
Portland, Oregon 97201

There are a number of strategies available to the investigator interested in determining the genetic basis for drug responsiveness. Many such methods are primarily utilized to demonstrate the existence of such control. In virtually all cases, genetic control is found to be present: thus, its existence may safely be assumed. Lately, pharmacogenetic strategies have been directed toward more immediately useful goals, including the development of genetic animal models, and the identification of specific genes important in the determination of drug responses.

This paper will discuss some of the many behaviors asserted to be indicative of drug reinforcement. Using these traits, the more powerful pharmacogenetic methods will be reviewed. Since pharmacogenetic studies of ethanol-related responses have been far more numerous than those for other drugs, the examples discussed will be drawn from the ethanol literature.

INDICES OF DRUG REINFORCEMENT

Several behavioral endpoints have been suggested as useful indicators of the reinforcing efficacy of psychoactive drugs.[1] Many, but not all, of these have been employed to study genetic determinants of ethanol reinforcement in rodents. In a recent review, we discussed pharmacogenetic studies examining: conditioned place preference for ethanol-associated locations; taste aversion for novel flavors conditioned by ethanol in-

[a] This research was supported by grants from the Department of Veterans Affairs, and PHS Grants AA06243, AA06498, and AA08621, and NIDA Contract 271-90-7405.
[e] Address all correspondence to Dr. Crabbe at the Veterans Center.

jection; locomotor stimulation by ethanol, and the development of sensitization to this response with chronic administration; and oral preference for and acceptance of ethanol solutions.[2] While ethanol in general appears not to be as potent a reinforcer for rodents as other abused drugs, there is a substantial pharmacogenetic literature evidencing genetic contributions to individual differences in sensitivity to ethanol reinforcement.

PHARMACOGENETIC METHODS

Several pharmacogenetic methods have been brought to bear on the question of ethanol's reinforcing effects. Perhaps the oldest technique in the arsenal of the pharmacogeneticist is *selective breeding*. By mating sensitive animals with each other generation after generation, and similarly intermating insensitive animals, selected lines have been created which differ widely in sensitivity to most drugs of abuse, including ethanol, opiates, benzodiazepines, cocaine, and nicotine.[3] Since selected lines differ predominantly in genes which are influential in determining the selected response, other differences between the lines (*e.g.*, neurochemical or pharmacological) can offer clues to drug mechanisms. A second method frequently employed is the examination of several *inbred strains*. Differences among the many available inbred strains of mice or rats are indicative of genetic influence, and can be used to establish genetic action on multiple drug-related traits. A third group of methods focuses on the analysis of *single genes*. Mutants have been studied for drug sensitivity, and where the genes bearing such mutants have known chromosomal locations, such studies have offered preliminary links reaching from the genome to behavior. The most recent innovations in pharmacogenetic research have combined the latter two methods with the explicit goal of gene mapping. These strategies combine mapping with the ability to develop genetic characterizations of individual mouse strains through molecular biological techniques such as identification of restriction fragment length polymorphisms. Examples of each of these methods will be discussed.

STUDIES WITH SELECTED LINES

We have used the technique of selective breeding to develop the Withdrawal Seizure Prone (WSP) line of mice, which displays genetic susceptibility to severe handling-induced convulsions after three days of chronic exposure to ethanol vapor. In parallel, the Withdrawal Seizure Resistant (WSR) line has been developed to display minimal convulsions.[4] The WSP line has become so sensitive to ethanol withdrawal that a rebound elevation of handling convulsions over baseline values can be seen 6–10 h after an acute injection of 4 g/kg ethanol.[5] This acute withdrawal reaction is also seen after injection of several other central nervous system depressants, which suggests common genetic control of the neurobiological mechanisms underlying withdrawal hyperexcitability.[6] We have recently found that WSP (but not WSR) mice given N-methyl-D-aspartate injections during acute ethanol withdrawal show further exacerbations of handling-induced convulsion severity (see also ref. 7), suggesting that excitatory amino acid systems may exert important influences on drug withdrawal states (see FIG. 1). In collaboration with Dr. Aaron Janowsky, we are currently using the technique of genetic selection to develop mouse lines which differ in MK-801 binding in brain. These

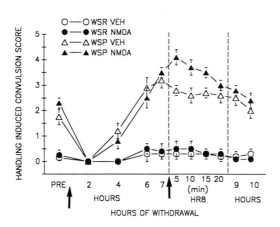

FIGURE 1. Effects of *N*-methyl-D-aspartate on handling induced convulsions in Withdrawal Seizure Prone (WSP) and Resistant (WSR) mice. VEH = vehicle, NMDA = 30 mg/kg NMDA. At the time of the first arrow, all mice were injected ip with 4 g/kg ethanol. Handling-induced convulsions were scored at hours 2, 4, 6, and 7. At the second arrow (hour 8) mice were injected with VEH (*open symbols*) or NMDA (*filled symbols*) and scored 5, 10, 15, and 20 min later, and again at hours 9 and 10. Mean ± SE shown where SE exceeds symbol size.

animals could prove to be extremely useful in exploring the relationships between brain excitatory amino acid function and drug-related traits.

In a recent study, WSP and WSR mice were tested for sensitivity to ethanol in a place-conditioning procedure. The apparatus was a chamber with two different interchangeable floor textures (hole and grid). After one habituation session in which mice were given saline and exposed in the apparatus to a neutral (paper) floor for 5 min, 8 conditioning trials were given. On alternate days, the mice were exposed for 5 min after injection to either the grid floor or the hole floor. An injection of 2 g/kg ethanol was consistently paired with one floor type, and saline with the other. Separate groups were counterbalanced for specific pairing. On the next day (test day), a 45-min preference test was given after saline injection. The floor of the apparatus was half grid and half hole on this trial. Mean ± SE seconds/minute spent on the grid floor side during the preference test were analyzed by ANOVA.

Results are given in TABLE 1. Mice who experienced ethanol on the grid floor during training spent significantly more time on the grid floor on the test day than mice who experienced saline on the grid floor ($F_{1,44}$ = 6.4, p < .05), indicating a conditioned place preference. There was no significant overall difference between selected lines (F < 1), but there was a significant Line x Conditioning Group interaction ($F_{1,44}$ = 5.2, p < .05). This occurred because WSP mice showed conditioned preference for the ethanol-associated floor ($F_{1,22}$ = 9.6, p < .01), while WSR mice did not (F < 1). These results suggest that mice selectively bred for severe withdrawal seizures show greater sensitivity to the rewarding effects of ethanol in the place-conditioning paradigm. *Ipso facto*, genes which determine ethanol withdrawal severity appear to be involved in the rewarding effects of ethanol.

In another selective breeding project, we have developed lines of mice sensitive (FAST) or resistant (SLOW) to the locomotor stimulant effects of ethanol, in hopes that a genetic animal model based on this behavioral response might shed light on ethanol's reinforcing properties.[8] Mice are tested for a 4-min period in an open field on two consecutive days, first 2–6 min after injection of 2.0 g/kg ethanol, and then, during this same time period, after saline injection. After 17 selected generations, the FAST and SLOW lines had diverged considerably in their acute stimulant response.[9]

TABLE 1. Mean Seconds per Minute (± SE) Spent on Grid Floor during 45-Minute Preference Test

Conditioning Group	Selected Line	
	WSP	WSR
Ethanol on grid floor	38.0 ± 3.2[a]	33.8 ± 2.1
Saline on grid floor	25.6 ± 2.4	33.2 ± 2.5

[a] $p < .01$ for comparison with WSP-Saline Group.

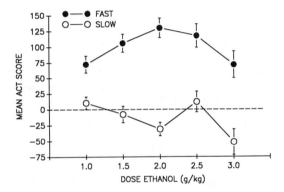

FIGURE 2. Locomotor activity dose-response curves (ACT = difference between ethanol and saline scores) for FAST (*filled circles*) and SLOW (*open circles*) mice given ethanol on Day 1 and saline on Day 2 at the indicated doses, 2 min before a 4-min test. Lines differ significantly ($p < .01$) at all doses. (Data adapted from reference 8).

Substantial differences in sensitivity can be seen across a range of low to moderate ethanol doses (see FIG. 2). When these mice are chronically administered ethanol, rather than developing tolerance, their locomotor responses show a progressive enhancement, characterized as sensitization.[10] They also show genetic differences (FAST > SLOW) in acute sensitivity to other alcohols and pentobarbital, but not to *d*-amphetamine or caffeine,[11] or to MK-801 (unpublished).

Using similar techniques, we have bred COLD and HOT mice to be sensitive or insensitive, respectively, to acute ethanol hypothermia. These mice were tested in three tasks purported to assess ethanol's hedonic properties: place conditioning, taste conditioning, and preference drinking.[12] HOT mice were more sensitive than COLD mice to develop both conditioned preference for ethanol-associated cues (place conditioning) and conditioned aversion for ethanol-paired flavor cues (taste aversion). They also drank less ethanol solution than COLD mice. In general, HOT mice seem to be more sensitive to ethanol-associated stimuli than COLD mice, suggesting that these three tasks all may assess the same motivational effects of ethanol.[12]

Studies such as these are representative of our beginning attempts to use the powerful genetic method of selective breeding to identify neurochemical and neuropharmacological substrates of drug reinforcement. Studies with other selected lines directed toward this goal are also appearing with greater frequency.[2] For example, rats selected for oral preference have been shown to self-administer ethanol by intragastric infusion.[13] Future use of selected lines may be expected to increase.

STUDIES WITH INBRED STRAINS

Among the earliest systematic pharmacogenetic studies were the pioneering observations of McClearn and Rodgers that mice from a number of highly inbred (therefore,
genetically distinct) strains showed marked differences in their propensity to drink
ethanol/tap water solutions. Some strains have been consistently characterized since
the first published report[14] as alcohol preferrers (C57BL/6) while others are alcohol
avoiders (DBA/2 and BALB/c). These traits are consistently expressed in a number of
different behavioral paradigms. For example, McClearn[15] showed that ethanol acceptance under thirst motivation, when measured as intake during a single day of preference testing, showed a strain distribution pattern that was highly correlated with
strain preferences expressed after weeks of preference drinking. We measured alcohol
acceptance in a larger panel consisting of 19 inbred strains.[16] The general correspondence of results in these three studies demonstrates a uniquely powerful feature of
working with inbred strains: since inbred genotypes are genetically fixed, work performed in different laboratories, studying the same strains, may be directly compared,
even across a time spanning more than 30 years. While there are some factors limiting
the generalizability of results with inbred strains,[17] this method will be more frequently employed in the future in the context of gene mapping, discussed in the last
section of this paper.

SINGLE-GENE METHODS

As the studies mentioned thus far would seem to indicate, demonstrating genetic
influence on a drug-related trait of interest is generally an easy task. Far more difficult
is the discovery of *which* genes may be important, and what their function may be.
The most straightforward approach to identifying individual genes of importance is
to take advantage of naturally occurring mutations where they affect a trait of interest.
Rats of the Brattleboro strain are heterozygous ($+/di$) or homozygous recessive (di/di)
at a locus which results in a neurophysin sequence with a single deletion.[18] In the
homozygotes, the abnormal neurophysin results in a total failure to synthesize a functional brain or pituitary vasopressin,[19] and the animals display a marked diabetes insipidus.[20] When Brattleboro rats were offered the choice between 2.2% ethanol in tap
water and tap water for 8 days, the di/di animals showed the expected polydipsia compared to $di/+$ heterozygotes with normal fluid intake.[21] However, they showed a significantly reduced preference for ethanol (see TABLE 2). Since vasopressin was hypothesized to regulate ethanol responding, we attempted to restore preference independent
of the diabetes insipidus by administering des-9-Glycinamide-[Arginine[8]] vasopressin
(DGAVP), a peptide analog of vasopressin with markedly reduced antidiuretic effects.
DGAVP restored normal levels of preference for ethanol: however, any doses of
DGAVP which restored preference also had antidiuretic effects, and water intake was
also reduced.

To resolve this difficulty, we turned to another available mutant, the oligosyndac-
tylic mouse ($Os/+$: the homozygous Os/Os condition is lethal). These animals have a
mild to severe diabetes insipidus depending upon presence of one or more recessive
modifiers.[22] The diabetes is caused by reduced kidney size and numbers of glomeruli;
compensatory hypertrophy of the nephrons cannot restore normal kidney function.[23] Furthermore, these mice have normal or elevated hypothalamic vasopressin

TABLE 2. Effects of DGAVP on Fluid Intake and Ethanol Preference in Brattleboro Rats[a]

Genotype	Concentration of DGAVP (μg/μl)	Average Daily Fluid Intake (ml)	Median Daily Preference (%)
di/di	0	159.9 ± 4.7	38
	0.1	53.5 ± 5.0*	76*
	1.0	33.3 ± 5.5*	68*
di/+	0	28.2 ± 1.4	85
	1.0	22.3 ± 0.7*	67

[a] Rats were offered 2.2% ethanol versus tap water for 8 days. DGAVP was administered via subcutaneously implanted osmotic minipumps at the indicated concentrations (release rate: 1 μl/h). Average Daily Fluid Intake = ethanol + water. Preference was calculated as ethanol as % total.

[b] Significantly differs from corresponding di/di or di/+ placebo group by at least $p < .05$ by two-tailed randomization test. Data are from reference 21.

levels.[24] When we offered these animals ethanol versus tap water, they showed highly elevated fluid intake, and significant reductions in ethanol preference.[25] There was a highly significant negative correlation between total fluid intake and ethanol preference. These studies demonstrate the highly significant influence that single genes can exert on drug-related traits.

As interest in pharmacogenetic strategies grows, methods combining the more simplistically presented alternatives discussed above have come into the forefront. One example is given. Using standard techniques for developing inbred strains, a specific variety of inbreds may be produced, called Recombinant Inbred strains. More details of their special features and uses will be given in a companion paper in this volume.[26] C57BL/6J and DBA/2J inbred mice differ markedly in almost all responses to alcohol and other drugs of abuse.[3] This, plus their general genetic diversity, makes their use

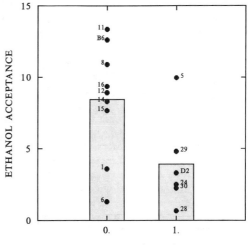

FIGURE 3. Distribution of BXD RI Recombinant Inbred strains for ethanol acceptance drinking. Ethanol intake (g/kg) during 24 h under thirst motivation for C57BL/6J (B6), DBA/2J (D2) and BXD RI strains (BXD number shown) are plotted. Strains shown with a score of 0 bear the B6 allele for the Brp-12 (LTW-4) locus on Chromosome 1, while those with a score of 1 bear the D2 allele.

as parent strains for a Recombinant Inbred series (the BXD RIs) ideal for gene mapping studies. In an early study, we characterized some of the BXD RI strains and the two parent strains for ethanol acceptance drinking. Some strains showed high acceptance, like C57BL/6J, while some strains were ethanol avoiders, like DBA/2J. These results (see FIG. 3) indicate the influence of a single gene on the trait, ethanol acceptance.[27] The strain distribution pattern (SDP: that is, which strains resembled C57 and which DBA) was compared to existing SDPs for genes which had been mapped to known chromosomal locations, and closely matched that for the gene encoding an abundant brain protein, LTW-4.[16] This linkage was also evident in a panel of standard inbred strains typed for LTW-4 and tested for ethanol acceptance.[15] While it does not appear that the LTW-4 protein product is closely enough linked to the preference-related trait to be a functionally related gene, recent application of Quantitative Trait Loci mapping methods[28] tentatively identified a number of other genes in this chromosome region which are also linked, and one of them could prove to be of functional significance.

CONCLUSIONS

This brief survey indicates that there are a number of pharmacogenetic methods available to explore the neurobiological basis for traits related to drug reinforcement. The classical methods of inbred strain analysis and development of genetic animal models specifically tooled for particular characteristics will continue to be of value. More exciting, however, is the potential for moving to the genomic level in analyses of drug reinforcement. The BXD RI panel of strains, in particular, will show rapid development in the density of their chromosomal map as they are characterized for restriction fragment length polymorphisms (RFLPs). The linkage of traits and particular RFLPs may be expected to lead to the identification of functionally important genes, which may then be studied using the powerful tools of molecular biology. In addition, the continued profusion of cloned genes coding for relevant neurotransmitter receptors and transporters will be exploited to elucidate the neurobiology of drug reinforcement.

SUMMARY

In this paper, we present examples of some of the several behaviors which have been taken to indicate the reinforcing efficacy of drugs, including ethanol. Efforts to identify the genetic determinants of these behaviors have employed diverse pharmacogenetic methods. For example, we have used selective breeding to develop mice selected for severe or attenuated ethanol withdrawal and have found that Withdrawal Seizure Prone mice show a greater conditioned preference for ethanol-associated locations than the selected Withdrawal Seizure Resistant line. Similarly, HOT mice, selected for insensitivity to ethanol-induced hypothermia, had greater conditioned place preference after ethanol training than COLD mice, selected for ethanol hypothermic sensitivity. We have also developed selected mouse lines responsive or unresponsive to ethanol-stimulated locomotor activity. These FAST and SLOW lines develop sensitization rather than tolerance to ethanol-induced activity. Using inbred strains of mice, others had shown that strains differed in preference for drinking ethanol solutions. We found that these strains also differed in acceptance of ethanol. Single-gene techniques have been used to show that preference drinking is significantly altered in mutant rodent strains lacking hypothalamic vasopressin, or with nephrogenic diabetes insipidus. In a specific panel of Recombinant Inbred mouse strains, we found that a single gene appeared to control a significant portion of the variance in preference drinking. These examples show that traits putatively related to drug reinforcement show substantial genetic control. Specifically, single-gene methods show promise of identification and mapping of genes related to drug reinforcement.

ACKNOWLEDGMENTS

The authors thank Dorcas Malott and Fred Risinger for assistance with the place conditioning studies.

REFERENCES

1. BOZARTH, M. A. 1987. An overview of assessing drug reinforcement. *In* Methods of Assessing the Reinforcing Properties of Abused Drugs. M. A. Bozarth, Ed.: 635–658. Springer-Verlag. New York.
2. PHILLIPS, T. J. & J. C. CRABBE. 1991. Behavioral studies of genetic differences in alcohol action. *In* The Genetic Basis of Alcohol and Drug Actions. J. C. Crabbe & R. A. Harris, Eds.: 25–104. Plenum Publishing Corporation. New York.
3. CRABBE, J. C. & R. A. HARRIS, EDS. 1991. The Genetic Basis of Alcohol and Drug Actions. Plenum Publishing Corporation. New York.
4. CRABBE, J. C., A. KOSOBUD, E. R. YOUNG, B. R. TAM & J. D. McSWIGAN. 1985. Bidirectional selection for susceptibility to ethanol withdrawal seizures in *Mus musculus*. Behav. Genet. **15:** 521–536.
5. KOSOBUD, A. & J. C. CRABBE. 1986. Ethanol withdrawal in mice bred to be genetically prone (WSP) or resistant (WSR) to ethanol withdrawal seizures. J. Pharmacol. Exp. Ther. **238:** 170–177.
6. CRABBE, J. C., C. D. MERRILL & J. K. BELKNAP. 1991. Acute dependence on depressant drugs is determined by common genes in mice. J. Pharmacol. Exp. Ther. **257:** 663–667.
7. GRANT, K. A., P. VALVERIUS, M. HUDSPITH & B. TABAKOFF. 1990. Ethanol withdrawal seizures and the NMDA receptor complex. Eur. J. Pharmacol. **176:** 289–296.
8. WISE, R. A. & M. A. BOZARTH. 1987. A psychomotor stimulant theory of addiction. Psychol. Rev. **94:** 469–492.
9. PHILLIPS, T. J., S. BURKHART-KASCH, E. TERDAL & J. C. CRABBE. 1991. Response to selection for EtOH-induced locomotor activation: Genetic analyses and selection response characterization. Psychopharmacology **103:** 557–566.
10. PHILLIPS, T. J., S. BURKHART-KASCH & J. C. CRABBE. 1991. Locomotor activity response to chronic ethanol treatment in selectively bred FAST and SLOW mice. Alcohol and Alcoholism (Suppl 1). In press.
11. PHILLIPS, T. J., S. BURKHART-KASCH, C. C. GWIAZDON & J. C. CRABBE. 1992. Locomotor responses of FAST and SLOW mice to several alcohols and drugs of abuse. Ann. N.Y. Acad. Sci. **654:** 499–501. This volume.
12. CUNNINGHAM, C. L., C. L. HALLETT, D. R. NIEHUS, J. S. HUNTER, L. NOUTH & F. O. RISINGER. Assessment of ethanol's hedonic effects in mice selectively bred for sensitivity to ethanol-induced hypothermia. Psychopharmacology. In press.
13. WALLER, M. B., W. J. McBRIDE, G. J. GATTO, L. LUMENG & T.-K. LI. 1984. Intragastric self-infusion of ethanol by ethanol-preferring and -nonpreferring lines of rats. Science **225:** 78–80.
14. McCLEARN, G. E. & D. A. RODGERS. 1959. Differences in preference among inbred strains of mice. Quart. J. Stud. Alcohol **20:** 691–695.

15. McCLEARN, G. E. 1968. The use of strain rank orders in assessing equivalence of techniques. Behav. Res. Methods Instrum. 1: 49–51.
16. GOLDMAN, D., R. G. LISTER & J. C. CRABBE. 1987. Mapping of a putative genetic locus determining ethanol intake in the mouse. Brain Res. 420: 220–226.
17. HARRIS, R. A. & J. C. CRABBE. 1992. Genetic animal models: A user's guide. In Neuromethods Vol. 22: Animal Models of Drug Addiction. A. A. Boulton, G. B. Baker & P. H. Wu, Eds. Humana Press, Inc. New York. In press.
18. SCHMALE, H. & D. RICHTER. 1984. Single base deletion in the vasopressin gene is the cause of diabetes insipidus in Brattleboro rats. Nature 308: 705–709.
19. DORSA, D. M. & L. C. BOTTEMILLER. 1982. Age-related changes of vasopressin content of microdissected areas of rat brain. Brain Res. 242: 151–156.
20. VALTIN, H. H., K. SCHROEDER, K. BERNISCHKE & H. SOKOL. 1962. Familial hypothalamic diabetes insipidus in the rat. Nature 196: 1109–1110.
21. RIGTER, H. & J. C. CRABBE. 1985. Vasopressin and ethanol preference. I. Effects of vasopressin and the fragment DGAVP on altered ethanol preference in Brattleboro diabetes insipidus rats. Peptides 6: 669–676.
22. FALCONER, D. S., M. LATYSZEWSKI & J. H. ISAACSON. 1964. Diabetes insipidus associated with oligosyndactylism in the mouse. Genet. Res. 5: 473–488.
23. NAIK, D. & H. VALTIN. 1969. Hereditary vasopressin-resistant urinary concentrating defects in mice. Am. J. Physiol. 217: 1183–1190.
24. NAIK, D. & H. KOBAYASHI. 1971. Neurohypophysial hormones in the pars nervosa of the mouse with hereditary nephrogenic diabetes insipidus. Neuroendocrinology 7: 322–328.
25. CRABBE, J. C. & H. RIGTER. 1985. Vasopressin and ethanol preference. II. Altered preference in two strains of diabetes insipidus rats and nephrogenic diabetes insipidus mice. Peptides 6: 677–683.
26. BELKNAP, J. K. & J. C. CRABBE. 1992. Chromosome mapping of genes affecting morphine and amphetamine response in BXD recombinant inbred mice. Ann. N.Y. Acad. Sci. 654: 311–323. This volume.
27. CRABBE, J. C., A. KOSOBUD, E. YOUNG & J. JANOWSKY. 1983. Polygenic and single-gene determination of response to ethanol in BXD/Ty recombinant inbred mouse strains. Neurobehav. Toxicol. Teratol. 5: 181–187.
28. GORA-MASLAK, G., G. E. McCLEARN, J. C. CRABBE, T. J. PHILLIPS, J. K. BELKNAP & R. PLOMIN. 1991. Use of recombinant inbred strains to identify quantitative trait loci in psychopharmacology. Psychopharmacology 104: 413–424.

Chromosome Mapping of Gene Loci Affecting Morphine and Amphetamine Responses in BXD Recombinant Inbred Mice[a]

J. K. BELKNAP[b] AND J. C. CRABBE[b,c]

Research Service (151W), VA Medical Center and
[b] Department of Medical Psychology
[c] Department of Pharmacology
Oregon Health Sciences University
3181 S.W. Sam Jackson Park Road
Portland, Oregon 97201-3098

GENE MAPPING

A genetic map is made up of the locations of gene loci on individual chromosomes. Among vertebrates, genetic maps have been most extensively developed for two species: mice and humans.[1] One of the more exciting discoveries to emerge from this effort is the surprising degree of homology (conservation) that appears to exist between the human and mouse genomes.[1,2] Close to 40% of the mouse genome can be matched to conserved regions of the human genome (syntenic conservation). Of this percentage, almost half shows linkage conservation, which involves homologous genes in the same linear order along the length of a chromosome in both species.

The construction of genetic maps, especially in the mouse, has relied heavily on two genetic phenomena: linkage and crossing-over.[3] Linkage refers to the tendency of gene loci on the same chromosome to be inherited together (to be associated) as they are transmitted from one generation to the next. In contrast, gene loci on different chromosomes are inherited independently (no linkage). Thus, if an individual inherits a particular gene from one parent (say, the father), there is a much increased probability of also inheriting all the other paternal genes on that same chromosome because of linkage. This is because the chromosome is in many ways the physical "unit" of heredity, and is usually transmitted intact from parent to offspring. However, there are important exceptions, where portions of a chromosome are occasionally recombined by crossing-over.

Crossing-over refers to the mutual exchange (recombination) of genetic material between two strands of the same chromosome during meiosis. The site of crossing-over along the length of any one chromosome is largely random. Moreover, the probability

[a] This work was supported by NIDA Contracts 271-90-7405, 271-87-8120, PHS Grants AA08621, DA05228, and two Merit Review grants from the Department of Veterans Affairs.

311

of crossing-over is greater over a long segment of a chromosome compared to a short one. Therefore, crossing-over is far more likely to recombine widely separated loci (loose linkage) than those located very close together (close linkage). Put more precisely, the frequency of recombination between two loci is a direct function of their map distance apart.[3] For this reason, the unit of map distance, termed the centi-Morgan (cM), is defined as a 1% frequency of recombination. This unit is named in honor of T. H. Morgan, who constructed the first genetic map in Drosophila. The mouse has 20 chromosomes, with an average length per chromosome of about 70 cM. Each cM represents about one million DNA base pairs, or roughly 15–20 gene loci.

RECOMBINANT INBRED (RI) STRAINS

Recombinant inbred (RI) strains are derived form an F2 cross between two parental (progenitor) inbred strains, followed by brother × sister inbreeding for at least 20 generations.[4] All members of a given inbred strain are genetically identical, and they are homozygous at each gene locus. They are called RI strains because, during their development, the parental chromosomes are recombined several times through crossing-over, yielding a unique pattern of recombinations of the parental chromosomes in each RI strain. An estimated average of about 3 cross-over events have occurred per chromosome.[5] The result is that the RI strains represent chance recombinations of the parental chromosomes in a fixed (inbred) state.[4] RI strains lend themselves to genetic mapping largely because of the relatively large number of loci that have been previously mapped (marker loci) through many years of cumulative effort.[4,6] There are about two dozen series (sets) of RI strains, each derived from a unique pair of parental inbred strains.[6]

The B×D RI series was derived from an F2 cross between two progenitor (parental) inbred strains, C57BL/6J (B6) and DBA/2J (D2). The resulting F2 individuals were intermated at random to form a large number of mating pairs, *each one* the beginning of a new inbred strain. Taylor[5,6] derived and maintains this RI series, which now consists of 24 strains. Maximal inbreeding (brother by sister) has been maintained for at least 70 generations within each of the B×D RI strains. Each RI strain is homozygous for either the B6 allele or the D2 allele at each locus. For chromosome mapping purposes, the B×D RI series is probably the best suited compared to other RI series when a combination of the following desirable attributes is taken into account. These are 1) number of available RI strains (n = 24), 2) number of mapped marker gene loci (over 400), 3) large genetic differences between progenitor strains, and 4) availability from an established supplier (The Jackson Laboratory).

The RI strains were originally developed as a tool in detecting and mapping a single gene locus with a major (very large) effect on a trait of interest.[4,5] These are known as major gene loci, in contrast to minor gene loci, with much smaller effects. For example, the albino locus has a major gene influence on coat color in many species; individuals homozygous for the recessive allele are albino. In the mouse, this locus (called the c locus) has been mapped to the 41 cM region of chromosome 7. When RI strain means on a given trait are found to be bimodally distributed (*i.e.*, some RI strains resemble one parent strain and some resemble the other parent, and none are intermediate), this is presumptive evidence for control of that trait by a single gene locus with a major influence.[4,7] Using the albino locus as an example, one would expect half of the strains to be albino, and half nonalbino, and none intermediate, if the two parent strains were albino and nonalbino, respectively. Normally, Mendelian ratios of 3:1 (dominance) or 1:2:1 (no dominance) would be expected for a major gene locus, as exemplified by Mendel's peas. However, because RI strains are highly inbred, there can be no heterozygotes. Thus, the expected Mendelian ratio is 1:1 among RI strains.

The major gene approach was extensively applied in the 1970s to a number of measures of morphine, amphetamine, and ethanol sensitivity in the C×B (Bailey) RI series, made up of seven RI strains derived from the BALB/cBy and C57BL/6By parental strains (reviewed by Broadhurst,[8] Shuster,[9] and Belknap and O'Toole[10]). Most traits were unimodal rather than bimodal, indicating polygene (several minor genes) rather than major gene control. Since pharmacological traits under major gene influence are rather unusual, few measures were amenable to the major gene mapping approach. One study that was successful provided evidence of a major gene influence on ethanol-induced reductions in locomotor activity.[11] A bimodal distribution was seen among the C×B RI strains, suggesting a major gene influence. The existence of a major gene was confirmed by work with congenic strains and in a backcross population. This locus, named *Eam* (ethanol activity modifier), was mapped to chromosome 4, in a region now known as the *H-16* region. It is interesting that in the B×D series, Gora-Maslak et al.[12] also found evidence for a locus affecting ethanol-induced reductions in activity in this same chromosome region (*Ly-20* locus).

In contrast to major gene loci, minor gene loci produce effects too small to force a bimodal distribution in the trait under study. The latter are often referred to as quantitative trait loci (QTL), because they are presumed to underlie quantitative traits, or those that are continuously rather than bimodally distributed.[12,13] Quantitative (or polygenic) traits, because they are usually determined by several minor loci (QTL), are generally unimodally normally distributed. A recent advance in the use of RI strains for genetic mapping is the QTL approach, so named because it seeks to map minor as well as major gene loci.[12,13] While used by plant geneticists for the past decade, this method has only recently been used in mammals, where it is well suited to mouse RI strains, especially the B×D RI series.[12,13]

THE QUANTITATIVE TRAIT LOCI (QTL) APPROACH

The QTL approach seeks to discover significant associations between a quantitative (continuous) trait and one or more previously mapped marker gene loci. When found, these are suggestive of linkage between a QTL affecting the quantitative trait, and a marker locus of known map location. Statistically, this can be approached in several ways, but the most straight-forward is to use the correlation coefficient (r) between the B×D RI strain means for the trait of interest and a series of marker loci as an initial screen for candidate QTLs.[12-14] For this purpose, each marker locus is scored as a 0 if the C57BL/6J (B6) allele is present, and a 1 if the DBA/2J (D2) allele is present, for each of the B×D RI strains. A significant correlation between a trait of interest and a marker locus suggests that a QTL affecting the trait of interest is located in the same chromosome region as the marker, *i.e.*, they are linked. A correlation of zero indicates no linkage, while a correlation of 1.0 would suggest very close linkage (no recombinations). The square of the correlation coefficient (r^2 or R^2) gives the proportion of the genetic variance accounted for by a marker locus. In this paper, we wish to illustrate this technique with several traits studied in B×D RI mice related to amphetamine and morphine sensitivity.

AMPHETAMINE-INDUCED HYPERTHERMIA

Seale et al.[15] studied 10 B×D RI strains, both progenitor strains and their F1 cross for maximal hyperthermia within one hour after a single 20 mg/kg i.p. dose of d-amphetamine sulfate. DBA/2J (D2) mice became markedly hyperthermic (+1.8°C), while C57BL/6J (B6) mice showed a much smaller response (+0.4°C) under the same conditions. Seven of the B×D RI strains responded as did the D2 parent, while the other three B×D strains resembled the B6 strain in their response. No strains were intermediate (FIG. 1). This markedly bimodal pattern of hyperthermic responses strongly suggests a single major gene locus effect on amphetamine hyperthermia.[15] No attempt to map this locus was made at the time of the original report. Gora-Maslak et al.[12] subjected the data presented by Seale et al.[15] to quantitative trait loci (QTL) analysis using the 173 marker loci available at the time, and found significant associations with several marker loci. The most important by far was the Lamb-2 locus on chromosome 1. We now review and update these initial findings.

We subjected these data to quantitative trait loci (QTL) analyses by correlating the hyperthermic response means for the 10 B×D strains with the allelic distribution of 360 marker gene loci of known chromosome map location. These markers were ob-

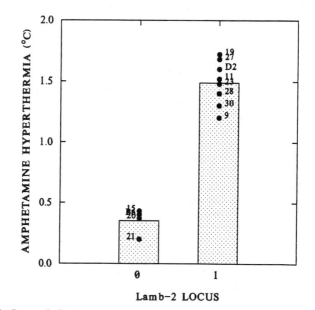

FIGURE 1. Bar graph showing the hyperthermic response of the mean of those strains possessing the C57BL/6J (B6) allele (*left bar*), and those possessing the DBA/2J (D2) allele (*right bar*) at the Lamb-2 locus on chromosome 1. Superimposed on the bars is a plot of the individual strain means. Each number refers to the strain numbers, *e.g.* strain B×D-21 is symbolized as "21." The correlation (r) between amphetamine hyperthermia and the two allelic groups, scored as a 0 (B6 allele) or a 1 (D2 allele), was 0.96 ($p < .00002$, $n = 10$ strains). This is the same p value obtained from a t-test between the two allelic groups of strains. The hyperthermia data were from Seale et al.[15]

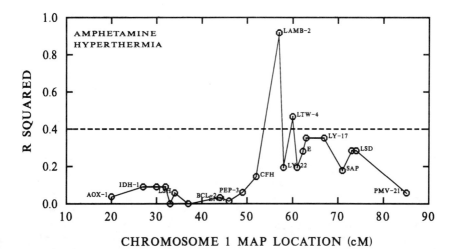

CHROMOSOME 1 MAP LOCATION (cM)

FIGURE 2. Plot of the associations (R^2) of each marker locus on chromosome 1 with amphetamine hyperthermia in 10 B×D RI strains (data from Seale *et al.*[15]). The known linear order of mapped marker loci is shown along the X axis. Each correlation coefficient (r) was calculated using the strain means for amphetamine hyperthermia and scores of 0 (C57BL/6 allele) or 1 (DBA/2 allele) for the same B×D strains at each marker locus. Squaring the correlation coefficient (R^2) yields the proportion of the total genetic variance for amphetamine hyperthermia accounted for by each marker locus. The horizontal dotted line represents the $p < .05$ significance threshold. Map locations were obtained from the linkage map of Davisson and Roderick.[25] A major gene effect is evident in the region of the *Lamb-2* locus, accounting for 92% of the genetic variance ($r = 0.96$).

tained from the recent compilation of B×D marker loci reported by Taylor[6] and updated more recently (Taylor, 1991, unpublished). The results of the QTL analysis for amphetamine hyperthermia revealed several marker loci with significant ($p < .05$) associations out of a total of 360. These were clustered on segments of four chromosomes. By far the largest and most important association was with the *Lamb-2* locus on chromosome 1 (57 cM), with a correlation of 0.96 (R^2 of 0.92, $p < .00002$, $n = 10$ strains). These results are shown in FIGURE 2 for the markers on chromosome 1 in terms of R^2 (square of the correlation coefficient). The very high correlation with *Lamb-2* strongly suggests close linkage between a gene locus with a major influence on amphetamine hyperthermia and the *Lamb-2* locus. The significance level of the correlation is the same as given by a *t*-test between those strains bearing the B6 allele and those bearing the D2 allele for the trait of interest. This is shown graphically in FIGURE 1 for the *Lamb-2* locus. This presumed major gene is probably only a few centiMorgans (cM) from *Lamb-2* (FIG. 2).

The above example is quite unusual, in that major gene effects are more the exception than the rule for drug response traits at the organismic level. But this example does illustrate that the QTL approach can map major genes when they are encountered. More typical are traits largely determined by several minor gene loci (QTL), each with relatively smaller effects on the trait of interest, as exemplified below.

SOME STATISTICAL CONCERNS

Before proceeding further with QTL analyses, we need to come to grips with a statistical problem inherent in this and all other RI gene mapping approaches. Because of the many correlation coefficients that were calculated for each measure in the B×D QTL analysis ($n = 360$), it is expected that some of them will be significant due to chance at the $p < .05$ level. We have discussed elsewhere the predicted number of chance correlations and their probability distribution.[14] There are two primary avenues for dealing with this concern. First, confirmation of the B×D data can (and should) be sought by using other genetic models. One suggestion[14] is to use the B×D data as a screen to identify a handful of candidate QTL map locations, which then would be specifically tested in other RI series, standard inbred (non-RI) strains, congenic lines, or by linkage analysis in F2 or backcross populations. We used standard inbred (non-RI) strains for this purpose in some of our work described below. Second, if the B×D data are to stand alone, without confirmation from other genetic models, then a correction is needed for the multiple correlations calculated for the marker loci. The simplest way to do this is the Bonferroni correction, whereby the observed level of significance for individual marker loci are multiplied by the number of independent determinations. We have estimated the latter to be 52, the average number of progenitor chromosome segments (linked regions) remaining intact (not recombined) in the B×D RI strains, and is thus our best estimate of the number of independent linkage units in this genetic model.[14] Thus, only significance levels approaching $p < .001$ (uncorrected) will emerge as $p < .05$ after correction (.001 × 52). Employing this correction gives $p < .05$ against *even one* fortuitous correlation arising anywhere in the genome covered by the marker loci. Thus, only significance levels of about $p < .001$ (uncorrected) for individual marker loci should be taken seriously as indicating linkage from the B×D data alone. For a study involving 20 RI strains, this requires correlations no smaller than 0.68. For the amphetamine hyperthermia data discussed above, the correlation (association) with the *Lamb-2* locus was r = 0.96, or $p < .00002$. When this p value is Bonferroni corrected (multiplied by 52), a p value of .001 results, a highly significant result.

VOLUNTARY MORPHINE CONSUMPTION

Two-bottle choice (preference) drinking studies have been an appealing model of drug self-administration largely because the method is straight-forward, nonstressful, noninvasive, and lends itself to chronic studies. This approach is also amenable to screening the large numbers of animals often required in genetic studies. However, a major problem is that taste factors are potential confounds in assessing the "rewarding" effects of drugs subject to abuse, since most such compounds have quinine-like bitter aversive tastes. In the case of morphine, mice will reject such compounds when dissolved in their drinking fluid, so a positive incentive, such as saccharin, must often be used to mask the bitter taste of morphine and induce the intake of pharmacologically significant amounts of the drug.[16,17]

Horowitz[16] studied nine inbred mouse strains presented with a two-bottle choice between morphine (0.375 mg/ml) in 0.06% saccharin in one bottle vs. plain tap water in the other. A very wide range of preference ratios resulted among the nine inbred strains from a low of 4% (DBA/2) to a high of 98% (C57BL/6). Since all strains were reared and treated in the same manner, these dramatically large strain differences can be presumed to be predominantly genetic in origin.[7] In the morphine-saccharin preferring C57BL/6J (B6) strain, daily consumption of morphine averaged 140 mg/kg. Under these conditions, some of the animals had fatal overdoses, and most exhibited signs of physical dependence when challenged with naloxone. In contrast, the DBA/2J (D2) strain consumed less than 10 mg/kg per day under the same conditions, and showed no apparent drug effects. We have recently replicated these findings using 0.2% saccharin, the maximally preferred concentration for both strains, and have also shown that these two strains do not differ appreciably in consumption of quinine-saccharin solutions, which stands in marked contrast to the large differences seen with morphine-saccharin solutions.[17] Quinine-saccharin served as a control for the taste of morphine-saccharin mixtures, since morphine and quinine are reputed to have similar bitter (alkaloid) tastes.[18] These findings suggest that the pharmacological effects of morphine, rather than its gustatatory effects, were the principal determiner of these very large strain differences in voluntary morphine consumption. These findings led us to pursue studies with the B×D RI series derived from the B6 and D2 strains.

Individual mice from 20 of the B×D RI and both parental (progenitor) strains were studied under two-bottle choice conditions.[19] For confirmation purposes, 15 standard (non-RI) inbred strains were also tested using a similar protocol. One of the bottles always contained water. In the other bottle, 0.2% saccharin was presented first for 5 days, followed by progressively increasing concentrations of quinine sulfate (0.1 to 0.4 mg/ml) in 0.2% saccharin over a 13-day period, followed by gradually increasing concentrations of morphine sulfate (0.3 to 0.7 mg/ml), also in 0.2% saccharin, in a parallel manner.[19] These concentrations of quinine were chosen because they lead to approximately equal preference ratios with water compared to the morphine concentrations employed. For each mouse, the maximum intake of quinine (mg/kg/day) was subtracted from the maximum intake of morphine (mg/kg/day) assessed under the same conditions. This is referred to as the corrected morphine intake. Since the amount of voluntary fluid intake (mls/day) and preference ratios with water were virtually the same for morphine compared to quinine for the entire data set, this largely corrects for the saccharin presented with both alkakoids. The methods and results for the B×D RI strains have been previously described.[19] QTL analysis for morphine-saccharin and quinine-saccharin have been previously reported,[12] but corrected morphine consumption has not.

The results for the QTL analyses for corrected morphine consumption are shown in TABLE 1. In the B×D series, significant ($p < .05$) associations were seen for seven chromosome regions, each indexed by seven marker loci. Of these, sufficient data for confirmation testing with the standard (non-RI) inbreds was available for only three of these chromosome regions. For confirmation purposes, we used only those standard inbred strains possessing the same allele as either the B6 or D2 strains, and required at least three strains per allele. Correlations between corrected morphine consumption and the marker loci were calculated in the same manner as the B×D data. Confirmation testing of these three chromosome regions showed two of them to be not supported, and one supported (TABLE 1). The supported site was the Es-1 region of chromosome 8, which showed a correlation of -0.45 ($p < .05$) among the B×D strains, and -0.59 ($p < .01$) among the 15 standard inbred strains. What about the four chromosome regions where sufficient data were lacking for confirmation testing (TABLE 1)? Since the missing data concern the alleles possessed by the standard inbred strains at four marker loci, it is likely that much of the needed data will eventually be

TABLE 1. Significantly Associated Marker Loci for Corrected Morphine Consumption (mg/kg/day) in the BXD RI Series under Two-bottle Choice (vs. Water) Conditions (left column)[a]

BXD Associated Marker Loci (correlation)	Location (chromosome, cM)	Standard Inbred Strain Associations
Fabpi (0.49)	3, 72?	NA
Lyb-8 (0.47), Gpi-1 (0.47),	7, 10–16	Gpi-1 (0.30, $p < .15$, $n = 15$)
Abpa (0.47), D7rp2 (0.53)		D7rp2 (0.10, $p < .35$, $n = 11$)
Zpf-4 (−0.50), Es-1 (−0.45)	8, 35?	Es-1 (−0.59,* $p < .01$, $n = 15$)
Xmv-15 (−0.52)	9, 30?	NA
Mpmv-5 (−0.60*)	10, ?	NA
D12nyu2 (0.47), Ah (0.61*)	12, 3–10	Ah (−0.47, $p < .90$, $n = 15$)
Xmv-29 (0.52)	18, ?	NA

[a] The correlation coefficients are given in parentheses. Only those loci significantly associated in the BXD series (*left column*) were analyzed with the standard inbred data (*right column*) whenever possible. NA indicates insufficient data for analysis among the standard inbreds due to missing allelic information. * $p < .01$.

reported in the literature, allowing confirmation testing to be carried out at some future time. Thus, the presently reported B×D data represent one piece of an incomplete puzzle, with other pieces likely to emerge in future work.

It will be of interest to compare this measure of drug reinforcement with other measures assessed in these same strains. Conditioned place preference and i.v. self-administration studies with morphine have begun in our and other laboratories. Additionally, two-bottle choice studies with amphetamine, cocaine, and ethanol are planned using B×D RI mice.

MORPHINE-INDUCED ANALGESIA, HYPOTHERMIA, HYPOACTIVITY, AND STRAUB TAIL

These same B×D strains and progenitors have recently been tested on a battery of morphine-sensitive measures in our laboratory, including analgesia (hot plate), open field activity, hypothermia, and Straub tail, and dose-response curves were constructed for each strain and measure. The procedure was to administer a single dose of morphine sulfate, i.p., and to assess four different measures at various times after injection. Morphine-induced analgesia (hot plate, 52.5°C) was assessed at 28 min after injection, followed by ambulatory activity (line crossings on an elevated open field), Straub tail (an index of muscular rigidity) and body temperature (rectal probe) at 30–33 minutes postinjection using methods described elsewhere.[20,21] Independent groups of eight mice per strain received either saline or 8, 16 or 32 mg/kg, i.p., of morphine sulfate. Straub tail was scored during open field testing by means of a 3-point rating scale: 0, no effect; 1, tail lifted to between 45 and 90 degrees from the floor; 2, tail arched beyond 90 degrees (over the animal's back). Body temperature was assessed just prior to injection (baseline) and immediately following the open field test by means of a rectal probe.

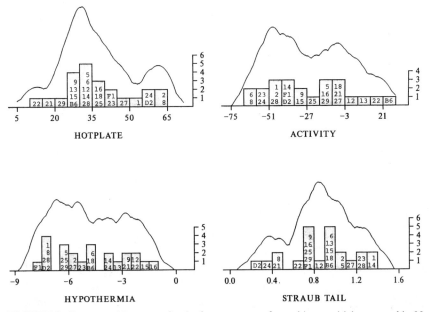

FIGURE 3. Frequency histograms for the four measures of morphine sensitivity assessed in 20 of the B×D RI strains, both progenitor strains (B6 or D2) and their F1. Each B×D RI strain is identified by its strain number, *e.g.*, B×D-12 is shown as "12." Also shown are the nonparametric Epanechnikov kernel density functions for the same data, which depict the distributions somewhat more accurately than the inherently discontinuous frequency histograms.[26] The window width setting, in standard units, was 0.27. The test for bimodality proposed by Belknap *et al.*[14] for RI data showed that the bimodal hypotheses provided a significantly better fit than the unimodal hypothesis for morphine-induced activity, suggesting a major gene influence.

In the analyses presented below, we used the slope of the dose-response curve based on the linear regression of scores for each measure (Y) on the log of the dose (X), with a y intercept of zero. Hot plate raw scores (hind paw-lift or shake) were first converted to the percent of maximum possible effect (%MPE) to more closely approximate a normal distribution. For activity and body temperature, the raw scores were first converted to the percent change from saline values prior to analysis. For Straub tail, the raw scores were used without transformation. For most strains, the dose of morphine was positively related to analgesia and Straub tail scores, but negatively related to activity and body temperature scores.

The results are shown in FIGURE 3. Of the four measures, the distribution for morphine-induced changes in activity fit a bimodal distribution significantly better than a unimodal one, based on the test proposed by Belknap *et al.*[14] for B×D RI data. This suggests a major gene effect for this measure of morphine sensitivity. The F1 hybrid scored essentially the same as the D2 strain, indicating dominance for morphine-induced hypoactivity on an elevated open field. In contrast, the B6 progenitor strain showed a dose-related increase in activity (FIGURE 3).

QTL analysis for the four morphine sensitivity measures are shown in TABLE 2. Sev-

TABLE 2. Significantly Associated Marker Loci ($p < .05$) for Four Measures of Morphine Sensitivity in 20 BXD RI Strains[a]

	Chromosome	Hot Plate	Activity	Hypothermia	Straub Tail
Lsd	1			−.51	
Psp	2	.46			
D17Tu51	3	−.58*			
Ms15-1	4	−.52	.44		
Fla	5				−.57*
Svp-2	7		−.47		
B	7	−.48	.52		
Defcr	8		.59*		
Bv-1	8				−.53
Cdt	9	−.54			
d	9				−.45
Mpmv-5	10	.50		−.73**	
Xmmv-3	11	−.46			.54
Es-3	11				−.47
Pmv-42	15				−.54
Pmv-35	17				−.68**
Xmmv-15	17			−.56*	.50
Ly-10	19	.48	−.50		
Cyp2c	19		−.48		

[a] Where a series of closely linked marker loci were significantly associated, only the marker showing the highest correlation is shown. For all marker loci, a 0 was assigned to the B6 allele, and a 1 to the D2 allele. * $p < .01$, and ** $p < .001$ for each marker (uncorrected).

eral chromosome regions were significantly associated with each of the sensitivity measures. Confirmatory analyses with another genetic model have yet to be carried out, so the results must be viewed with caution for the reasons noted above. However, it is interesting to note that two of the correlations reached the $p < .001$ level, which when Bonferroni corrected yield $p < .05$ against even one fortuitous correlation arising for the entire set of marker loci. These two are the Mpmv-5 region of chromosome 10 for hypothermia ($r = -0.73$), and the Pmv-35 region of chromosome 17 for Straub tail ($r = -0.68$).

The correlation coefficients among these measures are shown in FIGURE 4. Analgesia, hypothermia and activity induced by morphine were significantly intercorrelated in the expected directions, e.g., analgesia is negatively correlated with morphine-induced changes in activity and body temperature. Since the correlations are based on strain means, they can be presumed to be predominantly genetic in origin, i.e., they are estimates of genetic correlations.[22] Thus, the significant correlations suggest a considerable degree of common genetic influences affecting sensitivity to morphine-induced analgesia, hypothermia, and activity. However, no significant correlations were seen between these three and the fourth measure, Straub tail, an index of muscular rigidity (FIG. 4).

It is interesting to note that in the earlier literature involving B6 and D2 strains (reviewed by Belknap and O'Toole[10]), many of these authors concluded that hot plate analgesia and activity are genetically dissociated from one another in these two strains,

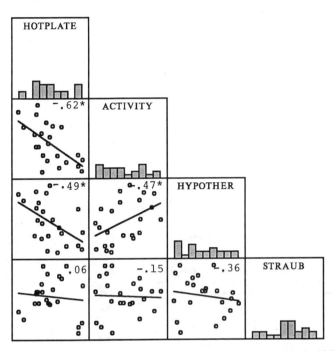

FIGURE 4. Scatterplots for the four measures of morphine sensitivity taken in 20 B×D and both progenitor strains. The correlation coefficients for the 20 B×D strains (parental strains omitted) are also shown among these measures. For each strain and measure, dose-response curves were constructed for saline or 8, 16 and 32 mg/kg morphine sulfate, i.p., and the regression slopes used as the index of sensitivity.

implying that they are independently genetically determined. The B×D RI strain data indicate that these two measures are not genetically independent in the B6 and D2 strains. Instead, they have common genetic influences resulting in a significantly negative genetic correlation (-0.62, $p < .01$), as shown in FIGURE 4.

K_D and B_{max} values for ^{3}H-naloxone binding in whole brain homogenates are now being determined, with data for 16 of the B×D strains collected thus far. K_D values are significantly correlated in the expected direction with hotplate (-0.70) and activity (0.60), while B_{max} values are not significantly correlated with any of the four morphine sensitivity measures at this stage in data collection. Brain morphine concentrations are also being determined on these same strains.

CONCLUSIONS

An important objective of the RI approach is to generate hypotheses concerning map locations by providing a handful of viable candidate QTL sites for further testing using other linkage or association methods. Thus, the RI strains serve as a very useful initial screen for QTL associations. Because the study of 20 RI strains represents only

20 genotypes, the B×D results by themselves can only map loci with relatively large (major) effects. For loci with smaller effects, such as those observed for voluntary morphine drinking, other genetic models should be employed for confirmation purposes. Such models could include other inbred or RI series, congenic lines,[4] or studies employing RFLP markers in individual F2 or backcross mice.[23] The latter is especially powerful, since the number of genotypes available for test is limited only by the number of individual mice that can be tested. However, a strength of the RI and standard inbred strain approach lies in the almost limitless replicability of the genotypes involved. Thus, knowledge gained in the future can be directly compared and accumulated with the wealth of data collected in the past on what is essentially the same genotypes, except for new mutations.[13,24]

REFERENCES

1. SEARLE, A. G., J. PETERS, M. F. LYON, J. G. HALL, E. P. EVANS, J. H. EDWARDS & V. J. BUCKLE. 1989. Chromosome maps of man and mouse. IV. Ann. Hum. Genet. **53:** 89–140.
2. NADEAU, J. & A. H. REINER. 1989. Linkage and synteny homologies in mouse and man. *In* Genetic Variants and Strains of the Laboratory Mouse, 2nd edit. M. F. Lyon & A. G. Searle, Eds.: 506–536. Oxford University Press. Oxford.
3. GREEN, M. C. 1981. Gene mapping. *In* The Mouse in Biomedical Research, Vol I. H. L. Foster, J. D. Small & J. G. Fox, Eds.: 105–117. Academic Press. New York.
4. BAILEY, D. W. 1981. Recombinant inbred strains and bilineal congenic strains. *In* The Mouse in Biomedical Research, Vol I. H. L. Foster, J. D. Small & J. G. Fox, Eds.: 223–239. Academic Press. New York.
5. TAYLOR, B. A. 1978. Recombinant inbred strains: Use in gene mapping. *In* Origins of Inbred Mice. H. C. Morse, Eds.: 423–438. Academic Press. New York.
6. TAYLOR, B. A. 1989. Recombinant inbred strains. *In* Genetic Variants and Strains of the Laboratory Mouse, 2nd edit. M. F. Lyon & A. G. Searle, Eds.: 773–789. Oxford University Press. Oxford.
7. MCCLEARN, G. E. 1992. The tools of pharmacogenetics. *In* The Genetic Basis of Alcohol and Drug Actions. R. A. Harris & J. C. Crabbe, Eds. Plenum. New York.
8. BROADHURST, P. L. 1978. Drugs and the Inheritance of Behavior. Plenum Press. New York.
9. SHUSTER, L. 1986. Genetic markers of drug abuse in mouse models. *In* Genetic and Biological Markers in Drug Abuse and Alcoholism. M. C. Braude & H. M. Chao, Eds.: 71–85. NIDA Research Monograph No. 66, GSGPO. Washington, D.C.
10. BELKNAP, J. K. & L. A. O'TOOLE. 1991. Studies of genetic differences in response to opioid drugs. *In* The Genetic Basis of Alcohol and Drug Actions. R. A. Harris & J. C. Crabbe, Eds.: 225–252. Plenum. New York.
11. OLIVERIO, A. & B. E. ELEFTHERIOU. 1976. Motor activity and alcohol: A genetic investigation in the mouse. Physiol. Behav. **16:** 577–581.
12. GORA-MASLAK, G., G. E. MCCLEARN, J. C. CRABBE, T. J. PHILLIPS, J. K. BELKNAP & R. PLOMIN. 1991. Use of recombinant inbred strains to identify quantitative trait loci in psychopharmacology. Psychopharmacology **104:** 413–424.
13. PLOMIN, R., G. E. MCCLEARN & G. GORA-MASLAK. 1991. Use of recombinant inbred strains to detect quantitative trait loci associated with behavior. Behav. Genet. **21:** 99–116.
14. BELKNAP, J. K., J. C. CRABBE, R. PLOMIN, G. E. MCCLEARN, K. E. SAMPSON, L. A. O'TOOLE & G. GORA-MASLAK. 1992. Single locus control of saccharin intake in B×D/Ty recombinant inbred mice: Some methodological implications for RI strain analysis. Behav. Genet. **22:** 81–100.
15. SEALE, T. W., J. M. CARNEY, P. JOHNSON & O. M. RENNERT. 1985. Inheritance of amphetamine-induced thermoregulatory responses in inbred mice. Pharmacol. Biochem. Behav. **23:** 373–377.
16. HOROWITZ, G. P. 1981. Pharmacogenetic models and behavioral responses to opiates. *In*

Development of animal models as pharmacogenetic tools. G. E. McClearn, R. A. Deitrich & V. G. Erwin, Eds. USDHH-NIAAA Research Monograph No. 6. U. S. Government Printing Office. Washington, D.C.

17. BELKNAP, J. K. 1990. Physical dependence induced by the voluntary consumption or morphine in inbred mice. Pharmacol. Biochem. Behav. **35:** 311–315.

18. FORGIE, M. L., B. L. BEYERSTEIN & B. K. ALEXANDER. 1988. Contributions of taste factors and gender to opioid preference in C57BL and DBA mice. Psychopharmacology **95:** 237–244.

19. PHILLIPS, T. J., J. K. BELKNAP & J. C. CRABBE. 1991. Use of voluntary morphine consumption in recombinant inbred strains to access vulnerability to drug abuse at the genetic level. J. Addict. Dis. **10:** 73–87.

20. BELKNAP, J. K., B. NOORDEWIER & M. LAME. 1989. Genetic dissociation of multiple morphine effects among C57BL/6J, DBA/2J and C3H/HeJ inbred mouse strains. Physiol. Behav. **46:** 69–74.

21. BELKNAP, J. K., M. LAMÉ & P. W. DANIELSON. 1990. Inbred strain differences in morphine-induced analgesia with the hot plate assay: A reassessment. Behav. Genet. **20:** 333–338.

22. CRABBE, J. C., T. J. PHILLIPS, A. KOSOBUD & J. K. BELKNAP. 1990. Estimation of genetic correlation: Interpretation of experiments using selectively bred and inbred animals. Alcoholism: Clin. Exp. Res. **14:** 141–151.

23. LANDER, E. S. & D. BOTSTEIN. 1989. Mapping mendelian factors underlying quantitative traits using RFLP linkage maps. Genetics **121:** 185–199.

24. PLOMIN, R., G. E. McCLEARN, G. GORA-MASLAK & J. M. NEIDERHISER. 1991. An RI QTL cooperative data bank for recombinant inbred quantitative trait loci analyses. Letter to the editor, Behav. Genet. **21:** 97–98.

25. DAVISSON, M. T. & T. H. RODERICK. 1989. Linkage map. *In* Genetic Variants and Strains of the Laboratory Mouse, 2nd edit. M. F. Lyon & A. G. Searle, Eds.: 416–428. Oxford University Press. Oxford.

26. SILVERMAN, B. W. 1986. Density Estimation for Statistics and Data Analysis. Chapman and Hall. London.

Role of Neuronal Calcium Channels in Ethanol Dependence: From Cell Cultures to the Intact Animal[a]

JOHN LITTLETON, HILARY LITTLE,
AND RICHARD LAVERTY

Division of Biomedical Sciences
Kings College, Strand
London, WC2R 2LS, United Kingdom

Department of Pharmacology
Medical School, University of Bristol
Bristol BS8 1TD, United Kingdom

Department of Pharmacology
University of Otago Medical School
Dunedin, New Zealand

INTRODUCTION

In order to establish the neurochemical basis of drug-dependent states it is necessary to utilize model systems because of the difficulty inherent in studying human brain chemistry *in vivo*. This paper attempts to link mechanisms of ethanol dependence, first suggested by animal models, to neurochemical changes which can be observed in even simpler systems requiring only cultured cells of neuronal origin.

Several models of the kind where forced administration of alcohol can be shown to induce chemical dependence (as identified by a clear syndrome of physical withdrawal on removal of the drug) are now available. These include the administration of alcohol in liquid diets, pioneered in Gerhard Freund's laboratory[1] and alcohol administration by inhalation, pioneered in Dora Goldstein's laboratory.[2] These models appear to be accurate predictors of the utility of drug treatments of alcohol withdrawal in the clinic[3] and, in addition, they have provided a wealth of information about the potential neurochemical mechanisms of alcohol chemical dependence.

One type of explanation of the changes which lead to tolerance and chemical dependence on alcohol invokes adaptive changes in central neurons which overcome the inhibitory effects of alcohol by making these nerves intrinsically more excitable. While alcohol is still present in the brain this opposing effect can confer tolerance, but on removal of alcohol it would be expressed as neuronal hyperexcitability, and could cause the alcohol withdrawal syndrome.[4] For some years now we have been interested in the possibility that the mechanism for such an increase in intrinsic excitability of nerves

[a] Some of the work described in this review was supported by the Wellcome Trust.

could be a change in their sensitivity to calcium ions. This hypothesis was based on experiments using brain slices from rats which had been exposed chronically to alcohol by inhalation.[5] The characteristics of catecholamine release from these slices seemed at least fourfold more sensitive to Ca^{2+} than that from controls.[5]

Despite several years of work on this problem using intact animals we were unable to isolate the reason for the increased neuronal Ca^{2+} sensitivity associated with alcohol dependence. We reasoned however, that if it represented an adaptive response to alcohol *at the neuronal level*, we should be able to reproduce the effect in an isolated "neuronal" system, where it might be more amenable to study. Because our previous experiments had been on catecholamine release, we decided to use adrenal chromaffin cells (of bovine origin) as a simple model system. In this review we consider the value of this approach and attempt to relate the findings that we have made to those obtained in more conventional models using intact animals.

BOVINE ADRENAL CHROMAFFIN CELLS

Cells of the adrenal medulla originate from the embryological neural crest, and migrate away from the CNS to lie in the position in the abdominal cavity that they occupy in the adult. They are effectively undifferentiated neurons, and in consequence are pluripotential. When exposed to the right conditions they will express many different types of receptor proteins and can synthesize and release many different types of transmitter.[6] Their function in the intact animal is to release catecholamines on stimulation by acetylcholine. This transmitter is released from the splanchnic nerve and acts on nicotinic cholinoceptors on the medullary cells to cause release of catecholamines (mainly epinephrine in the intact animal).[6]

When bovine adrenal chromaffin cells (BACC) are maintained in primary culture they readily adhere to the culture plates and send out neuritic extensions from the cell bodies. They take up catecholamines from the medium as well as synthesizing these. They also synthesize and release GABA[7] and opioid peptides.[6] They still release catecholamines from the cell bodies on stimulation with nicotinic agonists such as carbachol, but many other receptors, including GABA_A receptors and opioid receptors, can modify this release, suggesting feedback control via these other transmitters which are co-released with catecholamines. For example, GABA, by an action on GABA_A receptors, can greatly inhibit the release of catecholamines from BACC associated with nicotinic receptor stimulation.[7]

In relation to the Ca^{2+} sensitivity of catecholamine release stimulated by carbachol, or by depolarization via K^+, BACC require similar external concentrations of Ca^{2+} for release by either stimulus. However the release induced by K^+ is much more sensitive to inhibition with dihydropyridine (DHP) calcium channel antagonists than is that induced by carbachol.[8] It seems likely that the generalized depolarization caused by K^+ is associated with Ca^{2+} entry through "L-type" voltage-operated calcium channels whereas the localized depolarizations caused by nicotinic agonists are associated with Ca^{2+} entry through other channel sub-types.

The BACC therefore seems to have all the "machinery" relevant to investigating alterations in Ca^{2+} sensitivity of the catecholamine release process, and it is relatively simple to keep these cells alive in primary culture for the sort of period (about 6 days) necessary to produce chemical dependence on alcohol in the intact laboratory animal. Incidentally, the BACC also has the machinery for studying neuronal adaptation to a variety of other drugs including cocaine and amphetamine (catecholamine uptake proteins), heroin (opioid receptor proteins), benzodiazepines ($GABA_A$ receptor proteins) and nicotine (nicotinic receptor proteins). In this review we will concentrate on the effects of alcohol in this system, but we are already investigating these other potential uses of BACC cultures.

EFFECTS OF ALCOHOL ON BACC CULTURES

Ethanol inhibits depolarization-induced catecholamine release from BACC by all stimuli, but that evoked by nicotinic receptor stimulation is much more sensitive to inhibition than that evoked by K^+.[9] The effects of GABA are also known to be greater on nicotinic receptor-mediated release[7] suggesting the possibility that, as in neurons, ethanol can potentiate GABA in BACC. Since GABA is co-released with catecholamines after nicotinic receptor stimulation the inhibitory effect of ethanol on catecholamine release might be indirect, via an increased inhibitory effect of GABA. The imidazodiazepine RO 15-4513 is known to be a highly potent inhibitor of the effects of ethanol on the $GABA_A$ receptor in brain.[10] In our experiments[11] it also potently inhibited the effect of ethanol on catecholamine release induced by carbachol (a nicotinic receptor agonist). We therefore believe that a major factor in the inhibitory effect of ethanol on the BACC in culture is a potentiating action at the $GABA_A$ receptor, but other actions are also probable.

In relation to the effect of the presence of ethanol on Ca^{2+} entry, the action of the drug on the $GABA_A$ receptor would of course be expected to inhibit the ability of depolarization to cause Ca^{2+} entry. In adrenal-derived PC 12 cells it has been shown that ethanol inhibits depolarization-induced $^{45}Ca^{2+}$ entry,[12] but this is probably by other mechanisms since these cells do not express $GABA_A$ receptors. We have investigated a number of depolarization-induced biochemical changes in BACC, including the K^+-induced breakdown of inositol phospholipids[13] (which will be relevant later). Ethanol inhibits them all, suggesting that it inhibits depolarization-induced changes at an early stage such as Ca^{2+} entry. These effects are similar to many of our previous observations in CNS neurons.

Maintaining BACC in culture with the presence of ethanol (200 mM) in the culture medium for 6 days did not appear to affect cell viability in any way.[9,14] After this period re-exposure of these cells to ethanol no longer inhibited the release of catecholamines evoked by carbachol.[9] The cells appeared to have developed almost complete tolerance to this inhibitory effect of ethanol. The mechanism for this dramatic change is unknown, but it presumably must represent an alteration in the effect of ethanol on the $GABA_A$ receptor protein. Such an alteration has been described in the CNS of alcohol-tolerant laboratory animals.

When cells which had been exposed chronically to ethanol were examined in the absence of the drug they showed several differences from controls. Their content of stored catecholamines was higher, as was their basal (unstimulated) release of catecholamines.[14] Taken together these findings suggest a higher than normal synthesis of catecholamines in these cells. On stimulation with carbachol the cells "withdrawn" from alcohol released a similar amount of catecholamines to that of controls[15] (although this now represented a lower *proportion* of the total stored). However on stimulation with K^+, particularly at high concentrations of K^+ and Ca^{2+}, the cells withdrawn from alcohol released a much greater amount of catecholamines (and even a greater *proportion* of stored catecholamines) than controls.[14] This was particularly reminiscent of our original finding of increased sensitivity of catecholamine release in brain slice preparations from ethanol-dependent animals.[5]

Since the K^+-depolarization–induced release of catecholamines from BACC was uniquely sensitive to DHP calcium channel antagonists,[8,9] the changes described in BACC maintained in culture medium containing ethanol could be explained by some increase in the number, or activity, of the "L-type" calcium channels. The increase in K^+-induced catecholamine release could indeed be inhibited by DHP calcium channel antagonists and could be reproduced by the DHP calcium channel "agonist," BAY K 8644.[9,14] This focused attention on the possibility that the increase in calcium "sensitivity" might be a consequence of changes in "L-type," or at least "DHP-sensitive," calcium channels. This can be assessed by studying the binding of radiolabeled DHPs to BACC membranes.

DOES EXPOSURE TO ETHANOL CAUSE AN INCREASE IN DHP BINDING IN BACC MEMBRANES?

The first experiments on [³H]DHP binding in adrenal-derived cells exposed to ethanol were carried out on PC 12 cells in Ivan Diamond's laboratory.[15] Exposure to 200 mM ethanol for 6 days caused about a 100% increase in the number of binding sites with no change in binding affinity.[15] We obtained very similar results in BACC in culture.[16] The increase in binding sites reaches a maximum after about 4–6 days and returns to normal levels within about 24 hours after removal of ethanol.[15] This time course fits several of the changes in cell excitability described earlier, and is fairly typical of the sort of change which is caused by alterations in *de novo* protein synthesis.

BACC have the "disadvantage" that they are genetically heterogenous, as compared for example with the PC 12 tumor cell line. The variability in the increase in DHP binding in the BACC cultures was high, but seemed to be much less if cell cultures obtained from the same animal were compared. This suggested that the alteration in DHP binding may be genetically controlled. Experiments using inhibitors of protein synthesis supported this possibility.[16] Lomofungin, a putative inhibitor of DNA transcription, inhibited the increase in DHP binding sites associated with growth in ethanol. The increase in DHP binding may therefore represent increased expression of the gene for the DHP-binding protein (probably the "L-type" calcium channel in these cells).

If this increase in DHP binding in response to ethanol is truly an adaptive response to the inhibitory effects of the drug on the activity of the BACC cultures, then it should not occur if the inhibitory effects of ethanol are blocked. Conversely it should also be produced by chronic exposure to other inhibitory drugs. Both predictions appear to be true. Concomitant exposure to RO 15-4513 (which prevents the acute inhibitory effects of ethanol on these cells) prevents the up-regulation of DHP binding sites caused by ethanol in BACC cultures.[11] Chronic exposure to anxiolytic drugs, which, like ethanol, reduce catecholamine release from BACC cultures, increase DHP binding with a similar time course.[17] The alteration in DHP binding may prove a generalized response to drugs which depress the effects of depolarization in these cells. By extension similar adaptation to depressant drugs may occur in neurons.

It remains to be seen what triggers this presumed adaptive increase in DHP binding. The most obvious possibility would appear to be a reduced intracellular Ca^{2+} concentration, which would be expected to result from an inhibition of depolarization-induced Ca^{2+} entry. However, this seems very unlikely, partly because ethanol *increases* cytosolic Ca^{2+} in these cells by releasing it from intracellular stores.[18] In addition, the DHP calcium channel antagonists themselves, do not lead to an increase in DHP binding sites. Indeed, when present with ethanol in BACC culture medium they *prevent* the increase in DHP binding which ethanol causes.[11] Current evidence suggests that some second messenger, perhaps related to inositol lipid breakdown, generated by membrane depolarization might be the controlling mechanism.[19]

The potential importance of the finding of an increase in the number of DHP binding sites rests entirely on the assumption that these represent functional voltage-operated calcium channels. This is not easy to prove, but there is now considerable circumstantial evidence for the proposition.

WHAT ARE THE FUNCTIONAL CONSEQUENCES OF AN INCREASE IN DHP BINDING SITES IN BACC CULTURES?

There are several changes in adrenal cells after chronic exposure to ethanol which could be functional consequences of an increase in "L-type" calcium channels. These include increased catecholamine release and inositol lipid breakdown on stimulation with K^+ or with BAY K 8644 in BACC cultures,[9,14,13] and increased depolarization-induced entry of $^{45}Ca^{2+}$ in PC 12 cells.[20] All of these are sensitive to inhibition by DHP calcium channel antagonists and all provide circumstantial evidence that a functional increase in DHP-sensitive voltage-operated calcium channels accompanies the increase in DHP binding sites on these cells.

All the evidence described above, however, relies on "experimental" manipulations of the cells. The "physiological" release of catecholamines by stimulation of nicotinic cholinoceptors is either unchanged or inhibited (depending on how the results are expressed) in the ethanol "withdrawn" cells. This hardly suggests that there would be any withdrawal hyperexcitability of these cells if similar changes occurred in the intact animal. This assumption may be incorrect; in the adrenal gland *in vivo* the cells are aggregated and may function more as a syncytium, with electrotonic spread of depolarization (via voltage-operated channels) from cell to cell being more important for overall excitability than it is in the disaggregated cell cultures.

Even this proposal is of little use if we wish to apply our findings in these neuron-like cultures to neurons in the CNS. Electrotonic spread of depolarization from neuron to neuron is of doubtful significance in the mammalian CNS. Because of these objections we have tried to think carefully what the physiological role of these "L-type" channels could be in the CNS, and whether there is a functional counterpart in the BACC cultures.

The "L-type" calcium channels are probably concentrated at the base of major dendrites on neurons in the CNS.[21] In this situation they are ideally placed to allow the spread of depolarization from dendrites over the surface of the soma, and to synchronize Ca^{2+} entry into the cell body with electrical activity in the nerve. This latter function could be important in second messenger functions, such as gene regulation and release of transmitters from the cell body (both of which will be important later). Returning to the "electrical" function of these channels, they would probably be of most importance in the spread of depolarization caused by the action of excitatory amino acids on receptors on the dendrites. We resolved to see whether BACC cultures responded to excitatory amino acids and, if so, whether this response was affected by maintenance of the cultures in ethanol.

Several amino acids, including glutamate, N-methyl D-aspartic acid (NMDA) and homocysteic acid, caused release of catecholamines from BACC in culture.[22] This effect was inhibited by micromolar concentrations of the NMDA receptor antagonists amino phosphonovalerate and MK 801, and was potentiated by glycine and by exclusion of Mg^{2+}. The effect thus bears all the hallmarks of an NMDA receptor-mediated response, and this is supported by our recent finding of specific saturable binding of [³H]MK 801 to membranes of cultured BACC.[23]

When BACC cultures were exposed to ethanol for 4–6 days and then stimulated with excitatory amino acids there was clear evidence of hyperexcitability.[22] This was most obvious under conditions where physiological concentrations of Mg^{2+} were present, or where the cells were partially depolarized with K^+ before stimulation.[22] The hyperexcitability could therefore be explained by an increased spread of depolarization overcoming the Mg^{2+} block of the NMDA receptor. This in turn might be a consequence of increased numbers of functional voltage-operated calcium channels. It is probably *not* explained by alterations in numbers of NMDA receptors because MK 801 binding was unchanged by growth of BACC in culture medium containing ethanol.[23]

CONCLUSIONS FROM EXPERIMENTS ON ADRENAL CELLS

Exposure of adrenal cells chronically to ethanol evokes an increase in DHP binding sites which seem to represent functional calcium channels on the cell membranes. This alteration has all the characteristics of an adaptive response to the initial inhibitory effect of the drug. It is probably caused by an increased expression of the calcium channel gene. The major consequences in an increase in the electrical excitability of the cells (increased responsivity to excitatory amino acids may be particularly relevant to neurons in the CNS) and an increase in Ca^{2+} entry to the cell body for second messenger functions.

DO NEURONS IN THE CNS ADAPT TO ETHANOL IN THE SAME WAY AS BACC?

The experiments on adrenal cells were begun in order to compare findings in these cells with our original observations on catecholamines in the brains of laboratory animals. There are a surprising number of similarities. Brain preparations from ethanol-dependent laboratory animals have increased catecholamine content and release more catecholamines both basally and when stimulated with K^+ depolarization.[5] All these effects were also seen in the culture system and, in both cases, increased numbers of functional calcium channels could be the cause (although so could several other changes).

The position of "L-type" calcium channels on dendrites rather than at nerve terminals suggests that increases in their number would be more likely to influence transmitter release from areas rich in cell bodies rather than areas rich in nerve terminals. Experiments comparing release of dopamine from slices of substantia nigra and from corpus striatum[24] suggested that the effect seen in preparations from ethanol dependent rats could be explained by increased DHP-sensitive calcium channels in the cell body region (substantia nigra in these experiments). Similar circumstantial evidence (enhanced effects of depolarization susceptible to modification DHP calcium channel antagonists or agonists) were found for several other biochemical parameters, including inositol lipid breakdown.[25]

All the evidence suggests that the increase in "calcium sensitivity" which we reported originally as associated with ethanol tolerance and dependence might be explained by an increase in "L-type" calcium channels in the CNS. [³H]DHP binding studies provide further support for this.[25] Rats made dependent on ethanol showed a c50% increase in numbers of DHP binding sites in membranes of cerebral cortex compared to controls. There was no change in binding affinity.[25] Subsequent experiments have shown that the increase in DHP binding begins after 2–3 days of ethanol administration and reaches a maximum (in cortex) after about 6 days (L. Guppy, unpublished). The numbers of DHP binding sites were also increased in all other excitable tissues studied,[26] the greatest change being in the heart (250% of control values). On withdrawal from ethanol the increase in DHP binding sites disappeared within about 24 hours (L. Guppy, unpublished), again showing similarity with the results from cell cultures.[12]

DO INCREASES IN DHP BINDING SITES CONFER ELECTRICAL EXCITABILITY ON BRAIN SLICES?

Most of our experiments directed toward this question utilize hippocampal slice preparations from laboratory animals that have been made dependent on ethanol *in vivo*. These slice preparations are then examined for evidence of hyperexcitability in the absence of ethanol *in vitro*, so this preparation represents a kind of "*ex vivo*" model of ethanol withdrawal. We have demonstrated a variety of direct manifestations of withdrawal hyperexcitability that follow a consistent sequence in this model.[27] The first evidence of change, in extracellular recordings from area CA1, was an increase in paired pulse potentiation accompanied by a decrease in recurrent inhibition. These were transient and had disappeared by about 4 hours into withdrawal, when decreases in thresholds for elicitation of spike activity were seen that lasted until 7 hours after "withdrawal" *in vitro*. These changes in excitability of the hippocampal slice *ex vivo* were not seen in preparations from animals that had been withdrawn 24 hours beforehand, suggesting that the model genuinely represents ethanol withdrawal excitability.

The synaptic changes that underlie this hyperexcitability could be a consequence of an increased responsivity to excitatory amino-acids similar to that which we described in bovine adrenal chromaffin cells, and this is now under study. We already have considerable evidence that it is at least partly a consequence of increased activity of L-type calcium channels (or at least DHP-sensitive calcium channels). All the indices of increased excitability of hippocampal slices could be reduced by the inclusion of calcium channel antagonists in the perfusing medium.[28] This effect was stereospecific, being seen with the (+) isomer of PN 200-110 that possesses calcium channel antagonist activity, but not the (−) isomer which is devoid of such activity. It was also selective, as the active compound did not alter the hyperexcitability produced by the GABA antagonist, bicuculline, in hippocampal slices from control animals.

In addition to the acute protective effects of calcium channel antagonists when present in the perfusate, the same drugs were active *in vivo*. The ability of concomitant treatment with DHP calcium channel antagonists to prevent the up-regulation in DHP binding sites caused by ethanol in BACC cultures has already been referred to. The drugs have similar effects in the intact animal. When DHP calcium channel antagonists were given at the same time as ethanol to laboratory animals, both the behavioral signs of withdrawal excitability and the development of tolerance were prevented.[29-31] In addition the numbers of DHP binding sites remained unaltered from control levels, showing that the up-regulation caused by ethanol had been prevented.[29,31] In these animals that had been treated with the DHP calcium channel antagonists all the signs of hyperexcitability in the hippocampal slice preparations were decreased.[32] During all these studies the DHP calcium channel antagonists were not given for at least 24 hours before testing so that residual levels of the drugs would not be sufficient (confirmed by direct measurements of their concentration in brain) to affect the results. Our interpretation is that treatments that prevent the up-regulation of calcium channels associated with chronic administration of ethanol also prevent chemical dependence and the hyperexcitability associated with ethanol withdrawal.

We believe that this is good evidence to support the idea that increases in DHP-sensitive calcium channels can confer an increase in electrical excitability on neurons which becomes apparent in ethanol withdrawal. Definitive evidence is now being obtained from intracellular recording from neurons in the hippocampal slice preparations from ethanol-dependent animals.

CAN INCREASES IN CALCIUM CHANNELS IN THE CNS EXPLAIN THE ALCOHOL PHYSICAL WITHDRAWAL SYNDROME IN THE INTACT ANIMAL?

The alcohol physical withdrawal syndrome includes tremors and convulsions, which are relatively easy to assess in laboratory animals.[2] Using models of alcohol dependence which rely on the forced administration of the drug it has been possible to show a marked inhibitory effect of calcium channel antagonists on these signs of withdrawal.[33] This effect shows the same stereospecificity as the blockade of calcium channels and the inhibition of hyperexcitability in the hippocampal slice preparation that we described in the last section. In addition, the DHP calcium channel "agonist" BAY K 8644 both prevents the protective effect of calcium channel antagonists and mimics the seizures seen in alcohol withdrawal.[34] These are not generalized effects of the DHP drugs. The calcium channel antagonists show little anti-convulsant activity in a variety of other tests on laboratory rodents.

As with the experiments on brain slices, it has proved possible to prevent the increase in DHP binding sites by concomitant administration of DHPs with alcohol. The same regime which prevented the *ex vivo* hyperexcitability in brain slices also prevents both tolerance and the physical signs of withdrawal in the intact animal.[29-31] We feel this is good evidence for a causal association between the increase in DHP binding sites in the CNS which occurs on chronic treatment with alcohol and the signs of withdrawal that follow its removal.

The last piece of evidence in the intact animal relates to the genetic control of calcium channel expression which we suspected from our experiments on cell cultures. The severity of the alcohol physical withdrawal syndrome is strongly genetically influenced in laboratory animals. For example, in John Crabbe's laboratory, mice from an originally homogeneous stock have been selected for the severity of alcohol withdrawal for 26 generations.[35] The resulting two lines are characterized as "withdrawal seizure prone" (WSP) or "withdrawal seizure resistant" (WSR) and differ very greatly in their severity of alcohol withdrawal. When both lines were exposed to alcohol by inhalation for 3 days the WSP line up-regulated DHP binding sites (whole brain) by 125% whereas the WSR mice showed only a 25% increase in this parameter.[35] This genetic difference was not confined to brain, similar genetic differences were seen in the hearts of these animals (L. Guppy, unpublished).

In these experiments the difference in DHP binding between lines could not be a *consequence* of the differences in withdrawal severity because the animals were killed while still intoxicated. This seems strong evidence that genetic differences in the extent of DHP binding protein up-regulation in response to alcohol influence the severity of alcohol withdrawal. The genetic differences in withdrawal severity in these lines generalize to other depressant drugs, including benzodiazepines and barbiturates, suggesting a similar mechanism for withdrawal from these depressant drugs. The fact that genetic differences in DHP binding regulation can be detected in peripheral tissues also offers the possibility that tests assessing the extent of this change may be introduced into clinical medicine. (Though heart muscle is not the ideal tissue to biopsy!)

CONCLUSIONS

Adrenal chromaffin cells in primary culture mimic many of the properties of mature neurons, not only in the way they are affected acutely by drugs, but also in the way they respond to the long-term presence of drugs. Experiments on these cells suggest that there may be a very primitive mechanism of adaptation to depressant drugs which involves an increase in the number of "L-type" calcium channels on the cell surface. This finding seems to extend to animal models, at least of alcohol dependence and possibly of opiate dependence and benzodiazepine dependence also. In the intact CNS the immediate effect of such an up-regulation of "L-type" calcium channels may be to increase electrical excitability of neurons to excitatory transmitters such as glutamate. However, several longer term consequences, for example on gene regulation, would also be expected.

In conclusion the use of this particular cell culture model of drug dependence certainly seems to provide information which can be applied to animal models. Whether the findings can be extended into the clinical setting remains uncertain, but preliminary observations, *e.g.*, the protective effects of calcium channel antagonists in clinical alcohol withdrawal detoxification, are encouraging.[36]

REFERENCES

1. FREUND, G. 1969. Alcohol withdrawal syndrome in mice. Arch. Neurol. **21:** 315.
2. GOLDSTEIN, D. B. & N. PAL. 1971. Alcohol dependence produced in mice by inhalation. Grading the withdrawal reaction. Science **172:** 288–290.
3. GOLDSTEIN, D. B. 1973. Alcohol withdrawal reactions in mice. Effects of drugs that modify neurotransmission. J. Pharm. Exp. Ther. **190:** 1–9.
4. LITTLETON, J. M. 1983. Tolerance and physical dependence on alcohol at the level of synaptic membranes: A review. J. Royal Soc. Med. **76:** 593–601.
5. LYNCH, M. A. & J. M. LITTLETON. 1983. Possible association of alcohol tolerance with increased synaptic calcium sensitivity. Nature **303:** 175–176.

6. LIVITT, B. G. 1984. Adrenal medullary chromaffin cells in vitro. Phys. Rev. **64**: 1103–1161.
7. KATAOKA, Y., Y. GUTMAN, A. GUIDOTTI, P. PANULA, J. WROBLEWSKI & D. COSENZA-MURPHY. 1987. Intrinsic GABA-ergic system in adrenal chromaffin cells. Proc. Natl. Acad. Sci. USA **81**: 3218–3222.
8. BOARDER, M. R., D. MARRIOTT & M. ADAMS. 1987. Stimulus-secretion in cultured chromaffin cells. Dependency on external sodium and on DHP-sensitive calcium channels. Biochem. Pharmacol. **36**: 163–167.
9. HARPER, J. C. & J. M. LITTLETON. 1990. Development of tolerance to ethanol in cultured adrenal chromaffin cells. Alcoholism Clin. Exp. Res. **14**: 508–512.
10. SUZDAK, P. D., J. R. GLOWA, J. N. CRAWLEY, R. D. SCHWARTZ, P. SKOLNICK & S. M. PAUL. 1986. A selective imidazodiazepine antagonist of ethanol in the rat. Science **234**: 1243–1247.
11. BRENNAN, C. H., A. LEWIS & J. M. LITTLETON. 1989. Membrane receptors involved in up-regulation of calcium channels in bovine adrenal chromaffin cells chronically exposed to ethanol. Neuropharmacology **28**: 1303–1307.
12. MESSING, R. O., C. L. CARPENTER, I. DIAMOND & D. A. GREENBERG. 1986. Ethanol regulates calcium channels in clonal cells. Proc. Natl. Acad. Sci. USA **83**: 6213–6215.
13. BRENNAN, C. H. 1990. The role of dihydropyridine-sensitive calcium channels in alterations of cell excitability associated with ethanol dependence. University of London Ph.D. thesis.
14. HARPER, J. C. & J. M. LITTLETON. 1991. Characteristics of catecholamine release from adrenal chromaffin cells cultured in medium containing ethanol. 1 Spontaneous and K+ induced release. Alcohol & Alcoholism **26**: 25–32.
15. HARPER, J. C. & J. M. LITTLETON. 1991. Characteristics of catecholamine release from adrenal chromaffin cells cultured in medium containing ethanol. II. Carbachol and veratrine-induced release. Alcohol & Alcoholism **26**: 33–38.
16. HARPER, J. C., C. H. BRENNAN & J. M. LITTLETON. 1989. Genetic up-regulation of calcium channels in a cell culture model of ethanol dependence. Neuropharmacology **28**: 1299–1302.
17. BRENNAN, C. H. & J. M. LITTLETON. 1991. Chronic exposure to anxiolytic drugs working by different mechanisms causes up-regulation of dihydropyridine binding sites on cultured bovine adrenal chromaffin cells. Neuropharmacology **30**: 199–205.
18. RABE, C. S. & F. F. WEIGHT. 1988. Effects of ethanol on neurotransmitter release and intracellular calcium concentration in PC12 cells. J. Pharmacol. Exp. Ther. **244**: 417–422.
19. BRENNAN, C. H. & J. M. LITTLETON. 1990. Second messenger systems involved in genetic regulation of Ca^{2+} channels in adrenal chromaffin cells. Neuropharmacology **29**: 689–693.
20. GREENBERG, D. A., C. L. CARPENTER & R. O. MESSING. 1987. Ethanol-induced component of 45 Ca^{2+} uptake in PC 12 cells is sensitive to Ca^{2+} channel modulating drugs. Brain Res. **410**: 143–146.
21. WESTENBROEK, R. E., M. AHLIJANIAN & W. A. CATTERALL. 1991. Clustering of L-type calcium channels at the base of major dendrites in hippocampal pyramidal neurons. Nature **347**: 281–284.
22. CWYNARSKI, K., O. BOUCHENAFA, C. H. BRENNAN & J. M. LITTLETON. 1989. Bovine adrenal cells grown in culture medium containing ethanol show hyperexcitability to glutamate. Alcohol & Alcoholism **24**: 370.
23. BOUCHENAFA, O., R. LAVERTY, C. RUHE, R. DAVIES & J. LITTLETON. 1991. The hyperresponsivity to excitatory amino acids shown by bovine adrenal cells withdrawn from ethanol is prevented by calcium acetyl homotaurinate. Alcohol & Alcoholism **26**: 237.
24. PAGONIS, C. & J. M. LITTLETON. 1987. The calcium antagonist PN 200-110 inhibits [3H]-dopamine release from nigral but not striatal slices from ethanol-dependent rats. Br. J. Pharmacol. **91**: 416P.
25. DOLIN, S. J., H. J. LITTLE, M. J. HUDSPITH, C. PAGONIS & J. LITTLETON. 1987. Increased dihydropyridine-sensitive calcium channels in rat brain may underlie ethanol physical dependence. Neuropharmacology **26**: 275–280.
26. GUPPY, L. & J. M. LITTLETON. 1988. Increased [3H]DHP binding sites in brain heart and smooth muscle of ethanol dependent rats. Br. J. Pharmacol. **92**: 662P.
27. WHITTINGTON, M. A. & H. J. LITTLE. 1990. Patterns of changes in field potentials in the

isolated hippocampal slice on withdrawal from chronic ethanol treatment of mice in vivo. Brain Res. **523:** 237–244.

28. WHITTINGTON, M. A. & H. J. LITTLE. 1991. A calcium channel antagonist stereoselectively decreases the electro-physiological changes in the isolated hippocampal slice seen during ethanol withdrawal. Br. J. Pharmacol. **103:** 1313–1320.

29. WHITTINGTON, M. A., R. J. SIAREY, T. L. PATCH, A. R. BUTTERWORTH, S. J. DOLIN & H. J. LITTLE. 1991. Chronic dihydropyridine treatment can reverse the behavioural consequences and prevent the adaptations to chronic ethanol. Br. J. Pharmacol. **103:** 1669–1676.

30. WU, P. H., T. PHAM & C. A. NARANJO. 1987. Nifedipine delays the acquisition of tolerance to ethanol. Eur. J. Pharmacol. **139:** 233–236.

31. DOLIN, S. J. & H. J. LITTLE. 1989. Are changes in neuronal calcium channels involved in ethanol tolerance? J. Pharmacol. Exp. Ther. **150:** 985–991.

32. WHITTINGTON, M. A. & H. J. LITTLE. 1991. Nitrendipine, given during drinking, decreases the electrophysiological changes in the isolated hippocampal slice, seen during ethanol withdrawal. Br. J. Pharmacol. **103:** 1677–1684.

33. LITTLE, H. J., S. J. DOLIN & M. J. HALSEY. 1986. Calcium channel antagonists decrease the ethanol withdrawal syndrome in rats. Life Sci. **39:** 2059–2065.

34. LITTLETON, J. M., H. J. LITTLE & M. A. WHITTINGTON. 1990. Effects of dihydropyridine calcium channel antagonists in ethanol withdrawal; doses required, stereospecificity and actions of BAY K 8644. Psychopharmacology **100:** 387–392.

35. BRENNAN, C. H., J. CRABBE & J. M. LITTLETON. 1990. Genetic regulation of dihydropyridine sensitive calcium channels in brain may determine susceptibility to ethanol physical dependence. Neuropharmacology **29:** 429–432.

36. KOPPI, S., G. EBERHARDT, R. HALLER & P. KONIG. 1987. Calcium channel blocking agent in the treatment of acute ethanol withdrawal-caroverine versus meprobamate in a randomised double blind study. Neuropsychobiology **17:** 49–52.

Neurobiology of Conditioning to Drugs of Abuse

JANE STEWART

Center for Studies in Behavioral Neurobiology
Department of Psychology, Concordia University
1455 de Maisonneuve Boulevard W.
Montréal, Québec, Canada H3G 1M8

INTRODUCTION

Conditioning is a form of associative learning about the co-occurrence of two stimulus events. If one stimulus reliably predicts the occurrence of a second, and if each of them can activate some neural elements in common, a change will occur in the ability of the first, the conditional stimulus (CS), to activate processes originally activated only by the second, the unconditioned stimulus (UCS). If the UCS elicits measurable changes in behavior or neural activity, then evidence that the relation between the CS and the UCS has been learned is found in the ability of the CS alone to elicit some of the changes originally produced by the UCS. This phenomenon was originally demonstrated by Pavlov who studied the conditioning of food-elicited salivation and digestive responses to neutral environmental stimuli. UCSs such as food that have motivational significance for an animal elicit a wide variety of responses including autonomic and regulatory responses, consummatory responses and investigatory and approach responses. If the UCS elicits general approach or avoidance, then the CS will come to elicit general approach or avoidance as well. Advantage has been taken of this by those studying the positive motivational properties of drugs of abuse in the paradigm known as the conditioned place preference in which one of two distinctive places is repeatedly paired with a drug injection and the other with saline. On a test for conditioning when no drug is given, an increase in the time that the animal chooses to spend in the place previously paired with the drug injection is taken as a measure of conditioning of affective processes or motivation.

The effects of a CS can also be measured by the way it changes the response to the UCS and to other stimuli in the environment. If, for example, the occurrence of a receptive female rat, a motivationally positive stimulus for the male, is signaled by a CS, then the initiation and completion of copulation will occur more quickly.[1] The CS appears to activate sexual arousal which in turn facilitates the response to the female and the performance of copulation itself.

In the context of conditioning to drugs of abuse, I mention these points for two reasons. The first is that drugs of abuse, as do other motivationally important UCS, have many central nervous system actions. Only some of them are related to their abuse potential. CSs repeatedly paired with drugs of abuse gain the power to elicit many of the actions originally elicited by the drugs themselves, so-called conditioned drug effects. I will argue that drug-paired CSs have the potential to alter subsequent drug-related behaviors in two ways: by modifying the effects of drugs taken in their presence, and by eliciting conditioned effects that may contribute to relapse to drug-taking in drug-free individuals. In order to understand the contribution of conditioning to drug-related behaviors it will be important to determine which conditioned effects of drugs actually contribute to their abuse and how CSs gain the ability to control or modify the expression of drug actions.

CONDITIONED DRUG EFFECTS

Pavlov[2] reporting on the experiments of a certain Dr. Krylov of the Tashkent Bacteriological Laboratory wrote:

> It is well known that the first effect of a hypodermic injection of morphine (in the dog) is to produce nausea with profuse secretion of saliva, followed by vomiting, and then profound sleep. Dr. Krylov, however, observed when the injections were repeated regularly that after 5 or 6 days the preliminaries of injection were in themselves sufficient to produce all these symptoms—nausea, secretion of saliva, vomiting and sleep. Under these circumstances the symptoms are now the effect, not of the morphine acting through the blood stream directly on the vomiting centre, but of **all the external stimuli which previously had preceded the injection of morphine** . . .

Pavlov continued,

> . . . in the most striking cases all the symptoms could be produced by the dog simply seeing the experimenter. Where such a stimulus was insufficient it was necessary to open the box containing the syringe, to crop the fur over a small area of skin and wipe with alcohol, and perhaps even to inject some harmless fluid before the symptoms could be obtained.

In the years since these observations were made, conditioned drug effects have been demonstrated to a wide range of centrally acting drugs and the potential importance of such effects for an understanding of the long-lasting consequences of drug use has been raised by numerous investigators.[3-6] But although we continue to give lip-service to this view, little has been done to truly advance our understanding of these matters. There are steady advances in knowledge of the mechanisms of actions of various drugs of abuse; we are beginning to identify which actions of drugs are related to their abuse potential; and yet almost nothing is known about the mechanisms underlying the conditioning of these actions of drugs and how conditioned stimuli act to influence drug-taking behavior. What we lack are neural models to help us think about ways in which conditioned environmental stimuli can come to elicit drug effects or to modify the actions of drugs themselves.

If Conditioning Is to Occur to the Effects of Drugs, Conditional Stimuli Must Have Access to the Central Neural Elements Underlying Those Effects

Drugs may have effects on several response systems both within the central nervous system (CNS) and in the periphery. Some of the observed effects of drugs are produced directly by their action on central nervous system elements, whereas others are produced by their actions in the periphery. It is often found that drugs produce opposing changes depending on the time after injection and the dose administered. A high dose of morphine, for example, may produce hypothermia followed by hyperthermia. It is important when trying to think about conditioned drug effects to realize that such biphasic effects could arise either from the output of two independent CNS systems, each directly activated by a drug, or from the output of a single CNS system responding to compensate for the initial drug action. The nature and direction of a conditioned drug effect, or conditioned response (CR), therefore, will not be easily predicted from the observed drug effects, but will depend on our knowledge of which CNS response systems are actually activated. If, as stated above, conditioning of a drug effect depends on the access of the neural elements excited by the CS to those CNS elements activated either directly or indirectly by the drug, it will be necessary to know how the drug effects are produced. Some conditioned drug effects will mimic the observed drug effect (so-called drug-like CRs) whereas others will oppose the observed drug effect (so-called drug-opposite CRs). In a recent issue of TIPS, B. Max,[7] though apparently interested in such effects, remarked scornfully that the problem with people working in the field is that they wanted to eat their cake and have it too; in other words, we wanted our conditioned drug effects both ways. We don't want them both ways, they are both ways, just as drug effects often are!

Conditioning Procedures and Tests for the Effects of CSs

In studies of conditioned drug effects in animals, it has become standard to include at least three groups: a group which during the conditioning phase receives the drug on several occasions in the presence of a distinctive set of environmental stimuli (CSs) and saline in the absence of these stimuli (a PAIRED group), a group that receives saline in the presence of the distinctive stimuli and the drug injection in their absence (an UNPAIRED group), and a group that receives saline in both conditions (a CONTROL group).

In a standard test for conditioning, all groups are presented with the CS in the absence of drug and the responses to the CS are compared. In a test for CS control of drug actions, all groups are given the drug in the presence of the CS and effects of the drug are compared. CS may act to diminish or to enhance the effect of a drug; the former can be referred to as the CS control of tolerance and the latter the CS control of sensitization.

CONDITIONING AND THE BEHAVIORAL ACTIVATING EFFECTS OF STIMULANT AND OPIOID DRUGS

Common Neural Elements Underlie Some of the Behavioral Actions of Stimulant and Opioid Drugs

Systemic injections of either amphetamine or cocaine lead to increased behavioral activation, locomotor activity and at higher doses to stereotypy, which with repeated injections shows sensitization.[8] These effects are mediated by actions on the mesolimbic and striatal dopamine (DA) neurons where amphetamine increases extracellular DA by direct release and reuptake blockade, and cocaine by reuptake blockade.

Acute systemic injections of medium to high doses of morphine produce in rats depressant effects followed by excitatory effects. These are seen in the initial motor depression followed by heightened locomotor activity. With repeated intermittent injection the depressant actions show rapid tolerance revealing only the excitatory effects. The locomotor-activating effects of morphine can be elicited independently of the depressant actions, as shown by the direct application of morphine to the cell body regions of the mesolimbic and striatal dopamine (DA) neurons. Here morphine and other opioids act to increase firing in DA neurons thereby increasing extracellular dopamine in both cell body and terminal regions. As has been discussed in previous papers presented at this meeting, repeated injections of opioids lead, as do those of amphetamine and cocaine, to sensitization of the behavioral activating effects which appears to be mediated by long-term functional changes in the midbrain DA neurons.[9]

When systemic injections of drugs from either class are repeatedly paired with a set of environmental stimuli (CSs), increased locomotor activity is seen in the presence of these CSs when they are presented alone, that is, behavioral activation is elicited by the CSs. When repeated exposure to these drugs is paired exclusively with a set of environmental stimuli, the behavioral sensitization to the drugs is manifested only in the presence of these stimuli, that is, the expression of sensitization comes under CS control.[10]

This set of findings should be of particular interest to those interested in the motivational effects of stimulant and opioid drugs and to the long-term consequences of their use. The mesolimbic DA system appears to be a behavioral facilitatory system. Activity in this system promotes forward locomotion, enhances the behavioral effectiveness of positive incentive stimuli, and appears to underlie the motivational or rewarding properties of stimulant and opioid drugs as well as those of more natural positive incentives.[11] Sensitized functioning within this system could serve to enhance the response to stimuli having neural access to it. The fact that CSs are able to modulate the behavioral sensitization to drugs and to elicit drug-like behavioral activation in the absence of drugs implies that CSs may gain access directly to the facilitation system itself, *i.e.*, the mesolimbic DA system, or to those response systems activated by it, or to both. These possibilities are shown in the diagram in FIGURE 1. This diagram shows stimuli serving as CSs to have weak, but direct access to the facilitation system. There is evidence for this from studies of responses of DA neurons to novel sensory stimuli.[12-15] Though these effects would normally habituate with repeated presenta-

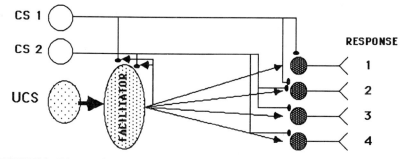

FIGURE 1. Diagram showing possible ways in which a conditional stimulus (CS) could gain access to neural units activated by an unconditioned stimulus (UCS). CSs neurons are shown to have weak, but direct access to a behavioral facilitation system normally activated by the UCS. The CSs are also shown to have access to some response units normally activated by the UCS via the facilitator. Changes in the behavioral effectiveness of a CS could be mediated by neural changes at either site through the co-occurrence of the CS and UCS (see text).

tion, when a CS is paired with a UCS that activates the facilitator, the ability of the CS to activate the facilitator is strengthened or reinforced. In addition, the CS are shown to have access to certain response units normally activated by the UCS via the facilitator. Through repeated paired presentations of the CS and UCS, the capability of the CS to activate these responses would be strengthened by co-occurrence of activity in the CS neurons and the facilitator neurons. Either one or both of these mechanisms could underlie the conditioning of behavioral activation produced by the effects of drugs on the facilitator. Whether either or both of these effects underlies conditioned effects produced by a particular drug should depend on how that drug interacts with the DA facilitatory system to produce its unconditioned behavioral activational effect.

Increased extracellular DA from midbrain DA neurons is common to the actions of morphine, amphetamine and cocaine. Increased extracellular DA at terminals is responsible for the behavioral activation produced by amphetamine and cocaine and, at least in part, for that produced by morphine; increased extracellular DA in the cell body region, appears to initiate processes responsible for the development of sensitization to these drugs, but we have not as yet identified the role of DA in conditioned activity to these drugs or in the CS control of the expression of behavioral sensitization to these drugs. As we explore what is known about conditioned effects, it is important to keep in mind how increased extracellular DA levels are achieved in the case of each drug. Morphine acts to increase DA cell firing causing impulse-dependent release. Cocaine interferes with the reuptake of DA, but release depends on impulses initiated by other means. In both cases the opportunity for concurrent activity in CS neurons and the DA neurons would exist making it possible that CS could come to activate DA neurons directly. The situation is less clear, however, for amphetamine which causes release directly, independent of firing in the DA neuron. In all three cases the possibility for CS-UCS interactions exist in the terminal regions of the DA neurons, either pre- or post-synaptically.

Loci for the Development of Behavioral Sensitization and for Conditioned Stimulus Control

The locomotor activity elicited and the sensitization that develops when morphine is applied directly into the ventral tegmental area (VTA) can be brought under CS control. We showed that animals given pairings of the distinctive environment of an activity box and intra-VTA morphine (PAIRED) were more active in that environment compared to animals that received the same morphine injections elsewhere (UN-PAIRED), or no morphine in either environment (CONTROL), when placed in it following placebo injections. Moreover, on a test for sensitization when all animals received intra-VTA morphine, only group PAIRED showed sensitization to the effects of morphine.[16] Thus it appeared that repeated activation of the mesolimbic DA system in the presence of a specific set of environmental stimuli was a sufficient condition for the development of drug-induced conditioned activity and conditioned control of the expression of sensitized responding to intra-VTA morphine. We later showed that animals preexposed to systemic injections of amphetamine in the activity boxes were significantly more active in this environment on tests for cross-sensitization to morphine given either systemically or intra-VTA than were animals in either an UNPAIRED or CONTROL group.[17]

In an attempt to specify where the effects of the CS might interact with the unconditioned effects of these drugs to allow for conditioned activity and CS control of sensitization, we studied the development of sensitization to the effects of amphetamine injected directly into the VTA or the nucleus accumbens (NAC) using a conditioning paradigm.[18] Sensitization developed following repeated VTA amphetamine injections, as reported previously,[19] but there was no evidence for conditioned activity or for CS control of the expression of sensitization; sensitization did not develop following repeated NAC injections[19,20] nor was there evidence for conditioning. In this case, DA release and reuptake blockade from the somatodendritic region of the neurons, though sufficient for the development of sensitization, appeared not to engage the neural circuitry in a manner that allowed the integration of sensory information necessary for the development of CS control. In addition, excessive post-synaptic DA receptor stimulation in the NAC alone, led neither to conditioning of activity nor sensitization even though the animals were very active during drug exposure. These experiments are summarized in TABLE 1. It can be seen that only when DA neurons are activated to release DA from both somatodendritic regions and from their terminals allowing for feedback from postsynaptic regions can the interaction between sensory and drug-produced signals occur that is necessary for CSs to gain control of behavior. What we do not know is whether the CSs paired with these types of drug actions gain access, either directly or indirectly, to the DA cells. There is the possibility that the activity seen when the CS is presented alone or with drug is due to CS modification of activity in DA neurons *per se*, to learned modifications in circuits no longer DA-dependent, or to both.

There are several studies of the effects of DA antagonists on the CS control of sensitization and on conditioned activity that have tried to address this question. Pimozide, a non-selective antagonist, has been reported to block the development of conditioned activity based on amphetamine or cocaine, but not to block its expression; the effects on CS control of sensitization were not tested in these experiments.[21,22] In another experiment, however, conditioned circling based on amphetamine was found to be attenuated by both SCH-23390 and the D_2 blocker metoclopramide.[23] Weiss et al.[24] reported that haloperidol blocked the development, but not the expression of sensitization to cocaine, both of which were CS-dependent. Gold et al.[25] showed that the expression of conditioned activity to amphetamine was blocked by 6-hydroxydopamine (6-OHDA) lesions of the mesolimbic DA system. These results suggest that DA neuron activity can be involved in both the development and expression of con-

TABLE 1. Summary of Data from Sensitization Experiments Using Systemic and Intracranial Injections of Amphetamine and Morphine

Preexposure Drug	DA Release		Animal Active	Behavioral Sensitization	Conditioned Stimulus Control
	Cell Body	Terminal			
Amphetamine i.p.	+	+	+	+	+
Amphetamine VTA	+	−	−	+	−
Amphetamine NAC	−	+	+	−	−
Morphine i.p.	+	+	+	+	+
Morphine VTA	+	+	+	+	+
Morphine NAC	Non-DA–dependent		+	−	?

ditioned activity based on stimulant drugs such as amphetamine and cocaine, but that under some conditions the conditioned activity can be DA-independent. Interestingly, the findings with the direct agonist, apomorphine, suggest that the conditioned response is DA-independent. It has been shown that in the unilaterally 6-OHDA–lesioned rat, the direct DA receptor agonist, apomorphine, produces strong conditioned contralateral turning which was not blocked by haloperidol.[26,27] It is not clear from these studies, however, how apomorphine has its effects on turning in the unilaterally 6-OHDA–lesioned animal. It is possible that the remaining intact contralateral DA system or residual fibers on the lesioned side are involved. The fact that the unconditioned and the conditioned effects were obtained with .05 mg/kg apomorphine, an autoreceptor selective dose, which could increase contralateral turning by inhibiting firing and DA release on the non-lesioned side, and that the conditioned effects were most obvious six weeks post surgery, at a time when compensatory changes in remaining fibers would have occurred, supports this idea.

There is a growing literature on conditioning and sensitization in normal animals with direct DA agonists including the mixed D_1/D_2 agonist, apomorphine.[28,29] Mattingly[30] has shown recently that sensitization to apomorphine, as has previously been shown for amphetamine[23,31,32] is blocked by the D_1 antagonist, SCH-23390, but not by a selective D_2 antagonist. The D_2 selective agonist, bromocriptine[33] also leads to sensitization that is completely under CS control and is not blocked by the D_1 antagonist. It appears that sensitization and conditioning induced by these direct acting drugs may be mediated differently from each other and from that found with the indirectly acting stimulants. For example, there is no cross-sensitization between bromocriptine and cocaine or heroin.[34] Although considerable work will be required for an understanding of the bases of these differences, it does appear that there are conditioned changes that are dependent on the DA system for their expression and others that are not. It may be that CSs gain access to circuits involved in the activation of DA neurons at the somatodendritic region or in the release of DA directly from terminals, and to circuits that are modulated by DA during learning, but that once modified are DA-independent. Conditioned behavioral facilitation produced by CS-pairings with drugs such as morphine, amphetamine, and cocaine probably involve both types of circuits. The situation may be different in the case of direct DA agonists which do not cause DA release either directly or indirectly.

A Possible Role for Excitatory Amino Acid Receptors in Conditioned Behavioral Activation

It has been reported[35] that systemic injections of the noncompetitive N-methyl-D-aspartate (NMDA) receptor antagonist, MK801, block the development of sensitization to both amphetamine and cocaine implicating the actions of excitatory amino acids (EAA) at NMDA receptors in the plastic changes brought about by repeated drug administration. Because of the known role of NMDA receptors in several instances of learning, we considered that MK801 might be acting by blocking conditioning of behavioral activation rather than the development of sensitization *per se*. Using the two sets of the usual three groups, PAIRED, UNPAIRED and CONTROL, one pretreated with MK801 and the other with saline during the conditioning phase, we showed that in the MK801-pretreated groups there was no evidence for conditioned activity on the test for conditioning, nor was there any evidence for sensitization when these animals were tested with amphetamine alone.[36] We can say from this experiment that MK801 blocked the development of conditioned activity, however, we cannot determine whether sensitization was blocked independently from conditioning, or whether MK801 interfered with the effectiveness of amphetamine as a UCS (but see ref. 37). In order to do this, a sensitization paradigm that does not allow for the possibility of conditioned effects must be used. Experiments are currently under way in our laboratory to explore this question. The idea, however, that MK801 interferes with conditioning of the drug effect is supported by the results of a recently reported experiment[38] in which it was found, using a morphine treatment regimen known to produce environment-specific analgesic tolerance,[39] that MK801 blocked the development of tolerance to the analgesic effects of morphine, without affecting analgesia *per se*.

A ROLE FOR CONDITIONED DRUG EFFECTS IN DRUG-TAKING

It has long been proposed that conditioned drug effects play a role in relapse to drug-taking in experienced, drug-free individuals. Two kinds of conditioned effects have been proposed to play such a role: drug-opposite effects or those associated with withdrawal, and drug-like effects. Drug-opposite conditioned effects are said to precipitate drug-taking by creating aversive symptoms resembling withdrawal,[3,6] whereas drug-like effects are said to create a positive motivational state, enhancing the incentive value of drug-related stimuli, and thereby increasing the probability of drug-related thoughts and actions.[5] Both types of conditioned effects have been shown to occur. However, studies done in animals in search of evidence that conditioned aversive effects lead to drug-taking have been unsuccessful (see ref. 5 for a review and ref. 39). On the other hand, numerous studies have shown that animals seek out places associated with drugs and respond persistently to stimuli associated with them. Conditioning of the unconditioned reinforcing and behavioral activating effects of opioid and stimulant drugs occurs readily. These unconditioned drug effects are mediated at least in part by the mesolimbic DA system and that activity in this system is increased by natural incentives and in turn enhances the effectiveness of incentive stimuli. These observations taken together lead logically to the hypothesis that CSs associated with these drugs might increase activity in this system and thus serve to increase the probability of drug-taking behaviors.

Conditioned Drug Effects in Withdrawal and after Abstinence

In an early study of the conditioned effects of opioids, it was shown in rats that presentation of a CS that had been paired repeatedly with morphine could reverse the decrease in body temperature that accompanies withdrawal from morphine.[41] Animals were maintained on high doses of morphine and then the drug was abruptly withdrawn. Core temperature was measured every 12 hours over three subsequent days. Presentation of the bell CS was able to reverse the withdrawal precipitated hypothermia. In a subsequent study the conditioning of body temperature changes produced by morphine was observed both during the period of repeated daily morphine injections and after a period of abstinence.[42] Groups of animals were given injections of either 0, 5, 25, or escalating to 100 mg/kg morphine i.p. The daily routine was to measure temperature at 09:00h in the home cage (HC), to transport the animals to a distinctive preinjection environment (PreINJ) at 10:00h, to measure their temperature there at 11:00h, to transport them to a distinctively different injection environment (INJ) at 12:00h and to give the daily injection immediately. Temperature was measured at 12:45 and at 14:15h in the injection environment. During the conditioning phase, animals in the morphine treatment groups were hypothermic at 11:00h in PreINJ compared to control group animals and compared to themselves at 11:00h in the HC. This effect, seen 23 hours after the previous morphine injection, suggested a withdrawal-like hypothermia which was subsequently shown to be precipitated by the time of day and to be exaggerated by the PreINJ room cues. Following a period of abstinence, this preINJ hypothermia was no longer evident, but when animals were placed in INJ and given saline, body temperature rose and marked hyperthermia relative to control group animals was seen at 12:45h and 14:15h. This experiment demonstrates that CSs previously paired with morphine injections caused conditioned hyperthermia (an excitatory drug-like CR) in drug-free animals after a prolonged period of abstinence. A very similar pattern of results was obtained when amphetamine was used as the drug for conditioning.[43]

An interesting parallel to these findings was found in a recent study on conditioned heart rate changes to ethanol.[44] Volunteer social drinkers were given discriminative conditioning to ethanol using a combination of a distinctive room and a flavored drink as CSs. During the period of conditioning, subjects were brought into one of the rooms and then given a flavored drink containing ethanol; in the other room a different flavored drink contained no ethanol. Heart rate rose in response to ethanol and remained higher than that of control subjects over the 30 minute test period. On the tests for conditioning, subjects were presented with each of the CSs alone or in combination. Presentation of the Room alone led to a decrease in heart rate from baseline. Presentation of the Flavored Drink (in a neutral room) led to a sharp increase in heart rate; the combination of cues Room then Drink led to changes that were similar to the Room alone. This study points out that not only can opposite conditioned responses be obtained, but that different elements of the stimulus complex may lead to different conditioned responses. In this case the stimulus most proximal to and that best predicted the ethanol led to a response that mimicked the unconditioned effect of the drug. It would have been interesting to see what would have happened to the two responses as the time between the original conditioning trials and the tests increased.

Conditioned Drug Effects after Extinction and the Problem of Reinstatement

Repeated presentation of a CS in the absence of the unconditioned stimulus leads to the reduction and elimination of the CR. This phenomenon, known as extinction, has been the basis of various therapies aimed at eliminating conditioned drug effects;[45] the assumption being that conditioned drug effects play a role in drug-taking and in relapse to drug-taking after abstinence. CRs are known to be resistant to change and are not eliminated without extinction training. Furthermore, extinction is a fragile process and does not erase the original learning. Extinguished responses are found to recover "spontaneously" with the passage of time and to be easily reinstated by a single CS-UCS pairing. Bouton[46] has shown in a series of experiments that extinction makes behavior especially sensitive to the background or context in which extinction occurs. A response may appear to be eliminated by extinction trials in one context, only to be fully reinstated in another. Contextual cues as diverse as physical environments, drug states and emotions can reinstate the ability of CSs to elicit CRs.

In our studies of the CS control of the expression of sensitization of the locomotor effects of amphetamine[47] and morphine,[48] we studied the effects of extinction training on previously established CS control of sensitization. The three standard groups were used in each experiment (groups PAIRED, UNPAIRED, and CONTROL). Conditioned activity and CS control of sensitization were both evident on tests made following CS-drug pairings. A series of extinction sessions followed during which all groups were tested repeatedly in the activity boxes, but after being given saline injections only both in the activity boxes and in the home cages. By the last day of extinction there were no differences in activity between groups, *i.e.*, no evidence of conditioning. On the tests for sensitization which followed, however, in which all animals were given drug before going into the activity boxes, sensitized responding was reinstated. In the case of morphine, animals in group PAIRED were once again significantly more active than animals in the other two groups. Interestingly in the case of amphetamine, both group PAIRED and UNPAIRED were now more active than CONTROL, suggesting that the extinction sessions had eliminated the inhibition of the expression of sensitization previously seen in group UNPAIRED when tested in the CS-environment.

These findings are reminiscent of those from experiments on reinstatement of drug self-administration. In these experiments it is found that, following a period of extinction in which responding is no longer reinforced, noncontingent injections of the drug reinstate drug-taking behavior, suggesting that the drug reinstates the effectiveness of drug-related stimuli, or CSs.[49-52] These findings show that, in spite of extensive extinction experience in which conditioned stimuli are repeatedly presented in the absence of drug, the effectiveness of such stimuli is easily reinstated by simple re-exposure to the drug in their presence. There is also good reason to think that exposure to other similarly acting drugs and to stressors, both of which show cross-sensitization (see ref. 53), and the arousal of strong positive emotions could all act to reinstate the effectiveness of these stimuli.

REFERENCES

1. ZAMBLE, E., G. M. HADAD, J. B. MITCHELL & T. R. H. CUTMORE. 1985. Pavlovian conditioning of sexual arousal: First- and second-order effects. J. Exp. Psychol. (Anim. Behav.) 11: 598–610.
2. PAVLOV, I. P. 1926. Conditioned reflexes. Dover Press. New York.
3. SIEGEL, S. 1977. Learning and psychopharmacology. In Psychopharmacology in the Practice of Medicine. M. E. Jarvik, Ed.: 59–70. Appleton-Century-Crofts. New York.
4. SOLOMON, R. L. & J. D. CORBIT. 1974. An opponent-process theory of motivation: I. Temporal dynamics of affect. Psychol. Rev. 81: 119–145.
5. STEWART, J., H. DE WIT & R. EIKELBOOM. 1984. Role of unconditioned and conditioned drug effects in the self-administration of opiates and stimulants. Psychol. Rev. 91: 251–268.
6. WIKLER, A. & F. PESCOR. 1967. Classical conditioning of a morphine abstinence phenomenon, reinforcement of opioid drinking behavior, and "relapse" in morphine-addicted rats. Psychopharmacologia 10: 255–284.
7. MAX, B. 1990. This and that: Drug tolerance and great expectations. TIPS 11: 401–404.
8. ROBINSON, T. E. & J. B. BECKER. 1986. Enduring changes in brain and behavior produced by chronic amphetamine administration: A review and evaluation of animal models of amphetamine psychosis. Brain Res. Rev. 11: 157–198.

9. KALIVAS, P. W. 1985. Sensitization to repeated enkephalin administration into the ventral tegmental area of the rat: II. Involvement of the mesolimbic dopamine system. J. Pharmacol. Exp. Ther. **235**: 544–550.

10. STEWART, J. & P. VEZINA. 1988. Conditioning and behavioral sensitization. *In* Sensitization in the Nervous System. P. W. Kalivas & C. D. Barnes, Eds.: 207–224. Telford Press. Caldwell, NJ.

11. WISE, R. A. & M. A. BOZARTH. 1987. A psychomotor stimulant theory of addiction. Psychol. Rev. **94**: 469–492.

12. FREEMAN, A. S. & B. S. BUNNEY. 1987. Activity of A9 and A10 dopaminergic neurons in unrestrained rats: Further characterization and effects of apomorphine and cholecystokinin. Brain Res. **405**: 46–55.

13. KELLER, R. W., E. M. STRIKER & M. J. ZIGMOND. 1983. Environmental stimuli but not homeostatic challenges produce apparent increases in dopaminergic activity in the striatum: An analysis by in vivo voltametry. Brain Res. **279**: 159–170.

14. LOUILOT, A., M. LEMOAL & H. SIMON. 1986. Differential reactivity of dopaminergic neurons in the nucleus accumbens in response to different behavioral situations: An in vivo voltammetric study in the free moving rat. Brain Res. **397**: 395–400.

15. ROMO, R. & W. SCHULTZ. 1990. Dopamine neurons of the monkey midbrain: Contingencies of responses to active touch during self-initiated arm movements. J. Neurophysiol. **63**: 592–606.

16. VEZINA, P. & J. STEWART. 1984. Conditioning and place-specific sensitization of increases in activity induced by morphine in the VTA. Pharmacol. Biochem. Behav. **20**: 925–934.

17. STEWART, J. & P. VEZINA. 1987. Environment-specific enhancement of the hyperactivity induced by systemic or intra-VTA morphine injections of rats pre-exposed to amphetamine. Psychobiology **15**: 144–153.

18. VEZINA, P. & J. STEWART. 1990. Amphetamine administered to the ventral tegmental area but not to the nucleus accumbens sensitizes rats to systemic morphine: Lack of conditioned effects. Brain Res. **516**: 99–106.

19. KALIVAS, P. W. & B. WEBER. 1988. Amphetamine injection into the ventral mesencephalon sensitizes rats to peripheral amphetamine and cocaine. J. Pharmacol. Exp. Ther. **245**: 1095–1102.

20. DOUGHERTY, JR., G. G. & E. H. ELLINWOOD, JR. 1981. Chronic D-amphetamine in nucleus accumbens: Lack of tolerance or reverse tolerance to locomotor activity. Life Sci. **28**: 2295–2298.

21. BENINGER, R. J. & B. L. HAHN. 1983. Pimozide blocks establishment but not expression of amphetamine-produced environment-specific conditioning. Science **220**: 1304–1306.

22. BENINGER, R. J. & R. S. HERZ. 1986. Pimozide blocks establishment but not expression of cocaine-produced environment-specific conditioning. Life Sci. **38**: 1425–1431.

23. DREW, K. L. & S. D. GLICK. 1990. Role of D-1 and D-2 receptor stimulation in sensitization to amphetamine-induced circling behavior and in expression and extinction of the Pavlovian conditioned response. Psychopharmacology **101**: 465–471.

24. WEISS, S. R. B., R. M. POST, A. PERT, R. WOODWARD & D. MURMAN. 1989. Context-dependent cocaine sensitization: Differential effect of haloperidol on development versus expression. Pharmacol. Biochem. Behav. **34**: 655–661.

25. GOLD, L. H., N. R. SWERDLOW & G. F. KOOB. 1988. The role of mesolimbic dopamine in conditioned locomotion produced by amphetamine. Behav. Neurosci. **102**: 544–552.

26. BURUNAT, E., R. CASTRO, M. D. DIAZ-PALAREA & M. RODRIGUEZ. 1987. Conditioned response to apomorphine in nigro-striatal system-lesioned rats: The origin of undrugged rotational response. Life Sci. **41**: 1861–1866.

27. CAREY, R. J. 1990. Dopamine receptors mediate drug-induced but not Pavlovian conditioned contralateral rotation in the unilateral 6-OHDA animal model. Brain Res. **515**: 292–298.

28. MATTINGLY, B. A. & J. E. GOTSICK. 1989. Conditioning and experiential factors affecting the development of sensitization to apomorphine. Behav. Neurosci. **103**: 1311–1317.

29. MATTINGLY, B. A. & J. K. ROWLETT. 1989. Effects of repeated apomorphine and haloperidol treatments on subsequent behavioral sensitivity to apomorphine. Pharmacol. Biochem. Behav. **34**: 345–347.

30. MATTINGLY, B. A., J. K. ROWLETT, J. GRAFF & G. LOVELL. 1990. Effects of selective dopamine antagonists on the development of behavioral sensitization to apomorphine. Soc. Neurosci. Abst. **16:** 253.
31. STEWART, J. & P. VEZINA. 1989. Microinjections of SCH-23390 into the ventral tegmental area and substantia nigra pars reticulata attenuate the development of sensitization to the locomotor activating effects of systemic amphetamine. Brain Res. **495:** 401–406.
32. VEZINA, P. & J. STEWART. 1989. The effect of dopamine receptor blockade on the development of sensitization to the locomotor activating effects of amphetamine and morphine. Brain Res. **499:** 108–120.
33. HOFFMAN, D. C. & R. A. WISE. 1990. Failure to observe cross-sensitization between the locomotor-activating effects of bromocriptine and cocaine or bromocriptine and heroin. Abst. Can. Coll. Neuropharm.
34. WISE, R. A., Personal Communication.
35. KARLER, R., L. D. CALDER, I. A. CHAUDHRY & S. A. TURKANIS. 1989. Blockade of "reverse tolerance" to cocaine and amphetamine by MK-801. Life Sci. **45:** 599–606.
36. STEWART, J. & J. P. DRUHAN. 1991. The non-competitive NMDA antagonist, MK801, blocks the development of conditioned activity to amphetamine (AMPH). Soc. Neurosci. Abst.
37. WEIHMULLER, F. B., S. J. O'DELL, B. N. COLE & J. F. MARSHALL. MK-801 attenuates the dopamine-releasing but not the behavioral effects of methamphetamine: An in vivo microdialysis study. Brain Res. **549:** 230–235.
38. TRUJILLO, K. A. & H. AKIL. 1991. Inhibition of morphine tolerance and dependence by the NMDA receptor antagonist MK801. Science **251:** 85–87.
39. SIEGEL, S. 1975. Evidence from rats that morphine tolerance is a learned response. J. Comp. Physiol. Psychol. **89:** 498–506.
40. SOBRERO, A. P. & M. E. BOUTON. 1989. Effects of stimuli present during oral morphine administration on withdrawal and subsequent consumption. Psychobiology **17:** 179–190.
41. ROFFMAN, M., C. REDDY & H. LAL. 1973. Control of morphine-withdrawal hypothermia by conditional stimuli. Psychopharmacologia **29:** 197–201.
42. EIKELBOOM, R. & J. STEWART. 1979. Conditioned temperature effects using morphine as the unconditioned stimulus. Psychopharmacology **61:** 31–38.
43. EIKELBOOM, R. & J. STEWART. 1981. Conditioned temperature effects using amphetamine as the unconditioned stimulus. Psychopharmacology **75:** 96–97.
44. STAIGER, P. K. & J. M. WHITE. 1988. Conditioned alcohol-like and alcohol-opposite responses in humans. Psychopharmacology **95:** 87–91.
45. CHILDRESS, A., A. MCLELLAN & C. O'BRIEN. 1986. Abstinent opiate abusers exhibit conditioned craving, conditioned withdrawal, and reductions in both through extinction. Br. J. Addiction **81:** 655–660.
46. BOUTON, M. E. & D. SWARTZENTRUBER. 1991. Sources of relapse after extinction in Pavlovian and instrumental learning. Clin. Psychol. Rev. **11:** 123–140.
47. STEWART, J. & P. VEZINA. 1991. Extinction procedures abolish conditioned stimulus control but spare sensitized responding to amphetamine. Behav. Pharmacol. **2:** 65–71.
48. STEWART, J., Unpublished data.
49. DE WIT, H. & J. STEWART. 1981. Reinstatement of cocaine-reinforced responding in the rat. Psychopharmacology **75:** 134–143.
50. DE WIT, H. & J. STEWART. 1983. Drug reinstatement of heroin-reinforced responding in the rat. Psychopharmacology **79:** 29–31.
51. STEWART, J. 1984. Reinstatement of heroin and cocaine self-administration behavior in the rat by intracerebral application of morphine in the ventral tegmental area. Pharmacol. Biochem. Behav. **20:** 917–923.
52. STEWART, J. & P. VEZINA. 1988. A comparison of the effects of intra-accumbens injections of amphetamine and morphine on reinstatement of heroin intravenous self-administration behavior. Brain Res. **457:** 287–294.
53. KALIVAS, P. W. & J. STEWART. 1991. Dopamine transmission in the initiation and expression of drug- and stress-induced sensitization of motor activity. Brain Res. Rev. **16:** 223–244.

Conditioning of Opioid Reinforcement: Neuroanatomical and Neurochemical Substrates

TONI S. SHIPPENBERG, A. HERZ, R. SPANAGEL,
R. BALS-KUBIK, AND C. STEIN

Department of Neuropharmacology
Max-Planck Institute for Psychiatry
Am Klopferspitz 18a
D-8033 Martinsried, Germany

INTRODUCTION

The conditioned place preference paradigm has been used to examine the incentive motivational effects of opioids and other psychoactive drugs.[1,2] Using this procedure, it has been shown that μ-opioid receptor agonists function as conditioned reinforcers in experimental animals, eliciting approach and subsequent preferences for environmental stimuli previously associated with their administration.[1-3] In contrast, $\varkappa$-opioid receptor agonists, which produce aversive and dysphoric effects in humans,[4] induce conditioned aversions for stimuli associated with their administration.[1,3,5] Several lines of evidence[1,4,5] suggest that the ability of opioids and other drugs to function as rewarding or aversive stimuli is a critical factor in determining their abuse liability.

The mesolimbic dopamine (DA) system, which arises in the midbrain ventral tegmental area (VTA),[6] has been implicated in the mediation of the rewarding effects of intracranial self-stimulation, natural rewards such as food and water, and of several drugs of abuse.[2,5] Recent studies suggest that this DA system may also be an important site for both the conditioned reinforcing and aversive effects of opioids.[5,7] Furthermore, as will become apparent, there is evidence that tonically active endogenous opioid systems modulate the basal activity of mesolimbic DA neurons and that alterations in these systems may, in fact, have marked effects on motivation.

BACKGROUND

The existence of three opioid receptor types (μ, δ, and $\varkappa$) within the CNS is well-documented.[8] Subtypes for each of these receptors have also been postulated. With regard to the mesolimbic system, the VTA is rich in μ-opioid receptors and contains only a modest amount of $\varkappa$ receptors. In contrast, the nucleus accumbens (NAC), a terminal projection site of VTA A10 DA neurons, contains μ-, as well as δ- and $\varkappa$-binding sites.[9,10] The distribution of the various receptor types within this region is, however, heterogenous.

Since the initial discovery of the enkephalins (ENKs), a number of endogenous opioid peptides have been isolated. These opioid peptides are derived from one of three precursor molecules. Representative peptides from each are β-endorphin (END), methionine- and leucine- ENK, and dynorphin (DYN), respectively.[11] Of particular interest to the present discussion are END and DYN. END neurons, located in the mediobasal hypothalamus, project to various limbic structures including both the VTA and the NAC. Both DYN fibers and perikarya are found in the NAC, but are minimal in the VTA.[9,11]

END binds with higher affinity to μ than δ receptors and is postulated to be the endogenous ligand for this opioid receptor type. In contrast, the ENKs and DYN bind preferentially to δ and $\varkappa$ receptors, respectively, and are presumed to be endogenous ligands for these receptor types. It is important, however, to note that these peptides bind with varying affinities to other opioid receptor types. Therefore, each can potentially interact with other opioid receptor types and their net effects will be determined by the ratio of the various opioid receptor types present in a particular brain region.

CONDITIONED REINFORCING EFFECTS OF OPIOID AGONISTS

The recent availability of ligands selective for each of the opioid receptor types has contributed greatly to the understanding of the neural substrates mediating the conditioned reinforcing and aversive effects of opioids.

μ- and δ-Opioid Agonists

The administration of morphine or other preferential μ-receptor agonists, when paired with a previously neutral environment, produces dose-related preferences for that environment in the absence of drug.[3] Similar conditioning is observed in response to the selective μ-opioid receptor agonist D-Ala,[2] N-methyl-Phe,[4] Gly[5]-ol-ENK (DAMGO) suggesting that such effects are mediated by μ-opioid receptors.[12] Indeed, the selective blockade of μ but not δ receptors abolishes the reinforcing effects of these agents.[3,12] As shown in FIGURE 1, conditioned place preferences are also observed in response to the selective δ-opioid receptor agonist D-Pen[2], D-Pen[5] ENK (DPDPE). However, pretreatment with δ- but not μ-receptor antagonists abolishes these effects suggesting that: 1) the conditioned reinforcing effects of opioids result from the activation of either μ or δ receptors and 2) the activation of either receptor type is sufficient for the induction of these effects.

Conditioned place preferences are also observed following the central administration of endogenous opioid peptides such as ENK or END. In contrast, however, to other opioid agonists, the reinforcing effects of END (FIG. 1) as well as the ability of this peptide to stimulate DA release in the NAC (see below) require the concurrent activation of both μ and δ receptors.[14] Such findings are of particular interest in view of recent evidence suggesting the existence of an opioid receptor complex upon which this peptide may act within the CNS to produce its effects.[15]

$\varkappa$-Opioid Agonists

In contrast to μ- or δ-receptor agonists, $\varkappa$ agonists produce conditioned aversions

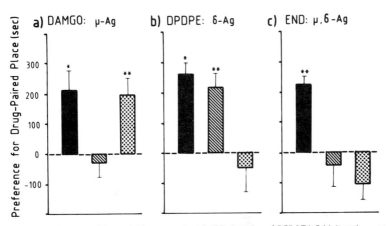

FIGURE 1. Influence of the opioid antagonists CTOP (▨) and ICI 174,864 (▦) upon the place conditioning produced by DAMGO (a), DPDPE (b), and END (c). The doses of antagonists used in these studies were, by themselves, ineffective as conditioning stimuli. Asterisks denote a significant difference from the vehicle-pretreated control group (■). (Adapted from ref. 12.)

for an environment previously paired with their administration.[3,5] The potency of these agents in producing these effects parallels differences in their binding affinity to the x receptor indicating a specific role for this receptor type. For all opioid agonists tested, the doses effective in producing place conditioning are substantially lower following the intracerebral as compared to the systemic route of administration suggesting a central site of action.

Neuroanatomical Basis of Opioid-Agonist–Induced Conditioning

Initial evidence for an involvement of the mesolimbic system in mediating the conditioned reinforcing effects of opioids was derived from studies in which μ or δ agonists were microinjected into discrete brain areas and a map of those sites producing conditioned place preferences generated (FIG. 2).[1,5,7,16] More recently, we have used this technique to determine the location of those receptors upon which highly selective x agonists (*e.g.*, U50,488H, U-69593) act to produce their conditioned aversive effects.[5,7,17] These studies are summarized in FIGURE 3. As can be seen, the activation of opioid receptors in: 1) the VTA, 2) those structures which are terminal projection sites of VTA DA neurons, or 3) structures which feedback upon the VTA is sufficient for the conditioning of opioid-induced aversion: other injection sites are without effect. In contrast, the highly selective μ agonist, DAMGO, only produces conditioned reinforcing effects when injected into the VTA.

Data regarding the influence of 6-hydroxydopamine (6-OHDA) lesions of the NAC provide more definitive evidence for an involvement of the mesolimbic system in the conditioned reinforcing effects of opioids and suggest a specific role for DA neurons projecting from the VTA to the NAC, therein. Thus, several studies[17,18] have shown that the selective depletion of DA in this brain region results in an abolition of the

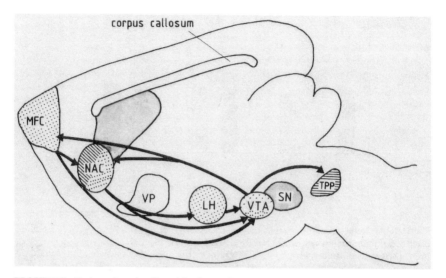

FIGURE 2. Brain regions implicated in the mediation of the reinforcing and aversive effects of opioid agonists as revealed by microinjection and lesion studies. Data represent the results obtained with the μ agonists DAMGO and morphine and the $\varkappa$ agonist U-50,488H. (+++) and (:::) indicate significant conditioning following injections of μ and $\varkappa$ agonists, respectively. Shaded regions depict ineffective injection sites. Slashed regions indicate attenuation of opioid conditioning following neurotoxic lesions to these areas (6-OHDA: NAC; ibotenic acid: TPP). (Adapted from refs. 5 and 9.)

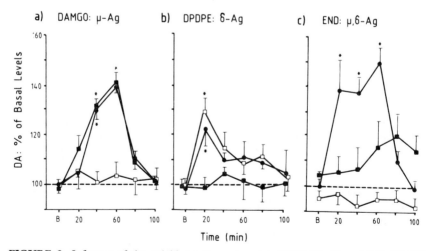

FIGURE 3. Influence of the opioid receptor antagonists CTOP (□—□) and ICI 174,864 (■—■) upon the DA-releasing effects of opioid peptides: DAMGO (a), DPDPE (b), and END (c) as revealed by *in vivo* microdialysis. Opioid ligands were administered ICV and the effects upon DA release (percentage of mean basal values) in the NAC are shown. Asterisks denote a significant difference from control vehicle-treated animals (●—●). (Adapted from refs. 14 and 27.)

conditioned reinforcing effects of systemically administered μ-opioid receptor agonists. Recent studies from this laboratory[19] have shown that lesions which result in a 40%–60% reduction in NAC DA also abolish the conditioned aversive effects of a systemically applied $\varkappa$-opioid agonist. In contrast, an equivalent reduction of DA in either the medial prefrontal cortex or caudate/putamen fails to modify the reinforcing or aversive properties of opioid agonists. As such, these data indicate that the activity of DA neurons projecting to the NAC, in contrast to either mesocortical or mesostriatal DA neurons, is required for the incentive motivational effects of both μ- and $\varkappa$-opioid agonists. Furthermore, the inability of such lesions to modify the conditioning produced by several other drugs demonstrates that the effects of such lesions do not result from an impairment of those processes which are necessary for the acquisition or performance of a conditioned response.[21]

There are also data, although more limited, suggesting an involvement of serotonin (5-HT) neurons located in or projecting to the NAC in mediating the conditioned reinforcing effects of opioids. Thus, 5,7-dihydroxytryptamine (DHT) lesions of the NAC were shown to attenuate the conditioned place preferences produced by morphine.[20,21] Interestingly, this manipulation does not modify the conditioned place aversions produced by $\varkappa$-opioid receptor agonists.[21] Therefore, although it appears that the functional activity of both DA and 5-HT neurons within the mesolimbic system is necessary for the conditioning of opioid reinforcement, the conditioned aversive effects of opioids are 5-HT independent. Interestingly, 5-HT$_3$ receptor antagonists abolish both the conditioned reinforcing effects of morphine and its ability to increase DA release in the NAC (see below) suggesting that the effects of 5,7-DHT lesions and 5-HT-antagonists upon morphine conditioning may be secondary to changes in DA.[22,23] This could result either from the destruction of μ-opioid receptors on 5-HT neurons projecting to the NAC or via the disruption of 5-HT input to the VTA. Although speculative, either explanation would account for the apparent involvement of both DA and 5-HT neurons in the effects of μ but not $\varkappa$ agonists.

Influence of Opioid Agonists on Mesolimbic DA Neurons

In contrast to their inhibitory effects in other brain regions, μ opioid receptor agonists stimulate the activity of mesolimbic DA neurons. Thus, systemically applied morphine increases the firing rate of VTA DA neurons and its unilateral microinjection into the VTA induces contralateral rotation.[24,25] More recently, using the technique of *in vivo* microdialysis, several studies[26–28] have shown that morphine and other μ-opioid receptor agonists administered either systemically or via the intracerebroventricular (ICV) route preferentially stimulate DA release and metabolism in the NAC. A similar increase is observed in response to the ICV administration of the selective δ-opioid receptor agonist DPDPE.[27] However, as shown in FIGURE 3a–b, this effect, unlike that of the μ receptor agonist DAMGO, is only blocked by the selective δ-receptor antagonist ICI, 174,864. Thus, the activation of either μ or δ receptors can stimulate DA release. Importantly, for all opioids tested, the doses producing such effects are identical to those which elicit conditioned reinforcement suggesting that opioid-induced increases in DA neuronal activity and the resulting increase in NAC DA release underlie such effects.[3,5,13]

As mentioned previously, the ICV administration of END, again, at doses which produce conditioned place preferences, markedly increases DA release and metabolism

(FIG. 3c). However, the blockade of either μ or δ receptors is sufficient to attenuate these effects suggesting that the activation of both receptor types underlies the actions of this peptide.[12,14]

Data derived from both *in vivo* and *in vitro* studies have shown that κ agonists, which have conditioned aversive effects, inhibit DA release and metabolism in the NAC.[26,27,29] A similar effect is observed in response to a metabolically stable analog of DYN, the postulated endogenous ligand for the κ receptor.[27] In most cases, a biphasic dose-response relationship is seen. Thus, at low doses, κ agonists inhibit DA release whereas higher doses are without significant effect. This finding is of potential interest in view of the postulated existence of multiple κ-opioid receptor subtypes[7] and may, in fact, reflect activation of another κ subtype, which opposes those actions resulting from activation of the higher affinity κ-binding site. It is also of particular relevance to the present discussion since identical dose-response curves are obtained in studies of the conditioned aversive properties of these agents. Thus, low doses of U-50488H, U-69593 or the DYN analog E-2078, which inhibit DA release, produce conditioned place aversions whereas higher doses are without significant effect.[3,27,30]

The data just reviewed demonstrate that μ/δ-versus κ-opioid agonists differentially modulate DA neurotransmission in the mesolimbic system and, when viewed in the context of lesion studies[18,19] (see above), suggest that the opposing actions of μ- and δ-versus κ-opioid agonists on mesolimbic DA neurons underlie the conditioned reinforcing and aversive effects of these agents.

In view of the apparent relationship between the DA-releasing effects of opioids and their conditioned reinforcing effects, we have sought to identify the site of action of opioid ligands in affecting DA release.[30] As shown in FIGURE 4A, infusion of DAMGO into the VTA stimulates DA release. Again, there is a good correlation between the doses of DAMGO which affect release and those which produce conditioned reinforcement following their intra-VTA application.[5] Infusion of equivalent concentrations of this μ agonist into the NAC, via the dialysis probe is, however, without effect. Infusion of the selective κ opioid agonist U-69593 into the NAC results in a marked inhibition of DA release and the characteristic biphasic dose-effect curve is obtained.[30] In contrast, the intra-VTA applied κ agonist fails to modify DA release. Although additional studies are needed, such data demonstrate the presence of anatomically distinct and functionally opposing opioid receptors which modulate DA neuronal activity: the activation of μ-opioid receptors in the vicinity of DA perikarya stimulates DA release whereas activation of κ receptors at the level of the DA nerve terminal inhibits such release. With regard to the VTA, an involvement of 5-HT and/or GABA in the actions of μ-opioid agonists appears likely.

OPIOID ANTAGONIST-INDUCED CONDITIONING

Numerous studies have shown that systemic or ICV administration of the opioid antagonist naloxone produces conditioned place aversions in drug-naive animals.[32] Such findings are particularly interesting in view of early clinical studies[33] indicating aversive effects of opioid antagonists in human subjects and suggest the existence of a tonically active endogenous opioid "reward" pathway, the blockade of which can induce aversive states. Place aversions are also produced by the selective μ-opioid receptor antagonist CTOP but not by the δ antagonist ICI, 174,864 suggesting that this pathway is μ-opioidergic. Interestingly, and in contrast to μ or δ antagonists, the se-

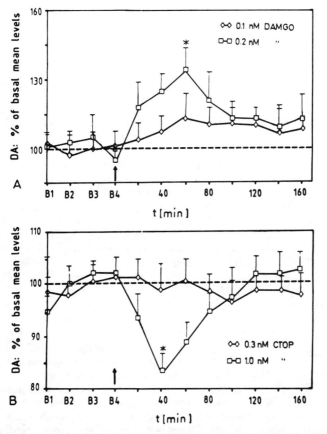

FIGURE 4. Influence of intra-VTA infusion of the selective μ opioid receptor agonist DAMGO (**A**) or the selective μ-opioid receptor antagonist CTOP (**B**) upon basal DA release in the NAC. Asterisks denote a significant difference from vehicle-treated controls. (Adapted from ref. 31.)

lective $\varkappa$ antagonist nor-binaltorphimine produces conditioned reinforcing effects in most but not all animals tested. Therefore, there may, in certain individuals, be a tonically active $\varkappa$ (*e.g.*, DYN) opioid system and the activation of both μ and $\varkappa$ systems may be necessary for the maintenance of neutral motivational states.

Neural Substrates Mediating the Aversive Effects of Opioid Antagonists

Evidence that END is the substrate upon which opioid antagonists act to produce their aversive effects has been derived from a study[34] in which the mediobasal hypothalamus, the primary site of END synthesis in the CNS,[7] was lesioned. This manipulation, which reduces the content of END but not ENK, attenuates the place aversions produced by systemically applied naloxone. It does not modify the conditioning produced by opioid agonists. Such findings indicate that there is a tonically active END system and when the activity of this system is disrupted (*e.g.*, by the administration of opioid antagonists), aversive states ensue.

What then is the location of the opioid receptors upon which naloxone and μ receptor antagonists act to produce their conditioned aversive effects? Preliminary studies[35] in which the antagonists CTOP and naloxone were microinjected into regions comprising the three major ascending DA systems show that the blockade of μ-opioid receptors in the VTA results in marked conditioned place aversions. Such findings are consistent with the presence of both END fibers and μ-opioid receptors in this brain region and suggest that the VTA may, in fact, be one component of the tonically active END "reward" pathway.

The question then arises as to the role of the VTA, and the DA neurons therein, in mediating the conditioned aversive effects of systemically administered opioid antagonists. Although the above data demonstrate that the blockade of VTA opioid receptors is sufficient to produce place aversions, they do not enable determination of whether this action is necessary for the expression of these effects. Furthermore, they provide no information as to whether those DA neurons which have been implicated in the conditioned reinforcing (and aversive) effects of opioid agonists also mediate the conditioned aversive effects of opioid antagonists.

At present, data regarding the first issue are lacking. However, there is both direct and indirect evidence that DA neurons may, in fact, be necessary for the expression of all opioid-induced conditioning. Firstly, several studies[1,5,36] have shown that the chronic blockade of D_1 but not D_2 DA receptors during conditioning attenuates the place conditioning produced by opioid agonists, as well as that produced by naloxone. Such findings indicate that D_1 receptor activity is necessary for opioid ligand-induced place conditioning. Furthermore, the finding[36] that the acute administration of D_1 antagonists produces place aversions suggests that: 1) the tonic release of DA and the activation of D_1 receptors is necessary for the maintenance of neutral motivational states and 2) opioid-induced increases or decreases in the activation of this DA receptor type may underlie their conditioned reinforcing and aversive properties. The D_1 receptors underlying such effects have subsequently been localized to the NAC suggesting that this tonically active DA pathway is, in fact, the same as that upon which opioid agonists act to produce reinforcement and aversion.[35,37]

Recent data[5,35] regarding the effects of 6-OHDA lesions of the NAC upon naloxone-induced place conditioning provide additional information regarding the role of mesolimbic DA neurons in mediating the aversive effects of opioid antagonists. In contrast to the effects of such lesions upon opioid agonist–induced conditioning, such treatment attenuates, but does not abolish, the aversive effects of systemic naloxone. NAC lesions do, however, abolish the aversive effects produced by the intra-VTA application of opioid antagonists.[35] Although such data must be interpreted cautiously, they suggest, that in contrast to opioid agonists, both mesolimbic DA-dependent and DA-independent components underlie the aversive effects of opioid antagonists. As such, disruption of both components would be necessary for the abolition of the conditioned aversive effects of systemically administered antagonists.

Influence of Opioid Antagonists Upon DA Release

If the aversive effects of opioid antagonists result, in part, from the blockade of an endogenous opioid "reward" pathway which modulates mesolimbic DA neuronal activity, then an effect of these agents upon basal DA release should be evident. Although previous microdialysis studies[14,26,27] examining the influence of opioid antagonists applied systemically or ICV have failed to obtain such, a marked inhibition of DA release can be observed when μ-opioid receptor antagonists are infused directly into the VTA[31] (FIG. 4B). In contrast, equivalent concentrations infused into the NAC are without effect. Such findings are in line with the postulated involvement of mesolimbic DA neurons in mediating the aversive effects of μ opioid antagonists and provide direct evidence for the existence of a tonically active endogenous opioid system in the VTA which regulates the basal activity of this system. Thus, opioid agonists such as morphine, by increasing the activity of this endogenous opioid "reward" pathway, increase DA release in the NAC and produce reinforcing states. μ-opioid antagonists inhibit the activity of this system. This action and the resulting decrease in NAC DA release would appear to underlie the aversive effects of intra-VTA applied naloxone and CTOP. They also play an important, but not sole role in mediating the effects of systemically-administered antagonists.

Surprisingly, infusion of the selective $\varkappa$ antagonist nor-binaltorphimine into the NAC can also affect DA release.[31] In this case, however, a marked stimulation of release in the NAC is observed. Therefore, it would appear that there is, in fact, an opposing tonically active $\varkappa$-opioidergic system (DYN) located in the NAC which inhibits the activity of mesolimbic DA neurons. It is the activation of this system which plays a critical role in mediating the aversive effects of endogenous and exogenous $\varkappa$ agonists. Furthermore, the ability of μ or $\varkappa$ antagonists to modify DA release in naive animals suggest that the activation of both μ- and $\varkappa$-opioid receptors by endogenous opioid systems functions to regulate the activity of DA neurons and that alterations in either opioid system may have profound effects on incentive motivational states.

CONCLUSIONS

Several lines of evidence indicate the existence of endogenous "reward" pathways within the brain upon which drugs and other stimuli act to produce their rewarding effects. The results of place conditioning and microdialysis studies suggest that DA neurons projecting from the VTA to the NAC are an essential component of one such reward pathway and that increases or decreases in the activity of this DA system underlie the reinforcing and aversive effects of opioids.

It is also apparent that endogenous μ and $\varkappa$ opioid systems located in the VTA and NAC, respectively, regulate the activity of mesolimbic DA neurons. The tonic activation of both systems is necessary for maintaining the basal activity of this reward pathway. Such findings are intriguing in view of the hypothesis,[38] put forth over a decade ago, that a deficiency in an endogenous opioid peptide may predispose opioid-seeking behavior in some individuals. Furthermore, they suggest the possibility that increased sensitivity to the rewarding effects of opioids may result from a decrease in the activity of an endogenous μ-opioid peptide system (*e.g.*, END) in the VTA or an increased activity of the $\varkappa$ (DYN) system located in the NAC.

REFERENCES

1. CARR, G. D., H. C. FIBIGER & A. G. PHILLIPS. 1989. Conditioned place preference as a

measure of drug reward. *In* The Neuropharmacological Basis of Reward. J. M. Liebman & S. J. Cooper, Eds.: 264–319. Oxford Press. New York.
2. HOFFMAN, D. C. 1989. Brain Res. Bull. **23:** 373–387.
3. MUCHA, R. F. & A. HERZ. 1985. Psychopharmacology **86:** 274–280.
4. PFEIFFER, A., V. BRANTL, A. HERZ & H. M. EMRICH. 1986. Science **233:** 744–746.
5. SHIPPENBERG, T. S. & R. BALS-KUBIK. 1991. Motivational aspects of opioids: Neurochemical and neuroanatomical substrates. *In* The Neurobiology of Opioids. O. F. X. Almeida & T. S. Shippenberg, Eds.: 331–350. Springer-Verlag. New York.
6. UNGERSTADT, U. 1971. Acta. Physiol. Scand. (Suppl.) **367:** 1–48.
7. MARTIN, W. R. 1984. Pharmacol. Rev. **35:** 283–323.
8. PAUL, D., C. G. PICK, L. A. TIVE & G. W. PASTERNACK. 1991. J. Pharmacol. Exp. Ther. **257:** 1–7.
9. WATSON, S. J., K. J. TRUJILLO, J. P. HERMAN & H. AKIL. 1989. Neuroanatomical and neurochemical substrates of drug-seeking behavior: Overview and future directions. *In* Molecular and Cellular Aspects of the Drug Addictions. A. Goldstein, Ed.: 29–92. Springer-Verlag. New York.
10. MANSOUR, A., H. KHACHATURIAN, M. E. LEWIS, H. AKIL & S. J. WATSON. 1987. J. Neurosci. **7:** 2445–2464.
11. SCHAFER, M. K., R. DAY, S. J. WATSON & H. AKIL. 1991. Distribution of opioids in brain and peripheral tissues. *In* The Neurobiology of Opioids. O.F.X. Almeida & T. S. Shippenberg, Eds.: 53–71. Springer-Verlag. New York.
12. BALS-KUBIK, R., T. S. SHIPPENBERG & A. HERZ. 1990. Eur. J. Pharmacol. **175:** 63–69.
13. SHIPPENBERG, T. S., R. BALS-KUBIK & A. HERZ. 1987. Brain Res. **436:** 234–239.
14. SPANAGEL, R., A. HERZ & T. S. SHIPPENBERG. 1990. Eur. J. Pharmacol. **190:** 177–184.
15. SCHOFFELMEER, A. N., Y. H. YAO & E. J. SIMON. 1989. Eur. J. Pharmacol. **149:** 179–186.
16. BECHARA, A. & D. VAN DER KOOY. 1989. J. Neurosci. **9:** 3400–3409.
17. BOZARTH, M. A. & R. A. WISE. 1981. Life Sci. **29:** 1881–1886.
18. SPYRAKI, C., H. C. FIBIGER & A. G. PHILLIPS. 1983. Psychopharmacology **79:** 278–283.
19. SHIPPENBERG, T. S., R. BALS-KUBIK & A. HERZ. Unpublished observations.
20. SPYRAKI, C., G. G. NOMIKOS, P. PALANOPOULU & Z. DAIFOTIS. 1988. Behav. Brain Res. **29:** 127–134.
21. SHIPPENBERG, T. S., R. SPANAGEL & A. HERZ. 1990. Psychopharmacology **101**(Suppl.): 202.
22. CARBONI, E., E. ACQUAS, P. LEONE & G. DI CHIARA. 1989. Psychopharmacology **97:** 175–179.
23. CARBONI, E., E. ACQUAS, R. FRAU & G. DI CHIARA. 1989. Eur. J. Pharmacol. **164:** 515–519.
24. MATTHEWS, R. T. & D. C. GERMAN. 1984. Neuroscience **11:** 617–626.
25. HOMES, L., M. A. BOZARTH & R. A. WISE. 1983. Brain Res. Bull. **11:** 295–298.
26. DI CHIARA, G. & A. IMPERATO. 1988. J. Pharmacol. Exp. Ther. **244:** 1067–1080.
27. SPANAGEL, R., A. HERZ & T. S. SHIPPENBERG. 1990. J. Neurochem. **55:** 1734–1740.
28. BROWN, E. E., J. M. FINLAY, J. F. WONG, G. DAMSA & H. C. FIBIGER. 1991. J. Pharmacol. Exp. Ther. **256:** 119–126.
29. MULDER, A. H., G. WARDEH, R. HOGGENBOOM & A. FRANKHUYZEN. 1989. Neuropeptides **14:** 99–114.
30. BALS-KUBIK, R., A. HERZ & T. S. SHIPPENBERG. 1989. Psychopharmacology **98:** 203–206.
31. SPANAGEL, R., A. HERZ & T. S. SHIPPENBERG. Proc. Natl. Acad. Sci. USA. In press.
32. MUCHA, R. & S. D. IVERSEN. 1984. Psychopharmacology **82:** 241–247.
33. GREVERT, P. & A. GOLDSTEIN. 1977. Proc. Natl. Acad. Sci. USA **73:** 1291–1294.
34. MUCHA, R., M. J. MILLAN & A. HERZ. 1985. Psychopharmacology **86:** 281–285.
35. SHIPPENBERG, T. S. & R. BALS-KUBIK. Unpublished observations.
36. SHIPPENBERG, T. S. & A. HERZ. 1988. Eur. J. Pharmacol. **151:** 233–242.
37. SHIPPENBERG, T. S., R. BALS-KUBIK, A. HUBER & A. HERZ. 1991. Psychopharmacology **103:** 209–214.
38. GOLDSTEIN, A. 1976. Science **193:** 1081–1086.

Potential Involvement of Anxiety in the Neurobiology of Cocaine[a]

NICK E. GOEDERS[b]

Departments of Pharmacology & Therapeutics and Psychiatry
Louisiana State University Medical Center
Shreveport, Louisiana 71130

Humans often report profound subjective feelings of well-being and a decrease in anxiety following initial cocaine use.[1,2] However, chronic use or the administration of high doses of the drug can be anxiogenic.[3,4] Cocaine has even been reported to precipitate episodes of panic attack in some individuals.[5-7] Furthermore, benzodiazepines (BZDs) are useful in the emergency room for the treatment of convulsions which are often apparent following an acute cocaine overdose.[8,9] Finally, some of the major symptoms associated with cocaine withdrawal also often include severe anxiety, restlessness, and agitation.[2,9,10] However, although BZDs are not usually recommended as the treatment of first choice for cocaine withdrawal because of the concern that the use of these drugs might result in a secondary dependence,[11] the experiments described below were designed to investigate the effects of cocaine on binding sites in the rat brain potentially associated with stress since anxiety appears to be involved in the etiology of cocaine use and withdrawal in humans. The role for BZDs in the behavioral effects of the drug were also assessed.

EFFECTS OF COCAINE ON CORTICOTROPIN-RELEASING FACTOR (CRF) BINDING IN THE RAT BRAIN

CRF has been reported to be involved in a variety of human neuropsychiatric disorders, including both depression and anxiety.[12,13] CRF administration also produces anxiogenic responses in rats,[14] that can be attenuated with the benzodiazepine receptor agonist, chlordiazepoxide (CDP), in both conflict[15,16] and acoustic startle[17] tests. Acute cocaine administration has been demonstrated to increase plasma levels of adrenocorticotropin (ACTH), β-endorphin and corticosterone,[18,19] and the effects of the drug on ACTH secretion appear to evolve from a CRF-induced mechanism.[20] Cocaine has also been reported to stimulate the release of CRF from rat hypothalamic organ culture systems *in vitro*.[21] These data suggest that the anxiety and/or the depression associated with cocaine use in humans may result in part through the actions of the drug on CRF release. The following experiments were therefore designed to investigate

[a] This work was supported by USPHS Grants DAO4293 and DAO6013 from the National Institute on Drug Abuse.
[b] Address correspondence to Dr. Goeders at the Department of Pharmacology & Therapeutics, P.O. Box 33932; Tel.: (318) 674-7863; Fax: (318) 674-7857.

357

the effects of chronic cocaine administration on CRF receptors labeled in the rat brain using quantitative receptor autoradiography.[22] The potential role for dopamine (DA) in these effects was assessed following intraventricular injections of 6-hydroxydopamine (6-OHDA).

Twenty-four adult male Fisher 344 strain rats received intracerebroventricular (icv) 6-OHDA or sham injections following desmethylimipramine (DMI) pretreatment (to protect noradrenergic neurons) according to previously reported procedures.[23,24] After 2 weeks, the 24 lesioned or sham-treated rats were divided into two equal groups. The first group of rats received daily injections of cocaine hydrochloride (20 mg/kg, ip), while the animals in the second group were injected with an equivalent volume of saline (1 ml/kg, ip). Twenty minutes after the 15th injection, the rats were anesthetized and sacrificed by cardiac perfusion. The brains were rapidly removed, embedded in brain paste and frozen onto brass microtome chucks over dry ice. Ten micron coronal sections were cut in a cryostat microtome, and the sections were thaw-mounted onto chrome alum/gelatin-subbed slides and stored at $-20°C$. CRF-binding sites were measured autoradiographically using $[^{125}I]Try^0$-ovine CRF according to previously reported procedures.[25,26] The extent of the lesion was assessed autoradiographically using $[^3H]$mazindol.[23,27]

6-OHDA infusions into the lateral ventricles resulted in significant decreases in dopaminergic uptake sites labeled with $[^3H]$mazindol in specific brain regions without affecting noradrenergic uptake sites.[22,23,28] Statistically significant increases in CRF receptors labeled with $[^{125}I]Try^0$-ovine CRF were observed throughout the nigrostriatal and mesocortical (but not mesolimbic) dopaminergic systems following 6-OHDA. However, this apparent up-regulation of CRF receptors was also seen in brain regions with less DA innervation (e.g., anterior hypothalamus, medial forebrain bundle, hippocampus) that were likely not affected by the lesion. Even so, these data suggest that CRF secretion may be partially under the control of dopaminergic activity. In contrast to the effects of 6-OHDA, cocaine resulted in a statistically significant decrease in CRF receptor labeling exclusively in brain areas associated with terminal fields for the mesocorticolimbic dopaminergic system, although increases in binding were seen in the substantia nigra and ventral tegmental area (VTA). A cocaine-induced increase in the release of CRF in the mesocorticolimbic system could account for this apparent down-regulation of CRF receptor binding. Finally, all of these cocaine-induced effects on CRF receptor binding were attenuated in the animals that received 6-OHDA two weeks prior to the initiation of chronic cocaine administration, suggesting that the effects of cocaine on CRF receptor binding may be mediated to a large extent through dopaminergic neuronal activity.[22]

EFFECTS OF COCAINE ON BZD RECEPTOR BINDING IN THE RAT BRAIN

Forty-two adult male Fisher 344 strain rats were assigned to seven different treatment conditions. The animals in the first group (n = 6) were injected daily with saline (1 ml/kg, ip) for fifteen days and were sacrificed 20 min following the final injection. The animals in the other six groups were sacrificed 20 min, 2 days or 14 days following the 15th daily injection of cocaine (20 or 40 mg/kg, ip; n = 3 groups of 6 rats per dose) as described above to investigate the persistence of the effects of chronic cocaine intoxication on BZD receptors in discrete brain loci.[28] The brains were rapidly removed and prepared for quantitative autoradiography as described above. BZD receptors were visualized using [^{3}H]Ro 15-1788 under standard conditions.[23,29-31] In the second experiment, 24 rats received icv injections of 6-OHDA (n = 12) or vehicle (n = 12) 14 days prior to the initiation of chronic cocaine or saline injections as described above to determine the potential role for DA in the effects of cocaine on BZD receptors. These 6-OHDA and sham-treated animals were divided into two equal groups receiving either daily injections of saline (1 ml/kg, ip) or cocaine hydrochloride (20 mg/kg, ip) for 15 days and were sacrificed 20 min following the 15th injection, and the brains were removed and prepared for quantitative autoradiography.

Chronic cocaine administration for 15 days resulted in differential effects on BZD receptors in various regions of the rat brain.[28,32] In general, cocaine decreased BZD binding in terminal fields for the mesocorticolimbic dopaminergic system, while increasing labeling in terminal fields for the nigro-striatal system. BZD receptor labeling was significantly reduced in the medial prefrontal cortex (MPC) following 20 mg/kg cocaine when the animals were sacrificed 20 min or 2 days after the final injection. This reduction in binding persisted for up to 2 weeks with the 40 mg/kg dose. Similar effects were observed in the nucleus accumbens (NAC), although binding returned to near control levels after 14 days with either dose. In contrast, cocaine significantly increased BZD receptor labeling in the caudate nucleus when the animals were sacrificed 20 min following the final injection. Opposite effects were also observed in brain regions containing the cell bodies for the nigro-striatal and mesocorticolimbic dopaminergic systems, respectively. In the substantia nigra, BZD receptor labeling was decreased 20 min and 2 days following the final injection. In contrast, while no significant changes were observed in the VTA 20 min after the final injection with either dose of cocaine, BZD receptor labeling was increased at 2 and 14 days. Since statistically significant decreases in BZD receptor binding in the MPC and increases in the VTA were still observed 2 weeks following the final injection, BZD receptors in these brain regions may be especially sensitive to the effects of cocaine. Moreover, statistical significance was only achieved in the VTA of rats sacrificed 2 or 14 days later, and the trend at 14 days was toward increasing effects, suggesting that the effects of cocaine on BZD receptor labeling in this brain region increase once exposure to the drug is terminated. On the other hand, 6-OHDA administration generally produced opposite effects on BZD binding when compared to the effects of cocaine. The lesion resulted in significant increases in BZD receptor binding in the MPC and NAC and significant decreases in the caudate nucleus, substantia nigra and VTA. Furthermore, 6-OHDA attenuated the cocaine-induced changes in BZD receptor binding observed in the MPC and caudate nucleus of the sham-treated animals. The neurotoxin also increased BZD receptor labeling more in the NAC and decreased labeling more in the VTA of the cocaine- than the saline-treated animals. These data strongly suggest an important role for DA in the regulation of BZD receptors, especially with respect to the effects of cocaine.[28] The effects of cocaine on BZD receptor binding were attenuated in terminal fields for the mesocorticolimbic and nigro-striatal dopaminergic systems, while BZD receptor labeling in brain regions associated with the cell bodies for both systems was decreased in both saline- and cocaine-treated animals following pretreatment with 6-OHDA.

EFFECTS OF BZDS ON INTRAVENOUS COCAINE SELF-ADMINISTRATION IN RATS

Since cocaine appears to affect CRF and BZD binding in the rat brain, suggesting a potential role for anxiety in the neurobiology of the drug, the next experiments were designed to determine if BZDs would alter the reinforcing efficacy of cocaine. The first study tested the effects of systemic pretreatment with the BZD agonist, CDP, on intravenous cocaine self-administration in rats.[33] In these experiments, 16 adult male Fisher 344 strain rats were trained to self-administer cocaine (0.5 or 1.0 mg/kg, iv) during daily 2.5 hour sessions conducted 5 days per week. The rats were trained to respond under a fixed-ratio 4 limited hold 300-sec (FR4 LH300) schedule of reinforcement where cocaine delivery was contingent on the animal pressing the response lever 3 additional times within 5 min from the first response. Pretreatment (15 min) with low doses (0.3 to 1.0 mg/kg, ip) of CDP produced small increases in drug-intake with 0.5 mg/kg cocaine, while higher doses (10 mg/kg, ip) significantly decreased drug-intake in all rats tested. The effects of CDP on self-administration were attenuated when the concentration of cocaine was increased to 1.0 mg/kg, suggesting that CDP was opposing rather than augmenting the pharmacological effects of cocaine. However, since the decreases in drug-intake may have resulted from a non-specific effect on the ability of the rats to respond with higher doses of CDP, the following study was initiated.

This experiment was designed to investigate the effectiveness and specificity of alprazolam on intravenous cocaine self-administration.[34] Alprazolam was studied since this drug has been proven to be clinically effective in the treatment of anxiety and panic attacks[35] and has been proposed to be useful in the treatment of some types of depression.[36-38] Cocaine use and withdrawal have also been associated with anxiety, depression and even panic attacks in some cases.[2,5,6,9,10] Alprazolam was tested in adult male Wistar rats under a multiple schedule of intravenous cocaine presentation and food reinforcement. Cocaine (0.25 or 0.5 mg/kg, iv) was available during the first hour of the session under a FR4 schedule of reinforcement. During the second hour, food presentation (45 mg pellets) was available under a discrete-trial FR10 schedule of reinforcement. The animals were pretreated with alprazolam (0, 0.25, 0.5, 1.0, 2.0, and 4.0 mg/kg, ip) 30 min prior to the start of the behavioral session. Initial exposure to alprazolam resulted in non-specific decreases in both cocaine- and food-maintained responding. However, the animals quickly became tolerant to the effects of the drug on food reinforced responding upon subsequent testing. On the other hand, dose-related decreases in cocaine self-administration (0.5 mg/kg) were maintained throughout testing with alprazolam. Furthermore, significant increases in drug-intake were observed in some animals with 0.25 mg/kg cocaine following pretreatment with low doses of alprazolam (e.g., 0.25 or 0.5 mg/kg, ip), suggesting that the animals were attempting to overcome a drug-induced blockade of the reinforcing properties of cocaine. These data also suggest that pharmacological effects inherent to alprazolam (i.e., anxiolytic?) specifically altered cocaine reinforcement without affecting responding maintained by food.

GENERAL DISCUSSION

It is well documented that cocaine administration augments dopaminergic neurotransmission by increasing the concentration of the neurotransmitter in the synapse[39-42] via an inhibition of DA reuptake.[43] Cocaine can also serve as a potent reinforcer in humans as well as non-human animals.[44-46] Receptor binding studies have suggested that the cocaine binding site for reinforcement is localized at the DA uptake site since the affinity of cocaine and related drugs for the DA transporter is highly correlated with the reinforcing efficacy of these drugs.[43,47] Intravenous self-administration studies have implicated the mesocorticolimbic, but not the nigro-striatal, dopaminergic system in cocaine reinforcement in rats since DA depletion within brain regions associated with this system attenuate drug-intake[48-51] and since DA levels in the NAC measured using *in vivo* microdialysis increase during self-administration.[41,52,53] The mesocortical dopaminergic system may also be important in the initiation of cocaine reinforcement processes in rats since the drug is self-administered directly into the MPC, but not into the NAC or VTA.[54-56] More recent investigations have suggested that dopaminergic activity within the MPC is also important for the acquisition of intravenous cocaine self-administration in rats.[57] The effects of cocaine on CRF and BZD receptor binding within the mesocorticolimbic dopaminergic system reported above may be reflective of the behavioral effects of the drug. More specifically, BZD receptors within the mesocorticolimbic dopaminergic system appear to be involved in cocaine reinforcement processes. For example, comparisons between rats that self-administered cocaine and animals that received identical yoked-infusions of the drug for 30 days demonstrated that BZD receptor labeling was significantly increased in the MPC and NAC of the self-administration animals.[58] In addition, CDP and alprazolam decrease intravenous cocaine self-administration in rats,[33,34] possibly by reducing the reinforcing efficacy of the drug. More recently, we have found that the discrete intracranial infusion of small doses of CDP (50 to 100 pmol) into the MPC results in a transient increase in intravenous cocaine self-administration,[59] demonstrating the direct involvement of BZD receptors localized in brain regions associated with the mesocortical dopaminergic system in cocaine reinforcement processes. The results of the experiments described above suggest that the neurobiological responses to cocaine are different in the mesocorticolimbic dopaminergic system when compared to other brain loci. The MPC and VTA were the only regions where the effects on BZD receptors were observed 14 days following chronic exposure to cocaine. Mesocorticolimbic brain regions were also the only sites examined where cocaine affected CRF binding.

However, response-contingent and response-independent cocaine administration can result in different behavioral and neurobiological effects.[58,60] In fact, while daily non-contingent injections of cocaine resulted in a decrease in BZD receptor labeling in the NAC and MPC in the experiments presented above, increases in BZD receptor binding in these same brain regions have been observed in animals trained to self-administer cocaine when compared to littermates receiving yoked infusions of the drug.[58] Recently, we reported that response-independent cocaine administered using a schedule identical to that used in the receptor autoradiography experiments described above resulted in defensive withdrawal behavior with an increase in plasma corticosterone in rats,[61] indicating an anxiogenic response.[62-64] Acute injections of cocaine produce comparable behavioral and neuroendocrine effects which can be reversed by pretreating the animals with CDP.[65] Other investigators have reported similar cocaine-induced anxiogenic responses. In drug discrimination studies, cocaine will generalize to a pentylenetetrazol discriminative stimulus, suggesting that non-contingent cocaine administration and/or withdrawal produces an anxiogenic stimulus in rats,[66-68] which is also blocked with diazepam but not haloperidol.[68] Anxiogenic behavior has also been reported in mice tested in a black/white two-compartment model of anxiety[69] and in rats tested in the conditioned suppression of drinking conflict model[70] following acute injections of cocaine, during chronic administration[70] and during withdrawal.[69,70] Finally, Ettenberg and Geist[71] recently reported that cocaine resulted in both reinforcing and anxiogenic behavior in rats trained to self-administer the drug by traversing the length of a straight alley. Following repeated testing, the latency to enter the goal box where intravenous cocaine infusions were delivered gradually increased, suggesting a pro-conflict or anxiogenic response. Diazepam pretreatment reduced the latency to enter the goal box,[71] suggesting that the anxiogenic effects following repeated cocaine administration in this paradigm were mediated through BZD receptors. These data suggest a potential involvement of BZD (and possibly CRF) receptors in brain regions associated with the mesocorticolimbic dopaminergic system not only in cocaine reinforcement, but also in cocaine-induced anxiety.

Other stressors also appear to selectively activate the mesocortical dopaminergic system. It is well documented that dopaminergic neuronal activity measured *in vitro* in the prefrontal cortex is selectively activated following electric footshock in rodents,[72-75] and that these stress-induced increases in DA turnover can be inhibited or reversed by pretreating the animals with diazepam[76-78] or by microinjections of the γ-aminobutyric acid$_B$ agonist, baclofen, into the VTA.[79] *In vivo* microdialysis studies have recently validated these earlier reports and demonstrated that footshock stress activates DA in the MPC to a much greater degree than in either the NAC or striatum.[80] Recent data also suggest that both cocaine and footshock stress appear to selectively activate the mesocortical dopaminergic system and that these effects may be additive.[81] The anxiogenic BZD receptor inverse agonist, FG 7142, also selectively increases DA turnover in the prefrontal cortex, while agonists decrease turnover, suggesting that BZD recognition sites exert a selective and powerful modulatory influence on the mesocorticolimbic DA system.[82] These data suggest that the changes in receptor binding reported above may be related to a regulatory role for BZD binding sites within the mesocorticolimbic DA system which is mediated through the cocaine-induced activation of dopaminergic neuronal activity in the MPC and, possibly, the NAC.

Recently, it has been reported that vulnerability to intravenous amphetamine self-administration in rats is associated with the animal's reactivity to a novel environment,[83,84] suggesting that physiological responses to stress may be predictive of individual abuse liability. Further studies demonstrated that environmental conditions[85] or even exogenous infusions of corticosterone[86] can increase the likelihood that a rat will acquire self-administration of low doses of amphetamine, suggesting that changes in activity within the hypothalamic-pituitary-adrenal (HPA) axis may be involved in the abuse liability of stimulant drugs. These reports are consistent with the behavioral data presented above demonstrating a specific decrease in cocaine self-administration following pretreatment with the BZD receptor agonists CDP or alprazolam[33,34] at doses which do not affect food-maintained responding.[34] In non-laboratory settings, social users of cocaine are often able to control their drug-intake and, therefore, do not escalate their patterns of use to levels that increase the risk of dependency and toxicity.[87] These data suggest that factors in addition to cocaine's reinforcing properties may determine why some individuals can remain casual recreational users of the drug while others progress to compulsive drug use. In fact, a subpopulation of chronic cocaine users may actually be self-medicating to regulate painful feelings and psychiatric symptoms via their drug use.[88-90] A better understanding of environmental events that can potentially influence self-administration may result in the more effective and efficient treatment of cocaine addiction and withdrawal. Based on the data reviewed above, changes in the amount or severity of and/or individual reactivity to environmental stress or anxiety may be one factor which predisposes some individuals to engage in compulsive drug use.

ACKNOWLEDGMENTS

The author would like to thank Ms. Marcia McNulty and Mr. Glenn Guerin for their expert technical assistance.

REFERENCES

1. GAWIN, F. H. & E. H. ELLINWOOD. 1988. Cocaine and other stimulants: Actions, abuse, and treatment. New Engl. J. Med. **318**: 1173–1182.
2. GAWIN, F. H. & E. H. ELLINWOOD. 1989. Cocaine dependence. Ann. Rev. Med. **40**: 149–161.
3. COHEN, S. 1975. Cocaine. J. Am. Med. Assoc. **231**: 74–75.
4. RESNICK, R. B., R. S. KESTENBAUM & L. K. SCHWARTZ. 1977. Acute systemic effects of cocaine in man: A controlled study of intranasal and intravenous routes of administration. In Cocaine and Other Stimulants. E. H. Ellinwood, Jr. & M. M. Kilbey, Eds.: 615–628. Plenum Press. New York.
5. ANTHONY, J. C., A. Y. TIEN & K. R. PETRONIS. 1989. Epidemiologic evidence on cocaine use and panic attacks. Am. J. Epidemiol. **129**: 543–549.
6. ARONSON, T. A. & T. J. CRAIG. 1986. Cocaine precipitation of panic disorder. Am. J. Psychiatry **143**: 643–645.
7. WASHTON, A. M. & M. S. GOLD. 1984. Chronic cocaine abuse: Evidence for adverse effects on health and functioning. Psychiatric Ann. **14**: 733–739.
8. GAY, G. R. 1981. You've come a long way baby! Coke time for the new American Lady of the eighties. J. Psychoactive Drugs **13**: 297–318.
9. TARR, J. E. & M. MACKLIN. 1987. Cocaine. Ped. Clin. N. Am. **34**: 319–331.
10. CROWLEY, T. J. 1987. Clinical issues in cocaine abuse. In Cocaine: Clinical and Biobehavioral Aspects. S. Fisher, A. Raskin & E. H. Uhlenhuth, Eds.: 193–211. Oxford University Press. New York.
11. WESSON, D. R. & D. E. SMITH. 1985. Cocaine: Treatment perspectives. In Cocaine Use in America: Epidemiologic and Clinical Perspectives. N. J. Kozel & N. J. Adams, Eds.: 193–202. NIDA Research Monograph **61**, DHHS publication number (ADM) 85-1414. U.S. Government Printing Office. Washington, D.C.
12. GOLD, P. W., G. CHROUSOS, C. KELLNER, R. POST, A. ROY, P. AUGERINO, H. SCHULTE, E. OLDFIELD & D. L. LORIAUX. 1984. Psychiatric implications of basic and clinical studies with corticotropin-releasing factor. Am. J. Psychiatry **141**: 619–627.
13. NEMEROFF, C. B. 1988. The role of corticotropin-releasing factor in the pathogenesis of major depression. Pharmacopsychiatry **21**: 76–82.
14. KOOB, G. F. 1985. Stress, corticotropin-releasing factor, and behavior. Perspect. Behav. Med. **2**: 39–52.
15. BRITTON, K. T., J. MORGAN, J. RIVIER, W. VALE & G. F. KOOB. 1985. Chlordiazepoxide attenuates response suppression induced by corticotropin-releasing factor in the conflict test. Psychopharmacology **86**: 170–174.
16. BRITTON, K. T., G. LEE & G. F. KOOB. 1988. Corticotropin-releasing factor and amphetamine exaggerate partial agonist properties of benzodiazepine Ro 15-1788 in the conflict test. Psychopharmacology **94**: 306–311.
17. SWERDLOW, N. R., M. A. GEYER, W. W. VALE & G. F. KOOB. 1986. Corticotropin-releasing factor potentiates acoustic startle in rats: Blockade by chlordiazepoxide. Psychopharmacology **88**: 147–152.
18. FORMAN, L. J. & S. ESTILOW. 1988. Cocaine influences beta-endorphin levels and release. Life Sci. **43**: 309–315.
19. MOLDOW, R. L. & A. J. FISCHMAN. 1987. Cocaine induced secretion of ACTH, beta-endorphin, and corticosterone. Peptides **8**: 819–822.
20. RIVIER, C. & W. VALE. 1987. Cocaine stimulates adrenocorticotropin (ACTH) secretion through a corticotropin-releasing factor (CRF)-mediated mechanism. Brain Res. **422**: 403–406.

21. CALOGERO, A. E., W. T. GALLUCCI, M. A. KLING, G. P. CHROUSOS & P. W. GOLD. 1989. Cocaine stimulates rat hypothalamic corticotropin-releasing hormone secretion in vitro. Brain Res. **505:** 7–11.
22. GOEDERS, N. E., O. J. BIENVENU & E. B. DE SOUZA. 1990. Chronic cocaine administration alters corticotropin-releasing factor receptors in the rat brain. Brain Res. **531:** 322–328.
23. GOEDERS, N., V. BELL, A. GUIDROZ & M. MCNULTY. 1990. Dopaminergic involvement in the cocaine-induced up-regulation of benzodiazepine receptors in the rat caudate nucleus. Brain Res. **515:** 1–8.
24. ONN, S., T. W. BERGER, E. M. STRICKER & M. J. ZIGMOND. 1986. Effects of intraventricular 6-hydroxydopamine on the dopaminergic innervation of striatum: Histochemical and neurochemical analysis. Brain Res. **376:** 8–19.
25. DE SOUZA, E. B., M. H. PERRIN, T. R. INSEL, J. RIVIER, W. W. VALE & M. J. KUHAR. 1984. Corticotropin-releasing factor receptors in rat forebrain: Autoradiographic identification. Science **224:** 1449–1451.
26. DE SOUZA, E. B., T. R. INSEL, M. H. PERRIN, J. RIVIER, W. W. VALE & M. J. KUHAR. 1985. Corticotropin-releasing factor receptors are widely distributed within the rat central nervous system: An autoradiographic study. J. Neurosci. **5:** 3189–3203.
27. JAVITCH, J. A., S. M. STRITTMATTER & S. H. SNYDER. 1985. Differential visualization of dopamine and norepinephrine uptake sites in rat brain using [³H]mazindol autoradiography. J. Neurosci. **5:** 1513–1521.
28. GOEDERS, N. E. 1991. Cocaine differentially affects benzodiazepine receptors in discrete regions of the rat brain: Persistence and potential mechanisms mediating these effects. J. Pharmacol. Exp. Ther. **259:** 574–581.
29. YOUNG, W. S. III & M. J. KUHAR. 1979. A new method for receptor autoradiography: [³H]Opioid receptors in rat brain. Brain Res. **179:** 255–270.
30. YOUNG, W. S. III, D. L. NIEHOFF, M. J. KUHAR, B. BEER & A. S. LIPPA. 1981. Multiple benzodiazepine receptor localization by light microscopic radiohistochemistry. J. Pharmacol. Exp. Ther. **216:** 425–430.
31. GOEDERS, N. E. & M. J. KUHAR. 1985. Benzodiazepine receptor binding *in vivo* with [³H]-Ro 15-1788. Life Sci. **37:** 345–355.
32. GOEDERS, N. E. 1990. The effects of chronic cocaine administration on brain neurotransmitter receptors. Drug Dev. Res. **20:** 349–357.
33. GOEDERS, N. E., M. A. MCNULTY, S. MIRKIS & K. H. MCALLISTER. 1989. Chlordiazepoxide alters intravenous cocaine self-administration in rats. Pharmacol. Biochem. Behav. **33:** 859–866.
34. GOEDERS, N. E., M. A. MCNULTY & G. F. GUERIN. 1991. Effects of alprazolam on intravenous cocaine self-administration in rats. Neurosci. Abstr. **17:** 1426.
35. CHOUINARD, G., L. ANNABLE, R. FONTAINE & L. SOLYOM. 1982. Alprazolam in the treatment of generalized anxiety and panic disorders: A double-blind placebo-controlled study. Psychopharmacology **77:** 229–233.
36. DAWSON, G. W., S. G. JUE & R. N. BROGDEN. 1984. Alprazolam. A review of its pharmacodynamic properties and efficacy in the treatment of anxiety and depression. Drugs **27:** 132–147.
37. FEIGHNER, J. P., G. C. ADEN, L. F. FABRE, K. RICKELS & W. T. SMITH. 1983. Comparison of alprazolam, imipramine and placebo in the treatment of depression. J. Am. Med. Assoc. **249:** 3057–3064.
38. RICKELS, K., J. P. FEIGHNER & W. T. SMITH. 1985. Alprazolam, amitriptyline, doxepin and placebo in the treatment of depression. Arch. Gen. Psychiatry **42:** 134–141.
39. CHURCH, W. H., J. B. JUSTICE, JR. & J. B. BYRD. 1987. Extracellular dopamine in rat striatum following uptake inhibition by cocaine, nomifensine and benztropine. Eur. J. Pharmacol. **139:** 345–348.
40. BRADBERRY, C. W. & R. H. ROTH. 1989. Cocaine increases extracellular dopamine in rat nucleus accumbens and ventral tegmental area as shown by in vivo dialysis. Neurosci. Lett. **103:** 97–102.
41. PETTIT, H. O. & J. B. JUSTICE, JR. 1989. Dopamine in the nucleus accumbens during cocaine self-administration as studied by in vivo microdialysis. Pharmacol. Biochem. Behav. **34:** 899–904.

42. KALIVAS, P. W. & P. DUFFY. 1990. Effect of acute and daily cocaine treatment on extracellular dopamine in the nucleus accumbens. Synapse **5**: 48–58.
43. RITZ, M. C., R. J. LAMB, S. R. GOLDBERG & M. J. KUHAR. 1987. Cocaine receptors on dopamine transporters are related to self-administration of cocaine. Science **237**: 1219–1223.
44. FISCHMAN, M. W. 1987. Cocaine and the amphetamines. *In* Psychopharmacology: The Third Generation of Progress. H. Y. Meltzer, Ed.: 1543–1553. Raven Press. New York.
45. JOHANSON, C. E. 1984. Assessment of the dependence potential of cocaine in animals. *In* Cocaine: Pharmacology, Effects and Treatment of Abuse. J. Grabowski, Ed.: 54–71. NIDA Research Monograph **50**, DHHS publication number (ADM)84-1326. U. S. Government Printing Office. Washington, D.C.
46. WOODS, J. H., G. D. WINGER & C. P. FRANCE. 1987. Reinforcing and discriminative stimulus effects of cocaine: Analysis of pharmacological mechanisms. *In* Cocaine: Clinical and Biobehavioral Aspects. S. Fisher, A. Raskin & E. H. Uhlenhuth, Eds.: 21–65. Oxford University Press. New York.
47. BERGMAN, J., B. K. MADRAS, S. E. JOHNSON & R. D. SPEALMAN. 1989. Effects of cocaine and related drugs in nonhuman primates. III. Self-administration by squirrel monkeys. J. Pharmacol. Exp. Ther. **251**: 150–155.
48. ROBERTS, D. C. S., M. E. CORCORAN & H. C. FIBIGER. 1977. On the role of ascending catecholaminergic systems in intravenous self-administration of cocaine. Pharmacol. Biochem. Behav. **6**: 615–620.
49. ROBERTS, D. C. S., G. F. KOOB, P. KLONOFF & H. C. FIBIGER. 1980. Extinction and recovery of cocaine self-administration following 6-hydroxydopamine lesions of the nucleus accumbens. Pharmacol. Biochem. Behav. **12**: 781–787.
50. ROBERTS, D. C. S. & G. F. KOOB. 1982. Disruption of cocaine self-administration following 6-hydroxydopamine lesions of the ventral tegmental area in rats. Pharmacol. Biochem. Behav. **17**: 901–904.
51. PETTIT, H. O., A. ETTENBERG, F. E. BLOOM & G. F. KOOB. 1984. Destruction of dopamine in the nucleus accumbens selectively attenuates cocaine but not heroin self-administration in rats. Psychopharmacology **84**: 167–173.
52. PETTIT, H. O., H. PAN, L. H. PARSONS & J. B. JUSTICE, JR. 1990. Extracellular concentrations of cocaine and dopamine are enhanced during chronic cocaine administration. J. Neurochem. **55**: 798–804.
53. PETTIT, H. O. & J. B. JUSTICE, JR. 1991. Effect of dose on cocaine self-administration behavior and dopamine levels in the nucleus accumbens. Brain Res. **539**: 94–102.
54. GOEDERS, N. E. & J. E. SMITH. 1983. Cortical dopaminergic involvement in cocaine reinforcement. Science **221**: 773–775.
55. GOEDERS, N. E. & J. E. SMITH. 1986. Reinforcing properties of cocaine in the medial prefrontal cortex: Primary action on presynaptic dopaminergic terminals. Pharmacol. Biochem. Behav. **25**: 191–199.
56. GOEDERS, N. E., S. I. DWORKIN & J. E. SMITH. 1986. Neuropharmacological assessment of cocaine self-administration into the medial prefrontal cortex. Pharmacol. Biochem. Behav. **24**: 1429–1440.
57. SCHENK, S., B. A. HORGER, R. PELTIER & K. SHELTON. 1991. Supersensitivity to the reinforcing effects of cocaine following 6-hydroxydopamine lesions to the medial prefrontal cortex in rats. Brain Res. **543**: 227–235.
58. GOEDERS, N. E., G. F. GUERIN, M. A. McNULTY, A. M. GUIDROZ & S. I. DWORKIN. 1991. Effects of self-administered cocaine on benzodiazepine receptors in the rat brain. FASEB J. **5**(3): A1562.
59. GUERIN, G. F. & N. E. GOEDERS. 1991. Effects of central chlordiazepoxide infusions on intravenous cocaine self-administration in rats. *In* Problems of Drug Dependence, 1991. U.S. Government Printing Office. Washington, D.C. In press.
60. GOEDERS, N. E., M. A. McNULTY, A. M. GUIDROZ & S. I. DWORKIN. 1990. Potential neurotoxic effects of self-administered cocaine on dopamine receptors. *In* Problems of Drug Dependence, 1989. L. S. Harris, Ed.: 504–505. NIDA Research Monograph **95**, DHHS publication number (ADM) 90-1663. U. S. Government Printing Office. Washington, D.C.

61. GOEDERS, N. E., G. F. GUERIN, X. M. YANG & A. J. DUNN. 1990. Anxiety or stress due to cocaine. Neurosci. Abstr. **16:** 581.
62. TAKAHASHI, L. K., N. H. KALIN, J. A. VANDEN BURGT & J. E. SHERMAN. 1989. Corticotropin-releasing factor modulates defensive-withdrawal and exploratory behavior in rats. Behav. Neurosci. **103:** 648–654.
63. BUTLER, P. D., J. M. WEISS, J. C. STOUT & C. B. NEMEROFF. 1990. Corticotropin-releasing factor produces fear-enhancing and behavioral activating effects following infusion into the locus ceruleus. J. Neurosci. **10:** 176–183.
64. YANG, X. M., A. L. GORMAN & A. J. DUNN. 1990. The involvement of central noradrenergic systems and corticotropin-releasing factor in defensive-withdrawal behavior in rats. J. Pharmacol. Exp. Ther. **255:** 1064–1070.
65. GORMAN, A. L., X. M. YANG, A. J. DUNN & N. E. GOEDERS. 1991. Anxiogenic effects of cocaine. Neurosci. Abstr. **17:** 1426.
66. SHEARMAN, G. T. & H. LAL. 1981. Discriminative stimulus properties of cocaine related to an anxiogenic action. Prog. Neuro-Psychopharmacol. **5:** 57–63.
67. WOOD, D. M. & H. LAL. 1987. Anxiogenic properties of cocaine withdrawal. Life Sci. **41:** 1431–1436.
68. WOOD, D. M., P. R. LARABY & H. LAL. 1989. A pentylenetetrazol-like stimulus during cocaine withdrawal: Blockade by diazepam but not haloperidol. Drug Dev. Res. **16:** 269–276.
69. COSTALL, B., M. E. KELLY, R. J. NAYLOR & E. S. ONAIVI. 1989. The actions of nicotine and cocaine in a mouse model of anxiety. Pharmacol. Biochem. Behav. **33:** 197–203.
70. FONTANA, D. J. & R. L. COMMISSARIS. 1989. Effects of cocaine on conflict behavior in the rat. Life Sci. **45:** 819–827.
71. ETTENBERG, A. & T. D. GEIST. 1991. Animal model for investigating the anxiogenic effects of self-administered cocaine. Psychopharmacol. **103:** 455–461.
72. THIERRY, A. M., J. P. TASSIN, G. BLANC & J. GLOWINSKI. 1976. Selective activation of the mesocortical dopaminergic system by stress. Nature (London) **263:** 242–244.
73. D'ANGIO, M., A. SERRANO, P. DRISCOLL & B. SCATTON. 1988. Stressful environmental stimuli increase extracellular DOPAC levels in the prefrontal cortex of hypoemotional (Roman high-avoidance) but not hyperemotional (Roman low-avoidance) rats. An in vivo voltammetric study. Brain Res. **451:** 237–247.
74. DEUTCH, A. Y., S. Y. TAM & R. H. ROTH. 1985. Footshock and conditioned stress increase 3,4-dihydroxyphenylacetic acid (DOPAC) in the ventral tegmental area but not substantia nigra. Brain Res. **333:** 143–146.
75. DEUTCH, A. Y., W. A. CLARK & R. H. ROTH. 1990. Prefrontal cortical dopamine depletion enhances the responsiveness of mesolimbic dopamine neurons to stress. Brain Res. **521:** 311–315.
76. FADDA, F., A. ARGIOLAS, M. R. MELIS, A. H. TISSARI, P. C. ONALI & G. L. GESSA. 1978. Stress-induced increase in 3,4-dihydroxyphenylacetic acid (DOPAC) levels in the cerebral cortex and in nucleus accumbens: Reversal by diazepam. Life Sci. **23:** 2219–2224.
77. LAVIELLE, S., J. P. TASSIN, A. M. THIERRY, G. BLANC, D. HERVÉ, C. BERTHÉLÉMY & J. GLOWINSKI. 1978. Blockade by benzodiazepines of the selective high increase in dopamine turnover induced by stress in mesocortical dopaminergic neurons of the rat. Brain Res. **168:** 585–594.
78. REINHARD, J. R., JR., M. J. BANNON & R. H. ROTH. 1982. Acceleration by stress of dopamine synthesis and metabolism in prefrontal cortex: Antagonism by diazepam. Naunyn Schmiedeberg's Arch. Pharmacol. **308:** 374–377.
79. KALIVAS, P. W., P. DUFFY & H. EBERHARDT. 1990. Modulation of A10 dopamine neurons by γ-aminobutyric acid agonists. J. Pharmacol. Exp. Ther. **253:** 858–866.
80. ABERCROMBIE, E. D., K. A. KEEFE, D. S. DIFRISCHIA & M. J. ZIGMOND. 1989. Differential effect of stress on in vivo dopamine release in striatum, nucleus accumbens, and medial prefrontal cortex. J. Neurochem. **52:** 1655–1658.
81. KALIVAS, P. W. & P. DUFFY. 1989. Similar effects of daily cocaine and stress on mesocorticolimbic dopamine neurotransmission in the rat. Biol. Psychiatry **25:** 913–928.
82. TAM, S. Y. & R. H. ROTH. 1989. Modulation of mesoprefrontal dopamine neurons by cen-

tral benzodiazepine receptors. I. Pharmacological characterization. J. Pharmacol. Exp. Ther. **252:** 989–996.
83. PIAZZA, P. V., J. M. DEMINIÈRE, M. LE MOAL & H. SIMON. 1989. Factors that predict individual vulnerability to amphetamine self-administration. Science **245:** 1511–1513.
84. PIAZZA, P. V., J. M. DEMINIÈRE, S. MACCARI, P. MORMÈDE, M. LE MOAL & H. SIMON. 1990. Individual reactivity to novelty predicts probability of amphetamine self-administration. Behav. Pharmacol. **1:** 339–345.
85. MACCARI, S., P. V. PIAZZA, J. M. DEMINIÈRE, V. LEMAIRE, P. MORMÈDE, H. SIMON, L. ANGELUCCI & M. LE MOAL. 1991. Life events-induced decrease of corticosteroid type I receptors is associated with reduced corticosterone feedback and enhanced vulnerability to amphetamine self-administration. Brain Res. **547:** 7–12.
86. PIAZZA, P. V., S. MACCARI, J. M. DEMINIÈRE, M. LE MOAL, P. MORMÈDE & H. SIMON. 1991. Corticosterone levels determine individual vulnerability to amphetamine self-administration. Proc. Natl. Acad. Sci. USA **88:** 2088–2092.
87. SIEGEL, R. K. 1984. Changing patterns of cocaine use: Longitudinal observations, consequences, and treatment. *In* Cocaine: Pharmacology, Effects and Treatment of Abuse. J. Grabowski, Ed.: 92–110. NIDA Research Monograph **50,** DHHS publication number (ADM) 84-1326. U.S. Government Printing Office. Washington, D.C.
88. KLEBER, H. D. & F. H. GAWIN. 1984. Cocaine abuse: A review of current and experimental treatments. *In* Cocaine: Pharmacology, Effects and Treatment of Abuse. J. Grabowski, Ed.: 111–129. NIDA Research Monograph **50,** DHHS publication number (ADM) 84-1326. U.S. Government Printing Office. Washington, D.C.
89. KHANTZIAN, E. J. 1985. The self-medication hypothesis of affective disorders: Focus on heroin and cocaine dependence. Am. J. Psychiatry **142:** 1259–1264.
90. GAWIN, F. H. 1986. New uses of antidepressants in cocaine abuse. Psychosomatics **27:** 24–29.

Behavioral and Pharmacological Determinants of Drug Abuse[a]

MICHAEL A. NADER

Department of Psychiatry
The University of Chicago
5841 S. Maryland Avenue
Chicago, Illinois 60637

THOMAS A. TATHAM

Department of Psychiatry
Uniformed Services University of the Health Sciences
4301 Jones Bridge Road
Bethesda, Maryland 20814-4799

JAMES E. BARRETT

Eli Lilly and Company
Lilly Research Laboratories
Lilly Corporate Center
Indianapolis, Indiana 46285

INTRODUCTION

While there is little doubt that the pharmacological properties of a drug play an important role in the initiation of a multitude of responses, it is also clear that several variables can significantly alter the effects of that drug both on intermediate processes and in its ultimate effects on behavior. This chapter focuses on some of the variables that have been shown to modify the behavioral effects of abused drugs. The emphasis is on describing certain conditions under which the effects of an abused drug are changed, often dramatically, by prior behavioral and/or pharmacological experience. Because these effects have been shown with a wide variety of abused drugs, are stable over lengthy periods of time, and are observed under a broad range of conditions, it would seem that these factors may have direct relevance for eventually understanding and being able to intercede in altering those conditions that lead to drug abuse.

Although several determinants of the behavioral effects of drugs have been described (*e.g.*, rate of responding in the absence of the drug, schedule of reinforcement and type of maintaining event), these variables typically are identifiable when assessing

[a] Preparation of this chapter was supported by NIDA grants DA-06828, DA-06829 and DA-02873.
[b] Address all correspondence to Michael A. Nader, Ph.D.; Tel.: (312) 702-6361; Fax: (312) 702-0857.

ongoing behavior.[1-3] The unique feature of historical influences on drug effects is that while conditions that have existed in the past may continue to exert a profound influence on the manner in which a drug affects behavior, the influence of that prior experience may not be apparent in behavior at the time the drug is administered.[4,5] The absence, as yet, of quantifiable details of behavior that reflect past experience poses special problems for being able to isolate and examine those variables that may contribute to the altered effects of the drugs. At the present time, very little is known about the historical factors and mechanisms responsible for modifying the effects of abused drugs on behavior. Additionally, it is also not clear whether the same variables that modify the behavioral effects of abused drugs also alter the likelihood of that drug being abused. Clearly, there are several issues left unresolved and many targets of inquiry. This chapter provides an overall summary of this area of research and addresses some avenues of research that could yield information on these issues.

EFFECTS OF HISTORY ON SCHEDULE-CONTROLLED BEHAVIOR

Food-maintained Behavior

Much of the work on the interactions of behavioral history with drug effects has been assessed on behaviors maintained by food presentation. Rather than present an exhaustive review of this literature, we will describe only select experiments that address certain methodological considerations. These considerations include the baseline schedule of reinforcement, the schedule used as the interpolated history and the use of appropriate control groups to better assess the changes in drug effects with changes in baseline rate of responding as a consequence of behavioral history. In addition, under some circumstances, the dosing regimen (*i.e.*, acute versus chronic) may reveal differences due to behavioral history that were not apparent from ongoing behavior.[6]

One of the most influential generalizations within behavioral pharmacology is that the rate-altering effects of many drugs can depend upon the ongoing rate of responding in the absence of drug.[7,8] With regards to behavioral history, it is important to distinguish between altered effects due to changes in baseline rates of responding as a consequence of behavioral history and more subtle changes that are not apparent from ongoing behavior in the absence of drugs. For example, Urbain *et al.*[9] trained separate groups of rats under either an interresponse times > 11-sec schedule (IRT > 11-sec), which engendered low rates of responding, or a fixed-ratio 40 schedule (FR 40), which generated high rates of responding. After 50 sessions under these schedules all rats responded under a fixed-interval 15-sec (FI 15-sec) schedule of food reinforcement. Prior to *d*-amphetamine administration, baseline FI response rates were different for the two groups. In general, *d*-amphetamine increased the lower rates emitted by rats with an IRT > 11-sec history, while decreasing the higher rates of responding of rats with an FR 40 history. The simplest explanation for these results is that the differential effects of *d*-amphetamine were rate-dependent and were a result of the persistent, differential response rates produced by low- versus high-rate schedule histories.

Investigators who have trained subjects under FI schedules know that response rates, in the absence of specific histories, can vary enormously. One of the questions regarding the Urbain *et al.*[9] results is whether the history would have modified *d*-.amphetamine's rate-altering effects in the absence of differences in baseline response rates. Nader and Thompson[10] trained pigeons under a similar protocol as that of Urbain *et al.*, except a third group of pigeons was included that was exposed to the FI schedule throughout. Prior to drug administration, pigeons with an FR 50 history had significantly higher response rates under an FI 90-sec schedule compared to pigeons with an IRT > 10-sec history, while the control group had intermediate response rates. However, it was observed that the control pigeons with the highest response rates had rates that were similar to pigeons with an FR history, and control pigeons with the lowest rates had rates similar to IRT > 10-sec-history pigeons. Thus, two groups of pigeons had nearly identical response rates under an FI 90-sec schedule, but different reinforcement schedule histories. When methadone was administered, low and intermediate doses significantly increased response rates of FR-history pigeons, while decreasing response rates of pigeons with similar rates but no FR history (FIG. 1). Thus, methadone's rate-altering effects were modified by the FR history, independent of baseline rates of responding.

It appears that behavior maintained under FI schedules is quite susceptible to historical influences in human[11,12] as well as nonhuman animals. Wanchisen *et al.*[13] examined whether another schedule that generates high rates of responding would influence FI performance to a similar degree as an FR history. Prior to training under an FI 30-sec schedule, four rats were trained under a variable-ratio 20 (VR 20) schedule for 30 sessions. Control rats were exposed to the FI 30-sec schedule throughout the experiment. For the first 20 sessions under the FI schedule, VR-history rats had higher response rates compared to FI controls. However, by session 30, VR-history subjects were responding at lower rates relative to rats trained only under the FI schedule. These results suggest that not all reinforcement schedule histories that generate high rates of responding influence FI performance similarly. Future research should address possible neurochemical or behavioral differences that exist between FR and VR histories that could account for the dissimilar effects. In the last section of this chapter we explore some behavioral and neurochemical mechanisms of action that could account for the

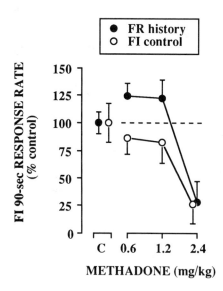

FIGURE 1. Fixed-interval 90-sec response rates (percent of control) as a function of methadone dose. One group of pigeons was trained under an FI 90-sec schedule throughout the experiment (*open circles*), while the other group had a history of responding under an FR 50 schedule of food presentation (*closed circles*). Drug-free baseline rates of responding were similar for both groups of pigeons. See text for complete description. (Adapted from ref. 10.)

long-lasting changes in behavior and possibly the behavioral effects of drugs following different histories.

The preceding section has shown that high- and low-rate schedule histories can have profound effects on FI response rates and on the rate-altering effects of drugs. As indicated previously, much of the research on the behavioral effects of reinforcement schedule history has utilized interval schedules (*e.g.*, refs. 6,9–14). Recently, Egli and Thompson[15] examined the influence of a fixed-interval history on methadone's effects on FR performance. In one experiment, the effects of methadone on responding under an FR 50 or FR 75 schedule of food reinforcement was assessed in pigeons with or without a history of responding under an FI 90-sec contingency. FIGURE 2 shows that methadone's rate-decreasing effects were attenuated by a history of responding under an FI contingency. In a second experiment, one group of pigeons was exposed to an alternative FR FI 90-sec schedule, in which the FR value varied weekly from 50, 75 or 200. Under alternative FR FI schedules, reinforcers may be earned under either the FR or FI schedule, whichever is satisfied first. Under the alternative FR 50 FI 90-sec or FR 75 FI 90-sec schedule, most reinforcers were earned under the FR contingency, while the majority of reinforcers were earned under the FI contingency when the schedule was alternative FR 200 FI 90-sec. Thus, this group received experience under the FI schedule when reinforcers were available under an alternative FR 200 FI 90-sec schedule. Responding by a second group of pigeons was maintained under an FR 50 or FR 75 schedule. For both groups of pigeons, an alternative FR 50 FI 90-sec or FR 75 FI 90-sec schedule was in effect when methadone was administered. Methadone decreased response rates in both groups, however, a "latent" methadone dose-dependent effect of the different histories was observed since subjects consistently exposed to the alternative schedule tended to earn more rein-

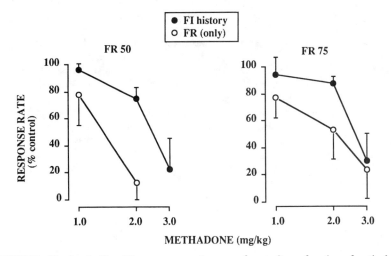

FIGURE 2. Fixed-ratio 50 or 75 response rates (percent of control) as a function of methadone dose. One group of pigeons was exposed to FR schedules throughout the experiment (*open circles*), while the other group had a history of responding under an FI 90-sec schedule of food presentation (*closed circles*). See text for complete description. (Adapted from ref. 15.)

forcers according to the FI contingency, despite comparable overall rates of responding. This study illustrates the subtle influence of nondrug exposure to drug testing conditions and demonstrates the occurrence of history effects with a more complex schedule than has been typically utilized in studies of behavioral history.

Behavior Maintained or Suppressed by Noxious Stimuli

A number of studies have demonstrated a reversal of the effects of d-amphetamine or morphine following exposure to a schedule in which responding was maintained by either response-produced electric shock or by a shock-postponement schedule. For example, the effects of d-amphetamine on punished behavior of squirrel monkeys, suppressed by shock presentation, was reversed following exposure to a shock-postponement or avoidance schedule.[16] Prior to the avoidance history, d-amphetamine only decreased responding, an outcome which is characteristic for this drug.[17,18] Following the interpolated experience with the avoidance schedule, however, d-amphetamine produced increases in responding that exceeded 300% of control performance. Importantly, rates of punished responding before and after exposure to the avoidance schedule did not differ, thereby ruling out a contribution of response rate to the altered effects of d-amphetamine. Bacotti and McKearney[19] also reported that training under an avoidance schedule yielded increases in punished responding with d-amphetamine, but that the effects of chlorpromazine were not modified by the avoidance history. This study raises the suggestion that only the effects of abused drugs might be modifiable by such interventions, but considerably more research must be done to address this possibility.

Another study found that the effects of morphine on responding maintained by a shock-postponement schedule could also be reversed by exposing squirrel monkeys to a schedule in which responding was maintained by response-produced shock.[20] Prior to training under the schedule of response-produced shock,[21] morphine only decreased responding under the avoidance schedule. However, following training under a schedule in which responding was maintained by a fixed-interval schedule of shock presentation, morphine increased responding under the avoidance schedule. This experiment employed separate manipulanda for the avoidance schedule and shock presentation conditions, thereby suggesting that the effects of a particular behavioral history are not limited to a particular response class.

These experiments, taken together with those summarized previously, indicate that behavioral experience can produce a dramatic modification of the way in which a drug of abuse affects behavior. Despite the generality of the finding across experimental conditions and drug classes, a great deal remains to be achieved. All of the studies summarized above involved analyses of the effects of a wide range of doses. There were no modifications of the extremes of the dose-response curve, a finding that might suggest the development of tolerance or sensitization.[22] For example, in the experiments involving noxious stimuli, the mid-range of the dose-response curve was simply modified from being either non-effective or rate-decreasing to rate-increasing with both morphine and d-amphetamine. Thus, the qualitative effects of the particular drug changed, suggesting a pharmacological mechanism other than one involving metabolic or pharmacokinetic processes. Studies described in a subsequent section of this chapter are providing increasing evidence that behavioral procedures similar to those described above can produce changes in receptor binding and neurotransmitter activity, as well as in other fundamental neuropharmacological processes. Thus, the possibility that behavioral experience may "drive" the more molecular neurochemical processes underlying the effects of an abused drug seems quite plausible.

Drug-maintained Behavior

There is clear evidence that behaviors maintained by drug reinforcers can be similar in rates and patterns to behaviors maintained by nondrug reinforcers.[23-26] While there is a growing volume of data on the effects of historical variables on food-maintained responding, little systematic work has been done with drug-maintained behavior. Because of their cost and the extensive training that is sometimes required, nonhuman primates are repeatedly used in self-administration experiments, despite the fact that prior experience may influence the behavioral effects of drugs. The top panels of FIGURE 3 show cumulative records from two rhesus monkeys responding under an FI 15-min schedule of cocaine presentation. The monkey whose data are depicted on the left had experience responding only under FI schedules, while the monkey whose record is shown on the right had a history of responding under FR schedules for several years. It appears that a history of responding under FR schedules can produce higher rates of responding under FI schedules of cocaine presentation. The lower panels of FIGURE 3 show responding by monkeys maintained by cocaine presentation under either an FR 100 (left) or FR 90 schedule. The monkey whose record is shown in the lower-right panel had several years of training under various FI schedules, whereas the monkey on the left has not had this experience. Note the scallop pattern of responding by the monkey with an FI history rather than the "break and run" pattern typically seen under FR schedules of reinforcement. Although the histories of these monkeys were not controlled in a systematic manner, it is clear that behavioral histories can modify the rate and pattern of drug-maintained behavior.

Under some circumstances, a particular reinforcement schedule history is necessary for the demonstration of reinforcement by a drug. For example, much of the early work on oral drug self-administration utilized schedule-induced polydipsia procedures,[27] in which intermittent food presentation induced large volumes of liquid intake (see refs. 28 and 29 for reviews). Schedule-induced polydipsia allowed for low doses of a drug to be consumed at high levels, thereby allowing for behaviorally active (and presumably reinforcing) doses to be self-administered. Falk and his colleagues have recently shown that certain histories may influence schedule-induced drug intakes and preferences.[30-34] For example, Tang *et al.*[34] reported that rats initially exposed to an FI 1-min schedule of food presentation with no water available, showed a retarded rate of acquisition and final level of schedule-induced polydipsia relative to a group that had water available from the outset. In another experiment,[32] rats initially made polydipsic with 0.9% NaCl, showed a retarded acquisition of 5% (v/v) ethanol polydipsia, suggesting that the initial substance that is available for consumption can influence subsequent levels of self-administration.

Choice for a drug reinforcer can also be modified by prior experience. Tang and Falk[33] allowed two groups of rats to drink 5% (v/v) ethanol from two drinking tubes in the chamber. After approximately 1 month under these conditions, one of the bottles was changed to 5% glucose ($n = 6$) and, for the second group, 0.7% glucose ($n = 6$). After several months, tests were conducted with different concentrations of glucose. When both groups were tested with a low concentration of glucose (0.7%)

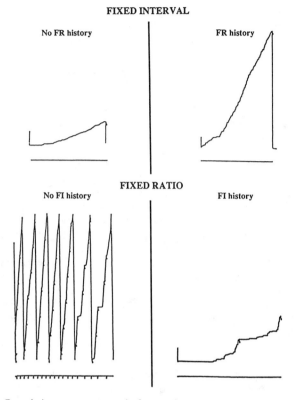

FIGURE 3. Cumulative response records for monkeys responding under fixed-interval (*top panel*) or fixed-ratio (*bottom panel*) schedules of cocaine presentation. *Top panels*: Fixed-interval 15-min performance maintained by cocaine 0.03 mg/kg/injection. The monkey whose record is depicted on the left was trained only under FI schedules of reinforcement, while the record on the right is from a monkey with a history (approximately 1 year) of responding under FR schedules of cocaine reinforcement. The cumulative record on the right is from the 60th session under the FI contingency. *Lower panels*: Fixed-ratio 100 (*left*) or 90 (*right*) performance maintained by cocaine 0.1 mg/kg/injection. The monkey whose record is depicted on the left was trained only under FR schedules of reinforcement. The record on the left represents performance under a multiple FR 100 schedule of food and cocaine presentation. Cocaine reinforcement is indicated by the deflection of the event pen. The record on the right is from a monkey with an extensive (approximately 3 years) history of responding under FI schedules of cocaine reinforcement. The cumulative record on the right is from the 91st session under the FR contingency. (Unpublished observations by M. A. Nader and W. L. Woolverton.)

versus 5% ethanol, both groups preferred the 5% ethanol solution. As glucose concentration was increased, 5% ethanol preference decreased for both groups. However, the decrease occurred earlier and more rapidly in the group with the history of 5% glucose exposure. Thus, while the differential treatments had no apparent effect on 5% ethanol consumption when it was the only solution or when it was the alternative to

0.7% glucose, the acceptance of 5% ethanol, in the presence of greater concentrations of glucose, was influenced by the behavioral histories of the subjects. Most recently, Falk and Tang[31] reported that pharmacological history can influence levels of schedule-induced polydipsia for certain drugs. Separate groups of rats had either water, cocaine (0.15 mg/ml) or ethanol (2.5% v/v) solutions available during daily 3-h sessions in which food was presented under a fixed-time 1-min (FT 1-min) schedule. Under the FT 1-min schedule, food was presented noncontingently every minute. All three groups became polydipsic and levels of liquid intake were not different for the groups. Similarly, when chlordiazepoxide (0.25 mg/ml) was substituted for the baseline liquids, total liquid intake was comparable for all groups when food was presented under the FT 1-min schedule. However, when single sessions of FT 3-min or FT 5-min were conducted, rats initially exposed to ethanol showed a higher level of chlordiazepoxide intake relative to the other two groups. Thus, intake for chlordiazepoxide depended not only on the subjects' drug history, but also on the schedule of food presentation (FT 1-min versus 3- or 5-min).

Pharmacological history also has been shown to modify the reinforcing effects of intravenously administered drugs.[35-37] For example, in one experiment,[38] responding by rhesus monkeys was initially maintained under a fixed-ratio 10 schedule of intravenous cocaine (33 μg/kg/injection) presentation. When responding was stable, various doses of the noncompetitive N-methyl-D-aspartate antagonists MK-801 and phencyclidine were evaluated during substitution tests. When substituted for cocaine, phencyclidine maintained responding in all monkeys, while no monkeys self-administered MK-801 above saline levels. After completing the MK-801 and phencyclidine dose-response curves, the baseline drug was changed from cocaine to phencyclidine (10 μg/kg/injection) and, after responding stabilized, the MK-801 dose-response curve was redetermined. Although no monkeys self-administered MK-801 when it was substituted for cocaine, MK-801 maintained responding above saline levels in three of four monkeys when it was substituted for phencyclidine. It has been suggested that one characteristic of pharmacological history that may modify the reinforcing effects of drugs using substitution procedures is overlapping discriminative stimulus effects with the baseline drug.[35] Taken together, these results provide further evidence for the substantial influence of pharmacological history on the reinforcing effects of drugs.

Recently, Piazza and colleagues have begun investigating individual differences in vulnerability to the acquisition of self-administration behavior.[39-42] Typically in these experiments, rats' responses to stress are initially assessed by examining locomotor behavior in a novel environment, with the subjects being divided into subgroups of low rate (LR) and high rate (HR) responders. In one experiment,[40] some rats from each group were injected with amphetamine under a regimen that has been shown to produce sensitization to amphetamine's behavioral effects (LR-amph, HR-amph), while the other subjects were injected with saline (LR-sal, HR-sal). Two days after the last injection, rats were surgically prepared with intravenous catheters and allowed to self-administer a low dose of amphetamine (10 μg/injection). HR rats that were treated with saline readily acquired amphetamine self-administration, whereas saline-treated LR rats did not. Thus, acquisition (*i.e.*, vulnerability) to low-dose amphetamine self-administration may be predicted by activity levels in a novel environment. In the groups of rats sensitized to some of amphetamine's behavioral effects (LR-amph, HR-amph), self-administration behavior was readily acquired, suggesting that repeated exposure to amphetamine may enhance the reinforcing effects of amphetamine in rats less likely to acquire self-administration (*i.e.*, LR rats). While these experiments did not systematically manipulate the animal's experimental history, they illustrate the possibility that behavior in one condition can predict the reinforcing effects of a drug under different conditions. It may be that a particular experimental history that increases (*e.g.*, anxiolytic drug treatment) or decreases (*e.g.*, inescapable shock) an animal's activity level in a novel environment may alter the reinforcing efficacy of a drug when it is available for self-administration.

In addition to reinforcing effects, a drug's discriminative stimulus effects, a measure of subjective effects by humans, may also influence drug use. Recently, the discriminative stimulus effects of drugs have been shown to be influenced by pharmacological history.[43] In that study, pigeons were trained to discriminate spiroxatrine, a compound with dopamine D_2 antagonist and serotonin 1A (5-HT_{1A}) agonist actions, from saline. The investigators found that in pigeons initially tested with buspirone, a compound with D_2 antagonist and 5-HT_{1A} agonist actions, prior to tests with more selective 5-HT_{1A} agonists, generalization would occur only with buspirone. In these pigeons, tests with the 5-HT_{1A} agonist 8-hydroxy-2-(di-*n*-propylamino)tetralin (8-OH-DPAT) occasioned only saline-appropriate responding. However, if the pigeons were first tested with 8-OH-DPAT, responding would be primarily on the drug-appropriate key following both 8-OH-DPAT and buspirone. These experiments indicate that pharmacological history can modify the discriminative stimulus effects of drugs. It will be interesting to determine whether pharmacological histories that modify the discriminative stimulus effects of a drug will similarly modify its reinforcing effects and vice versa.

In other cases, environmental stimuli that set the occasion for drug self-administration can acquire discriminative control over responding, such that their presence or absence influence the probability of drug-taking behavior (*cf.* ref. 44). For example, Wikler[45] suggested that previously neutral stimuli paired with opiate withdrawal can acquire conditioned aversive properties that may influence relapse to opiate addiction. In addition, previously neutral stimuli paired with drug reinforcers may become conditioned reinforcers that maintain drug-seeking behavior (*e.g.*, refs. 46–48). The use of these historical variables in drug abuse treatment has only recently been undertaken (see O'Brien *et al.*, this volume). The next section discusses experiments in which environmental stimuli, paired with drugs, were able to affect ongoing behavior in the absence of drugs.

Classical Conditioning and Drug Effects

In addition to the studies mentioned above in which stimuli paired with reinforcing doses of drugs can maintain behavior in the absence of the drug, other studies have shown that pairing drugs with other stimuli may play a potent role in determining the effects of that drug on schedule-controlled behavior. For example, Glowa and Barrett[49] trained pigeons under fixed-ratio schedules of grain presentation and injected them with either saline or various doses of *d*-amphetamine after the session. Whether the pigeons received saline or drug was signaled by different colored lights illuminating the grain magazine. Following training, responding was suppressed by visual stimuli correlated with postsession administration of *d*-amphetamine. Thus, while *d*-amphetamine was not administered before the session, the stimulus that was paired with *d*-amphetamine appeared to influence behavior in a manner that is consistent with *d*-amphetamine–induced response rate decreases.

The findings of Glowa and Barrett[49] have been extended by Watanabe,[50] using a similar procedure except that *d*-amphetamine or saline were administered prior to behavioral sessions; administration of drug or saline was signaled by different colored ceiling lights. Responding by pigeons was maintained under a multiple FI 3-min, FR 30 schedule of food presentation. Occasionally, the pigeons were injected with saline prior to sessions in which the ceiling lights indicated drug administration. Watanabe[50] found that the drug-associated stimulus produced response-rate increases during the FI component in pigeons with low rates, while decreasing higher rate FR performance. In another experiment using pentobarbital, Watanabe[50] gave two groups of pigeons similar drug-stimulus pairings, but only one group was allowed to key peck during sessions. Only the pigeons with a history of responding following drug administration showed increases in responding when only the conditioned stimulus was presented. Thus, under some circumstances, modification of the effects of a stimulus by pairing with a drug may depend upon experiencing the drug's effects in the presence of that stimulus. These results are difficult to reconcile with those of Glowa and Barrett[49] in which pigeons were not directly exposed to drugs during conditioning sessions. Future research may show whether the discrepant findings are attributable to differences in 1) the conditioning drug (*d*-amphetamine versus pentobarbital); 2) the schedules of food reinforcement or 3) pre- versus post-session drug administration. Despite these unanswered questions, it is clear that environmental stimuli can acquire powerful effects on schedule-controlled responding as the result of classical conditioning procedures.

It has also been demonstrated that the discriminative stimulus effects of drugs may be conditioned to exteroceptive stimuli. For example, Spencer *et al.*[51] trained rats to press one lever after injections of saline and a different lever following clonidine injections. After the rats reliably discriminated clonidine from saline, discrimination training was suspended and classical conditioning sessions were begun in which anise oil was rubbed on the rat's nose prior to clonidine injections. When discrimination testing resumed, anise oil occasioned clonidine-lever responding, demonstrating that environmental stimuli may come to occasion, following classical conditioning, drug-like discriminative stimulus effects.

Studies of this sort will undoubtedly increase in frequency for they have important implications for clinical situations in which drugs are administered in the presence of salient stimuli. Although beyond the scope of this chapter, there is considerable evidence that drug-paired environments can control tolerance or sensitization to drug effects on non-schedule–controlled behaviors (*e.g.*, refs. 52 and 53; see ref. 54 for review). Considering the demonstration of the conditioning of drug effects to the odor of anise oil, and other demonstrations of altered physiological effects of drugs through pairings with other drugs and/or exteroceptive stimuli (*e.g.*, refs. 55 and 56), there exists an intriguing possibility that the reinforcing and discriminative stimulus effects of drugs could be altered through similar conditioning procedures. To the extent that the stimulus properties of drugs play an important role in determining the likelihood of self-administration, it may be possible to modulate a drug's abuse liability through classical conditioning procedures (for a more detailed discussion see chapters by Fibiger; Shippenberg; O'Brien *et al.*; Stewart; this volume).

MECHANISMS OF ACTION

Behavioral Mechanisms of Action

This chapter has attempted to document some of the more recent experiments on the interactions of behavioral history with drug effects. In this last section we will describe some potential mechanisms of action, both behavioral and neurochemical, that correlate with certain behavioral histories. A behavioral mechanism of action can be defined as ". . . a description of a drug's effect on a given behavioral system expressed in terms of some more general set of environmental principles regulating behavior"[57] (p. 5). Certainly several behavioral mechanisms may influence ongoing behavior and the identification of a possible behavioral mechanism suggests only one factor that may contribute to the behavioral effects of drugs.[58] Although the present review is by no means exhaustive, it should be clear from the studies described that behavioral history can modify the effects of drugs from several pharmacological classes, including amphetamine, morphine, methadone, pentobarbital, chlordiazepoxide and ethanol. It is important to note that these drugs can all be classified as drugs of abuse. The behavioral effects of nonabused compounds, such as chlorpromazine, appear not to be altered by behavioral history.[19] This suggests that one characteristic of drugs of abuse are that their behavioral effects are malleable. Many of the drugs that are not abused seem to have more unitary effects on behavior, i.e., rate-decreasing effects, while drugs of abuse have a wide spectrum of behavioral effects. Conditions that tap this variability in drug effects may contribute significantly to a drug's abuse potential.

An example of an experiment that was designed to systematically evaluate potential behavioral mechanisms for the altered effects of a drug following a particular history is given by Barrett and Witkin.[5] In that study, the authors addressed the issue of what aspect of the shock-avoidance history resulted in increases in punished responding following d-amphetamine. That is, were the changes in d-amphetamine's effects on punished responding due to shock delivery per se or due to the specific avoidance contingencies? Initially, the effects of d-amphetamine on punished responding were assessed in two monkeys. Following completion of the dose-response curves, one monkey was exposed to an avoidance schedule, while a second monkey received response-independent shocks that could not be postponed by responding (yoked subject). That is, the yoked monkey received the same number and temporal distribution of shocks, but could not avoid them. After 2–3 weeks, both monkeys were returned to the punishment schedule and the d-amphetamine dose-response curves were redetermined. Prior to the avoidance or response-independent shock histories, d-amphetamine only decreased punished responding. After the interpolated history, d-amphetamine increased punished responding by the monkey with the avoidance history, but not the yoked monkey, suggesting that the avoidance contingency was necessary for d-amphetamine-induced increases in punished responding. Barrett and Witkin[5] also reported that while response rates under the punishment contingency did not change following the avoidance or response-independent shock history, response duration did. Following an avoidance history, response duration under the punishment contingency decreased, while response duration remained approximately the same following a history of response-independent shocks. Although it cannot be concluded from this experiment, it is possible that changes in response duration may have indirectly contributed to the amphetamine-induced increases in punished responding (cf. ref. 5). Studies designed to examine particular aspects of an organism's behavioral history may allow for the identification of the variables that influence subsequent behavior.

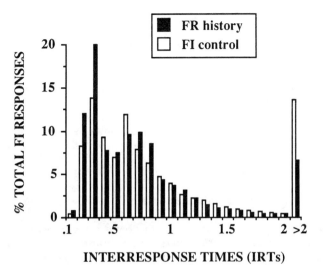

FIGURE 4. Interresponse time distributions for two groups ($n = 4$–6/group) of pigeons responding under an FI 90-sec schedule of food presentation. Control rates were similar for both groups. One group of pigeons had previous experience under an FR 50 schedule (*closed bar*), while the second group was trained exclusively under an FI 90-sec schedule (*open bars*). See text for complete description. (Unpublished data from experiment by Nader and Thompson.[10])

It is possible that some aspect of behavior is influenced by prior schedule history, even in the absence of changes in response rates, as shown by the Barrett and Witkin[5] results with response duration. This same analysis may be used to elucidate a possible influence of an FR history on the rate-altering effects of methadone that were reported earlier.[10] In that study, methadone increased FI response rates of pigeons with an FR history at doses that decreased comparable response rates by pigeons without an FR history (see Fig. 1). Figure 4 shows interresponse time (IRT) distributions for the two groups of pigeons, prior to drug administration. It is important to note that while response rates were approximately equal (38 r/min), the pattern of responding was different. Responding by pigeons with an FR history was characterized by more frequent short IRTs and fewer long IRTs relative to control subjects. This difference in IRT distributions between the groups may be what Egli and Thompson[15] have referred to as "latent history effects," and may account for the differences seen in the behavioral effects of methadone between FR-history subjects and control pigeons with similar response rates but no prior exposure to FR schedules.

Neurochemical Mechanisms of Action: Food-maintained Behavior

Although no studies specifically examining the effects of behavioral history on neurochemical levels have been undertaken, several investigators have examined neurochemical correlates of operant behavior that may be relevant to more molecular mechanisms of drug action related to the history effects described above (see refs. 59–63 for reviews). Using food-maintained responding of pigeons, Barrett and Hoffmann[64] reported that cerebrospinal fluid metabolite levels for serotonin and dopamine were different in animals responding under a fixed-interval schedule compared to levels when responding was maintained under a fixed-ratio schedule. It is certainly possible that one effect of a history of responding under a particular schedule of reinforcement is to produce long-lasting changes in neurochemical function. Thus, one possible mechanism for the altered behavioral effects of drugs following an FR or IRT > t-sec history may involve either changes in basal levels (i.e., drug free) or changes in drug-induced metabolite levels. Future research will undoubtedly examine further whether the neurochemical changes induced by the drug are altered following interpolated histories (see ref. 60).

Behavior Maintained or Suppressed by Noxious Stimuli

Properly controlled studies have shown that behavioral contingencies can produce distinct changes in neurochemistry and that such changes reflect the impact of environmental variables (cf. ref. 59). For example, Smith, Dworkin and their colleagues have designed experiments using triads of rats, to allow for an evaluation of the role of contingent versus noncontingent presentation of a reinforcing or noxious stimulus.[61] In one experiment, serotonin turnover was increased in the frontal cortex, while serotonin and dopamine turnover was decreased in the hypothalamus, of rats exposed to a punishment contingency compared to animals that received response-independent shocks.[65] Thus, dopamine and serotonin levels were influenced by the punishment contingency, not simply by a history of shock presentation. Neuroanatomical changes have also been reported following exposure to punishment contingencies. Izenwasser et al.[66] reported that benzodiazepine binding was increased in the cerebellum of rats that received shock contingent on a lever press (punishment) compared to rats that received response-independent shocks. These results provide neurochemical and neuroanatomical support for the behavioral results described above.[5]

There is also evidence that neurochemical and neuroanatomical changes can occur as a consequence of avoidance responding. Vogt et al.[67] have demonstrated that neurochemical changes can be induced in parts of the limbic system during the acquisition, maintenance and extinction of discriminative avoidance training of rabbits. Muscarinic ACh receptor binding was evaluated using quantitative autoradiography of binding sites correlated with [3H]-oxotremorine-M or [3H]-pipenzepine and the changes did not occur in a yoked group of animals. While these results do not provide direct evidence for a molecular change that may account for a drug's altered effects following an avoidance history, it is clear that distinct changes in neurochemistry may occur as a result of particular contingencies involving noxious stimuli.

Drug-maintained Behavior

Kalivas and Duffy[68] examined the effects of stress on neurotransmitter levels and on the effects of cocaine. In one experiment, rats were administered cocaine (15 mg/kg) or saline for 3 consecutive days in their homecage. This dosing regimen has been shown to produce behavioral sensitization to cocaine.[69] In a second experiment, separate groups of rats were exposed to daily footshock (0.3 mA) or sham shocks for 10 consecutive days. Ten to 14 days after these four pretreatments, all rats were exposed to acute footshock or sham shock, prior to decapitation. The authors reported substantial differences in levels of dopamine and dopamine metabolites dihydroxyphenylacetic acid (DOPAC) and homovanillic acid (HVA), between cocaine-treated and saline-treated rats and between shock- and sham-treated rats, in the medial prefrontal cortex, nucleus accumbens and in the mesocorticolimbic (A10) dopamine region. Interestingly, Kalivas and Duffy[68] found that daily exposure to mild footshock stress and daily cocaine injections produced similar changes in dopamine levels and dopamine metabolism, suggesting a similar mechanism of action. Furthermore, these authors reported that chronic exposure to stress enhanced the motor stimulant effects of cocaine. It is possible that the effects on dopamine and its metabolites following chronic stress may account for the rapid acquisition of stimulant self-administration reported by Piazza *et al.*[40] It is clear that stress alters levels of dopamine and its metabolites. Whether these stress-induced changes can account for changes in the effects of amphetamine on punished responding[16] is for future investigation.

CONCLUSIONS

This chapter began by describing environmental, behavioral and pharmacological variables that interact with certain behavioral histories that may subsequently influence the reinforcing and discriminative stimulus effects of drugs and concluded by describing potential mechanisms of action for some of these variables. It is clear that historical factors can alter the behavioral effects of drugs, and that these altered effects may modify subsequent drug self-administration. Thus, a better understanding of historical variables may be important in understanding the etiology, maintenance, treatment and prevention of drug abuse. While this chapter has focused on experiments involving nonhuman animals, it should be pointed out that experiments utilizing human subjects may benefit from a better understanding of the influences of historical variables. For example, discrepancies in results using operant behavior of human and animal subjects may be better explained in terms of environmental or pharmacological variables, rather than uniquely human processes, such as verbal behavior.[70] Furthermore, Wanchisen[71] has suggested that clinicians interested in changing a clients' well-learned (and apparently inappropriate) behavior may benefit from studies examining the sensitivity of particular reinforcement schedules to historical influences. While historical variables are typically controlled for rather than systematically studied, this area of research may provide a better understanding of the determinants of behavior.

ACKNOWLEDGMENT

The authors thank Susan H. Nader for her comments on an earlier version of this manuscript.

REFERENCES

1. BARRETT, J. E. & J. L. KATZ. 1981. Drug effects on behaviors maintained by different events. *In* Advances in Behavioral Pharmacology. T. Thompson, P. B. Dews & W. A. McKim, Eds. Vol. **3:** 119–168. Academic Press. New York.

2. KELLEHER, R. T. & W. H. MORSE. 1968. Determinants of the specificity of the behavioral effects of drugs. Ergeb. Physiol. Biol. Chem. Exp. Pharmakol. **60:** 1–56.
3. MCKEARNEY, J. W. & J. E. BARRETT. 1978. Schedule-controlled behavior and the effects of drugs. *In* Contemporary Research in Behavioral Pharmacology. D. E. Blackman & D. J. Sanger, Eds.: 1–60. Plenum Press. New York.
4. BARRETT, J. E. 1986. Behavioral history: Residual influences on subsequent behavior and drug effects. *In* Developmental Behavioral Pharmacology. N. A. Krasnegor, D. B. Gray & T. Thompson, Eds. Vol. **5:** 99–114. Lawrence Erlbaum Assoc. Hillsdale, NJ.
5. BARRETT, J. E. & J. M. WITKIN. 1986. The role of behavioral and pharmacological history in determining the effects of abused drugs. *In* Behavioral Analysis of Drug Dependence. S. R. Goldberg & I. P. Stolerman, Eds.: 195–223. Academic Press. New York.
6. NADER, M. A. & T. THOMPSON. 1987. Interaction of methadone, reinforcement history and variable-interval performance. J. Exp. Anal. Behav. **48:** 303–315.
7. DEWS, P. B. 1958. Studies on behavior, IV. Stimulant actions of methamphetamine. J. Pharmacol. Exp. Ther. **122:** 137–147.
8. DEWS, P. B. & G. R. WENGER. 1977. Rate-dependency of the behavioral effects of amphetamine. *In* Advances in Behavioral Pharmacology. T. Thompson & P. B. Dews, Eds. Vol. **1:** 167–227. Academic Press. New York.
9. URBAIN, C., A. POLING, J. MILLAM & T. THOMPSON. 1978. *d*-Amphetamine and fixed-interval performance: Effects of operant history. J. Exp. Anal. Behav. **29:** 385–392.
10. NADER, M. A. & T. THOMPSON. 1989. Interaction of reinforcement history with methadone on responding maintained under a fixed-interval schedule. Pharmacol. Biochem. Behav. **32:** 643–649.
11. WEINER, H. 1964. Conditioning history and human fixed-interval performance. J. Exp. Anal. Behav. **7:** 383–385.
12. WEINER, H. 1969. Controlling human fixed-interval performance. J. Exp. Anal. Behav. **12:** 349–373.
13. WANCHISEN, B. A., T. A. TATHAM & S. E. MOONEY. 1989. Variable-ratio conditioning history produces high- and low-rate fixed-interval performance in rats. J. Exp. Anal. Behav. **52:** 167–179.
14. POLING, A., K. KRAFFT & L. CHAPMAN. 1980. *d*-Amphetamine, operant history, and variable-interval performance. Pharmacol. Biochem. Behav. **12:** 559–562.
15. EGLI, M. & T. THOMPSON. 1989. Effects of methadone on alternative fixed-ratio fixed-interval performance: Latent influences of schedule-controlled responding. J. Exp. Anal. Behav. **52:** 141–153.
16. BARRETT, J. E. 1977. Behavioral history as a determinant of the effects of *d*-amphetamine on punished behavior. Science **198:** 67–69.
17. GELLER, I. & J. SEIFTER. 1960. The effects of meprobamate, barbiturates, *d*-amphetamine and promazine on experimentally-induced conflict in the rat. Psychopharmacologia **1:** 482–492.
18. HANSON, H. M., J. J. WITOSLAWSKI & E. H. CAMPBELL. 1967. Drug effects in squirrel monkeys trained on a multiple schedule with a punishment contingency. J. Exp. Anal. Behav. **10:** 565–569.
19. BACOTTI, A. V. & J. W. MCKEARNEY. 1979. Prior and ongoing experience as determinants of the effects of *d*-amphetamine and chlorpromazine on punished behavior. J. Pharmacol. Exp. Ther. **211:** 80–85.
20. BARRETT, J. E. & J. A. STANLEY. 1980. Prior behavioral experience can reverse the effects of morphine. Psychopharmacology **81:** 107–110.
21. MORSE, W. H. & R. T. KELLEHER. 1977. Determinants of reinforcement and punishment. *In* Handbook of Operant Behavior. W. K. Honig & J. E. R. Staddon, Eds.: 174–200. Prentice-Hall. New York.
22. BARRETT, J. E., J. R. GLOWA & M. A. NADER. 1989. Behavioral and pharmacological history as determinants of tolerance- and sensitization-like phenomena in drug action. *In* Psychoactive Drugs. A. J. Goudie & M. Emmett-Oglesby, Eds.: 181–219. Humana Press, Inc. Clifton, NJ.

23. GRIFFITHS, R. R., G. E. BIGELOW & J. E. HENNINGFIELD. 1980. Similarities in animal and human drug-taking behavior. *In* Advances in Substance Abuse. N. K. Mello, Ed. Vol. **1**: 1–90. JAI Press. Greenwich, CT.
24. JOHANSON, C. E. 1978. Drugs as reinforcers. *In* Contemporary Research in Behavioral Pharmacology. D. E. Blackman & D. J. Sanger, Eds.: 325–390. Plenum Press. New York.
25. SPEALMAN, R. D. & S. R. GOLDBERG. 1978. Drug self-administration by laboratory animals: Control by schedules of reinforcement. Annu. Rev. Pharmacol. Toxicol. **18**: 313–339.
26. WOOLVERTON, W. L. & M. A. NADER. 1990. Experimental evaluation of the reinforcing effects of drugs. *In* Testing and Evaluation of Drugs of Abuse. M. W. Adler, Ed.: 165–192. Wiley-Liss, Inc. New York.
27. FALK, J. L. 1961. Production of polydipsia in normal rats by an intermittent food schedule. Science **133**: 195–196.
28. MEISCH, R. A. 1977. Ethanol self-administration: Infrahuman studies. *In* Advances in Behavioral Pharmacology. T. Thompson & P. B. Dews, Eds. Vol. **1**: 35–84. Academic Press. New York.
29. SAMSON, H. H. 1987. Initiation of ethanol-maintained behavior. A comparison of animal models and their implications to human drinking. *In* Advances in Behavioral Pharmacology. T. Thompson, P. B. Dews & J. E. Barrett, Eds. Vol. **6**: 221–248. Lawrence Erlbaum Assoc. Hillsdale, NJ.
30. FALK, J. L. & M. TANG. 1989a. Schedule induction of drug intake: Differential responsiveness to agents with abuse potential. J. Pharmacol. Exp. Ther. **249**: 143–148.
31. FALK, J. L. & M. TANG. 1989b. Schedule-induced chlordiazepoxide intake: Differential effect of cocaine and ethanol histories. Pharmacol. Biochem. Behav. **33**: 393–396.
32. TANG, M. & J. L. FALK. 1986. Ethanol polydipsic choice: Effects of alternative fluid polydipsic history. Alcohol **3**: 361–365.
33. TANG, M. & J. L. FALK. 1988. Preference history prevents schedule-induced preferential ethanol acceptance. Alcohol **5**: 399–402.
34. TANG, M., S. L. WILLIAMS & J. L. FALK. 1988. Prior schedule exposure reduces the acquisition of schedule-induced polydipsia. Physiol. Behav. **44**: 817–820.
35. BERGMAN, J. & C. E. JOHANSON. 1985. The reinforcing properties of diazepam under several conditions in the rhesus monkey. Psychopharmacology **86**: 108–113.
36. SCHLICHTING, U. U., S. R. GOLDBERG, W. WUTTKE & F. HOFFMEISTER. 1970. *d*-Amphetamine self-administration by rhesus monkeys with different self-administration histories. Excerpta Med. Internatl. Congress **220**: 62–69.
37. YOUNG, A. M., S. HERLING & J. H. WOODS. 1981. History of drug exposure as a determinant of drug self-administration. *In* Behavioral Pharmacology of Human Drug Dependence. T. Thompson & C. E. Johanson, Eds. NIDA Research Monograph No. **37**: 75–89. Government Printing Office. Washington, D.C.
38. BEARDSLEY, P. M., B. A. HAYES & R. L. BALSTER. 1990. The self-administration of MK-801 can depend upon drug-reinforcement history, and its discriminative stimulus properties are phencyclidine-like in rhesus monkeys. J. Pharmacol. Exp. Ther. **252**: 953–959.
39. DEMINIÈRE, J. M., P. V. PIAZZA, M. LE MOAL & H. SIMON. 1989. Experimental approach to individual vulnerability to psychostimulant addiction. Neurosci. Biobehav. Rev. **13**: 141–147.
40. PIAZZA, P. V., J-M. DEMINIÈRE, M. LE MOAL & H. SIMON. 1989. Factors that predict vulnerability to amphetamine self-administration. Science **245**: 1511–1513.
41. PIAZZA, P. V., J-M. DEMINIÈRE, S. MACCARI, P. MORMÈDE, M. LE MOAL & H. SIMON. 1990. Individual reactivity to novelty predicts probability of amphetamine self-administration. Behav. Pharmacol. **1**: 339–345.
42. PIAZZA, P. V., S. MACCARI, J-M. DEMINIÈRE, M. LE MOAL, P. MORMÈDE & H. SIMON. 1991. Corticosterone levels determine individual vulnerability to amphetamine self-administration. Proc. Natl. Acad. Sci. USA **88**: 2088–2092.
43. BARRETT, J. E. & S. OLMSTEAD. 1989. Spiroxatrine as a discriminative stimulus: Effects depend on pharmacological history. Drug Devel. Res. **16**: 365–374.
44. PICKENS, R., R. A. MEISCH & T. THOMPSON. 1978. Drug self-administration: An analysis

of the reinforcing effects of drugs. *In* Handbook of Psychopharmacology. L. L. Iversen, S. D. Iversen & S. H. Snyder, Eds. Vol. **12:** 1–37. Plenum Publishing Co. New York.

45. WIKLER, A. 1961. On the nature of addiction and habituation. Br. J. Addict. **57:** 73–79.
46. GOLDBERG, S. R., W. H. MORSE & D. M. GOLDBERG. 1976. Behavior maintained under a second-order schedule by intramuscular injection of morphine or cocaine in rhesus monkeys. J. Pharmacol. Exp. Ther. **199:** 278–286.
47. KATZ, J. L. 1980. Second-order schedules of intramuscular injection in the squirrel monkey: Comparison with food presentation and effects of *d*-amphetamine and promazine. J. Pharmacol. Exp. Ther. **212:** 405–411.
48. SCHUSTER, C. R. & J. H. WOODS. 1968. The conditioned reinforcing effects of stimuli associated with morphine reinforcement. Int. J. Addict. **3:** 223–230.
49. GLOWA, J. R. & J. E. BARRETT. 1983. Response suppression by visual stimuli paired with postsession *d*-amphetamine injections in the pigeon. J. Exp. Anal. Behav. **39:** 165–173.
50. WATANABE, S. 1990. Isodirectional conditioning effects of *d*-amphetamine and pentobarbital on schedule-controlled operant behavior in pigeons. Pharmacol. Biochem. Behav. **36:** 157–161.
51. SPENCER, D. G., JR., S. YADEN & H. LAL. 1988. Behavioral and physiological detection of classically-conditioned blood pressure reduction. Psychopharmacology **95:** 25–28.
52. BRIDGER, W. H., S. R. SCHIFF, S. S. COOPER, W. PAREDES & G. A. BARR. 1982. Classical conditioning of cocaine's stimulatory effects. Psychopharmacol. Bull. **18:** 210–213.
53. VEZINA, P. & J. STEWART. 1984. Conditioning and place-specific sensitization of increases in activity induced by morphine in the VTA. Pharmacol. Biochem. Behav. **20:** 925–934.
54. SIEGEL, S. 1983. Classical conditioning, drug tolerance, and drug dependence. *In* Research Advances in Alcohol and Drug Problems. Y. Israel, F. B. Glaser, H. Kalant, R. E. Popham, W. Schmidt & R. G. Smart, Eds. Vol. **7:** 207–246. Plenum Publishing Co. New York.
55. SIEGEL, S. 1975. Evidence from rats that morphine tolerance is a learned response. J. Comp. Physiol. Psychol. **89:** 498–506.
56. SIEGEL, S. 1978. Tolerance to the hyperthermic effect of morphine in the rat is a learned response. J. Comp. Physiol. Psychol. **92:** 1137–1149.
57. THOMPSON, T. 1984. Behavioral mechanisms of drug dependence. *In* Advances in Behavioral Pharmacology. T. Thompson, P. B. Dews & J. E. Barrett, Eds. Vol. **4:** 1–45. Academic Press. New York.
58. KATZ, J. L. 1990. Effects of drugs on stimulus control of behavior under schedules of reinforcement. *In* Advances in Behavioral Pharmacology. J. E. Barrett, T. Thompson & P. B. Dews, Eds. Vol. **7:** 13–38. Lawrence Erlbaum Assoc. Hillsdale, NJ.
59. BARRETT, J. E. 1991. Behavioral neurochemistry: Application of neurochemical and neuropharmacological techniques to the study of operant behavior. *In* Techniques in the Behavior and Neural Sciences: Experimental Analysis of Behavior. I. H. Iversen & K. A. Lattal, Eds. Vol. **6:** 79–115. Elsevier. New York.
60. BARRETT, J. E. & M. A. NADER. 1990. Neurochemical correlates of behavioral processes. Drug Devel. Res. **20:** 313–335.
61. DWORKIN, S. I. & J. E. SMITH. 1989. Assessment of neurochemical correlates of operant behavior. *In* Neuromethods. A. A. Boulton, G. B. Baker & A. J. Greenshaw, Eds. Vol. **13:** 741–785. Humana Press, Inc. Clifton, NJ.
62. SEIDEN, L. S., R. C. MACPHAIL & M. W. OGLESBY. 1975. Catecholamines and drug-behavior interactions. Fed. Proc. **34:** 1823–1831.
63. SPARBER, S. B. 1975. Neurochemical changes associated with schedule-controlled behavior. Fed. Proc. **34:** 1802–1812.
64. BARRETT, J. E. & S. M. HOFFMANN. 1991. Neurochemical changes correlated with behavior maintained under fixed-interval and fixed-ratio schedules of reinforcement. J. Exp. Anal. Behav. **56:** 395–405.
65. MIYAUCHI, T., S. I. DWORKIN, C. Co & J. E. SMITH. 1988. Specific effects of punishment on amino acid turnover in discrete brain regions. Pharmacol. Biochem. Behav. **31:** 523–531.
66. IZENWASSER, S., M. J. BLAKE, N. E. GOEDERS & S. I. DWORKIN. 1989. Punishment

modifies the effects of chlordiazepoxide and benzodiazepine receptors. Pharmacol. Biochem. Behav. **32:** 743–748.

67. VOGT, B. A., M. GABRIEL, L. J. VOGT, A. POREMBA, E. L. JENSEN, Y. KUBOTA & E. KANG. 1991. Muscarinic receptor binding increases in anterior thalamus and cingulate cortex during discriminative avoidance training. J. Neurosci. **11:** 1508–1514.
68. KALIVAS, P. W. & P. DUFFY. 1989. Similar effects of daily cocaine and stress on mesocorticolimbic dopamine neurotransmission in the rat. Biol. Psychiatry **25:** 913–928.
69. KALIVAS, P. W., P. DUFFY, L. A. DUMARS & C. SKINNER. 1988. Neurochemical and behavioral effects of acute and daily cocaine. J. Pharmacol. Exp. Ther. **245:** 485–492.
70. WANCHISEN, B. A. & T. A. TATHAM. 1991. Behavioral history: A promising challenge in explaining and controlling human operant behavior. Behav. Anal. **14:** 139–144.
71. WANCHISEN, B. A. 1990. Forgetting the lessons of history. Behav. Anal. **13:** 31–38.

Conditioned Sensitization to the Psychomotor Stimulant Cocaine

ROBERT M. POST,[a] SUSAN R. B. WEISS,
DAVID FONTANA,[b,c] AND AGU PERT

Biological Psychiatry Branch
National Institute of Mental Health
Building 10, Room 3N212
9000 Rockville Pike
Bethesda, Maryland 20892

INTRODUCTION

Increased behavioral and convulsive responsivity to cocaine (sensitization and kindling, respectively) has been recognized since the early 1930s,[1-3] although it was not until the 1970s and 1980s that this began to be explored systematically.[4-7] The phenomenon of behavioral sensitization has also been demonstrated to be associated with the environmental context in which a drug is repeatedly administered. That is, enhanced responsivity to cocaine is more readily elicited if an animal is pretreated and tested in the same environment compared with an animal treated and tested in different environments. For example, we administered cocaine (10 mg/kg) to one group of rats in a Plexiglas cage situated on an activity monitor (test cage) and gave a second injection of saline to these rats when they were removed from the test cage; we treated a second group of rats with a saline injection in the test cage, and the same dose of cocaine (10 mg/kg) upon leaving the test environment.[8] After repeating this procedure for 10 days, robust behavioral sensitization was observed only in the animals that had received cocaine in the context of the test cage, and not in those receiving equal doses of cocaine in their home cage (and then challenged in the test environment).

Similar results showing context-dependent sensitization were observed by Hinson and Poulos,[9] who also found that sensitization could be extinguished by repeated injections of saline in the test environment. In our study,[8] the test cage cocaine-treated animals were also significantly more responsive to a saline challenge than the animals treated with cocaine in the home cage. This degree of locomotor activation was minimal, however, compared to that achieved with the cocaine challenge, suggesting that

[a] Address correspondence to: Robert M. Post, M.D., Chief, Biological Psychiatry Branch; Fax: (301) 402-0052.
[b] This work has been partially supported by a post-doctoral training fellowship from the MacArthur Foundation Mental Health Research Network I (Psychobiology of Depression) for Dr. Fontana at the NIMH.
[c] Current position: Syntex Corporation/Institute of Pharmacology, Palo Alto, CA 94303.

the interoceptive cues and cocaine's effects contribute to the total stimulus complex to which an animal is conditioned.

CONTEXT-DEPENDENT COCAINE SENSITIZATION: SINGLE VERSUS MULTIPLE INJECTIONS

Considering the powerful contribution of conditioning to cocaine-induced behavioral sensitization, we have initiated a program to explore in detail its neuropharmacological and neuroanatomical substrates. In order to facilitate this process, we employed a novel one-day conditioning paradigm, in which one group of animals received a high dose of cocaine (40 mg/kg) in the test environment (and saline in the home cage), a second group received cocaine in the home cage (and saline in the test cage), and a third group received saline in both environments. Following the differential day 1 pretreatments, all 3 groups were challenged with a low dose of cocaine (10 mg/kg) in the test cage on day 2. As illustrated in FIGURE 1, only those animals pretreated with cocaine in the test cage showed increased locomotor activation compared to the saline-pretreated controls. That is, the animals that received cocaine in the home cage, and had equal exposure to the test environment, did not differ from those that received only saline.

Thus, in this one-day cocaine-induced behavioral sensitization (CIBS) paradigm, all of the day 2 increased behavioral responsivity to cocaine is attributable to the conditioned component (*i.e.*, that involving the interaction with environmental context) of CIBS and not to the cocaine injection itself. It is noteworthy that in other paradigms context-independent cocaine sensitization can be revealed as well. For example, injecting animals with high doses of cocaine (40 mg/kg) for 3 consecutive days (or more) results in a context-independent as well as a context-enhanced sensitization. Interest-

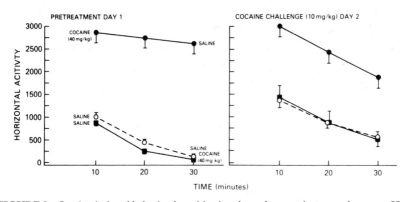

FIGURE 1. Cocaine-induced behavioral sensitization depends on environmental context. Horizontal locomotor activity is illustrated for three groups of rats (*n* = 10/group) receiving the following day-1 pretreatments: cocaine in the test-cage and saline in the home cage (●); saline in the test-cage and cocaine in the home cage (■); saline in both cages (○) (*left*). Horizontal activity is illustrated for these three groups following a cocaine challenge (10 mg/kg). Only the rats that received cocaine in the test-apparatus on day 1 showed sensitization to cocaine on day 2 (*right*).

ingly, the context-independent sensitization is not consistently observed following this procedure, and is less long-lasting than context-dependent sensitization (see FIG. 3 in Post et al.[10]; Tandeciarz, Weiss, Pert and Post, unpublished data). Other researchers have also observed a context-independent sensitization to cocaine or other psychomotor stimulants.[11-13]

The parametric aspects of this progression and evolution are schematically illustrated in FIGURE 2. This figure presents a matrix of cocaine effects where differences in behavioral responsivity are achieved on the basis of either greater dosage or greater numbers of injections; context-dependent components can contribute exclusively to some occurrences of behavioral sensitization as in the one day paradigm, but perhaps only partially in other paradigms such as those involving chronic and high dose administration. The data summarized in this table are convergent with the findings of

COCAINE		EFFECT							
Number of Injections	Dose mg/kg i.p.	Behavioral Sensitization Duration	Activity Context Dep.	Activity Context Indep.	Stereotypy Context Dep.	Stereotypy Context Indep.	Saline Conditioning	Sensitization Neuroleptic Independent	Seizure Kindling	Death
↑↑↑	COC₆₅								++	++
x10 days	COC₁₆₀ subcut. (K. Gale)	++		++		++		++		
✦✦✦✦✦✦✦✦✦	COC₁₀	++ months	++	0			++			
↑↑↑	COC₄₀	+	0	++	++	++	±			
↑	COC₄₀	++ days	++	0	0	0	0	0		
↑↑↑	COC₂₀	0 0	0	0	0	+				
✦✦✦	COC₁₀	0 0	0	0	0	0				
✦	COC₁₀	0 0								

FIGURE 2. Size and number of arrows indicate dose of cocaine and number of administrations. COC, cocaine; subscript, dose in mg/kg administered once daily i.p. except in the study of Gale,[11] when doses were subcutaneous; 0, no effect; ±, equivocal; +, moderate effect; ++, marked or definite effect. Effects of cocaine increase are more persistent with increases in either dose or number of repetitions. The highest doses also become less dependent on environmental context and conditioning, and are associated with seizures, kindling and lethality. Thus, effects shift from dopaminergic-mediated behavioral sensitization (motor endpoints) to local anesthetic-mediated kindling (seizure endpoints) as the dose is increased.

Mattingly and Gotsick[14] who demonstrated similar context-dependent and context-independent components of sensitization to apomorphine. Finally, context effects do not appear to play a major role in the development of kindled seizures which result from repeated administration of high doses of cocaine, presumably involving cocaine's local anesthetic mechanisms.[4,15-16]

In addition to the dose and frequency of repetition variables highlighted in FIGURE 2, a variety of other variables appear to be important to the eventual magnitude and persistence of behavioral sensitization. These include interval between doses (*e.g.*, intermittent compared to continuous administration), degree of control over injections (self- versus other-administered), degree of similarity of environmental context conditions and test environment,[17] and finally time-dependent phenomenon. Dafters and Odber[18] found that environment-specific morphine tolerance was acquired when low doses and long interdose intervals were used. Tiffany *et al.*[19] also found an effect of interdose interval on associative tolerance to morphine. Antelman[20] raises the possibility that some stress or drug effects may increase over time independent of repeated administration. Moreover, Dr. Antelman's most recent work[21] demonstrates that the magnitude of the initial drug challenge or stressor may determine the direction of the time-dependent behavioral effects, *i.e.* either increased (sensitization) or decreased (tolerance) responsivity over time. The dose-effect matrix illustrated in FIGURE 2 highlights the possibility that cocaine sensitization is an evolving process dependent on a variety of drug and context variables, and foreshadows the theme noted later in this manuscript that pharmacological interventions and anatomical substrates critical to the development versus expression of cocaine-induced behavioral sensitization may differ as a function of when they are employed in the course of evolution of sensitized behaviors.

CROSS SENSITIZATION TO AND FROM COCAINE: MECHANISTIC IMPLICATIONS

From Cocaine to Other Drugs

The ability of the one-day high-dose cocaine treatment to produce context-dependent behavioral sensitization can be probed with a variety of challenge drugs. As illustrated in TABLE 1, cocaine-pretreated animals are more responsive to cocaine, procaine, cocaine methiodide, MK-801, and the selective D_2 agonist quinpirole, but not to lidocaine, caffeine, the selective D_1 agonist 6-chloro-APB, or the selective reuptake blockers GBR 12909 (DA), fluoxetine (5HT), or xylamine (NE). The effects with procaine suggest that some components of cocaine's local anesthetic actions may be contributing to context-dependent sensitization. The similar data with cocaine methiodide (Pert, unpublished data), which is a polar cocaine compound that does not cross the blood-brain barrier, suggest that peripheral components of cocaine's actions may also contribute to the sensitization. It is of interest, however, that in contrast to procaine, the local anesthetic lidocaine does not reveal this effect.

A similar lack of cross sensitization is observed from cocaine to caffeine, which is a motor stimulant that does not act primarily by increasing dopaminergic mechanisms. In addition, the lack of cross sensitization to agents which selectively block the reuptake of dopamine (GBR 12909), serotonin (fluoxetine) and norepinephrine (xylamine) (Pert, unpublished observations) suggests greater complexity and specificity of the drug cue, or drug effect, necessary to elicit context-dependent cocaine-induced be-

TABLE 1. Cross Sensitization from Cocaine to Other Drugs

Cocaine (Day 1) to ⟶ Drug (Day 2)	Sensitization Observed	
	(Yes + +)	(No − −)
Stimulant		
Caffeine		− −
Local Anesthetics		
Lidocaine		− −
Procaine	+ +	
Cocaine-Methiodide	+ +	
Dopamine agonists		
(D_1) 6-chloro-APB		− −
(D_2) Quinpirole	+ +	
(D_1, D_2) Apomorphine	+ +	
Glutamate antagonist		
MK-801	+ +	
Selective blockers of reuptake		
GBR 12909 (DA)		− −
Fluoxetine (5HT)		− −
Xylamine (NE)		− −

havioral sensitization than had previously been surmised. Thus, it appears that psychomotor activation per se, local anesthetic cuing, or increased dopamine at the synapse are not sufficient to elicit context-dependent behavioral sensitization induced by cocaine. In addition, there appear to be minor alterations in the environmental context that will or will not convey the conditioned aspects of sensitization, as Weiss et al.[17] have documented that the degree of similarity in pretreatment and test environment can be an important variable in the degree of behavioral sensitization achieved. These data suggest that subtleties in the context cues and in the interoceptive cuing achieved by neurotransmitter selective agents may both be important in the development of the conditioned component of CIBS.

From Other Drugs to Cocaine

This notion is further supported by the view that differential dopaminergic pretreatments are necessary to elicit behavioral sensitization upon challenge with cocaine on day 2 (see TABLE 2). That is, pretreatment with either a D_1 (6-chloro-APB) or D_2 (quinpirole) agonist alone is insufficient to produce cross-sensitization to cocaine. However, administration of a combination of a D_1 plus a D_2 agonist (6-chloro-APB [1 mg/kg] quinpirole [1 mg/kg]) on day 1 does produce cross sensitization to cocaine on day 2. These data are convergent with data presented below that pretreatment with either a D_1 or D_2 selective antagonist is able to block the development of cocaine-induced behavioral sensitization.

Thus, combined activation of D_1 and D_2 receptors may be necessary for the induc-

TABLE 2. Cross Sensitization from Drug to Cocaine Challenge

	Sensitization to Cocaine Challenge	
Pretreatment: Day 1	(Yes + +)	(No − −)
Stimulant		
Caffeine —▶		− −
Local Anesthetics		
Procaine —▶	+ +	
Lidocaine —▶		− −
Dopamine Agonists		
Quinpirole (D₂) —▶		− −
6-chloro-APB (D₁) —▶		− −
6-chloro-APB plus		
Quinpirole (D₁ plus D₂) —▶	+ +	
NMDA antagonist		
MK-801 —▶	+ +	

tion (development) of cocaine sensitization through dopaminergic mechanisms. However, local anesthetic cues achieved by procaine (but not lidocaine) are also sufficient to produce cross sensitization to cocaine. The induction of motor activity per se with caffeine on day 1 is not adequate.

DIFFERENTIAL PHARMACOLOGY OF THE DEVELOPMENT VERSUS EXPRESSION OF COCAINE-INDUCED BEHAVIORAL SENSITIZATION

As summarized in TABLE 3, neuroleptics administered prior to the cocaine pretreatment on day 1 are able to block the development of cocaine-induced behavioral sensitization (CIBS). However, if the animals are pretreated with cocaine on day 1 and then administered neuroleptics prior to the day 2 challenge, the expression of CIBS is not affected. This dissociation has been observed with the nonselective dopamine blocker haloperidol, the selective D_2 antagonist raclopride, or the D_1 antagonist SCH 23390. This pharmacological dysjunction as a function of stage of evolution of cocaine-induced behavioral sensitization parallels previous data with different agents with repeated stimulant administration showing that neuroleptics block the development but not the expression of conditioned locomotor activity.[23–25] Taken together these data suggest that dopaminergic mechanisms involving both D_1 and D_2 receptors may be critically involved in the acquisition of the cocaine-induced conditioned behavioral sensitization, but may not be as important for its expression. This conclusion must be tempered, however, by the possibility that conditioning enhances dopaminergic functions. If this is the case (see below), and if the doses of neuroleptics used in these studies did not achieve a total blockade of DA receptors, then a behavioral differential between the conditioned and unconditioned groups would still be expected following DA blockers.

This ineffectiveness in the blockade of the expression of CIBS occurs at the same

TABLE 3. Differential Drug Effects on the Development vs. Expression of Context-Dependent Cocaine Sensitization in the One Day, High Dose Paradigm

Treatment	Block[a] Day 1 Hyper-activity	Block[b] Development	Block[c] Expression	References
Haloperidol				
0.2 mg/kg	+ +	+ +	− −	Weiss et al.[17]
0.5 mg/kg	+ +	+ +	− −	
0.5 mg/kg	+ +	+ +	(+ +)[d]	Weiss et al., 1991 (unpub. obs.)
Raclopride (D₂)	+ +	+ +	− −	Fontana et al., 1990 (unpub. obs.)
SCH 23390 (D₁)	+ +	+ +	− −	
Sulpiride (D₂)	− −	+ +		
Clonidine (α₂)	− −	+ +	+ +	Weiss et al., 1989 (unpub. obs.)
Diazepam	+ +	+ +	+ +	Weiss et al.[17]
Carbamazepine	− −	− −	− −	Weiss et al.[16] & unpub. obs.
MDL-72222 (5HT₃ antagonist)	( )	− −	+ +	Pert et al., 1991 (unpub. obs.)
ECS	( )	+ +	( )	Pert et al., 1991 (unpub. obs.)
N. accumbens lesions	− −	+ +[e]		Post et al.[22]; Weiss et al., 1990 (unpub. obs.)
Amygdala lesions	− −	+ +[e]		

^{a} Treatment effects on Day 1 activity produced by cocaine (40 mg/kg).
^{b} Effect of pretreatment given on Day 1 on cocaine challenge (10 mg/kg) given on Day 2.
^{c} Effect of pretreatment given on Day 2 on cocaine challenge (10 mg/kg) given on Day 2.
^{d} Haloperidol at this dose may suppress all activity.
^{e} Lesions preceded sensitization, so blockade could be of development or expression.

doses of neuroleptics that are effective in blocking the development of CIBS when they are administered prior to the day 1 challenge. At the very least, these findings seem to suggest that some aspects of the sensitization process are more sensitive to disruption by pharmacological interventions than others. Elsewhere we have discussed the potential importance of these data for modeling neuroleptic refractoriness in some psychotic states,[26–28] but these data may as well be relevant to issues of cocaine-induced craving and their potential conditioned components which also may not be amenable to blockade with neuroleptics once they are well engendered.

It is noteworthy that inhibition of locomotor activity on day 1 is not the critical factor determining whether the development of CIBS is in fact disrupted. This is demonstrated by the finding that the D₂ antagonist sulpiride administered on day 1 is able to block the development of CIBS even though it is unable to interfere with locomotor activation in response to the high dose cocaine. In contrast with the situation with neuroleptics which are able to block the development but not the expression of cocaine-induced behavioral sensitization, clonidine and diazepam are able to block both components of the syndrome.[10,17] (and Post *et al.*, unpublished data). Carbamazepine, however, is unable to block the development or the expression of cocaine-induced behavioral sensitization or the locomotor-activating effects of cocaine.[10,29] These data are of considerable interest in relation to the promising effects of carbamazepine in the treatment of cocaine craving and addiction (as summarized elsewhere[30]). This inability of carbamazepine to affect CIBS is a noteworthy contrast to its potent attenuating effects in the development of cocaine-induced kindled seizures in rodents[16] and intravenous self-administration in rhesus monkeys.[31] Thus, even though intravenous cocaine self-administration and cocaine-induced behavioral sensitization have both been presumed to involve dopaminergic mechanisms in the nucleus accumbens, the data with carbamazepine suggest a mechanistic dissociation of these two cocaine phenomena.

Pert and associates (1991 unpublished data), using the one-day cocaine sensitization paradigm, have found that MDL-72222, a $5HT_3$ antagonist, is unable to block the development of behavioral sensitization but is effective in blocking its expression. These data re-highlight the notion that the neurobiology of CIBS may differ as a function of stage of evolution and that some agents may be effective in the development (or acquisition) phase, but not in the later expression phase, and vice versa (see TABLE 3). Pert and associates have also found that administering electroconvulsive seizures immediately following removal from the activity chambers on day 1 (following cocaine [40 mg/kg] or saline) is able to block the development of CIBS. These data are of interest in relationship to a variety of examples where ECS has been demonstrated to interfere with the acquisition or consolidation of information in other learning and memory paradigms.

Taken together, the cross sensitization and blockade data in the one-day paradigm suggest that combined D_1 and D_2 agonist effects are necessary for the initiation of context-dependent CIBS, but once engendered CIBS can be elicited by mechanisms independent of dopamine receptors. That is, although D_2 agonists can reveal context-dependent CIBS, neuroleptics are unable to block its expression. Clonidine and a $5HT_3$ antagonist are able to block its expression, suggesting that $\alpha2$, $5HT_3$, and other mechanisms have become critical to the maintenance of context-dependent CIBS.

EFFECTS OF LESIONS ON THE DEVELOPMENT OF CIBS: DIFFERENTIAL IMPACT UPON SINGLE VERSUS MULTIPLE INJECTIONS

We have begun to elucidate the neuroanatomical substrates of the one-day cocaine-induced behavioral sensitization. Electrolytic lesions or 6-hydroxydopamine-induced depletion of dopamine in the amygdala blocked the development of cocaine-induced behavioral sensitization.[32] In addition, 6-hydroxydopamine (plus DMI)-induced depletion of dopamine in the nucleus accumbens blocked cocaine-induced behavioral sensitization, while electrolytic lesions of the dorsal and ventral hippocampus and deep cerebellar nuclei were without effect. In these studies the neurotoxin lesions of the nucleus accumbens and amygdala blocked the development of CIBS despite only a 60% reduction in DA and without altering the response to cocaine on day 1.

One possible interpretation of these observations is that lesions of the nucleus accumbens were able to block cocaine-induced behavioral sensitization by interfering with limbic-motor integration.[33] In contrast, the amygdala lesions may have blocked the CIBS because of interference with the associative or environmental context-dependent component of this paradigm. This effect of amygdala lesions on CIBS has been observed in four studies in our laboratory and is convergent with data from other laboratories emphasizing the critical role of the amygdala in fear conditioning and associative learning.[34-38]

However, just as the pharmacology of cocaine-induced behavioral sensitization appears to change as a function of stage of evolution, we have observed a similar evolution in the impact of anatomical lesions on the sensitization process. While the lesions of the amygdala blocked cocaine-induced behavioral sensitization in the one-day paradigm, they did not affect CIBS in the three-day paradigm in which animals experienced three consecutive days of cocaine-induced hyperactivity (40 mg/kg, i.p.) before challenge on day 4 with a low dose of cocaine (10 mg/kg).

These data may be interpretable from several perspectives. First, it is possible that intact structures are able to compensate eventually for the loss of the amygdala. For example, there may be a certain amount of redundancy in limbic mechanisms involved in the associative process. On the other hand, perhaps several different parallel processes are involved in conditioning as in other forms of learning. Mishkin and Appenzeller[39] have postulated that learning is determined by both "representational" memories which are highly dependent on limbic structures such as the amygdala and hippocampus and "habit" formation which may involve the striatum. In the case of CIBS, the repetition of drug and environmental associations may similarly allow the evaluation of one mechanism over another. Thus, pathways may become involved in the development of cocaine-induced behavioral sensitization that are no longer dependent on amygdala mechanisms to convey the environmental cues. While the lack of effect of amygdala lesions in the repeated cocaine administration paradigm has been replicated twice, the neuroanatomical substrates involved await further exploration. Given the postulated role of the caudate nucleus in other cognitive and learning models that mediate habit formation, this substrate deserves investigation. Other structures more directly involved in the outflow pathway mediating cocaine-induced locomotor activity achieved with behavioral sensitization also deserve exploration.

IMPACT OF COCAINE SENSITIZATION ON DOPAMINE OVERFLOW AS MEASURED BY *IN VIVO* DIALYSIS

Pert and associates have observed dose-dependent cocaine-induced increases in dopamine overflow in the striatum and nucleus accumbens, but not in the frontal cortex or the amygdala. These observations are of interest in relationship to the relative density of dopamine re-uptake sites, which is prominent in accumbens and striatum but not so in frontal cortex and amygdala.

Pert and associates have also observed increases in dopamine overflow in the striatum and nucleus accumbens of anesthetized rats following chronic cocaine administration (30 mg/kg i.p. × 7–10 days) compared with the saline injected controls. This effect might in part be accounted for by pharmacokinetic variables as cocaine is significantly elevated following chronic pretreatment when compared to saline-injected controls.[40-43]

Fontana, Pert, and associates[44] developed an *in vivo* dialysis system in awake, behaving animals so that context-dependent sensitization could be evaluated ruling out potential pharmacokinetic confounding variables. These investigators have found significantly increased dopamine overflow in the nucleus accumbens in animals pretreated with cocaine in the same environmental context compared to controls exposed to the same amount of cocaine in a different environmental context or saline controls. These observations represent the first evidence of increased dopamine overflow occurring in relation to the conditioned component of cocaine-induced behavioral sensitization. The *in vivo* dialysis data suggest that increased neuronal activity in dopaminergic neurons may mediate this increase in activity in context-conditioned animals, and not be observed in animals equally exposed to cocaine in a different environment. The studies represent the first in a series of explorations of the biochemistry of the conditioned components of CIBS and are convergent with other findings of the involvement of dopaminergic systems in other conditioning and associative learning paradigms.[34,36,37,45-48]

CLINICAL IMPLICATIONS

The foregoing analysis suggests that conditioned cocaine-induced behavioral sensitization is expressed through distinct biochemical, neuroanatomical, and neurotransmitter alterations. Context-dependent CIBS appears to evolve with time in its pharmacology and its anatomical substrates. A hypothetical schema of how this might occur is illustrated in FIGURE 3. Cocaine-induced increases in extracellular dopamine may be associated with the acute induction of the proto-oncogene c-fos through a D_1 receptor mechanism.[49-53] C-fos, fos-related antigens (fras), other oncogenes, and transcription factors may then program the cell for longer term adaptations such as increases in dynorphin[54,55] and neurotensin[55] and decreases in NPY and somatostatin.[56] Nestler and associates[57] have reported alterations in G proteins, phosphoproteins, and protein kinases in association with chronic but not acute cocaine administration. White and associates[58] have also shown transient induction of subsensitivity at dopamine auto-receptors and of longer-lasting increases in sensitivity of striatal post-synaptic D_1 receptors associated with chronic cocaine administration. Recently, Hitri *et al.*[59] have shown time-dependent alterations of dopamine uptake sites in rat brain, paralleling the longer-lasting alterations observed in human autopsy studies of cocaine abusers. Thus, repeated cocaine administration may be associated with a sequence of transient and longer-lasting biochemical changes, some of which provide the substrate for increased responsivity over time and others that might reflect compensatory or conditioned compensatory changes such as those postulated to underlie withdrawal and craving phenomena.[60-62] In another unrelated paradigm Weiss *et al.*[63] have demonstrated that compensatory biological changes can occur selectively in response to contingent presentation of a drug and not nonspecifically to the drug itself.

As revealed in the amygdala lesion studies mentioned above, different areas of brain may become involved with different components of cocaine-induced behavioral sensitization related to variables such as dose, repetition, and intermittency of administration. Similarly, the blockade of development but not expression of CIBS with neuroleptics suggests that neurotransmitter systems involved in the early encoding of CIBS may not be critical to its later expression. In this fashion, it would appear that the behavioral biology of CIBS may represent a moving target, one engaging a variety of direct and indirect neural mechanisms that may also be involved in learning and memory.

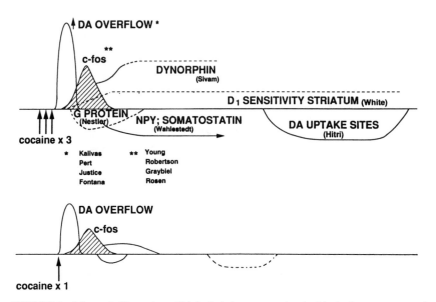

FIGURE 3. Schematic illustration of biological changes associated with single versus repeated cocaine administrations. Following a single injection of cocaine (*bottom*) short-lived changes can be observed in dopamine overflow as well as in the expression of the proto-oncogene c-fos. With repeated cocaine administration (*top*) the changes become more long lasting and involve additional neural and peptidergic substrates.

Given this analysis, the potential clinical complexities of trying to treat cocaine addiction and its associated conditioned and unconditioned aspects of craving become obvious. FIGURE 4 briefly schematizes some of the potential issues involved, again emphasizing the long-term and evolving nature of cocaine symptoms, vulnerabilities, and craving. Depending on the pattern of dose administration, its intermittency, chronicity and escalation, there may be tolerance or tachyphylaxis to cocaine's euphoric effects,[64] or sensitization to its activating and toxic effects. Considerable evidence points to a long-lasting sensitization manifest as vulnerability to reactivation of stimulant-induced paranoia even after many decades of abstinence. In addition repeated cocaine administration becomes increasingly associated with dysphoric elements (*i.e.*, anxiety, depression, and paranoia), some of which may represent direct sensitization phenomena and others which may reflect unconditioned or conditioned compensatory changes.[60,62]

Craving may then reflect these multiple components, and its strength may vary over time. After the initial positive cocaine experience, one might repeatedly seek to re-achieve the initial exquisite rush or euphoria. Even assuming no tachyphylaxis for this effect, re-experience of the same "high" might become increasingly difficult, as the addict, following chronic administration, may be starting from a more dysphoric baseline. Even after long-term abstinence and the normalization of this dysphoric baseline, conditioned cuing may be able to re-elicit withdrawal effects or craving depending on the circumstances.

Life-long vulnerability to relapse may be conveyed by the memory-like mechanisms

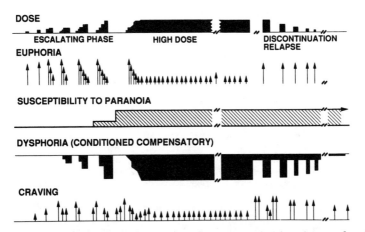

FIGURE 4. Hypothetical evolution of cocaine effects on mood and craving as a function of dose and repetition of drug administration. Initial euphoric effects diminish with rapidly repeated cocaine (tachyphylaxis), resulting in dosage escalation in an attempt to regain peak effects. An enhanced likelihood of aversive (paranoid or dysphoric) effects develops over time, associated with changes in baseline mood state as well as susceptibility to drug craving. With extended drug use, euphoric effects thus remain diminished while negative effects on mood and behavior become more "hard wired." Finally, attempts at discontinuation are associated with increased craving, negative mood states, and retriggering of previous cocaine effects upon relapse.

and conditioned components of cocaine-induced behavioral sensitization, some of which may be encoded at the level of gene expression and its downstream biochemical and neuroanatomical alterations. As the long-term consequences of cocaine self-administration and its underlying mechanisms become further elucidated, the development of more precise behavioral[65] and pharmacological treatment interventions should be greatly facilitated. The present analysis emphasizes the associative and conditioned components of cocaine-induced behavioral sensitization (CIBS). Conditioned aspects of CIBS appear to have a complex and evolving biochemistry, pharmacology, and anatomy. Their retriggering may play an important role in the addictive process and its treatment.

REFERENCES

1. Downs, A. W. & N. B. Eddy. 1932. J. Pharmacol. Exp. Ther. **46:** 199–200.
2. Downs, A. W. & N. B. Eddy. 1932. J. Pharmacol. Exp. Ther. **46:** 195.
3. Tatum, A. L. & M. H. Seevers. 1929. J. Pharmacol. Exp. Ther. **36:** 401–410.
4. Post, R. M., R. T. Kopanda & A. Lee. 1975. Life Sci. **17:** 943–950.
5. Post, R. M. & H. Rose. 1976. Nature **260:** 731–732.
6. Post, R. M. & N. R. Contel. 1983. *In* Stimulants: Neurochemical, Behavioral, and Clinical Perspective. I. Creese, Ed.: 169–203. Raven Press. New York.
7. Ellinwood, E. H., M. M. Kilbey, S. Castellani & C. Khoury. 1977. *In* Advances in Behavioral Biology, Vol. 21, Cocaine and Other Stimulants. E. H. Ellinwood & M. M. Kilbey, Eds.: 303–326. Plenum Press. New York.
8. Post, R. M., A. Lockfeld, K. M. Squillace & N. R. Contel. 1981. Life Sci. **28:** 755–760.

9. HINSON, R. E. & C. X. POULOS. 1981. Pharmacol. Biochem. Behav. **15:** 559–562.
10. POST, R. M., S. R. B. WEISS & A. PERT. 1991. *In* Cocaine: Pharmacology, Physiology, and Clinical Strategies. J. M. Lakoski, M. P. Galloway & F. J. White, Eds.: 115–161. Telford Press. New Jersey.
11. GALE, K. 1984. *In* NIDA Research Monograph Series 54, Mechanisms of Tolerance and Dependence. U.S. Government Printing Office. C. W. Sharp, Ed: 323–332. Washington, D.C.
12. SEGAL, D. S. 1975. *In* Advances in Biochemical Psychopharmacology XIII: Neurobiological Mechanisms of Adaptation and Behavior. A. J. Mandell, Ed.: 247–262. Raven Press. New York.
13. ROBINSON, T. E. & J. B. BECKER. 1986. Brain Res. Rev. **11:** 157–198.
14. MATTINGLY, B. A. & J. E. GOTSICK. 1989. Behav. Neurosci. **103:** 1311–1317.
15. POST, R. M., C. KENNEDY, M. SHINOHARA, K. SQUILLACE, M. MIYAOKA, S. SUDA, D. H. INGVAR & L. SOKOLOFF. 1984. Brain. Res. **324:** 295–303.
16. WEISS, S. R. B., R. M. POST, F. SZELE, R. WOODWARD & J. NIERENBERG. 1989. Brain Res. **497:** 72–79.
17. WEISS, S. R. B., R. M. POST, A. PERT, R. WOODWARD & D. MURMAN. 1989. Pharmacol. Biochem. Behav. **34:** 655–661.
18. DAFTERS, R. & J. ODBER. 1989. Behav. Neurosci. **103:** 1082–1090.
19. TIFFANY, S. T., P. M. MAUDE-GRIFFIN & D. J. DROBES. 1991. Behav. Neuroscience **105:** 49–61.
20. ANTELMAN, S. M. 1988. Drug Devel. Res. **14:** 1–30.
21. ANTELMAN, S. M. & A. R. CAGGIULA. 1990. Clin. Neuropharmacol. **13:** 585–586.
22. POST, R. M., S. R. B. WEISS, J. SMITH & A. PERT. 1987. Abstracts of the Society for Neuroscience 13-Ab. No. 185.7–661.
23. BENINGER, R. J. & B. L. HAHN. 1983. Science **220:** 1304–1306.
24. BENINGER, R. J. & R. S. HERZ. 1986. Life Sci. **38:** 1425–1431.
25. TADOKORO, S. & H. KURIBARA. 1986. Psychopharmacol. Bull. **22:** 757–762.
26. POST, R. M., S. R. B. WEISS & A. PERT. 1991. *In* The Mesolimbic Dopamine System: From Motivation to Action. P. Willner & J. Scheel-Kruger, Eds.: 443–472. John Wiley & Sons Ltd. Chichester, England.
27. POST, R. M. & S. R. B. WEISS. 1988. *In* Selected Models of Anxiety, Depression and Psychosis. P. Simon, P. Soubrie & D. Wildlocher, Eds.: 52–60. S. Karger. Basel.
28. POST, R. M. & S. R. B. WEISS. 1989. J. Clin. Psychiatry **50:** 23–30.
29. POST, R. M., S. R. B. WEISS & A. PERT. 1984. Prog. Neuropsychopharmacol. Biol. Psychiatry **8:** 425–434.
30. POST, R. M., S. R. B. WEISS & T. G. AIGNER. 1992. *In* Biological Basis of Substance Abuse. S. G. Korenman & J. Barchas, Eds. Oxford University Press. London. In press.
31. AIGNER, T., S. R. B. WEISS & R. M. POST. 1991. Abstracts, ACNP, p. 181.
32. WEISS, S. R. B., D. MURMAN, R. M. POST & A. PERT. 1986. Abstracts of the Society for Neuroscience 914-Ab. No. 249.13.
33. MOGENSON, G. J. 1987. Prog. Psychobiol. Physiol. Psychol. **12:** 117–170.
34. CADOR, M., T. W. ROBBINS & B. J. EVERITT. 1989. Neuroscience **30:** 77–86.
35. HITCHCOCK, J. & M. DAVIS. 1986. Behav. Neurosci. **100:** 11–22.
36. EVERITT, B. J., M. CADOR & T. W. ROBBINS. 1989. Neuroscience **30:** 63–75.
37. ROBBINS, T. W., M. CADOR, J. R. TAYLOR & B. J. EVERITT. 1989. Neurosci. Biobehav. Rev. **13:** 155–162.
38. MURRAY, E. A. & M. MISHKIN. 1985. Science **228:** 604–606.
39. MISHKIN, M. & T. APPENZELLER. 1987. Scientific Am. **256:** 80–89.
40. PAN, H. T., S. MENACHERRY & J. B. JUSTICE, JR. 1991. J. Neurochem. **56:** 1299–1306.
41. NG, J. P., G. W. HUBERT & J. B. JUSTICE, JR. 1991. J. Neurochem. **56:** 1485–1492.
42. PETTIT, H. O., H. T. PAN, L. H. PARSONS & J. B. JUSTICE, JR. 1990. J. Neurochem. **55:** 798–804.
43. PETTIT, H. O. & J. B. JUSTICE, JR. 1991. Brain Res. **539:** 94–102.
44. FONTANA, D. J., R. M. POST & A. PERT. 1991. Abstracts, Society for Neuroscience. Abs. No. 268.4.

45. PHILLIPS, A. G., C. D. BLAHA & H. C. FIBIGER. 1989. Neurosci. Biobehav. Rev. **13:** 99–104.
46. BENINGER, R. J. 1991. *In* The Mesolimbic Dopamine System: From Motivation to Action. P. Willner & J. Scheel-Krüger, Eds.: 273–299. John Wiley & Sons. Chichester, England.
47. CADOR, M., T. W. ROBBINS, B. J. EVERITT, H. SIMON, M. LE MOAL & L. STINUS. 1991. *In* The Mesolimbic Dopamine System: From Motivation to Action. P. Willner & J. Scheel-Krüger, Eds.: 225–250. John Wiley & Sons. Chichester, England.
48. PHILLIPS, A. G., J. G. PFAUS & C. D. BLAHA. 1991. *In* The Mesolimbic Dopamine System: From Motivation to Action. P. Willner & J. Scheel-Krüger, Eds.: 199–224. John Wiley & Sons. Chichester, England.
49. ROBERTSON, H. A., M. R. PETERSON, K. MURPHY & G. S. ROBERTSON. 1989. Brain Res. **503:** 346–349.
50. YOUNG, S. T., L. J. PORRINO & M. J. IADAROLA. 1989. Abstracts, Society for Neuroscience **15:** Abs. No. 432.5–1091.
51. YOUNG, S. T., L. J. PORRINO & M. J. IADAROLA. 1991. Proc. Natl. Acad. Sci. USA **88:** 1291–1295.
52. ROBERTSON, G. S., S. R. VINCENT & H. C. FIBIGER. 1990. Brain Res. **523:** 288–290.
53. GRAYBIEL, A. M., R. MORATALLA & H. A. ROBERTSON. 1990. Proc. Natl. Acad. Sci. USA **87:** 6912–6916.
54. SIVAM, S. P. 1989. J. Pharmacol. Exp. Ther. **250:** 818–824.
55. JOHNSON, M., L. G. BUSH, J. W. GIBB & G. R. HANSON. 1991. Biochem. Pharmacol. **41:** 649–652.
56. WAHLESTEDT, C., F. KAROUM, G. JASKIW, R. J. WYATT, D. LARHAMMAR, R. EKMAN & D. J. REIS. 1991. Proc. Natl. Acad. Sci. USA **88:** 2078–2082.
57. NESTLER, E. J., R. Z. TERWILLIGER, J. R. WALKER, K. A. SEVARINO & R. S. DUMAN. 1990. J. Neurochem. **55:** 1079–1082.
58. WHITE, F. J., D. J. HENRY, X.-T. HU, M. JEZIORSKI & J. M. ACKERMAN. 1991. *In* Cocaine: Pharmacology, Physiology and Clinical Strategies. J. M. Lakoski, M. P. Galloway & F. J. White, Eds.: 261–293. Telford Press, Inc. West Caldwell, NJ.
59. HITRI, A., M. E. CASANOVA, J. E. KLEINMAN & R. J. WYATT. 1991. Biol. Psychiatry **29:** 183a–184a.
60. SIEGEL, S. 1985. *In* Placebo: Clinical Phenomena and New Insights. L. White, B. Tursky & B. Schwartz, Eds.: 288–305. Guilford Press. New York.
61. MARKOU, A. T. & G. F. KOOB. 1991. Neuropsychopharmacology **4:** 17–26.
62. BLOOM, F. E. 1992. *In* Biological Basis of Substance Abuse. S. G. Korenman & J. Barchas, Eds. Oxford University Press. London. In press.
63. WEISS, S. R. B., K. HAAS & R. M. POST. 1991. Exp. Neurol. **114:** 300–306.
64. FOLTIN, R. W. & M. W. FISCHMAN. 1991. J. Pharmacol. Exp. Ther. **257:** 247–261.
65. O'BRIEN, C. P., A. R. CHILDRESS, I. O. ARNDT, A. T. MCLELLAN, G. E. WOODY & I. MAANY. 1988. J. Clin. Psychiatry **49:** 17–22.

Classical Conditioning in Drug-Dependent Humans[a]

CHARLES P. O'BRIEN, ANNA ROSE CHILDRESS,
A. THOMAS McLELLAN, AND RONALD EHRMAN

Addiction Research Center
University of Pennsylvania
3900 Chestnut Street
Philadelphia, Pennsylvania 19104-6178
and
Veterans Administration Medical Center
Philadelphia, Pennsylvania 19104

INTRODUCTION

Drugs that tend to be taken excessively produce prompt pleasant feelings in the user. In addition to producing reliable and rapid changes in affect (feelings), drugs of abuse produce changes in numerous organ systems such as cardiovascular, digestive and endocrine systems. Such pharmacological effects may not be perceptible to the drug user or these effects (*e.g.*, tachycardia) may simply contribute to an overall feeling of excitement. These changes occur repeatedly within the context of a drug-seeking and drug-using environment. Thus there are environmental cues that are consistently present before the user experiences the effects of the drug. Not only the appearance of the drug itself, but also the people, sights, sounds, odors and situations that often are associated with drug use can become predictors of the onset of drug effects. The user need not consciously be aware of these cues in order for an association to occur. With repetition, the cues may provoke a chain of behaviors leading to drug administration. The same stimuli may also begin to produce automatic changes in various organ systems *in advance* of the drug being received. These pre-drug effects in drug users can be demonstrated in a laboratory situation by giving experienced users a placebo when drug is expected. The observed non-pharmacological changes have been considered to be a form of learning and they have been the focus of study for many years.[1]

The learning factors involved in drug dependence have been examined from both respondent and operant conditioning perspectives. Environmental cues that have been associated with drug use in the past can evoke physiological changes (autonomic responses) that the experienced user interprets as drug-craving or withdrawal symptoms. These symptoms may, in turn, motivate voluntary drug-seeking (operant) behaviors.

[a] This work was supported by USPHS grants RO 1 DA 000586 and P50 DA 5186 and by the Department of Veterans Affairs. Portions of this review were previously presented at a NIDA technical review. This paper was presented in part at the 26th annual meeting of the Association for Research on Nervous and Mental Disease; see reference 47.

If the drug-seeker succeeds in finding the drug, the chain of behaviors is again reinforced by the pleasant drug-induced feelings (brain effects) and by the pharmacological effects produced by the drug on various other organ systems.

CYCLES OF REMISSION AND RELAPSE

Typical treatment of addiction requires a period of detoxification or gradual removal from the addicting drug by the administration of decreasing doses of the drug itself or by giving a replacement drug from a similar category. Detoxification is followed by rehabilitative measures usually involving group or individual counseling or psychotherapy. After leaving the hospital or rehabilitation center, the treated, drug-free former addict may report occasional unexpected episodes of a sudden compulsion or drive to obtain the drug. In these instances the desire for the drug may appear paradoxical. For example, the patient has completed a rehabilitation program; he has returned to his job; he is reunited with his family and he can present an apparently genuine and logical argument that he never intends to touch the drug again. And then, as one patient said, "I bumped into a guy that I used to do 'coke' with and my heart started pounding and I started shaking. Then I went on automatic pilot." While it is possible that some of these patients are making up stories to evade responsibility for the relapse, they appear sincere and there is a consistency to their reports. These relapse anecdotes suggest that there are involuntary factors involved and that learning produced by repetitive drug use may play a role in the mechanisms of relapse.

From the perspective of the clinician, cessation of drug use (detoxification) is just the beginning of treatment. Even a 28-day rehabilitation program has no impact unless there is some program to deal with the proneness to relapse when the former addict returns to his usual environment. As is the case with chronic medical illnesses such as arthritis, addictive behavior has a proclivity to return repeatedly, despite apparently successful short-term treatment. Even without treatment there are interruptions in regular drug taking. During the years of active drug use, there are often periods when the addict temporarily stops taking drugs. This may be by choice in an attempt to stop or reduce his drug use or by force such as when he is arrested. Detoxification may be accomplished by using medication to ease withdrawal symptoms or by abrupt stopping of the drug of abuse with no medication for withdrawal. However, detoxification even accompanied by brief rehabilitation treatment rarely has a lasting effect. True success is measured by the function of patients over the weeks, months and years after an initial detoxification.

The typical addict may continue drug use for years before seriously trying to break the habit by entering a treatment program. While the length of time before requesting treatment varies, the cumulative effects of daily compulsive drug use produce long-term changes in a person. These changes mean that the reactions of the drug user are different from the way they were before beginning drug use. Thus it is not surprising that the *reasons for relapse after treatment may be different from the reasons that caused the patient to begin using drugs*.[2] Both psychosocial and biological factors probably contribute to the phenomenon of relapse. A critical part of treatment is analyzing those factors that increase the likelihood of relapse after a period of abstinence.

In follow-up studies, we have examined the factors that have been associated with relapse. For drug-dependence disorders in general, multiple factors have been found to be important in influencing long-term outcome. The presence of a psychiatric disorder in addition to addiction significantly worsens prognosis[3] and clinical evidence suggests that social and economic conditions and drug availability in the community play a role. Withdrawal symptoms that persist for months[4] may also increase the risk of relapse. The combination of animal and human laboratory evidence plus clinical reports[1,5] suggest that learning factors also play a role in relapse.

STUDIES OF CONDITIONING PHENOMENA

One of the first scientists to study relapse among addicts was Abraham Wikler.[1] Wikler noted the similarity of certain relapse phenomena to Pavlovian conditioned responses.[1,6] Wikler observed withdrawal-like signs in opiate addicts who were participating in group therapy sessions in the Public Health Service Hospital in Lexington, KY during the 1940s. These patients had been completely drug free for at least several months and thus they shouldn't have had any signs of opiate withdrawal. But when they started talking about drugs in group therapy, Wikler observed yawning, sniffling and tearing of the eyes—signs of an opiate abstinence syndrome. Wikler was aware of studies from Pavlov's lab in the 1920s showing that the effects of morphine could be conditioned,[7] and he postulated that conditioning had occurred in his patients.

Wikler labeled this phenomenon "conditioned withdrawal," speculating that environmental stimuli had acquired the ability through classical conditioning to elicit many of the signs and symptoms of pharmacological withdrawal. He further hypothesized that cues formerly associated with drug effects or drug withdrawal symptoms might play an important role in triggering relapse to drug use in the abstinent opioid abuser. Wikler also pointed out that the adaptation to drugs could be conditioned, a phenomenon later explored in a series of elegant studies by Siegel on conditioning of drug tolerance.[9–12] Wikler developed a rat model for studying morphine withdrawal and in subsequent experiments[13–15] he demonstrated that withdrawal signs could be conditioned in rats. Goldberg and Schuster,[16] Davis and Smith,[17] and Siegel[9–12] and others[18,19] confirmed that many drugs from different pharmacological classes can produce conditioned responses in experimental animals. Conditioned opioid withdrawal responses have also been experimentally produced in human subjects.[5,20,21] See reference 22 for a detailed review of conditioned responses reported in animals and in humans.

CATEGORIES OF CONDITIONED RESPONSES

Studies in human subjects have demonstrated that conditioned responses (CRs) can be drug-like or drug-opposite depending on the circumstances.[23,24] We have attempted to classify these responses according to the proposed mechanism of their origin and the conditions under which they can be demonstrated:

Drug-opposite CRs
a. Conditioned withdrawal
b. Conditioned tolerance

Drug-like CRs
a. Conditioned euphoria ("needle-freak" phenomenon)
b. Placebo effects of drugs (under certain circumstances)

DRUG-OPPOSITE CONDITIONED RESPONSES

Repetitive use of the same drug can produce CRs that are opposite to the effects produced by the pharmacological action of the drug itself. For example, opiate injections produce *elevations* in skin temperature in human subjects, but stimuli that have repeatedly preceded opiate injections will reliably produce *reductions* in skin temperature when presented to experienced opiate users. This reduction in skin temperature begins before the person receives the drug. Thus it cannot be a pharmacological effect and it is presumed to be a conditioned response. There are many other examples of "drug-opposite" CRs which can be demonstrated by polygraphic measurement of physiological changes, by ratings of effects that subjects perceive (subjective effects) or by observer ratings of subject behavior. The drug-opposite responses can mimic the drug withdrawal syndrome. If these responses occur just before a dose of the drug is received, they subtract from the drug effect resulting in an attenuation of drug effects. The attenuation of drug effects produced by conditioned responses can be classed as a form of "tolerance" and it may form a partial explanation for the diminished drug effects commonly seen with repeated administration under similar circumstances of the same dose of a drug.[10]

One of the reasons given by opiate users for continuing opiate use is the avoidance of withdrawal symptoms. But viewing addiction as being motivated solely by avoidance of withdrawal symptoms is clearly incomplete. Further, the appearance of conditioned withdrawal symptoms in former drug users does not fully explain the high rate of relapse in former users. Although the phenomenon of *conditioned withdrawal* was the first type of conditioning considered by Wikler and is still closely associated with his name, Wikler also emphasized the importance of *reward* mechanisms in the maintenance of drug-taking behavior.[6] In opiate addicts, however, physical dependence and withdrawal symptoms are very common, especially in those applying for treatment. The presumed mechanism for the development of conditioned withdrawal is shown in FIGURE 1. Since in most opioid addicts, some withdrawal symptoms will occur several times per day, there may be thousands of pairings of environmental stimuli and withdrawal symptoms during the life of a patient before he seeks treatment. In the laboratory, we have shown that after as few as *seven* pairings between mild methadone withdrawal symptoms (unconditioned response, UR) and a neutral stimulus such as a peppermint odor (CS), humans begin to show signs of withdrawal (CR) when exposed to the odor alone.[20,21] These CRs have been found to be long-lasting in

---

Unconditioned Stimulus ⟶	**Unconditioned Response**
Opioid metabolized	*Rebound activity; adrenergic, cholinergic, etc.*
Receptors evacuated	*(tearing, rhinorrhea, tachycardia, nausea, diarrhea, etc.); drug-opposite effects*
Conditioning Stimulus ⟶	**Conditioned Response**
Drug-procuring or drug-using	*Mild version of above symptoms; drug-opposite*
environment: sights, sounds,	*effects*
smells, situations, fantasies	

FIGURE 1. Conditioned withdrawal (dependent subject).

an animal model[16] and they have been found to occur when the subject is re-exposed to the CS long after detoxification from drugs. This mechanism could, therefore, explain the stories reported by Wikler[13,14] and others[5] concerning onset of withdrawal symptoms when a drug-free patient returns to an environment in which withdrawal symptoms had occurred in the past. This mechanism would also explain the reactions of drug-free former addicts when shown, while in the laboratory, visual and auditory cues previously associated with past drug use.[5,25-27]

Conditioned tolerance is a term applied to another mechanism by which drug-opposite responses might be produced by conditioning. Siegel and others, in a series of experiments utilizing morphine, alcohol and insulin,[9-12,18,19] presented evidence that drug tolerance could be considered, at least in part, to be a classically conditioned phenomenon. As shown in FIGURE 2, the drug disturbs homeostatic equilibrium resulting in a reflex response against the drug as the organism attempts to regain equilibrium. This reflex response (UR, Unconditioned Response) counteracts the effects of the drug. The environmental cues (sights, smells, situations) repeatedly associated with drug procurement or injection provide a signal (CS) that, after repetition, can trigger homeostatic responses that are opposite to the effects of the drug (tolerance) in advance of the drug's being received. The conditioning of tolerance was termed "counter-adaptation" by Wikler.[8] Siegel's studies demonstrate that the learned aspects of tolerance follow the pattern of classically conditioned responses.

We have demonstrated apparent conditioned tolerance in a group of detoxified opiate addicts who were studied on four separate occasions under double-blind conditions.[28] The subjects received either *unsignaled* infusions of a moderate dose of opioid (4 mg hydromorphone) or a self-injection of the same dose. On the two other occasions, the subjects received an unsignaled infusion of saline or a self-injection of saline. When the opioid was given without warning by an infusion (unsignaled), the subjects showed a significantly greater physiological response to the drug than when the same dose was "expected" (self-injected). Our interpretation is that the unsignaled nature of the infusion of opioid prevented any warning that would have triggered the onset of drug-opposite or conditioned tolerance responses. On the occasions when the opioid was expected, the conditioned drug-opposite responses reduced the observed drug effect. This interpretation was supported by the saline self-injection occasion which showed greater drug-opposite responses presumably because there was no opiate in the injection to oppose the conditioned responses.

Conditioning clearly does not explain the entire phenomenon of tolerance, but the magnitude of the portion produced by conditioning may be significant. Siegel[29]

Unconditioned Stimulus	⟶	Unconditioned Response
Drug injection, Drug effects,		*Homeostatic response counter to drug effect*
Conditioning Stimulus	⟶	Conditioned Response
Sights, sounds, smells which signal that drug is about to appear		*Homeostatic responses counter to drug effects which in the absence of drug can be perceived as withdrawal*

FIGURE 2. Conditioned tolerance (dependent or non-dependent subject).

showed that situation-specific tolerance can protect against the deadly effects of an opiate overdose. When rats experienced with morphine received a high dose of the drug in an environment different from the conditions under which they had learned to expect morphine, rapid overdose signs ensued and death occurred in some animals. In contrast, another group of rats with the same experience of morphine exposure showed significantly less drug effect and no deaths when given the same high dose of morphine in the environment where morphine was "expected."

Conditioned drug-opposing (tolerance) responses can occur in opiate users who have only used intermittently and thus have never been physically dependent on opiates. This is because even intermittent users generally develop tolerance. Learned tolerance responses can develop according to the mechanism described in FIGURE 2. The learned tolerance responses will be evoked by drug related stimuli and they will be opposite to the effects of the drug, thus resembling opiate withdrawal responses. Similarly, a user such as a physician or pharmacist who has had enough opiates consistently available to avoid repeated episodes of withdrawal could still show conditioned withdrawal-like responses even though true pharmacological withdrawal had never occurred. In this situation, the learned tolerance would be based on a CR that is drug-opposite and physiologically similar to a withdrawal response. If the former addict encounters stimuli that were previously associated with drug use (CS), the CR would produce symptoms that may be perceived as "withdrawal-like." Typical drug users who *have* had repeated episodes of withdrawal in a specific environment will thus have *two mechanisms* for producing conditioned withdrawal-like symptoms: the first by the "conditioned withdrawal" paradigm described in FIGURE 1 and the second by the "conditioned tolerance" mechanism described in FIGURE 2.

DRUG-LIKE CONDITIONED RESPONSES

Conditioned *drug-like responses* can also be produced by pairing distinct stimuli with drug administration. After repeated pairing, the stimuli by themselves can produce drug-like effects.[22,30] Pavlov's original report[7] of morphine conditioning described a CR which resembled the unconditioned effects of morphine itself. Similar findings of "drug-like" conditioning have been reported by others in dogs[30-32] and in rats.[16,33,34] Drug-like conditioned effects have also been described in human studies.[5] Such a conditioning mechanism may form a partial explanation for what are known as the "placebo effects" of drugs. A variety of subjective and physiological responses have been reported when research subjects or patients are given an inert substance when they are expecting an active drug. The conditioning explanation presumes that drug-like or "placebo effects" have been conditioned by past exposure to drugs under similar circumstances. Our research over the years has provided clues as to which conditioning paradigms are most likely to produce either drug-like conditioned responses or drug-opposite responses. Confusion occurs in trying to understand these drug conditioned phenomena because both drug-like and drug-opposite effects can be learned. Both animal and human data suggest that stimulants such as amphetamine and cocaine are more likely to produce drug-like conditioned responses while opioids in human subjects produce more prominent drug-opposite responses, particularly in response to stimuli associated with pre-injection rituals. However, drug-like effects in opioid addicts in the laboratory have been demonstrated *after* self-injection.[5,35,36] Thus it is possible to observe opiate-opposite and opiate-like effects sequentially in the same opiate addict subject while he prepares and injects placebo material in the laboratory.

Drug-like effects are found clinically in patients known as "needle freaks."[37] Typically, these are individuals who may formerly have been physically dependent on opioids, but are currently using drugs intermittently or using low-potency opiate supplies. These "needle freaks" report *euphoria* from the act of self-injection and they have also been observed to show physiological signs such as pupillary constriction after injecting saline.[5] A similar finding was reported by Meyer and Mirin.[36] Some of these "needle freaks" have been detected among applicants applying for methadone treatment. Federal regulations limit the use of methadone maintenance (except in certain special cases) to individuals who are already physically dependent on opioids at the time of application for treatment. If there are no signs of withdrawal in an applicant for methadone, the opioid antagonist naloxone may be given as a diagnostic test for the presence of dependence.[38] Even a very small dose of naloxone will precipitate withdrawal symptoms in a person physically dependent on opioids. Occasionally, we have observed the naloxone injection to produce *mild euphoria instead of withdrawal* in applicants for methadone who claim to be addicts and who show the scars of chronic drug injections. Subsequently, we observed sedation and reports of euphoria when in the laboratory these subjects self-injected saline. Thus the euphoria observed after naloxone was not a pharmacological effect of naloxone, but likely a conditioned response to the injection procedure which served as a conditioned stimulus.[5]

There have been few direct observations using physiological and psychological monitoring of human addicts in the act of self-injecting addicting drugs. Our group reported a series of such studies[5,37,39] that described self-injections in detoxified opioid addicts being treated with the opioid antagonists cyclazocine or naltrexone. Several experimental protocols were used that involved maintaining patients on opiate antagonists that block the pharmacological effects of opioids. In one series of experiments, the patients were randomly assigned to self-injections with either saline or opioid; in others the patients were tested with both saline and opioid on different occasions. These experiments began with pre-naltrexone trials in which the subject's responses to unblocked opioid was compared to saline under double-blind conditions. Subsequently, we conducted "extinction trials" in which the subject repeatedly self-injected opioid or saline while being maintained on the opioid antagonist for up to six months. The findings were that saline self-injections were usually reported as pleasurable and identified as a low dose of opioid. This reaction to saline was assumed to be a drug-like conditioned response (placebo effect). The effect was greatest when the subjects injected themselves under naturalistic conditions resembling the patient's "shooting gallery" with the patient *expecting* to get "high." The drug-like effect was diminished but still present when the patient was placed alone in a more artificial setting, such as a recording chamber, with various electrodes and strain gauges attached.

We found that drug-like effects in most patients did not persist with repeated trials as did the drug-opposite effects described above. After several un-reinforced trials consisting of either saline injections or blocked opioid injections in patients pre-treated with an antagonist, the drug-like effects disappeared. The drug-opposite effects persisted in these patients, however.

Meyer and Mirin[36] used a different design and also observed conditioned opiate-like autonomic effects in human subjects. Their subjects were all recently detoxified inpatients who were given either naltrexone or naltrexone placebo under double-blind conditions. The subjects were then permitted to self-inject known amounts of heroin that they had earned by performing a simple operant task (pressing a lever). The subjects who received naltrexone placebo, in effect, had the opportunity to inject heroin unimpeded by naltrexone, and they injected it nearly the maximum number of times permitted by the protocol. However, the 22 subjects who received naltrexone had the rewarding effects of heroin blocked by this antagonist. Eleven of these subjects stopped injecting heroin after fewer than five trials, but the other 11 subjects took an average of 16 doses of heroin despite the presence of naltrexone. These 11 subjects were found to be different from those who stopped quickly in that they showed distinct autonomic changes during and after the injection procedure. These physiological responses resembled opiate effects and continued even after the first three blocked injections. The authors interpreted these autonomic changes (pupil, heart rate, and blood pressure) as conditioned opiate-like effects and they found that these autonomic changes had disappeared (extinguished) by the time the subjects decided to stop injecting. Unlike the outpatient studies described above, the Meyer and Mirin protocol did not require the subjects to continue to inject unless they wished to do so. Since they did not continue injecting past the point at which the patient's response to the procedure changed from positive to neutral, this probably explains why unpleasant or withdrawal-like symptoms were not reported.

Thus the evidence for conditioned opioid-like effects in humans is based on clinical anecdotes and on the laboratory studies involving self-injection described above. These CRs are elicited by the complex CS of pre-injection rituals and the act of self-injection. In most subjects the opioid-like CR is extinguished quickly and then withdrawal-like CRs are elicited by the same CSs that previously produced opioid-like effects.

SPECIFICITY

A question that arises concerns the specificity of responses to drug-related stimuli. Are these responses present in non-drug users? Ternes et al.[40] compared the reactions of opiate addicts to those of non-addicts viewing the same stimuli. It was found that non-addicts showed signs of arousal when viewing scenes of drug-taking behavior, but they showed rapid habituation compared to opiate addicts in the study who persisted in their arousal/withdrawal-like responses. Another study of specificity has just been completed among cocaine addicts. Ehrman et al.[40] compared the responses of cocaine addicts and normals to neutral stimuli, cocaine stimuli and opiate stimuli. The normals showed non-significant reactions to all sets of stimuli. The cocaine addicts showed significant responses only to the cocaine-related stimuli and not to the opiate-related stimuli.

Additional studies of the responses demonstrated by abstinent drug addicts have shown that they interact with negative mood states. Recent work from our laboratory has demonstrated that depression, anxiety and anger increase the responses in opiate addicts to opiate-related stimuli. After making these observations, Childress and colleagues designed an experiment in which negative mood states were elicited in addict volunteers using a hypnotic procedure.[41] In this study, negative mood states increased the response to drug cues and euphoric states reduced the response.

CLINICAL RELEVANCE

One way of assessing clinical importance is to determine whether modification of conditioned responses can influence the course of addiction. Using a variety of patient populations, we have attempted to extinguish or reduce presumed conditioned responses in patient volunteers and compare their clinical course with that of control patients who do not receive extinction therapy. We first studied the conditioned responses associated with chronic opioid use, speculating that some of these responses (particularly conditioned craving and withdrawal) could lead to drug use in the abstinent patient.[5,23,43-45] The responses that we targeted in our extinction program included subjective responses such as "craving," feelings of "high," and feelings of drug withdrawal. We also have studied the effects of the extinction program on autonomic responses such as changes in pulse, blood pressure, skin resistance and skin temperature. The procedure for modifying these responses was based on a process of systematic, gradual exposure to drug-associated cues without the possibility of reinforcement (actually receiving a drug). The general approach in this series of studies has been to first select cues that reliably elicit subjective and physiological responses in the target population, and then to attempt to reduce these responses through repeated, nonreinforced exposure (extinction).

We found that conditioned opiate-like responses extinguished rapidly in most patients, but responses that were opposite to the effects of opiates (withdrawal-like physiological responses and subjective craving) were very resistant to extinction.[35,39,46] We first studied detoxified and long-term drug-free patients, some of whom were therapeutic community graduates. We also studied methadone patients in a large scale treatment-outcome study employing extinction trials.[43,44] We found that drug-related stimuli were reliable elicitors of conditioned opioid-related responses, particularly conditioned craving and conditioned withdrawal, even in a methadone population. With 20 or more extinction sessions, conditioned craving was significantly reduced, but conditioned withdrawal signs and symptoms were still present in response to opiate-related cues.

RESPONSES TO COCAINE-RELATED STIMULI

Over the past several years, most of the patients applying for treatment in our program have been cocaine-dependent or they were cocaine abusers. Cocaine is cheap and widely available in Philadelphia. Most of our current research, therefore, is focused on cocaine dependence.[48,49] Cocaine use generally is episodic. Whether the user has stopped taking cocaine because of toxicity, incarceration, or admission to hospital for detoxification, there is a strong tendency to resume taking cocaine after a short abstinent period. When detoxified former cocaine users are confronted with stimuli previously associated with cocaine use, they report cocaine craving despite their expressed and apparently genuine intention to refrain from returning to drug use. Some report intense urges to use cocaine along with arousal and palpitations when they encounter stimuli as diverse as seeing a friend with whom they had used cocaine or seeing any powdery substance such as sugar or talcum powder. Some users interpret these responses as beginning to feel a cocaine "high" when they get close to the drug, but before it even enters their body. Detoxified former cocaine-dependent patients also experience similar responses when they encounter drug-buying locations, a pharmaceutical odor or almost anything that has been repeatedly associated with getting and using cocaine. These stimuli appear to act as a trigger for arousal and cocaine craving. After years of using cocaine, there are usually numerous stimuli within the patient's normal environment that have strong links to cocaine.

There are numerous studies in animals showing the conditioning of responses to cocaine and other stimulants.[49] In human cocaine-using subjects, we have conducted studies in the laboratory of reactivity to cocaine-related cues.[47,50] We found significant effects of cocaine-related stimuli as compared to control stimuli on autonomic measures such as skin temperature and skin resistance and on subjective measures such as feelings of craving, withdrawal or high. A subgroup of patients who had spent a period of 28 days for rehabilitation treatment in a hospital environment after detoxification from cocaine were also studied. All of these patients expressed the strong intention of remaining abstinent after leaving the hospital. The patients were shown cocaine and neutral stimuli on separate days in a balanced order while being monitored in a laboratory setting. The results were similar to patients recently detoxified; there was strong reaction to the cocaine cues and many of the rehabilitated patients reported surprise at the severity of their response. The additional 28 days of treatment had no apparent effect on the reactivity to cocaine-related cues.

It is of interest that not all patients in treatment for cocaine dependence showed reactivity to cocaine-related cues. At least one-third of these patients were adamant "non-responders," insisting that the cocaine-related stimuli triggered no craving, arousal or other responses. For these patients, physiological arousal (as reflected in either decreased skin temperature or a fall in GSR) was sometimes present, even though the patients denied perceiving any subjective reaction. The subjective and physiological data were analyzed for the total sample including those who reported no effects from the stimuli that we used. The average temperature reduction in response to cocaine-related stimuli for the entire unselected group (including "non-responders") was approximately 2.5 degrees Celsius. Among those classed as "responders," however, dramatic reductions of 5 to 8 degrees Celsius (in response to cocaine-related stimuli) were not uncommon.

CLASSIFICATION OF THE COCAINE-RELATED RESPONSES

Reactions to opiate-related stimuli among opiate abusers could be classified as drug-like or drug-opposite. This is because opiates affect several systems in specific ways. Opiate-like effects observed in our studies are rush, euphoria, pupillary constriction, slowing of the heart, lowered blood pressure, warming of the skin, and increased skin resistance. Withdrawal effects are the opposite of the preceding list plus yawning, tearing, sniffing, and nausea. Classification is much less clear among cocaine users. The physiological effects seen in abstinent former users when exposed to cocaine-related stimuli are decreased skin temperature, increased heart rate and increases in skin conductance. These are both the signs of stimulant drug effects and those of non-specific arousal. Some patients report high-like effects; others simply report craving or even "crash" feelings. Animal studies show clear conditioning of cocaine induced hyperactivity, a drug-like response. A most intriguing study of the CR for cocaine comes from direct brain studies using the micro-dialysis technique in the region of the nucleus accumbens in rats.[51] Increased dopamine was recorded in this region after each dose of intraperitoneal cocaine. The dopamine responses increased with successive cocaine doses (sensitization). After repeated exposure to cocaine injections, the animals were given a saline (placebo) injection under similar conditions on a different day. The response in the nucleus accumbens was a small but significant augmentation of dopamine, presumably conditioned by the prior experiences with cocaine. This work will have to be replicated, but it raises the possibility that the former cocaine-using patients experience a similar augmentation of limbic dopamine when they are exposed to cocaine-related stimuli. The peripheral measures of arousal would be consistent with this interpretation. The central dopamine increase could provide a priming effect in former users and precipitate a relapse to cocaine use.

COCAINE TREATMENT STUDY

Traditional treatment approaches have intuitively recognized the power of drug-associated stimuli. Therefore, abstinent patients are warned to avoid "people, places and things" associated with prior cocaine use. In reality, complete avoidance is very difficult, even in a well-motivated patient. Patients need additional tools for coping with and reducing drug craving. Our research treatment strategy consists of systematically exposing patients to stimuli that they are likely to see when they leave the treatment program.[47] We give patients repeated exposure to cocaine "reminders" while they are in a safe environment in an attempt to reduce the craving and arousal often triggered by these stimuli. This strategy complements an avoidance approach and it is a potentially useful adjunct to traditional abstinence-oriented treatment programs. This treatment approach is based on the view that cocaine "reminders" are classically conditioned stimuli that acquire their "reminder power" through repeated pairings with cocaine's pharmacologic effects over the natural course of a patient's drug use. By repeatedly exposing the patient to cocaine "reminders" without cocaine, it should be possible to reduce or extinguish the power of such cues to trigger the conditioned responses (arousal, craving, etc.) that could lead to drug use and relapse to addiction.

To prevent relapse, all categories of relapse-producing factors should be addressed including pharmacological, social, occupational, medical, legal, and family issues. If conditioning factors play a role in relapse, the influence of conditioning probably varies with the individual patient depending on the relative importance of other relapse-producing factors. Thus we have integrated the extinction procedure within the context of a treatment program that addresses a wide range of issues thought to be important to the recovering addict. Initial exposure to drug-related stimuli should be conducted in a protected therapeutic setting, to minimize the possibility of drug use in association with the strong craving/arousal triggered by the cocaine "reminders." The stimuli should be tied closely to the patient's cocaine history, particularly to their preferred mode of cocaine administration (intra-nasal, intravenous, or smoked).

Our early studies among cocaine subjects also taught us that the conditioned responses produced by cocaine could be highly varied and complex. When smoked or injected, cocaine results in a rapid onset of euphoria and pleasurable sensations, often followed, only a few minutes later, by dysphoria, nervousness, and extreme drug craving. These biphasic effects are further complicated by the appearance of toxic symptoms (suspiciousness, paranoia, etc.) after high doses, long binges, or even a long history of less frequent use. Finally, after termination of use, patients may complain of "crash" feelings, that may include depression, irritability and fatigue. Any of these affective and physiologic effects of cocaine could become conditioned to the many environmental stimuli consistently associated with cocaine use.

We recently completed a randomized trial of cocaine-dependent patients assigned to extinction or to a control group. This was an 8-week outpatient study. The results of this randomized clinical trial of passive cue exposure or extinction are being reported in detail elsewhere.[51] Briefly, the patients randomly assigned to extinction showed better retention in outpatient treatment and a higher proportion of clean urines than the control group. Both of these differences were significant at the 5% level. These results were encouraging because the extinction sessions were well-accepted by the patients and the technique can be applied by non-professional drug counselors. However despite the improved results, full extinction of the responses was not accomplished and relapses continued to occur although they were less common in the extinction group. Our results suggested to us that an active procedure should be tried to enhance the results of passive extinction.

ACTIVE PROCEDURES TO COMBAT CRAVING

Clearly, detoxified cocaine abusers can experience conditioned craving and arousal to cocaine reminder stimuli. These responses can be both intense and persistent, meaning that the abstinent cocaine abuser may be vulnerable long after detoxification is complete. Though the program of extinction described here is effective in reducing craving to cocaine-related stimuli presented in the context of the laboratory or clinic, patients can still report craving in the natural environment. We are currently evaluating two approaches to improve generalization from the lab to the street: 1) One approach is an attempt to increase the generalization of extinction by the use of even more realistic stimuli (*e.g.*, the sight of real cocaine) and stimulus contexts (*e.g.*, *in vivo* repeated exposures). Previously, we have been reluctant to employ *in vivo* exposures near "copping corners or shooting galleries" because of possible risk to both patients and clinical staff. Somewhat less dangerous stimuli could involve the patient's own home, or the use of "neighborhood" videos taped from a moving car. 2) A second approach involves the use of several other techniques in countering or reducing conditioned craving and arousal. These techniques include training of alternative behaviors (competing responses, thought blocking, relaxation response, *etc.*) as a useful adjunct to more conventional treatments for cocaine abuse, *e.g.*, counseling, therapy, and relapse-prevention techniques.

We are currently conducting a randomized clinical trial of active techniques to combat craving. The experimental treatment involves evoking responses to cocaine-related cues in the clinic and coaching the patient in the use of a behavioral technique to combat the response. Our pilot work suggests that this technique will be more successful than a passive cue exposure technique. The patient learns a set of active coping devices and has the opportunity to practice them in the clinic with the help of a therapist. This increases the patient's confidence that he can resist the responses which occur when he is confronted with cocaine cues in his natural environment. In addition, our new extinction procedures include 1) more individualized cocaine reminders to benefit patients who do not respond strongly to our standard test stimuli, and 2) more extinction sessions, in an attempt to more completely extinguish the persistent physiological arousal which occurs in response to cocaine cues.

Use of Response to Cocaine-related Cues as a Medication-screening Device

A potential application of the response to drug-related cues is the screening of new medications for aide in the maintenance of abstinence. For cocaine dependence, it is unlikely that any single treatment approach will be effective. We would like to find more effective medications and devise a way to combine the effects of various treatments such as medications and behavior therapy. Our group has just completed a preliminary study of the effects of a putative medication for cocaine dependence on the magnitude of the reaction to cocaine-related cues. The purpose was to determine whether potential medications could be tested for their effects on craving and arousal evoked by the drug-related cues in the laboratory. Medications that seemed to reduce the reaction to cocaine-related cues might then be tested in a controlled clinical trial to determine their overall clinical efficacy.

Patients volunteering for a trial of amantadine therapy were tested for their reactivity to cocaine cues before receiving either amantadine or placebo.[53] They were tested again after 7–10 days of stabilization on the medication (either amantadine or placebo). The two groups of patients had similar reactions to the cocaine cues on the first occasion, but after stabilization on the medication, the patients assigned to amantadine had significantly greater reactions to the cues than did the patients assigned to placebo. This effect may relate to the pro-dopamine activity of amantadine. The clinical significance of this finding is, of course, not clear at this time. In our efforts to develop predictors of successful medication for cocaine dependence, we will have to test many potential medications and correlate the findings in the test model with clinical outcome. Thus far the clinical outcome studies with amantadine are equivocal, but we are in the process of comparing the results of cue reactivity with the clinical outcome in specific patients.

SUMMARY

Repetitive use of psychoactive drugs produces a variety of learned behaviors. These can be classified in the laboratory according to an operant/classical paradigm, but *in vivo* the two types of learning overlap. The classically conditioned responses produced by drugs are complex and bi-directional. There has been progress in classifying and predicting the types of conditioned responses, but little is known of mechanisms. New techniques for understanding brain function such as micro-dialysis probes in animals and advanced imaging techniques (PET and SPECT) in human subjects may be utilized in conditioning paradigms to "open the black box."

Because the existence of conditioned responses in drug users is now well established, clinical studies have been instituted to determine whether modification of conditioned responses can influence clinical outcome. A recently completed study in cocaine addicts has produced evidence that outcome can be improved by a passive extinction technique over an 8-week outpatient treatment program.

REFERENCES

1. WIKLER, A. 1948. Recent progress in research on the neurophysiological basis of morphine addiction. Am. J. Psychiat. **105:** 329–338.
2. O'BRIEN, C. P., R. EHRMAN & J. TERNES. 1986. Classical conditioning in human opioid dependence. *In* Behavioral Analysis of Drug Dependence. S. Goldberg & I. Stolerman, Eds.: 329–356. Academic Press. San Diego, CA.
3. MCLELLAN, A. T., L. LUBORSKY, G. E. WOODY & C. P. O'BRIEN. 1983. Predicting response to alcohol and drug abuse treatment: Role of psychiatric severity. Arch. Gen. Psychiat. **40:** 620–625.

4. MARTIN, W. & D. JASINSKI. 1969. Physiological parameters of morphine dependence in man-tolerance, early abstinence and protracted abstinence. J. Psychiat. Res. **7:** 9–17.
5. O'BRIEN, C. P. 1975. Experimental analysis of conditioning factors in human narcotic addiction. Pharmacol. Rev. **27:** 535–543.
6. WIKLER, A. 1973. Dynamics of drug dependence: Implications of a conditioning theory for research and treatment. Arch. Gen. Psychiat. **28:** 611–616.
7. PAVLOV, I. P. 1927. *In* Conditioned Reflexes. G. Anrep, Ed. Oxford University Press. London.
8. WIKLER, A. 1973. Conditioning of successive adaptive responses to the initial effects of drugs. Conditional Reflex **8:** 193–210.
9. SIEGEL, S. 1975. Evidence from rats that morphine tolerance is a learned response. J. Comp. Physiol. Psychol. **89:** 498–506.
10. SIEGEL, S., R. HINSON & M. KRANK. 1978. The role of predrug signals in morphine analgesic tolerance: Support for a Pavlovian conditioning model of tolerance. J. Exp. Psychol.: Animal Behav. Processes **4:** 188–196.
11. SIEGEL, S. 1978. Morphine tolerance: Is there evidence for a conditioning model? Science **200:** 343–344.
12. SIEGEL, S., R. HINSON & M. KRANK. 1981. Morphine-induced attenuation of morphine tolerance. Science **212:** 1533–1534.
13. WIKLER, A. & F. PESCOR. 1967. Classical conditioning of a morphine abstinence phenomenon, reinforcement of opioid-drinking behavior and relapse in morphine-addicted rats. Psychopharmacologia **10:** 255–284.
14. WIKLER, A. 1968. Interaction of physical dependence and classical and operant conditioning in the genesis of relapse. *In* The Addictive States. 280–286.
15. WIKLER, A., F. PESCOR, D. MILLER & H. NORRELL. 1971. Persistent potency of a secondary (conditioned) reinforcer following withdrawal of morphine from physically dependent rats. Psychopharmacologia **20:** 103–117.
16. EIKELBOOM, R. & J. STEWART. 1982. The conditioning of drug-induced psychological responses. Psychol. Rev. **89:** 507–528.
17. DAVIS, W. N. & S. G. SMITH. 1974. Naloxone use to eliminate opiate-seeking behavior: Need for extinction of conditioned reinforced. Biol. Psychiat. **9:** 181–189.
18. POULOS, C. & H. CAPPELL. 1979. Conditioned tolerance to the hypothermic effect of ethyl alcohol. Science **206:** 1109.
19. POULOS, C. & R. HINSON. 1982. Pavlovian conditional tolerance to haldoperidol catalepsy: Evidence of dynamic adaptation in the dopaminergic system. Science **218:** 491–492.
20. O'BRIEN, C. P., T. J. O'BRIEN, J. MINTZ & J. P. BRADY. 1975. Conditioning of narcotic abstinence symptoms in human subjects. Drug Alcohol Dep. **1:** 115–123.
21. O'BRIEN, C. P., T. TEST, T. J. O'BRIEN, J. P. BRADY & B. WELLS. 1977. Conditioned narcotic withdrawal in humans. Science **195:** 1000–1001.
22. GRABOWSKI, J. C. & C. P. O'BRIEN. 1980. Conditioning factors in opiate use. *In* Advances in Substance Abuse. N. K. Mello, Ed. Vol. II. JAI Press.
23. O'BRIEN, C. P., R. EHRMAN & J. TERNES. 1986. Classical conditioning in human opioid dependence. *In* Behavioral Analysis of Drug Dependence. S. Goldberg & I. Stolerman, Eds.: 329–356. Academic Press. San Diego, CA.
24. O'BRIEN, C. P., A. R. CHILDRESS & A. T. MCLELLAN. 1988. Types of conditioning found in drug-dependent humans. Learning factors in drug dependent humans. Learning Factors in Drug Dependence NIDA Research Monograph Series, edited by B. Ray. DHHS publication number (ADM)88-1576: 44–61.
25. TEASDALE, J. 1973. Conditioned abstinence in narcotic addicts. Int. J. Addict. **8:** 273–292.
26. TERNES, J., C. O'BRIEN, J. GRABOWSKI, H. WELLERSTEIN & J. JORDAN-HAYES. 1980. Conditioned drug responses to naturalistic stimuli. Proceedings of the 41st Annual Meeting, Committee on Problems of Drug Dependence, NIDA Research Monograph No. **27:** 282–288.
27. SIDEROFF, S. & M. E. JARVIK. 1980. Conditioned responses to a video-tape showing heroin-related stimuli. Int. J. Addict. **15:** 529–536.
28. EHRMAN, R. N., J. T. TERNES, C. P. O'BRIEN & A. T. MCLELLAN. 1991. Conditioned tolerance in human opiate addicts. Psychopharmacology. In press.
29. SIEGEL, S., R. E. HINSON, M. S. KRANK & J. MCCULLY. 1982. Heroin "overdose" death: Contribution of drug-associated environmental cues. Science **216:** 436–437.

30. LYNCH, J. J., E. A. STEIN & A. P. FERTSIGER. 1973. An analysis of 70 years of morphine classical conditioning: Implications for clinical treatment of narcotic addiction. J. Nervous Mental Dis. 163: 147–158.

31. COLLINS, K. H. & A. L. TATUM. 1925. A conditioned salivary reflex established by chronic morphine poisoning. Am. J. Physiol. 74: 14–15.

32. RUSH, M. L., L. PEARSON & W. J. LANG. 1970. Conditional autonomic responses induced in dogs by atropine and morphine. Eur. J. Pharmacol. II: 22–28.

33. MIKSIC, S., N. SMITH, R. NUMAN & H. LAL. 1975. Acquisition and extinction of a conditioned hyperthermic response to a tone paired with morphine administration. Neuropsychobiology 1: 277–283.

34. NUMAN, R., N. SMITH & H. LAL. 1975. Reduction of morphine-withdrawal body shakes by a conditional stimulus in the rat. Psychopharmacol. Commun. 1: 295–303.

35. O'BRIEN, C., R. GREENSTEIN, J. TERNES, A. T. MCLELLAN & J. GRABOWSKI. 1980. Unreinforced self-injections: Effects on rituals and outcome in heroin addicts. Problems of Drug Dependence, NIDA Research Monograph 27: 275–281.

36. MEYER, R. E. & A. M. MIRIN. 1979. The heroin stimulus: Implications for a theory of addiction. Plenum Press. New York.

37. LEVINE, D. G. 1974. Needle freaks: Compulsive self-injections by drug users. Am. J. Psychiat. 131: 297–300.

38. BLACHLY, P. H. 1973. Naloxone for diagnosis in methadone programs. J. Am. Med. Assoc. 224: 334–335.

39. O'BRIEN, C. P., B. CHADDOCK, G. WOODY & R. GREENSTEIN. 1974. Systematic extinction of narcotic drug use using narcotic antagonists. Psychosom. Med. 36: 458.

40. TERNES, J., C. O'BRIEN, J. GRABOWSKI, H. WELLERSTEIN & J. JORDAN-HAYES. 1980. Conditioned drug responses to naturalistic stimuli. Problems of Drug Dependence, NIDA Research Monograph 27: 282–288.

41. EHRMAN, R., S. ROBBINS, A. R. CHILDRESS & C. P. O'BRIEN. 1992. Conditioned responses to cocaine-related stimuli in cocaine abuse patients. Psychopharmacology. In press.

42. CHILDRESS, A. E., R. EHRMAN, A. T. MCLELLAN, J. MACRAE, M. NATALE & C. P. O'BRIEN. 1992. Negative mood states trigger conditioned drug craving and arousal in opiate abuse patients. J. Sub. Abuse Treat. In press.

43. CHILDRESS, A. R., A. T. MCLELLAN & C. P. O'BRIEN. 1984. Measurement and extinction of conditioned withdrawal-like responses in opiate dependent patients. Problems of Drug Dependence, NIDA Research Monograph 49: 212–219. DHHS publication number (ADM)84-1316.

44. CHILDRESS, A. R., A. T. MCLELLAN & C. P. O'BRIEN. 1986b. Conditioned responses in a methadone population: A comparison of laboratory, clinic, and natural setting. J. Sub. Abuse Treat. 3: 173–179.

45. MCLELLAN, A. T., A. R. CHILDRESS, C. P. O'BRIEN & R. EHRMAN. 1986. Extinguishing conditioned responses during treatment for opiate dependence: Turning laboratory findings into clinical procedures. J. Sub. Abuse Treat. 3: 33–40.

46. CHILDRESS, A. R., A. T. MCLELLAN & C. P. O'BRIEN. 1986a. Abstinent opiate abusers exhibit conditioned craving, conditioned withdrawal and reductions in both through extinction. Br. J. Addict. 81: 655–660.

47. O'BRIEN, C. P., A. R. CHILDRESS, A. T. MCLELLAN & R. EHRMAN. 1990. The use of cue exposure as an aid in the prevention of relapse to cocaine or heroin dependence. Addict. Behav. 15(4): 355–365.

48. O'BRIEN, C. P., A. E. CHILDRESS, A. T. MCLELLAN & R. EHRMAN. 1992. A learning model of addiction. In Advances in Understanding the Addictive States. C. P. O'Brien & J. Jaffe, Eds. Association for Research in Nervous and Mental Disease 70: 157–177.

49. POST, R. M., S. WEISS, A. PERT & T. UHDE. 1987. Chronic cocaine administration: Sensitization and kindling effects. In Cocaine: Clinical and Biobehavioral Aspects: 109–173. Oxford University Press. London.

50. CHILDRESS, A. R., A. T. MCLELLAN, R. EHRMAN & C. P. O'BRIEN. 1987. Extinction of conditioned responses in abstinent cocaine or opioid users. Prob. Drug Depend. 76: 189–195.

51. KALIVAS, P. W. & P. DUFFY. 1990. Effect of acute and daily cocaine treatment on extra-cellular dopamine in the nucleus accumbens. Synapse **5:** 48–58.
52. CHILDRESS, A. R., R. EHRMAN, A. T. MCLELLAN & C. P. O'BRIEN. 1991. Clinical efficacy of cocaine cue extinction in the treatment of cocaine dependence: A randomized con-trolled outcome study. Submitted.
53. ROBBINS, S., R. EHRMAN, A. R. CHILDRESS & C. P. O'BRIEN. 1992. Using cue reactivity to screen medications for cocaine abuse: Amantadine hydrochloride. Addict. Behav. In press.

Behavioral Sensitization Induced by Psychostimulants or Stress: Search for a Molecular Basis and Evidence for a CRF-Dependent Phenomenon

M. CADOR,[a] S. DUMAS,[b] B. J. COLE,[c] J. MALLET,[b]
G. F. KOOB,[c] M. LE MOAL,[a] AND L. STINUS[a]

[a] U259, University of Bordeaux II
Rue Camille Saint-Saens
33077, Bordeaux Cedex, France

[b] N.B.C.M., Laboratoire de Neurobiologie Cellulaire et Moléculaire
Centre National de la Recherche Scientifique
Gif sur Yvette, 91198, France

[c] Department of Neuropharmacology
Scripps Clinic Research Institute
North Torrey Pines Road
La Jolla, California 92037

In humans, the repeated use of amphetamine (AMPH) produces a hypersensitivity to the psychotogenic effects of AMPH that persists for months to years after the cessation of drug use.[1] In animals, the repeated intermittent administration of AMPH produces an enduring enhancement in behaviors elicited by a subsequent exposure to AMPH.[2] Most importantly, these animals are not only hypersensitive to an amphetamine challenge but also show increased responsiveness to several other pharmacological agents or stressors.[3] This phenomenon, called sensitization or cross-sensitization, has been reported to last several months and has been proposed to model the longitudinal, progressive course of several psychiatric disorders.[4] At a neurobiological level, most interest has been devoted to the mesencephalic dopaminergic system (A9–A10) for two major reasons. First, the dopaminergic system has been involved in the psychostimulant and reinforcing properties of most drugs of abuse[5] and second it appears that a common property of any kind of "sensitizer" is to activate the mesencephalic dopaminergic system.[6]

For these reasons, efforts to elucidate the neuroanatomical and neurochemical substrates of behavioral sensitization have focused on potential modifications at the level of the dopaminergic neurons. Many data suggest that sensitization is accompanied by a prolonged change in the releasability of DA,[7] but the molecular bases of such changes have not been identified. The purpose of this study was to examine the effect of repeated amphetamine administration on potentially long-lasting modification of tyrosine hydroxylase gene expression, the limiting enzyme of dopamine synthesis, in animals repeatedly pretreated with amphetamine (10 injections, 3 mg/kg, 3 days apart). There was a 119% increase in TH mRNA expression in the ventral mesencephalon using a northern blot analysis three weeks after the last amphetamine injection and in basal conditions (no challenge; see FIG. 1). A western blot analysis performed in the same samples revealed a decreased total amount of the TH protein at the level of the DA cell bodies. These two results together suggest an increased synthesis and utilization of tyrosine hydroxylase.

In a second study, the relation between sensitization and CRF was explored since psychostimulant drugs significantly activate the hypothalamic-pituitary adrenal axis (HPA). The peptide CRF is the major activator of the HPA, and central administration of CRF, outside the HPA,[8] elicits autonomic, electrophysiologic and behavioral response similar to a stress response.[9-11] For these dual central and peripheral activities, CRF has been hypothesized to be a coordinator of central and peripheral response to a stressor.[12] Since stress shows cross-sensitization with amphetamine, the potential implication of CRF in the development of sensitization was examined. Administration

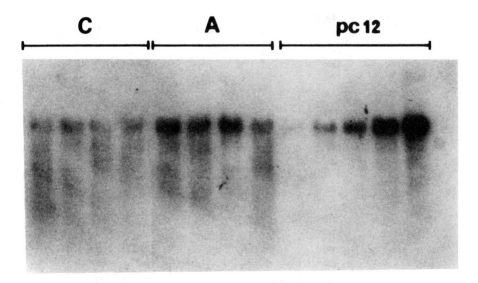

TH RNA

FIGURE 1. Northern blot analysis of TH mRNA. Ventral mesencephalon were dissected including substantia nigra and ventral tegmental area. Total RNA was extracted, electrophoresed (⅛ of total ventral mesencephalon), blotted and hybridized with a TH cDNA probe. Lanes **A** correspond to ⅛ of RNA from the ventral mesencephalon of 4 sensitized animals (10 injections of amphetamine 3 mg/kg, 3 days apart, 3 weeks before the northern blot analysis). Lanes **C** correspond to ⅛ of RNA from the ventral mesencephalon of 4 control animals (10 injections of saline, 3 days apart, 3 weeks before the northern blot analysis). Lanes **PC12** correspond to a serial dilution of total RNA extract from PC12 cells (5, 25, 50, 125, 250 ng).

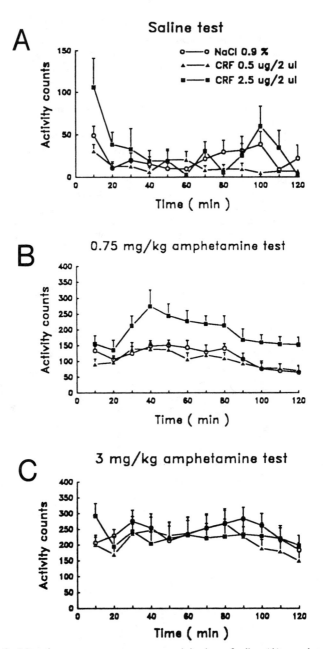

FIGURE 2. Mean locomotor response to a s.c. injection of saline (**A**), amphetamine 0.75 mg/kg (**B**) and 3 mg/kg (**C**) 1 week following repeated treatment with saline or CRF (0.5 or 2.5 μg/2 μl) i.c.v. (one injection per day during 5 days).

of the CRF antagonist prior to repeated restrained stress prevented the development of sensitization to the psychostimulant effects of a subsequent amphetamine challenge.[13] In a complementary experiment, the repeated exogenous application of CRF into the brain induced sensitization to the motor effect of amphetamine administered one week later (FIG. 2). Finally, since CRF is also implicated in the stimulation of the HPA axis, an attempt was made to block sensitization with an intravenous injection of a CRF antibody. The CRF antibody prevented the development of sensitization to subsequent administration of *d*-amphetamine.[14]

In conclusion, psychostimulant sensitization appears to be mediated by long-lasting changes in the dopaminergic system which can be observed at the molecular level. Furthermore, the hypothesized coordinator of the stress response, the peptide CRF, appears at least to participate in the development of sensitization through its central as well as its HPA axis stimulatory effect. These results suggest that sensitization should be regarded as a more general phenomenon involving participation of other neuronal systems as well as peripheral hormones in addition to the dopaminergic system.

REFERENCES

1. ANTELMAN, S. M. 1988. Stressor-induced sensitization to subsequent stress: Implications for the development and treatment of clinical disorders. *In* Sensitization in the Nervous System. P. W. Kalivas & C. D. Barnes, Eds.: 227–257. The Telford Press. Caldwell, NJ.
2. ROBINSON, T. E. & J. B. BECKER. 1986. Enduring changes in brain and behavior produced by chronic amphetamine administration: A review and evaluation of animal models of amphetamine psychosis. Brain Res. Rev. **11**: 157–198.
3. ANTELMAN, S. M., A. J. EICHLER, C. A. BLACK & D. KOCAN. 1980. Interchangeability of stress and amphetamine in sensitization. Science **207**: 329–331.
4. POST, R. M. & S. R. B. WEISS. 1988. Sensitization and kindling: Implications for the evolution of psychiatric symptomatology. *In* Sensitization in the Nervous System. P. W. Kalivas & C. D. Barnes, Eds.: 257–293. The Telford Press. Caldwell, NJ.
5. DI CHIARA, G. & A. IMPERATO. 1988. Drugs of abuse preferentially increase synaptic dopamine concentrations in the mesolimbic system of freely moving rats. Proc. Natl. Acad. Sci. **85**: 5274–5278.
6. KALIVAS, P. W., P. DUFFY, R. ABHOLD & R. P. DILTS. 1988. Sensitization of mesolimbic dopamine neurons by neuropeptides and stress. *In* Sensitization in the Nervous System. P. W. Kalivas & C. D. Barnes, Eds.: 119–145. The Telford Press. Caldwell, NJ.
7. ROBINSON, T. E., P. A. JURSON, J. A. BENNETT & K. M. BENTGEN. 1988. Persistent sensitization of dopamine neurotransmission in ventral striatum (nucleus accumbens) produced by prior experience with (+)-amphetamine: A microdialysis study in freely moving rats. Brain Res. **540**: 159–163.
8. OLSCHOWKA, J. A., T. L. O'DONOHUE, G. P. MUELLER & D. M. JACOBOWITZ. 1982. The distribution of corticotropin releasing factor-like immunoreactive neurons in rat brain. Peptides **3**: 995–1015.
9. SUTTON, R. E., G. F. KOOB, M. LE MOAL, J. RIVIER & W. VALE. 1982. Corticotropin releasing factor produces behavioural activation in rats. Nature **297**: 331–333.
10. BRITTON, K. T., G. F. KOOB & J. RIVIER. 1982. Intraventricular corticotropin releasing factor enhances behavioral effects of novelty. Life Sci. **31**: 363–367.
11. FISHER, L. A. 1989. CRF: Endocrine and autonomic integration of responses to stress. TINS. **10**: 189–193.
12. KOOB, G. F., K. T. BRITTON, A. TAZI & M. LE MOAL. 1989. Corticotropin releasing factor, stress and arousal. *In* Neuropeptides and Stress. Y. Tache, Ed.: 49–60. Springer-Verlag. New York.

13. COLE, B. J., M. CADOR, L. STINUS, J. RIVIER, W. VALE, G. F. KOOB & M. LE MOAL. 1990. Central administration of a CRF antagonist blocks the development of stress-induced behavioral sensitization. Brain Res. **512**: 343–346.
14. COLE, B. J., M. CADOR, L. STINUS, C. RIVIER, J. RIVIER, W. VALE, M. LE MOAL & G. F. KOOB. Critical role of the hypothalamic pituitary adrenal axis in amphetamine-induced sensitization of behavior. Life Sci. **47**: 1715–1720.

NMDA Receptor Complex Antagonists Have Ethanol-like Discriminative Stimulus Effects

GIANCARLO COLOMBO AND
KATHLEEN A. GRANT

Section on Receptor Mechanisms
Laboratory of Physiologic and Pharmacologic Studies
National Institute on Alcohol Abuse and Alcoholism
12501 Washington Avenue
Rockville, Maryland 20852

The N-methyl-D-aspartate receptor exists as a macromolecular complex with several sites that modulate the depolarizing actions of NMDA. The primary components of the complex are the NMDA recognition site, a strychnine-insensitive glycine site, and the receptor-coupled cation channel. Phencyclidine-like compounds, including the dibenzocycloheptenimine dizocilpine (MK-801) bind within the channel and block conductance in an uncompetitive manner. Drugs such as CPPene and CGS 19755 bind to the NMDA recognition site and block conductance in a competitive manner.[1]

Ethanol (10–50 mM) has been reported to antagonize cation conductance associated with the stimulation of NMDA receptors in both *in vitro* studies[2,3] and *in vivo* studies.[4] We have used a drug discrimination procedure to demonstrate that antagonism of NMDA neurotransmission results in stimulus effects that are perceptively similar to ethanol.[5] The following study examined whether NMDA antagonists that act either within the ionophore or at the NMDA recognition site have stimulus effects similar to ethanol, and if these similarities are influenced by the training dose of ethanol.

METHODS

Rats were trained to discriminate either 1.0, 1.5 or 2.0 g/kg ethanol (i.g.) from water (i.g.) in a chamber containing 2 levers and using food reinforcement. The ethanol or water was given 20 min prior to the onset of the session, and responding on the appropriate lever was reinforced under a fixed ratio 20 schedule. The session ended following 25 reinforcers or 30 min. The uncompetitive NMDA antagonist dizocilpine (MK-801) and the competitive antagonists CPPene and CGS 19755 were given (i.p.) 20 min and phencyclidine (PCP) was given (i.p.) 10 min prior to the start of the test sessions. Under test conditions, responding on either key was reinforced. Complete substitution was defined as 80% or greater ethanol-appropriate responding.

RESULTS AND DISCUSSION

The results of this study demonstrate in a third species[5] that antagonism of NMDA neurotransmission can result in stimulus effects that are perceived as similar to ethanol.

As shown in TABLE 1, at least one dose of the uncompetitive NMDA antagonists dizocilpine and PCP substituted for ethanol in every rat of each training dose group. The group data show that the dose determinations of both dizocilpine and PCP substitution for ethanol were affected by the training dose. In rats trained to discriminate 1.0 g/kg ethanol, dizocilpine resulted in only partial ethanol-appropriate responding, whereas in rats trained to discriminate 1.5 g/kg ethanol, dizocilpine completely substituted for ethanol. Finally, rats trained to discriminate 2.0 g/kg ethanol from water were the most sensitive to the discriminative stimulus effects of dizocilpine. These results suggest that the blockade of the NMDA channel by 1.0 g/kg ethanol is not a prominent characteristic of its stimulus effects; that increasing the training dose of ethanol to 1.5 g/kg enhances the NMDA channel-blockade characteristic of the ethanol cue;

TABLE 1. Average Responses Made on the Ethanol-Appropriate Lever

Antagonist	Dose (mg/kg)	Ethanol Training Dose		
		1.0 g/kg	1.5 g/kg	2.0 g/kg
Phencyclidine		$n = 5/5$	$n = 5/5$	$n = 3/3$
	0.3	17 ± 16	33 ± 23	
	1	41 ± 17	41 ± 17	
	1.7	71 ± 15	52 ± 17	25 ± 28
	3	77 ± 15	98 ± 2	50 ± 24
	5.6	100 ± 0		98 ± 2
Dizocilpine		$n = 5/5$	$n = 5/5$	$n = 4/4$
	0.03		8 ± 8	
	0.1	45 ± 19	17 ± 12	41 ± 19
	0.17	67 ± 17	46 ± 15	89 ± 7
	0.3	35 ± 21	98 ± 1	99 ± 1
CPPene		$n = 5/5$	$n = 4/6$	
	1	11 ± 10		
	3	30 ± 16	0 ± 0	
	5.6	79 ± 14	39 ± 18	
	10		76 ± 15	
CGS 19755		$n = 2/5$	$n = 3/6$	
	5.6	56 ± 30	0 ± 0	
	10	50 ± 33	60 ± 27	
	17	63 ± 28	42 ± 26	

The average responses were made following various doses of the uncompetitive NMDA antagonists dizocilpine and PCP and the competitive NMDA antagonists CPPene and CGS 19755 in rats trained to discriminate 1.0, 1.5, or 2.0 g/kg ethanol. Numbers in bold type indicate complete substitution for the ethanol stimulus (>80% responding on the ethanol lever). The ratio for the number of rats indicate the number of rats reporting substitution of the drug for ethanol at any dose tested (numerator) to the number of rats tested with the drug (denominator).

and that blockade of the NMDA channel is an easily discriminable, component part of the effects of 2.0 g/kg ethanol.

In contrast to dizocilpine, PCP substituted for all 3 training doses of ethanol. The main effect of increasing the training dose was to shift the dose-response determinations to the left. The differential abilities of PCP and dizocilpine to completely substitute for 1.0 g/kg ethanol may be due to an additional action of PCP and ethanol at another receptor system. Since the dizocilpine data indicate that the inhibition of the NMDA-associated channel is not a prominent discriminative stimulus effect of a low dose of ethanol, the substitution of PCP for 1.0 g/kg ethanol may be due to mutual action at the NMDA receptor channel complex and another receptor system, thereby allowing substitution of PCP for low doses of ethanol.

Administration of the competitive NMDA antagonists CPPene and CGS 19755 resulted in only partial substitution for 1.0 or 1.5 g/kg ethanol. The partial substitution was measured by the percentage of rats tested that met the criteria for substitution (at any dose tested) and by the average group data of response choice. The partial substitution appears to be due to the poor separation between the motor impairing and discriminative stimulus effects of the competitive antagonists which precludes testing higher doses of these antagonists that may result in exclusive ethanol-appropriate responding. The partial substitution data suggests that antagonism of NMDA recognition site is less effective at producing a discriminative stimulus similar to that of ethanol, when compared to effects of the NMDA channel blockers.

REFERENCES

1. WONG, E. H. F. & J. A. KEMP. 1991. Ann. Rev. Pharmacol. Toxicol. **31:** 401–425.
2. LOVINGER, D. M., G. WHITE & F. F. WEIGHT. 1989. Science **243:** 1721–1724.
3. HOFFMAN, P. L., C. S. RABE, F. MOSES & B. TABAKOFF. 1989. J. Neurochem. **52:** 1937–1940.
4. SIMSON, P. E., H. CRISWELL, K. JOHNSON, R. HICKS & G. BREESE. 1991. J. Pharm. Exp. Ther. **257:** 225–231.
5. GRANT, K. A., J. S. KNISELY, B. TABAKOFF, J. E. BARRETT & R. L. BALSTER. 1991. Behav. Pharmacol. **2:** 87–95.

Cocaine-induced Changes in Extracellular Levels of Striatal Dopamine Measured Concurrently by Microdialysis with HPLC-EC and Chronoamperometry

A. COURY,[a] C. D. BLAHA, L. J. ATKINSON,
AND A. G. PHILLIPS

Department of Psychology
University of British Columbia
Vancouver, B.C., Canada V6T 1Z4

INTRODUCTION

The study of the neurochemical effects of drugs of abuse such as cocaine was greatly facilitated by the use of *in vivo* microdialysis. Enhanced levels of dopamine (DA) in the nucleus accumbens and striatum following cocaine are now well established.[1-4] Chronoamperometry is a complementary *in vivo* technique, and its finer temporal resolution may permit better correlation between changes in extracellular DA levels and drug-seeking behavior.[5] In the present study both techniques were used bilaterally in the same brain to monitor dynamic changes in DA levels in the striatum in response to single injections of cocaine-HCl (10 mg/kg i.p.). In addition, levels of DOPAC and HVA were measured in the dialysates.

METHODS AND MATERIALS

Male Long-Evans rats (weight 450 g, $n = 5$, Charles River Canada, Inc., St. Constance, Québec) had a stearate-modified carbon paste electrode chronically implanted into the dorsal striatum and a guide cannula implanted above the contralateral striatum for subsequent insertion of the microdialysis probe. Animals were allowed to recover at least 48 hours prior to the day of the experiment. The stereotaxic coordinates used were: incisor bar, -3.3; chronoamperometry electrode: A/P, $+0.7$; M/L, $±3.3$; D/V, -4.0 (from dura); microdialysis guide cannula: A/P, $+0.7$; M/L, $±3.3$; D/V, -1.0 (from dura).

[a] Author to whom correspondence should be addressed; Tel.: (604) 822-2024; Fax: (604) 822-6923.

Microdialysis

The day before the experiment (18–24 h), the animals were briefly anesthetized with halothane to facilitate manual insertion of the microdialysis probe into the guide cannula at −7.2 mm from dura (4 mm exposed). This post-insertion period greatly reduces the contribution of DA from damaged cells. We have also verified in these conditions that the levels of DA are CA^{++}, TTX, and K^+ dependent. The animal was then placed into a test chamber and connected to a combined liquid swivel and electrical commutator. The probe was flushed overnight at 1.5 μl/min in a physiological perfusate made of 0.01 M sodium phosphate buffer (pH 7.4 with 1.3 mM Ca^{++}). On the day of the experiment, 15 min dialysis samples (1.5 μl/min) were collected and injected manually through an HPLC-EC system.

The dialysis probe has a concentric design consisting of semipermeable membrane (O.D. 340 μm, 60,000–65,000 MW cut-off, Filtral 12, Hospal), a PE50 inlet tubing, a fused silica outlet tubing (75 μm I.D. × 150 μm O.D.) and a 26 g stainless steel cannula. Epoxy (Devcon, 2 ton) was used to seal the joints and plug the dialysis membrane. The inlet tubing was connected to a Harvard 22 syringe pump. A typical *in vitro* recovery at 21 °C (1.5 μl/min) is 30% for DA and 22% for the metabolites.

HPLC-EC

The compounds were separated by microbore reverse chromatography, Beckman column (ODS 5 μm, 15 cm, 2 mm I.D.) using 0.083 M sodium acetate buffer pH 3.5 with 4.2% methanol. The glassy carbon working electrode was set at +0.65 V. The apparatus consisted of Waters 501 HPLC pump, Waters U6K injector and Waters 460 electrochemical detector. The data were analyzed using Maxima software.

Chronoamperometry

Chronoamperometric recordings (1s pulse vs. Ag/AgCl reference electrode) were taken at 30s intervals for the duration of the experiment. Baseline levels were established for both chronoamperometry and microdialysis during the hour prior to drug injection. Recording continued at least 5 hours following injection.

Statistics

Data were analyzed using a one-way analysis of variance with adjusted degrees of freedom (Huynh-Feldt) for using time as a repeated measure. Post-hoc analyses were conducted using the Dunnett test.

DISCUSSION

The present experiment was designed explicitly to compare and contrast measures of cocaine-induced changes in extracellular dopamine levels of the striatum by two *in vivo* analytical techniques, namely microdialysis with HPLC-EC and the electrochem-

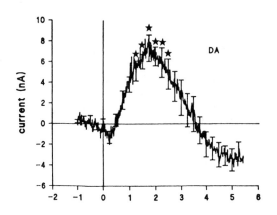

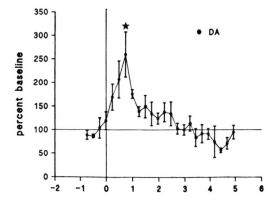

FIGURE 1. Time course of changes in dopamine, DOPAC, and HVA following an injection of cocaine hydrochloride (10 mg/kg i.p.) as measured by chronoamperometry (*upper panel*) or microdialysis (*middle and lower panels*). Data shown are means ± SEM from five rats. Mean basal values measured by HPLC-EC (not adjusted for recovery) were, DA = 1.8 ± 0.52 nM; DOPAC = 0.76 ± 0.16 μM; HVA = 0.36 ± 0.10 μM. * p < .05.

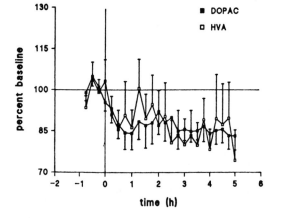

ical procedure of chronoamperometry with catecholamine selective stearate-modified carbon paste electrode.[6] Data obtained with both techniques provided clear evidence for a significant increase in extracellular levels of dopamine. The fact that the dopamine metabolites DOPAC and HVA were slightly attenuated below pre-drug baseline, provides independent confirmation that the stearate-modified electrode can measure the oxidation of dopamine unconfounded by DOPAC oxidation. Together, these two techniques confirm previous reports of cocaine-induced elevation of dopamine in the telencephalon.[1-4]

In addition to the similar qualitative nature of the data provided by microdialysis and chronoamperometry, there are several quantitative differences that are noteworthy. These relate primarily to the time course of the effect of cocaine, in particular the time to peak effect and the duration of action. The change in dopamine levels peaked more quickly when measured by microdialysis. Maximum change was reached in less than 45 min with microdialysis as compared to 100–105 min with chronoamperometry. Estimates of total duration of drug action were shorter with microdialysis than with chronoamperometry. The most probable explanation for these differences may lie in the size of the areas sampled by the two techniques. The microdialysis probe sampled a large cross section of the striatum with a 4 mm region of exposed membrane traversing a dorsal ventral tract. In contrast, the stearate-modified carbon paste electrode, being essentially planar and 200 μm in diameter sampled a much more restricted area of the dorsal striatum. These differences aside, the present findings confirm that both of these *in vivo* techniques can be used fruitfully to study the correlations between drug-induced changes in dopamine levels and behavior, in particular those changes that may accompany self-administration of drugs of abuse such as cocaine.

REFERENCES

1. HURD, Y. L. & U. UNGERSTEDT. 1989. Cocaine: An *in vivo* microdialysis evaluation of its acute action on dopamine transmission in rat striatum. Synapse **3:** 48–54.
2. KALIVAS, P. W., P. DUFFY, L. A. DUMARS & C. SKINNER. 1988. Behavioral and neurochemical effects of acute and daily cocaine administration in rats. J. Pharmacol. Exp. Ther. **245:** 485–492.
3. KALIVAS, P. W. & P. DUFFY. 1990. Effect of acute and daily cocaine treatment on extracellular dopamine in the nucleus accumbens. Synapse **5:** 48–58.
4. PETTIT, H. O., H. T. PAN, L. H. PARSONS & J. B. JUSTICE, JR. 1990. Extracellular concentrations of cocaine and dopamine are enhanced during chronic cocaine administration. J. Neurochem. **55:** 798–804.
5. NG, J. P., G. W. AUBERT & J. B. JUSTICE, JR. 1991. Increased stimulated release and uptake of dopamine in nucleus accumbens after repeated cocaine administration as measured by *in vivo* voltammetry. J. Neurochem. **5:** 1485–1492.
6. BLAHA, C. D. & M. E. JUNG. 1991. Electrochemical evaluation of stearate-modified graphite paste electrodes: Selective detection of dopamine is maintained after exposure to brain tissue. J. Electroanal. Chem. **310:** 317–334.

Behavioral Temperature Regulation during Withdrawal from Ethanol Dependency in Mice[a]

LARRY I. CRAWSHAW, CANDACE S. O'CONNOR,

AND DAVID L. HAYTEAS

Department of Biology and
Environmental Sciences and Resources Program
Portland State University
Portland, Oregon 97207

JOHN C. CRABBE

Veterans Administration Medical Center
Portland, Oregon 97201

Withdrawal reactions following ethanol dependence in humans are marked by definite changes in body temperature. Most patients exhibit hyperthermia, with body temperatures of up to 41°C. Experiments on laboratory rodents have yielded inconsistent results, and it is unclear whether the set-point of body temperature is altered during withdrawal from ethanol (see Kalant and Lê[1] for a literature summary). We herein report a series of experiments in which thermoregulatory variables were continuously monitored during a 24-h period following withdrawal from ethanol dependence.

Male HS mice were habituated to a temperature gradient for several hours and then implanted with intraperitoneal temperature transmitters. After recovery, the mice were exposed to ethanol vapor for 72 h. The ethanol concentration in the air during this period was increased from 4–9 mg·l^{-1}. At time zero, the mice were injected with a pyrazole (68.1 mg·kg^{-1}) and ethanol (1.5 g·kg^{-1}) solution. At 24 and 48 h, the pyrazole alone was administered. Control groups received either pyrazole or saline, but no ethanol vapor. The vapor dosing resulted in blood ethanol concentrations which increased from 0.64 ± 0.09 mg·ml^{-1} after 24 h to 1.89 ± 0.40 mg·ml^{-1} after 72 h. The mice were then placed in the temperature gradient (a submerged tube which was placed in an aquatic temperature gradient) which varied continuously from 10° to 43°C. The selected temperature was quantified by monitoring the position (and thus temperature) of the mice within the tubes. Core temperature was monitored via an antenna which was wrapped around the tube and received the output from the implanted transmitters.

The results of this experiment are depicted in FIGURE 1. The upper graph depicts the internal temperature of the three groups. During the first 10 h after the withdrawal from ethanol vapor, the internal temperatures of the three groups are very similar. The

[a] Supported by National Institute on Alcoholism and Alcohol Abuse Grant AA07592.

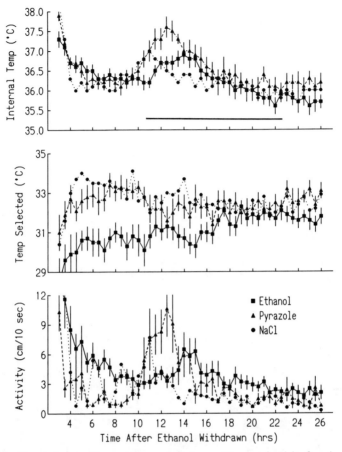

FIGURE 1. Changes in internal temperature, selected temperature, and activity for mice during withdrawal from ethanol dependence. Also shown are data from control mice injected with pyrazole and NaCl. The dark bar in the lower portion of the top graph indicates the period during which it would have been dark in the mouse colony.

selected temperature, however, is lower for the withdrawal group (30.2 ± 1.2°C) than for the saline (34.8 ± 0.6°C) or pyrazole (32.4 ± 0.8°C) controls. During some, but not all, of this period the activity is higher for the ethanol withdrawal group. Increases in activity and internal temperature were seen in all groups after about 10 h in the gradient. These increases corresponded with the usual time when lights were turned off in the mouse room. In a second set of experiments, "lights out" in the mouse room corresponded with the fifteenth hour after withdrawal. In this second group, the increased activity and internal temperature occurred 15 h after withdrawal from ethanol.

These experiments indicate that the regulated temperature is relatively stable during withdrawal from ethanol dependence. The mice undergoing withdrawal, however, select cooler temperatures. This indicates either an increased heat production, a decreased conductance, or both.

REFERENCE

1. KALANT, H. & A. D. Lê. 1984. Effects of ethanol on thermoregulation. Pharmacol. Ther. **23:** 313–364.

Methamphetamine-induced Conditioned Place Preference or Aversion Depending on Dose and Presence of Drug[a]

CHRISTOPHER L. CUNNINGHAM[b]

AND DeCARLO NOBLE

Department of Medical Psychology, L470
The Oregon Health Sciences University
3181 S.W. Sam Jackson Park Road
Portland, Oregon 97201-3098

Methamphetamine (METH) is characterized as having more pronounced central effects and less prominent peripheral actions than amphetamine.[1] Although METH is widely abused, the literature currently offers inconsistent evidence of its reinforcing efficacy in animals. For example, METH has been reported to have equivocal reinforcing properties as determined in IV self-administration studies.[2] In place conditioning studies, METH has been shown to have rewarding effects,[3] aversive effects or no effect.[4] The present experiments were designed to provide more information on the motivational properties of METH in the place conditioning paradigm using an inbred mouse strain known to be sensitive to the rewarding properties of morphine and ethanol.

METHOD AND RESULTS

The apparatus had two distinctive, interchangeable floor textures (grid or hole). After an habituation session (paper floor), DBA/2J mice were exposed to a differential conditioning procedure. One floor stimulus (CS+) was paired with IP injection of METH (0–16 mg/kg), whereas the other floor stimulus (CS−) was paired with saline. At each dose, one group received grid paired with METH and hole paired with saline (G+/H−); these contingencies were reversed for a second group (G−/H+) (n = 12–14/group). Dose 0 mice received saline on both floors. CS+ and CS− trials were given on alternate days and each trial lasted 15 min (total of 4 trials of each type). Experiments concluded with a preference test (without drug) in which the floor of the apparatus was half grid and half hole (position counterbalanced). In the second experi-

[a] This research was supported in part by NIAAA grant AA07468 awarded to C. Cunningham and NIDA Contract 271-90-7405 awarded to John Belknap.

[b] Author to whom correspondence should be addressed; Tel.: (503) 494-8464; Fax: (503) 494-6877.

TABLE 1. Mean Seconds per Minute (± SEM) Spent on Grid Floor during 30-min Preference Test

Experiment 1: Saline Test	± Methamphetamine Dose (mg/kg)				
	0	2	4	8	16ᵃ
Conditioning Group					
Grid + METH (G+/H−)	29.0 (3.8)	32.3 (3.2)	24.9 (1.8)	27.1 (2.8)	24.4 (1.9)
Grid + Saline (G−/H+)		30.9 (3.8)	26.6 (3.4)	33.9 (2.5)	32.9 (3.4)

Experiment 2: Saline Test	+ Methamphetamine Dose (mg/kg)					
	0	0.25	0.5ᵃ	1.0	2.0	8.0
Conditioning Group						
Grid + METH (G+/H−)	29.2 (3.0)	28.7 (3.3)	32.3 (2.1)	28.4 (1.9)	29.2 (3.7)	27.3 (2.2)
Grid + Saline (G−/H+)		21.9 (3.3)	21.3 (2.1)	32.4 (3.5)	33.5 (2.6)	31.5 (2.2)

Experiment 2: METH Test	+ Methamphetamine Dose (mg/kg)					
	0	0.25	0.5	1.0	2.0	8.0ᵃ
Conditioning Group						
Grid + METH (G+/H−)	29.5 (2.7)	31.3 (2.0)	26.4 (1.8)	23.9 (1.6)	21.6 (2.6)	14.7 (2.1)
Grid + Saline (G−/H+)		26.8 (3.1)	32.1 (3.0)	27.6 (2.9)	26.7 (3.1)	33.1 (2.2)

ᵃ Difference significant, $p < 0.05$, between conditioning groups at specified dose.

ment, a second preference test was given several days later after administration of METH at the conditioning dose. Test data were analyzed by comparing the amount of time (sec/min) spent on the grid floor by mice in the two conditioning groups at each dose.

METH evoked a dose-dependent increase in activity that was enhanced by repeated conditioning trials (data not shown). Preference test results are shown in TABLE 1. In saline tests, conditioned place preference was observed in mice conditioned with 0.5 mg/kg ($F[1,26] = 13.5$), whereas conditioned place aversion was evident at 16 mg/kg ($F[1,25] = 4.7$). No place conditioning was found in intermediate dose groups tested without drug. However, in tests with drug, reliable conditioned place aversion was seen at 8 mg/kg ($F[1,26] = 35.9$). Conditioned place preference was not observed at any dose during tests with drug.

DISCUSSION

Overall, these data suggest that METH has bivalent dose-dependent hedonic effects that are rewarding at low doses and aversive at high doses. Although no place conditioning was observed at intermediate doses in tests after saline, conditioned aversion was seen at 8 mg/kg when drug was present. The latter finding may be due either to associative or nonassociative processes. For example, it may be that interoceptive drug stimuli were a critical component of the CS associated with the drug's effect during conditioning; in the absence of drug, tactile floor cues may have been unable to activate the association with the drug's negative effects. Alternatively, drug may have augmented expression of conditioned aversion by providing an aversive source of motivation during testing. In other words, drug-induced dysphoria may have increased the difference in the hedonic values of the floor stimuli controlling spatial preference.

REFERENCES

1. HOFFMAN, B. B. & R. J. LEFKOWITZ. 1990. *In* Goodman and Gilman's The Pharmacological Basis of Therapeutics. A. G. Goodman, T. W. Wall, A. S. Niles & P. Taylor, Eds., 187–220. Pergamon Press. New York, NY.
2. YOKEL, R. A. 1987. *In* Methods of Assessing the Reinforcing Properties of Drugs. M. A. Bozarth, Ed., 1–33. Springer-Verlag. New York, NY.
3. DUNCAN, P. M., K. SAUNDERS & P. BYERLY. 1983. Soc. Neurosci. Abstr. **9**: 1146.
4. MARTIN, J. C. & E. H. ELLINWOOD. 1974. Psychopharmacologia (Berl.) **36**: 323–335.

Cocaine and Other Local Anesthetics Block Hippocampal Long-term Potentiation

T. V. DUNWIDDIE[a]

Department of Pharmacology, Box C236
University of Colorado Health Sciences Center
Denver, Colorado 80262

Veterans Administration Medical Center
4200 E. Ninth Avenue
Denver, Colorado 80262

D. SMITH

Neuroscience Program, Sperry Hall
Oberlin College
Oberlin, Ohio 44074

Considering the extensive research investigating the role of the catecholamines and particularly amphetamine's effects on learning and memory,[1-6] surprisingly little attention has been paid to the effects of a related psychomotor stimulant, cocaine. Because so little is known concerning the actions of cocaine on memory, we have investigated the effects of cocaine on hippocampal long-term potentiation (LTP), a putative learning mechanism by which information might be stored in the hippocampal formation. We studied LTP in transverse slices of rat hippocampus using standard electrophysiological recording techniques.[7] Extracellular recordings of population spikes in the CA1 regions were obtained using single barrel glass microelectrodes; responses were evoked by orthodromic stimulation of the Schaffer collateral and commissural afferents. All drugs were bath applied at known concentrations.

When slices were superfused with 30 μM cocaine for 10 min before a high frequency train of stimulation, LTP (measured 15 min post-train) was completely inhibited. FIGURE 1A illustrates averaged responses in a control slice, and in a slice that was treated with cocaine; FIGURE 1B illustrates mean data for all the slices treated with similar protocols. As can be seen, the short-term increase in the population spike response (termed post-tetanic potentiation, or PTP) was unaffected, but the potentiation in the cocaine-pretreated slice decayed back to control levels over the next 15–20 min.

In order to determine the mechanism underlying this effect of cocaine, we investigated the effects of a variety of agents that share some but not all of the pharmacological properties of cocaine. Other local anesthetic drugs (procaine, lidocaine) were

---

[a] Author to whom correspondence should be addressed at the Department of Pharmacology; Tel.: (303) 270-4222; Fax: (303) 270-7097.

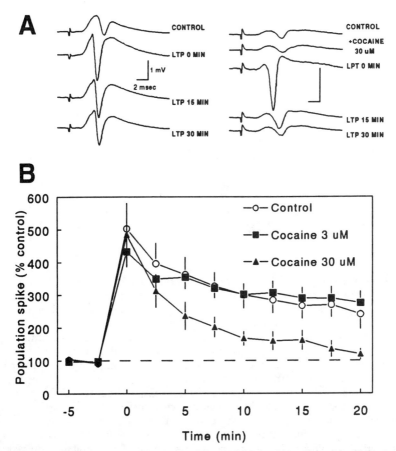

FIGURE 1. Effects of cocaine on electrically elicited LTP in the CA1 region of the hippocampal slice. **A** shows representative evoked potentials illustrating LTP in a control slice (*left*) and in a slice pretreated with 30 μM cocaine (*right*). Each trace is an average of 2–4 responses and shows the responses prior to the tetanizing stimulus (Control), immediately after stimulation (0 Min), and 15 and 30 minutes after tetanizing stimulation. In the cocaine condition (*right*), the second response (+Cocaine 30 μM) shows the change in the potential following 10 min of superfusion with 30 μM cocaine. **B** illustrates the effects of 3 and 30 μM cocaine on LTP. Cocaine was added to the perfusion medium 10 minutes before the delivery of the high frequency train and remained during the 20 minutes following stimulation. While 30 μM cocaine effectively blocked LTP, it had no effect on the initial PTP. Cocaine concentrations of 3 μM or less were ineffective in blocking LTP. Each point is the mean ± SEM for 20 slices (control) or 12 slices (3 and 30 μM cocaine).

also able to block LTP, but amphetamine did not (FIG. 2), suggesting that effects on catecholamine systems were unlikely to be important. However, concentrations of cocaine that were effective in blocking LTP had little effect upon evoked potentials; that is, they occurred in a range where local anesthetic effects were not particularly prominent. To determine whether local anesthetic effects *per se* were responsible for the block of LTP, we investigated the effects of cocaine on LTP_K, which is induced by su-

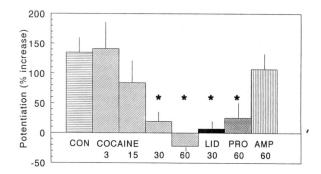

FIGURE 2. Bar graph showing the effects of cocaine, lidocaine (LID), procaine (PRO) and d-amphetamine (AMP) on LTP measured 20 minutes following a 100 Hz train of stimulation (n = 10 slices per condition). The drugs were superfused for 10 min prior to the stimulation train, and the concentrations are indicated below the bars in micromolar; * indicates treatments significantly different ($p < .05$) from the control (CON) condition.

perfusion with increased K^+ and tetraethylammonium (TEA)[8]; this treatment results in a significant and persistent increase in the population spike without requiring any electrical stimulation to elicit the potentiated response. Cocaine also blocked this form of LTP (potentiation was 113 ± 41% in controls, 13 ± 18% in 30 μM cocaine, $p <$ 0.05). These experiments suggested that cocaine was not blocking LTP because of its actions on electrical activity (*i.e.*, because of its local anesthetic actions), but rather because it was disrupting the biochemical mechanisms that underlie LTP. A likely hypothesis is suggested by the previous observations that a variety of local anesthetics are calmodulin (CaM) antagonists (*i.e.*, they inhibit CaM-stimulated calcium transport in erythrocytes[9]), and that CaM inhibitors such as trifluoperazine, calmidazolium, pimozide, block high frequency and calcium-induced LTP.[10,11]

At present, we think that the most likely possibility is that cocaine, like other local anesthetics, can block CaM activity and thereby reduce LTP by inhibiting the activity of CaM-dependent kinase which is thought to be essential in LTP. However, direct studies of the effects of cocaine on CaM and CaM-kinase will be essential to determine whether this is the case.

REFERENCES

1. Doty, B. & L. A. Doty. 1966. Psychopharmacologia 9: 234.
2. Krivanek, J. & J. L. McGaugh. 1969. Agents Actions 1: 36.
3. Evangelista, A. M. & L. Izquierdo. 1971. Psychopharmacologia 20: 42.
4. Delanoy, R. L., D. L. Tucci & P. E. Gold. 1982. Pharmacol. Biochem. Behav. 18: 137.
5. Gold, P. E. & S. F. Zornetzer. 1983. Behav. Neural. Biol. 38: 151.
6. Morimoto, K., S. Otani & G. V. Goddard. 1987. Brain Res. 407: 137.
7. Dunwiddie, T. & G. Lynch. 1978. J. Physiol. 226: 353.
8. Aniksztejn, L. & Y. Ben-Ari. 1991. Nature 349: 67.
9. Volpi, M., R. I. Sha'afi & M. B. Feinstein. 1981. Mol. Pharmacol. 20: 363.
10. Finn, R. C., M. Browning & G. Lynch. 1980. Neurosci. Lett. 19: 103.
11. Dunwiddie, T. V., N. L. Roberson & T. Worth. 1982. Pharmacol. Biochem. Behav. 17: 1257.

Effect of a Benzodiazepine Derivate Ro 15-4513 on Ethanol-Free Selection and CNS Mitochondrial Energetics in Rats

ENRIQUE EGAÑA, ANTONIO SALINAS,
AND MARÍA TERESA RAMIREZ

Faculty of Medicine
Institute of Experimental Medicine
Laboratory of Neurochemistry
University of Chile
Santiago 7, Chile

Ro 15-4513, a benzodiazepine (BDZ) partial inverse agonist, was studied using many parameters of its inhibition of the ethanol (EtOH) effect. It presumes that these effects, including the psychomotor, are partially due to alteration of the GABA/BDZ/Cl⁻ complex. The inhibitory actions were realized when the rats were injected with a fixed EtOH dose. The appetite for EtOH and sexual differences as well as effects on CNS mitochondrial energetics were not noticed.[1-7] The aims proposed for this study are as follows: 1) to study the Ro 15-4513 effect on the EtOH appetite in E.F.S. experiments; 2) to study the mitochondrial energetics of the CNS, particularly in areas involved in CNS EtOH metabolism, *i.e.*, neurochemical mechanisms related to "voluntary" intake and its ratio: e⁻ transport and oxidative phosphorylation (ADP/O).

MATERIALS AND METHODS

E.F.S. adult Wistar rats of both sexes treated separately were used ($n = 87$). Fluid intake was H_2O, and 3%, 12%, 18% and 25% EtOH solutions; daily intake was mea-

TABLE 1. Ro 15-4513 Effects on EtOH Intake in Male and Female Rats: Ethanol-Free Selection Experiments

	♂		♀	
Control E.F.S.	0.65 ± 0.02	} $p < 0.01$	0.85 ± 0.07	} $p < 0.009$
Plus Ro 15-4513	0.45 ± 0.03		0.43 ± 0.02	

E.F.S. comparison between control and Ro 15-4513 both sexes; males receive 10 mg and females 15 mg/kg rat/24 h, p.o. for 50 days. Number of rats (both sexes): each group 36. E.F.S. previous 50–60 days and EtOH plus Ro 15-4513 50 days. Ro 15-4513 showed maximum inhibition of EtOH intake at 10 mg in males and at 15 mg in females, respectively. Doses of 5, 10, and 15 mg were also studied in both sexes. Differences between normal and drug-treated animals were significant in both sexes.

TABLE 2. CNS (Hypothalamus) Mitochondrial Energetics: Electron Transport and Oxidative Phosphorylation (ADP/O) – Effect of Ro 15-4513

	Ethanol Free Selection Electron Transport				Oxidative Phosphorylation (ADP/O)		
	Control	Plus Ro 15-4513	p		Control	Plus Ro 15-4513	p
SITE I Glutamate/malate	132.5 ± 26.3	20.0 ± 1.5	<0.0025	♂	2.91 ± 0.08	2.40 ± 0.27	N.S.
SITE I Pyruvate/malate	87.7 ± 9.1	23.0 ± 0.7	<0.005		2.81 ± 0.25	2.50 ± 0.46	N.S.
SITE II Succinate	109.0 ± 15.2	21.1 ± 3.5	<0.05		2.0 ± 0.0	2.61 ± 0.57	N.S.
SITE I Glutamate/malate	92.2 ± 30.4	11.2 ± 7.1	<0.61	♀	2.15 ± 0.56	1.90 ± 1.05	N.S.
SITE I Pyruvate/malate	80.0 ± 26.9	11.0 ± 6.0	<0.60		2.14 ± 0.50	0.95 ± 0.76	N.S.
SITE II Succinate	86.4 ± 31.0	12.3 ± 8.0	<0.04		1.6 ± 0.03	0.71 ± 0.30	N.S.

General experimental protocol as in TABLE 1. Dose of Ro 15-4513 in males 10 mg and in females 15 mg. Electron transport was measured with a polarigraph (Gilson) expressed as nanoatom oxygen/mg mitochondrial protein/min. Oxidative phosphorylation (ADP/O) was measured in the presence of ADP 184 nM in the incubation media. The Site I substrates contained 10 mM glutamate/2 mM malate; pyruvate/malate in identical concentrations; Site II substrate was 10 mM succinate.

sured during the 50 days previous to treatment to compare to Ro 15-4513; treatment was for 40–60 days. Three groups received 5, 10 and 15 mg/kg rat/24 h (δ and $\female$). Mitochondrial energetics were studied in brain cortex, hypothalamus, and cerebellum. Mitochondria were prepared by fractionated centrifugation using the Crompton incubation medium. Electron transport was measured through O_2 uptake and expressed as nanoatom oxygen/mg mitochondrial protein/min. Site I substrates contained 10 mM glutamate/2 mM malate and pyruvate/malate in identical concentrations. The site II substrate was 10 mM succinate.

RESULTS

TABLE 1 shows the effects of Ro 15-4513 on E.F.S. and TABLE 2 shows the effects on hypothalamus mitochondrial energetics and ADP/O. Results on other areas of the CNS will be published elsewhere.

DISCUSSION

E.F.S. allows the study of: 1) Selective EtOH intake at several concentrations. The females were stronger drinkers than males which presumes a relationship with hypothalamus/pituitary/gonad (HPG) function as a drug collateral action; higher inhibitions were seen in males 10 mg vs. females 15 mg/kg rat/24 h. 2) Mitochondrial studies showed inhibition in E.F.S. electron transport; the ADP/O was not affected, *i.e.*, there was an uncoupled effect. Damage to the receptor-ligands of the GABA-BDZ-Cl$^-$ complex at cytoplasmatic (and mitochondrial) membranes is postulated as the cellular and molecular mechanism of Ro 15-4513 activity in CNS.

SUMMARY

1) Females are higher EtOH drinkers than males in E.F.S. experiments in rats. 2) Ro 15-4513 inhibited intake of EtOH. 3) Hypothalamus mitochondrial energetics, studied at Sites I and II, showed Ro 15-4513 inhibition of these parameters at different doses by sex: effects were seen in females at 15 mg and in males at 10 mg/kg rat/24 h. An uncoupled effect between electron transport and ADP/O was found.

ACKNOWLEDGMENT

We are grateful to the Research Laboratory of Hoffmann-La Roche, Basel, Switzerland, for the donation of the drug used in this research.

REFERENCES

1. GILL III, T. J., G. J. SMITH, R. W. WISSLER & K. W. KUNZ. 1989. The rat as an experimental animal. Science **245**: 269–276.
2. POLC, P. 1985. Interactions of partial inverse benzodiazepine agonist Ro 15-4513 and FG 7142 with ethanol in rats and cats. Br. J. Pharmacol. Proc. (Suppl.) **86**: 465.

3. BONETTI, E. P., W. P. BURKARD, M. GABL & H. MÖHLER. 1985. The partial inverse ben-zodiazepine agonist Ro 15-4513 antagonizes acute ethanol effects in mice and rats. Br. J. Pharmacol. Proc. (Suppl.) **86:** 463.
4. KOCH, H. P. 1988. The story of the anti-alcohol drug Ro 15-4513. Int. Pharmacy J. **2**(3): 3.
5. SUZDAK, P. D., J. R. GLOWA, J. N. CRAWLEY, R. D. SCHWARTZ, P. SKOLNICK & S. M. PAUL. 1986. A selective imidazobenzodiazepine antagonist of ethanol in the rat. Science **234:** 1243–1247.
6. BRITTON, K. T., C. L. EHLERS & G. F. KOOB. 1988. Is ethanol antagonist Ro 15-4513 se-lective for ethanol? Science **239:** 648–650.
7. SALINAS, A., R. CAVIEDES, O. ABARCA, L. HIDALGO & E. EGAÑA. 1989. Efecto sobre el apetito por etanol (EtOH de un benzodiazepina-derivado el Ro 15-4513 estudio de se-lección libre de etanol (S.L.E.). Arch. Biol. Med. Exp. **22**(4): R-432.

Effects of Chronic Ethanol Administration on Neurotensinergic Processes: Correlations with Tolerance in LS and SS Mice[a]

V. GENE ERWIN, A. D. CAMPBELL,
AND R. RADCLIFFE

Alcohol Research Center, School of Pharmacy
University of Colorado
Boulder, Colorado 80309-0297

Recent studies have shown that acute ethanol administration produces a dose-dependent decrease in neurotensin-immunoreactivity (NT-ir) levels in several brain regions of LS/Ibg (LS) and SS/Ibg (SS) mice.[1] These mice, selectively bred for differential sensitivity to ethanol, differ in brain NT receptor densities, suggesting that ethanol actions are mediated, in part, by neurotensinergic systems.[2,3] The present study examined the effects of chronic ethanol intake on NT levels and receptors. LS and SS mice were required to consume ethanol solutions (10% v/v for 4 days and 15% thereafter) in lieu of water; all animals received lab chow, *ad libitum*. Chronic ethanol consumption (ca. 15 g/kg/24 h) caused a marked tolerance to locomotor inhibitory and hypothermic (data not shown) effects of ethanol in LS mice, with maximum tolerance obtained after two weeks of treatment (FIG. 1). In chronically treated SS mice low-dose ethanol activation appeared to be increased; however, there was clear tolerance to ethanol-induced locomotor inhibition produced by higher doses of ethanol in these mice. Time-courses for acquisition and decay of tolerance were similar in LS and SS mice with return to control sensitivity complete in approximately 14 days after withdrawal (FIG. 1). Chronic ethanol treatment increased NT-ir levels up to 100% in nucleus accumbens and caudate putamen (data not shown), with maximum increases achieved after two weeks. The time-course for return of NT-ir levels to control values paralleled the time-course for disappearance in tolerance (FIG. 1). Binding characteristics for the high (NT$_H$)- and low (NT$_L$)-affinity NT receptors were markedly altered by chronic ethanol intake with apparent changes in K_d and B_{max} values as shown by Scatchard analyses (data not shown). Chronic ethanol treatment caused NT binding in ventral midbrain and entorhinal cortex to shift from a two-site binding model to a one-site model. ^{3}H-Neurotensin binding in the presence and absence of levocabastine, an inhibitor of low-affinity receptors, revealed that binding capacities as well as affinities were altered by chronic ethanol (FIG. 2). Receptor binding characteristics returned to control values in parallel with the disappearance of tolerance to ethanol. These results show that neuroadaptation to chronic ethanol exposure includes parallel

[a] This work was supported in part by USPHS Grants AA00079, AA07330, and AA03527.

441

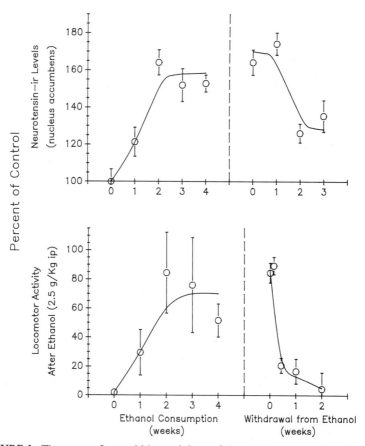

FIGURE 1. Time course for acquisition and decay of chronic tolerance to ethanol and corresponding changes in NT-ir levels in nucleus accumbens of LS mice. Mice were chronically treated with ethanol solutions for times indicated and as described in the text. After two weeks of chronic treatment mice were withdrawn at times indicated, then sacrificed, brains dissected and placed immediately in 0.01 N HCL. NT-ir was extracted and levels determined by specific radioimmunoassays as previously described.[1] NT-ir levels in control mice were 120.0 + 8.2 ng/g NA tissue. Separate groups of mice received ethanol (2 g/kg, i.p.) at times indicated and locomotor activity was measured as described previously (Erwin *et al.* 1990. Alcoholism: Clin. Exp. Res. **14**: 200–204). Locomotor activities in control mice were 2071 + 426 cm traveled/10 min.

changes in NT-ir levels and receptors. We propose that increased NT-ir levels may be caused by ethanol-induced increases in NT release in mesolimbic and striatal dopaminergic terminal fields, thus increasing NT synthesis and turnover. Prolonged increase in NT levels and turnover might produce the observed down-regulation of NT receptors. These results support the hypothesis that neurotensinergic processes mediate chronic as well as acute effects of ethanol.

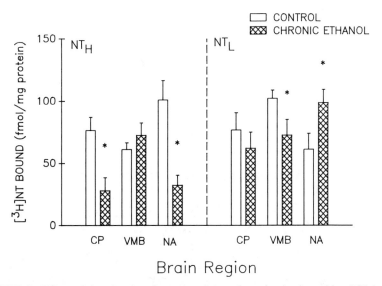

FIGURE 2. Effects of chronic ethanol consumption on levocabastine-insensitive (NT_H) and levocabastine-sensitive (NT_L) neurotensin-binding capacities in brain regions from LS mice. Mice were chronically treated with ethanol as described in FIG. 1. Homogenates from each dissected region were prepared, membranes isolated and specific [³H]-NT binding in the absence or presence of 0.05 mM levocabastine was performed as described previously[2] (also Kitabgi *et al.* 1970. Proc. Natl. Acad. Sci. USA 74: 1846–1850).

REFERENCES

1. ERWIN, V. G., B. C. JONES & R. RADCLIFFE. 1990. Low doses of ethanol reduce neurotensin levels in discrete brain regions from LS/Ibg and SS/Ibg mice. Alcoholism: Clin. Exp. Res. 14: 42–47.
2. ERWIN, V. G. & A. KORTE. 1988. Brain neurotensin receptors in mice bred for differences in sensitivity to ethanol. Alcohol 5: 195–201.
3. CAMPBELL, A. D. & V. G. ERWIN. 1991. Regional characterization of brain neurotensin receptor subtypes in LS and SS mice. Alcoholism: Clin. Exp. Res. 15: 1011–1017.

Sensitization and Individual Differences to IP Amphetamine, Cocaine, or Caffeine following Repeated Intra-cranial Amphetamine Infusions

M. S. HOOKS,[a] G. H. JONES,[b] B. J. LIEM,
AND J. B. JUSTICE, JR.

Department of Chemistry
Emory University
1515 Pierce Drive
Atlanta, Georgia 30322

The response to novelty has been shown to be predictive of both the initial locomotor response to amphetamine[3,6] (AMPH) and the rate at which rats sensitize to low locomotor–producing doses of the drug.[1,3] Subjects who show a high locomotor response in a novel environment (high responders: HR) show a larger initial locomotor response to AMPH and develop locomotor sensitization more rapidly following repeated AMPH than subjects who have a low locomotor response to a novel environment (low responders: LR). Recent evidence from our laboratory[2,3] and others[7] have suggested this may be due to differences in the reactivity of the mesolimbic dopamine system. For example, HR rats exhibit larger increases in extracellular dopamine in the nucleus accumbens (NACC) than LR rats following cocaine administration.[2] In addition, HR rats show a higher turnover in the NACC and medial frontal cortex (MFC) dopamine following exposure to novelty.[7] Repeated systemic administration of AMPH not only results in behavioral sensitization[9] including increased levels of locomotor activity and more intense behavioral stereotypies, including sniffing and biting, but also leads to increased levels of extracellular dopamine in the NACC.[8] In addition, repeated infusions of AMPH into the ventral tegmental area (VTA), the location of the dopamine cell bodies of the mesolimbic pathway, also produce an increased locomotor response to subsequent systemic administration of AMPH.[4] These findings suggest that changes in the mesolimbic dopamine projection play a role in AMPH sensitization and that variations in the activity of this system may also be responsible for individual differences in both the initial response[2,6] and the sensitization[1,3] to psychomotor stimulants.

[a] Author to whom correspondence should be addressed; Tel.: (404) 727-2629; Fax: (404) 727-3157.
[b] *Present address:* Department of Neuropsychopharmacology, Schering AG, Postfach 650311, D-1000 Berlin 65, Germany.

In the current experiment bilateral stainless-steel guide cannulae (22-gauge) were implanted to access either the NACC, AP +3.4 from bregma, Lat ±1.7, Vert −3.5 from dura with the incisor bar set at +5 mm; the VTA, AP −3.2, Lat ±0.5, Vert −7.6 from dura with the incisor bar set at +5 mm and the cannulae rotated 10°; or the MFC, AP +4.5, Lat ±0.7, Vert −1.0 from dura with incisor bar set at 5 mm.[5] Two days before the initial drug treatment, subjects were placed in individual photocell cages for a 3-h period. Subjects were divided into HR or LR based on whether their locomotor activity scores for the first hour were above or below the median locomotor activity for the subject sample.[1-3] Rats were assigned to one of two drug groups to receive repeated bilateral administration of either 0.0 or 3.0 μg/side of *d*-AMPH. Subjects were not tested the day before the initial drug treatment. On test days 1, 3, and 5 the rats were placed in the photocell cage for a 1.5-h habituation period prior to drug administration. Locomotor activity was measured for an additional 2 h after each infusion. On test days 2 and 4 animals received the appropriate dose of intra-cranial AMPH in the home cage to minimize possible environmental conditioning. On test day 9 all rats were administered IP 1 mg/kg of AMPH. All rats received 15 mg/kg of cocaine IP in the test-cage on test day 13. Rats received IP 20 mg/kg of caffeine in

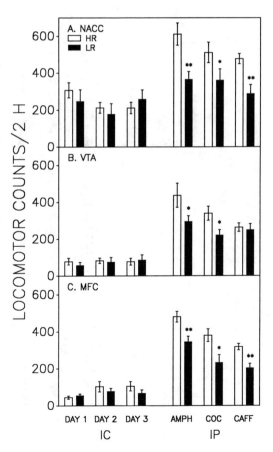

FIGURE 1. Comparison of HR and LR rats treated with 3.0 μg/side AMPH in the NACC, VTA or MFC and subsequent IP response to AMPH, cocaine and caffeine. Each group contained 9–10 subjects. No differences were observed between HR and LR rats following AMPH infusions into any of the three regions. HR NACC cannulated rats showed a greater locomotor activity to IP administered AMPH ($p <$ 0.0025), cocaine ($p < 0.05$), and caffeine ($p < 0.005$) than LR rats. In addition, HR VTA cannulated rats displayed greater locomotor activity compared to LR rats following IP administered AMPH ($p < 0.025$) and cocaine ($p < 0.01$). A Novelty × Time interaction was observed after caffeine ($p < 0.005$). HR MFC cannulated rats also exhibited a greater locomotor activity to IP administered AMPH ($p < 0.0025$), cocaine ($p < 0.01$) and caffeine ($p < 0.0005$) than LR rats. IP administered saline did not produce a difference between HR and LR rats in any of the regions. * $p < 0.05$, ** $p < 0.005$.

the test-cage on test day 17. Doses of drugs were chosen to produce roughly the same level of locomotor activity. All subjects received 0.9% saline (1 ml/kg) on test days 7, 11, and 15 in the test cage. No testing was performed on subjects on days 6, 8, 10, 12, 14, and 16.

As shown in FIGURE 1 no differences were observed between HR and LR rats following AMPH infusions into either the MFC, NACC, or VTA. However, there was a significant correlation between the locomotor response to novelty and the locomotor response to the initial treatment with intra-NACC AMPH. HR rats showed greater locomotor activity compared to LR rats following either IP AMPH, cocaine, or caffeine following AMPH pretreatment in either the NACC, MFC, or the VTA (FIG. 1). Repeated infusions of AMPH into the VTA increased the locomotor response to both IP AMPH and cocaine, but not to IP caffeine, while repeated infusions of AMPH into the NACC or MFC had no effect on locomotor response to any drug subsequently administered IP (FIG. 2).

In summary, the current experiment has demonstrated dissociations between the locomotor stimulating properties of AMPH infused directly into discrete regions of the mesolimbic dopamine system and sensitization to peripheral administration of var-

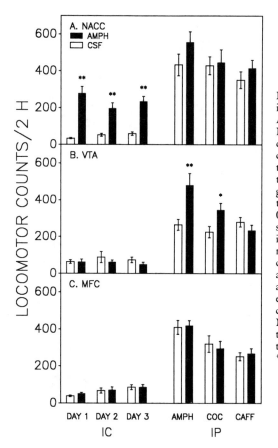

FIGURE 2. Comparison of rats infused with either 3.0 μg/side AMPH or CSF directly in the NACC, VTA or MFC and subsequent IP response to AMPH, cocaine and caffeine. Each group contained 18–20 rats. Infusions into the NACC of AMPH produced a greater amount of locomotor activity than CSF infusions ($p < 0.0001$) while no effect was observed after VTA or MFC AMPH infusions. While previous treatment with AMPH in the VTA increased locomotor response to IP administered AMPH ($p < 0.005$) and cocaine ($p < 0.025$), it had no effect on the locomotor response to caffeine. AMPH infusions in the NACC and MFC had no effect on the subsequent locomotor response to AMPH, cocaine or caffeine. * $p < 0.05$, ** $p < 0.005$.

ious locomotor stimulating drugs. Repeated infusions of AMPH into the NACC while producing profound increases in locomotor activity did not alter the subsequent response to systemically administered AMPH, cocaine, or caffeine. On the other hand, infusions of AMPH into the VTA which did not elicit increases in locomotor activity enhanced the subsequent locomotor activity response to both IP AMPH and cocaine. However, these VTA infusions did not alter the locomotor stimulating properties of IP caffeine which, in contrast to those of AMPH and cocaine, are not dependent on dopaminergic mechanisms of the NACC. Repeated infusions of AMPH into the MFC did not increase locomotor activity and did not affect the subsequent response to IP AMPH, cocaine, or caffeine.

The present results also indicate that the locomotor response to AMPH, cocaine, and caffeine can be predicted from the responsiveness to a novel environment. This effect does not seem to be dependent on one region of the mesolimbic dopamine system as pre-treatment with AMPH in either the VTA, NACC, or MFC, by enlarge, did not affect the individual differences in the response to IP administration of these locomotor stimulating drugs. Also, the response to novelty did not as readily predict the response to central administered AMPH. These data together with previous findings[2,3,7] show the lack of localization to one region of the mesolimbic dopamine pathway of individual differences in the response to psychomotor stimulants. Of course, it is likely that other neural systems may also contribute to the vulnerability of individuals to drugs of abuse.

REFERENCES

1. HOOKS, M. S., G. H. JONES, A. D. SMITH, D. B. NEILL & J. B. JUSTICE, JR. 1991. Pharmacol. Biochem. Behav. **38:** 467–470.
2. HOOKS, M. S., G. H. JONES, A. D. SMITH, D. B. NEILL & J. B. JUSTICE, JR. 1991. Synapse **9:** 121–128.
3. HOOKS, M. S., G. H. JONES, D. B. NEILL & J. B. JUSTICE, JR. 1992. Pharmacol. Biochem. Behav. **41:** 203–210.
4. KALIVAS, P. W. & B. WEBER. 1988. J. Pharmacol. Exp. Ther. **245:** 1095–1102.
5. PELLEGRINO, L. J., A. S. PELLEGRINO & A. J. CUSHMAN. 1979. A Stereotaxic Atlas of the Rat Brain. Plenum Press. New York.
6. PIAZZA, P. V., J. M. DEMINIERE, M. LE MOAL & H. SIMON. 1989. Science **29:** 1511–1513.
7. PIAZZA, P. V., F. ROGUE-PONT, J. M. DEMINIERE, M. KHAROUBY, M. LE MOAL & H. SIMON. 1990. Soc. Neurosci. Abstr. **243**.14.
8. ROBINSON, T. E., P. A. JURSON, J. A. BENNETT & K. M. BENTGEN. 1988. Brain Res. **462:** 211–222.
9. SEGAL, D. S. 1975. *In* Advances in Biochemical Psychopharmacology, Vol. 13. A. J. Mandell, Ed.: 247–266. Raven Press. New York.

Solubilization of the Cannabinoid Receptor from Rat Brain Membranes[a]

DEVIN B. HOUSTON AND ALLYN C. HOWLETT

Department of Pharmacological & Physiological Science
Saint Louis University Medical Center
St. Louis, Missouri 63104

The psychoactive component of marihuana, Δ^9-THC, and its highly potent analogs interact with the cannabinoid receptor in rat brain.[1] The cannabinoid receptor is coupled to the G protein G_i to inhibit adenylate cyclase activity in brain and neuronal cells.[2] As a first step in the purification of the cannabinoid receptor, we have solubilized the receptor from rat forebrain membranes using the zwitterionic detergent 3-[(3-cholamidopropyl)dimethylammonio]-1-propane sulfonate (CHAPS).

METHODS

Optimal solubilization is obtained with a detergent:protein ratio of 0.5 in the presence of 10 mM $MgCl_2$ for 30 min in the cold followed by a 5-min exposure to ice-cold petroleum ether. Subsequent centrifugation and aspiration of the aqueous layer yields cannabinoid-binding activity that is not reduced by filtration through a 0.2 μ filter. The soluble receptor is assayed in a manner similar to that described previously for membranes using the radioligand [^{3}H]CP-55940.[1] Bound and free radioligand were separated by filtration on individual 4 ml Sephadex G-50 columns. Void volumes containing ligand-bound receptor were collected for liquid scintillation counting.

RESULTS AND CONCLUSIONS

Binding of [^{3}H]CP-55940 to the solubilized cannabinoid receptor is saturable and reaches equilibrium within 90 min under the described conditions. A comparison of Scatchard analyses performed on membrane- and soluble-receptor binding reveal comparable affinities for [^{3}H]CP-55940, indicating that the solubilized receptor is similar to that in membranes in its ligand associative properties (FIG. 1). The solubilized receptor retains high-affinity agonist binding as evidenced by heterologous competition assays using the cannabinoid desacetyllevonantradol (DALN) (FIG. 2), exhibiting a K_i comparable to that for the membrane-bound receptor. Pharmacologically, the

[a] Research for this paper was supported by USPHS Grants R01-DA03690, R01-DA06312, and T32-NS07254.

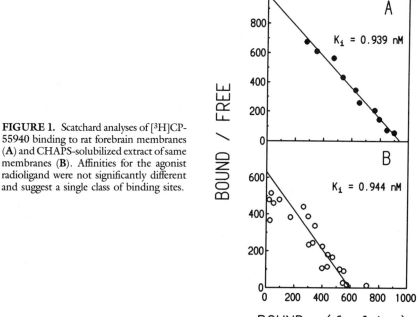

FIGURE 1. Scatchard analyses of [3H]CP-55940 binding to rat forebrain membranes (**A**) and CHAPS-solubilized extract of same membranes (**B**). Affinities for the agonist radioligand were not significantly different and suggest a single class of binding sites.

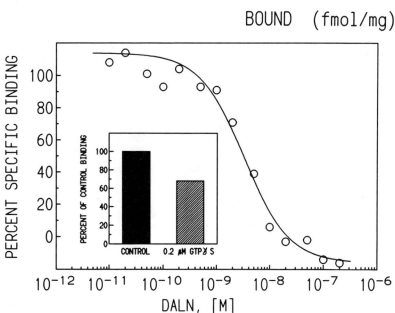

FIGURE 2. The agonist ligand desacetyllevonantradol (DALN) competes with [3H]CP-55940 in a dose-dependent manner for binding to the solubilized cannabinoid receptor. The presence of 200 nM GTPγS (*inset*) results in a 30% decrease in binding, indicating an association with G proteins.

potency order of various agonists (CP-55244 > DALN > Δ^9-THC > cannabinol >> cannabidiol) in binding to the soluble receptor is identical to that found with the membrane-bound receptor.

The GTP analog GTPγS decreases the binding of ligand without altering the ligand's affinity for the receptor (FIG. 2, *inset*), suggesting that the cannabinoid receptor is solubilized in the presence of its associated G protein(s).

The solubilization of the cannabinoid receptor will enable the purification of the receptor and its associated G protein(s), and will allow studies of cannabinoid receptor structure-activity relationships without the constraints of the membrane environment.

REFERENCES

1. DEVANE, W. A., F. A. DYSARZ, M. R. JOHNSON, L. S. MELVIN & A. C. HOWLETT. 1988. Determination and characterization of a cannabinoid receptor in rat brain. Mol. Pharmacol. **34:** 605–613.
2. HOWLETT, A. C., J. M. QUALY & L. K. KHACHATRIAN. 1986. Involvement of G_i in the inhibition of adenylate cyclase by cannabimimetic drugs. Mol. Pharmacol. **29:** 307–313.

Different Pharmacodynamics for Diazepam and Flunitrazepam?

J. INGUM,[a] R. BJØRKLUND,[b]
A. BJØRNEBOE,[a] AND J. MØRLAND[a]

[a] National Institute of Forensic Toxicology
P.O. Box 16 Gaustad
N-0320 Oslo, Norway

[b] Department of Physiology
National Institute of Occupational Health
P.O. Box 8149 Dep. 0033
Oslo, Norway

Recently, the existence of several benzodiazepine receptor subtypes has been reported, and it has been suggested that these subtypes may mediate the different psychodynamic and physiological effects of benzodiazepines.[1,2] In the present study we compared the psychomotor impairment after administration of ethanol and various doses of diazepam and flunitrazepam. The relative potency of the various treatments was examined, as well as the cross sensitivity between diazepam and flunitrazepam. The study was performed with a placebo-controlled, double blind design. Twelve volunteers (19–27 years) served as their own controls with intake of either 10 or 20 mg diazepam (mean maximal plasma concentration [C max] 1.0 and 2.0 μmol/l), 1 or 2 mg flunitrazepam (mean C max 0.02 and 0.04 μmol/l), 0.9 g ethanol/kg bodyweight (mean maximal blood ethanol concentration 0.071%) or placebo, respectively. The participants were tested with a simple and a choice reaction task before and several times during a period of 6 h after drug intake. Data analysis was performed by using the maximal impairments during a particular test day (Δ_{max} values) as detected by the variables simple and choice reaction time and number of errors, respectively. The ethanol dose caused the least performance impairment, followed by 10 mg diazepam. The most pronounced impairment was observed after 2 mg flunitrazepam, whereas 20 mg diazepam and 1 mg flunitrazepam were approximately equipotent on a group level. A factor analysis of the four benzodiazepine treatments with respect to reaction times of the simple and choice reaction tasks, was achieved to examine the cross sensitivity between diazepam and flunitrazepam. The four diazepam variables had loadings preferably on one of the factors extracted, whereas the four flunitrazepam variables had loadings preferably on the other (TABLE 1). Similar results were obtained when number of errors was included in the analysis. Thus, the results indicate a difference in individual sensitivity profiles to diazepam and flunitrazepam. This feature was still present after the results had been corrected for different concentrations between the individuals examined, and may, accordingly, suggest different pharmacodynamics for the two drugs. The diverse molecular structures of the monomers that form the GABA$_A$-benzodiazepine receptor indicate that different GABA$_A$ receptors may exhibit different binding properties for benzodiazepine ligands.[2] Thus, the present results may indicate somewhat different receptor affinity profiles of the two drugs.

TABLE 1. Factor Matrix after Varimax Rotation with the Δ_{max} Values of Choice Reaction Time (Δ_{max} CR) and Simple Reaction Time (Δ_{max} SR) following the Benzodiazepine Treatments as Factor Variables

Variable	Factor 1	Factor 2
Δ_{max} CR, 10dz	0.45	0.79
Δ_{max} SR, 10dz	0.55	0.75
Δ_{max} CR, 20dz	0.39	0.85
Δ_{max} SR, 20 dz	0.23	0.89
Δ_{max} CR, 1fn	0.91	0.29
Δ_{max} SR, 1fn	0.81	0.52
Δ_{max} CR, 2fn	0.89	0.33
Δ_{max} SR, 2fn	0.88	0.43

Abbreviations: 10dz, 10 mg diazepam; 20dz, 20 mg diazepam; 1fn, 1 mg flunitrazepam; 2fn, 2 mg flunitrazepam.

REFERENCES

1. PRITCHETT, D. P., H. LÜDDENS & P. H. SEEBURG. 1989. Type I and type II GABA$_A$-benzodiazepine receptors produced in transfected cells. Science **245:** 1389–1392.
2. SIEGHART, W. 1989. Multiplicity of GABA$_A$-benzodiazepine receptors. Trends Pharmacol. Sci. **10:** 407–411.

Effects of Withdrawal from Chronic Cocaine Administration on Behavior and β-Adrenergic and Serotonergic Brain Receptors in Rat[a]

ELIZABETH ANNE JOHNSON,[b,c,d]
IRVING J. GOODMAN,[e] YVONNE H. SHAHAN,[c]
AND ALBERT J. AZZARO[b,c,d]

Departments of [b] Behavioral Medicine/Psychiatry, [c] Neurology,
[d] Pharmacology/Toxicology, and [e] Psychology
West Virginia University, Health Science Center
Morgantown, West Virginia 26506

Chronic cocaine use has been shown to result in severe depression and anhedonia during abrupt withdrawal from the drug.[1] Little is known about the effects of withdrawal from chronic cocaine exposure on brain norepinephrine and serotonin transmission. However, desipramine, a tricyclic antidepressant, known to result in altered transmission in these pathways, is useful in treatment of cocaine withdrawal-induced depression in humans.[2] Therefore, the effects of withdrawal from chronic cocaine administration on behavior and on β-adrenergic (BETA) and serotonin₂ receptors (5-HT₂), a subset of brain serotonin receptors, were studied in frontal cortex (FC) and hippocampus (HIPP). Rats were administered cocaine (10 mg/kg, i.p.) daily for 15 days, then allowed to withdraw from the drug for 24, 48, or 72 hours ($n = 8$ for each group). Cocaine-treated rats exhibited a significantly slower rate of adaptation to a novel open field at 24 hours of withdrawal as measured by the rate of change of exploratory behavior over a 9-min period, when compared to saline controls (TABLE 1, Mann-Whitney test, $p < 0.05$). However, cocaine treated animals were not motor-retarded compared to saline controls (TABLE 1). This difference in behavior may reflect anxiogenic properties of cocaine withdrawal. Cocaine-treated animals also exhibited an increased amount of floating behavior (total seconds of float time measured over a 15-min period in the modified Porsolt swim-test[3]) compared to saline-treated rats at 48 h after withdrawal (TABLE 2, $p < 0.05$). This effect is a behavioral indication of depression in rats.[3]

Receptor binding studies in brains of cocaine and saline treated rats indicated small, time-dependent differences in FC and HIPP BETA receptor number (measured with [³H]CGP 12177), when compared to saline controls (TABLE 3). These changes did not achieve statistical significance. Likewise no significant differences were detected in

[a] This work was supported by the WVU Medical Corp. and NIH Biomedical Research Grant 2S07RR05433.

TABLE 1. Open-Field Exploratory Behavior

	Withdrawal		
	24 Hours	48 Hours	72 Hours
Cocaine-treated Rats			
Average distance traveled			
0–3 min (A)	196 ± 34	258 ± 28	225 ± 23
4–6 min	167 ± 17	208 ± 16	195 ± 34
7–9 min (B)	150 ± 30	159 ± 34	125 ± 33
0–9 min	514 ± 69	624 ± 63	545 ± 77
A-B	46 ± 22[a]	99 ± 23	101 ± 35
Time Visiting Zone 5	10 ± 5	5.0 ± 1.1	5.4 ± 1.3
	n = 8	n = 8	n = 8
Saline-treated Rats			
Average distance traveled			
0–3 min (A)	209 ± 20	257 ± 30	256 ± 19
4–6 min	153 ± 20	208 ± 23	203 ± 35
7–9 min (B)	94 ± 18	140 ± 28	165 ± 32
0–9 min	456 ± 50	604 ± 73	624 ± 81
A–B	115 ± 18	116 ± 24	91 ± 19
Time Visiting Zone 5	4 ± 2	5.1 ± 1.2	6.8 ± 1.6
	n = 8	n = 8	n = 8

[a] Different from saline controls, $p < 0.05$. Distance traveled in inches, in a novel open field 40 cm × 42.5 cm. Time in seconds. Zone 5 is the innermost zone of the field.

TABLE 2. Modified Porsolt Swim Test

	Withdrawal		
	24 Hours	48 Hours	72 Hours
Cocaine-treated Rats			
Struggle Time[a]			
0–5 min	78 ± 18	63 ± 15	88 ± 6
0–15 min	98 ± 25	74 ± 20	138 ± 23
Float Time			
0–5 min	112 ± 26	138 ± 27	115 ± 29
0–15 min	454 ± 80	579 ± 86*	415 ± 95
Dives	3.4 ± 1.2	4.0 ± 1	7 ± 2
Headshakes	22 ± 10	26 ± 9.0	47 ± 15
	n = 8	n = 8	n = 8
Saline-treated Rats			
Struggle Time			
0–5 min	91 ± 11	79 ± 12	78 ± 8
0–15 min	128 ± 37	174 ± 44	131 ± 34
Float Time			
0–5 min	96 ± 17	91 ± 18	117 ± 11
0–15 min	398 ± 77	351 ± 45	513 ± 69
Dives	4.0 ± 1	5 ± 1	4.0 ± 1
Headshakes	18 ± 8	31 ± 17	50 ± 12
	n = 8	n = 8	n = 8

[a] Struggle and float time in seconds ± SEM; * = $p < 0.05$ compared to saline.

TABLE 3. Results of Brain Receptor Assay

	Withdrawal		
	24 Hours	48 Hours	72 Hours
Brain β-Adrenergic Receptor Binding in Cocaine-treated Rats			
Frontal cortex	89.4% ± 3.5%	106% ± 4.2%	107% ± 6.2%
	$n = 8^a$	$n = 8$	$n = 8$
Hippocampus	103% ± 2.3%	117% ± 13%	93% ± 6.2%
	$n = 8$	$n = 8$	$n = 8$
Brain Serotonin$_2$ Receptor Binding in Cocaine-treated Rats			
Frontal cortex	100% ± 16%	89.2% ± 5.2%	120% ± 11%
	$n = 8$	$n = 8$	$n = 8$
Hippocampus	48% ± 10%	142% ± 26%	82% ± 17%
	$n = 8$	$n = 8$	$n = 8$

[a] n = number of animals analyzed, values represent percent of control specific binding at approximate Kd concentrations ligand: [^{3}H] CGP 12177 (0.2 or 0.25 nM) for β-adrenoceptors; [^{3}H]Ketanserin ([^{3}H]KET) (0.2 or 0.25 nM) for serotonin$_2$ receptors, plus or minus SEM. Rats were treated with cocaine 10 mg/kg i.p. daily for 15 days then allowed to withdraw the specified number of hours. Equal numbers of rats were treated with 0.4 ml sterile saline i.p. daily for 15 days and allowed to withdraw the specified number of hours. Control values for beta receptor binding were as follows, expressed as specific bound (moles/liter) [^{3}H] CGP 12177: FC, 1.71 × 10^{-11}M ± 0.11 × 10^{-11}M; HIPP, 7.48 × 10^{-12}M ± 0.58 × 10^{-12}M. Control values for serotonin$_2$ receptor binding were as follows, expressed as specific bound (moles/liter) [^{3}H]KET: FC, 1.16 × 10^{-11}M ± 0.06 × 10^{-11}M; HIPP 2.09 × 10^{-12}M ± 0.95 × 10^{-12}. Specific binding as a percent of total bound were as follows: [^{3}H]CGP12177; FC 90%, HIPP 79%: [^{3}H]KET; FC 59%, HIPP 21%.

FC 5-HT$_2$ receptors (measured with [^{3}H]Ketanserin, TABLE 3). In contrast, HIPP 5-HT$_2$ receptors were depressed at 24 h ($p < 0.05$) but returned to control levels at 48 h, and 72 h of withdrawal (TABLE 3).

These results indicate that rats treated with cocaine (10 mg/kg, i.p., for 15 days) and then withdrawn for 24, 48, or 72 h show behavioral signs of depression at 48 h and evidence of anxiety at 24 h. Our preliminary evidence also shows that some of these behavioral changes (anxiety) are temporally correlated with decreased hippocampal 5-HT$_2$ receptors at 24 h of withdrawal.

REFERENCES

1. GAWAIN, F. H. & H. D. KLEBER. 1986. Arch. Gen. Psych. **41:** 107–113.
2. GAWAIN, F. H., H. D. KLEBER, R. BYCK, B. J. ROUNSAVILLE, T. R. KOSTEN, P. I. JATLOW & C. MORGAN. 1989. Arch. Gen. Psych. **46:** 117–121.
3. WEISS, J. M., P. A. GOODMAN, B. G. LOSITO, S. CORRIGAN, J. M. CHARRY & W. H. BAILEY. 1981. Brain Res. Rev. **3:** 167–205.

Psychomotor Stimulant Effect of Cocaine Is Affected by Genetic Makeup and Experimental History

B. C. JONES,[a,c] A. D. CAMPBELL,[b]
R. A. RADCLIFFE,[b] AND V. G. ERWIN[b]

[a] Program in Biobehavioral Health
College of Health and Human Development
210 East Health and Human Development Building
The Pennsylvania State University
University Park, Pennsylvania 16802

[b] Alcohol Research Center
University of Colorado
Boulder, Colorado 80309

Cocaine has been shown to have differential locomotor stimulant effects in inbred strains[1] and selected lines[2,3] of mice. The selected lines were long-sleep (LS) and short-sleep (SS) mice, which were bred for differential sensitivity to the hypnotic effects of ethanol. In one study, LS were more activated by cocaine than were SS[2] while in the other study, LS were not stimulated by cocaine.[3] Because it has been shown that experiential history of the test subject may affect stimulant-sedative properties of psychoactive drugs,[4] and thus may be relevant to the differential results from the two studies above, we tested the locomotor-stimulant effects of cocaine in LS and SS mice exposed once previously, or not, to the test apparatus. Male LS and SS mice were tested on two consecutive days under one of two treatment-orders, saline (i.p.) on day 1, cocaine (15 mg/kg, i.p.) on day 2 or cocaine on day 1 followed by saline on day 2. Testing consisted of injecting the animals and immediately placing them into an automated open-field apparatus for 30 min, sampled in 5 min segments. Behaviors measured were total distance, rearings, stereotypy, and wall-seeking. In separate sets of experiments, whole brain cocaine levels at 5 min post-injection and cocaine receptors in forebrain were measured in LS and SS mice. FIGURE 1 presents LS and SS mean difference scores (cocaine scores minus saline scores) for distance traveled, 0–5 min post-injection. Order of treatment had a significant effect in LS but not in SS with LS more highly activated in the saline-cocaine order than in the cocaine-saline order. This same differential effect between LS and SS was observed 5–10 min and disappeared at 15 min post-injection. The other major behavioral effect was on wall-seeking, a putative measure of fear. In this case, SS were more affected by order of treatment than LS with cocaine-saline producing greater wall seeking than saline-cocaine. Brain cocaine levels measured at 5 min were higher in SS than in LS; order of treatment had no effect in either line. Because,

---

[c] Author to whom correspondence should be addressed.

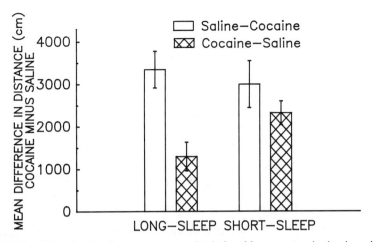

FIGURE 1. Effect of order of treatment on cocaine-induced locomotor activation in male LS and SS mice. All animals were tested on two consecutive days under one of two treatment orders, saline (i.p.) on day 1 and cocaine (15 mg/kg i.p.) on day 2 or cocaine on day 1 followed by saline on day 2. Data are reported as mean difference scores, cocaine minus saline, in cm for the first 5 min after injection.

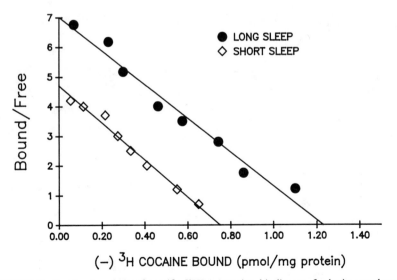

FIGURE 2. Scatchard analysis of specific [^{3}H]-(−)cocaine binding to forebrain membranes from LS and SS mice (typical experiment shown). Brains were sectioned at the optic chiasm and the anterior portion was prepared for receptor binding. Data were analyzed by the linear/nonlinear least squares regression analysis program, LIGAND.

under the saline-cocaine regimen, LS were as activated initially as SS, despite their evincing lower brain cocaine concentration, we proposed that there might be differential target tissue sensitivity between LS and SS. We therefore conducted a study of [³H]-cocaine binding to forebrain membranes in LS and SS. FIGURE 2 presents Scatchard analysis of [³H]-cocaine binding in LS and SS forebrain tissues and shows similar affinities between the two lines but higher densities (B_{max}) in LS. We conclude that pharmacokinetic and receptor characteristic measures are necessary, but not sufficient factors in determining cocaine actions on locomotor activity. The influence of novelty, for example, points to the probable importance of state of activity of a number of limbic and/or cortical circuits in determining cocaine actions.

REFERENCES

1. RUTH, J. A., E. A. ULLMAN & A. C. COLLINS. 1988. Pharmacol. Biochem. Behav. **29:** 157–162.
2. DeFIEBRE, C. M., J. A. RUTH & A. C. COLLINS. 1989. Pharmacol. Biochem. Behav. **34:** 887–893.
3. GEORGE, F. R. & M. C. RITZ. 1990. Psychopharmacology **101:** 18–22.
4. CONSROE, P. F., B. C. JONES & L. CHIN. 1975. Pharmacol. Biochem. Behav. **3:** 173–177.

Nifedipine Blocks the Development of Tolerance to the Anticonvulsant Effects of Ethanol

LISA E. KALYNCHUK,[a,c] SUNTANU DALAL,[a]
MICHAEL J. MANA,[b] AND JOHN P. J. PINEL[a]

[a] Department of Psychology
2136 West Mall, Kenny Building
University of British Columbia
Vancouver, B.C., Canada V6T 1Z4

[b] Department of Behavioral Neuroscience
University of Pittsburgh
Pittsburgh, Pennsylvania 15260

Chronic ethanol (ETOH) administration increases the number of dihydropyridine (DHP) binding sites on Ca^{2+} channels in rat cerebral cortex.[1] Administration of a DHP Ca^{2+} channel antagonist during ETOH exposure prevented this increase in binding sites and prevented the development of tolerance to ETOH-induced ataxia.[1] This suggests a causal relation between changes in DHP-sensitive Ca^{2+} channels and ETOH tolerance. In this experiment, the DHP antagonist nifedipine (NIF) prevented the development of tolerance to the anticonvulsant effects of ETOH in amygdala-kindled rats.

METHODS

A single bipolar electrode was implanted in the left basolateral amygdala of each of 32 male Long-Evans rats (380–560 g). The rats were subsequently kindled according to a previously described protocol.[2] Kindled rats respond to each stimulation with a clonic convulsion; the measure of convulsion severity was the duration of forelimb clonus. After kindling, the rats were stimulated once every 48 h: They were given, in succession, 4 no-drug baseline stimulations, 1 saline baseline stimulation, 1 ETOH baseline stimulation, 12 tolerance-development stimulations, and 2 test stimulations. One h prior to each of the tolerance-development stimulations, each rat received an injection of ETOH (1.5 g/kg) or isosaline, and 50 min later each rat received an injection of NIF (40 mg/kg) or vehicle (dimethyl sulfoxide, 0.5 ml/kg). Thus, there were four treatment groups: 1) ETOH ONLY ($n = 11$), 2) ETOH + NIF ($n = 9$), 3) SALINE ($n = 6$), and 4) NIF ONLY ($n = 6$). Each rat received ETOH 1 h prior to the first test stimulation; 7 days later this test was repeated.

---

[c] Author to whom correspondence should be addressed.

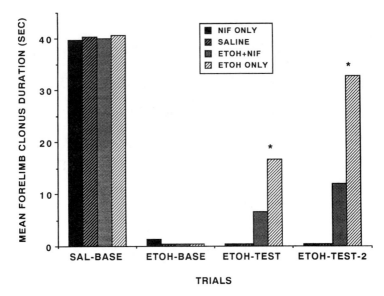

FIGURE 1. Mean forelimb clonus duration on key trials for the four treatment groups. The ETOH ONLY rats displayed significantly ($p < .05$) more forelimb clonus than the rats in the other three groups on both tolerance tests.

RESULTS

FIGURE 1 illustrates the inhibitory effect of NIF on the development of tolerance to the anticonvulsant effects of ETOH. As observed in previous studies,[3] forelimb clonus increased significantly from the ETOH baseline trial to the test trials for the ETOH ONLY rats, but neither the ETOH + NIF nor the two groups of control rats displayed a similar increase. Furthermore, the ETOH ONLY rats displayed significantly more forelimb clonus than the ETOH + NIF rats on both of the test trials. Of the 9 ETOH + NIF rats, only 1 displayed forelimb clonus on the first test trial and only 2, on the second. Thus, NIF prevented the development of tolerance to the anticonvulsant effects of ETOH in amygdala-kindled rats. This observation provides further support for the theory that DHP-sensitive Ca^{2+} channels mediate the development of tolerance to ETOH.

REFERENCES

1. DOLIN, S. J. & H. J. LITTLE. 1989. Are changes in neuronal calcium channels involved in ethanol tolerance? J. Pharmacol. Exp. Ther. **250:** 985–991.
2. PINEL, J. P. J., C. K. KIM & M. J. MANA. 1990. Contingent tolerance to the anticonvulsant effects of drugs on kindled convulsions. *In* Kindling 4. J. A. Wada, Ed. Plenum Press. New York.
3. PINEL, J. P. J., M. J. MANA & C. K. KIM. 1990. Development of tolerance to ethanol's anticonvulsant effect on kindled seizures. *In* Alcohol and Seizures. R. J. Porter, R. H. Mattson, J. A. Cramer & I. Diamond, Eds. F. A. Davis Company. Philadelphia.

Influence of Chronic Cocaine on Monoamine Neurotransmitters in Human Brain and Animal Model: Preliminary Observations

J. M. WILSON,[a,c] J. N. NOBREGA,[a,c] W. CORRIGALL,[b,c]
K. SHANNAK,[a] J. H. N. DECK,[b] AND S. J. KISH[a,c]

[a] Clarke Institute of Psychiatry
250 College Street
Toronto, Ontario, Canada M5T 1R8

[b] Addiction Research Foundation and
[c] University of Toronto
Toronto, Ontario, Canada

The increase in the illegal use of cocaine over the past decade has renewed interest in the potentially neurotoxic nature of this drug. Our study was undertaken in order to determine the brain neurochemical effects of cocaine exposure in the human and in an animal model of cocaine self-administration.

In the experimental animal study male Long-Evans rats (n = 6), implanted with chronic indwelling jugular catheters, had access to cocaine for 1 h per day, for 4 weeks (mean intake 8.6 ± 0.4 mg/kg i.v. per day), followed by 4 weeks withdrawal from the drug. The rats were killed by decapitation and the brains were removed and dissected into discrete areas. Levels of the monoamines dopamine, noradrenaline and serotonin were measured using HPLC and electrochemical detection and were compared with a group of control animals (n = 6) which underwent sham surgery for implantation of catheters and were exposed to the drug administration environment, but received no drug.

Striatal levels of dopamine and noradrenaline were not significantly different from those of control animals. However, the mean serotonin concentration was significantly elevated (+37%, $p < 0.05$, FIG. 1).

Levels of monoamines and metabolites were also measured in human autopsied basal ganglia of two chronic cocaine abusers (male, aged 26 and 35 years) who died as a result of cocaine toxicity and were known to have used cocaine for at least 1 year prior to death. They were compared with monoamine levels in identical brain areas of eight neurologically normal controls, matched with respect to age (30 ± 4 years) and post mortem time (12 ± 3 h).

In one human subject (C1), long-term cocaine exposure was associated with markedly reduced dopamine levels in striatum (−50 to −70%) but were within the control range in the substantia nigra (FIG. 2). In the second subject (C2), dopamine levels were reduced in the caudate (−50%) and putamen (−55%) but not in the nucleus ac-

461

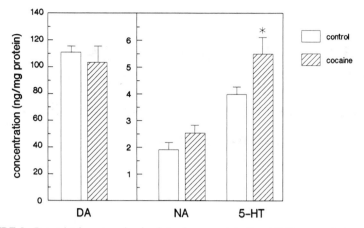

FIGURE 1. Rat striatal monoamine levels (ng/mg protein), (* $p < 0.05$, two-tailed t-test).

cumbens or substantia nigra. Levels of the other monoaminergic neurotransmitters and their metabolites were normal in the brain areas examined (data not shown).

Our data suggest that repeated self-administration of cocaine in the rat, at the dose chosen, does not produce permanent striatal dopaminergic damage. However, unlike the rat, the preliminary human data indicate that long-term cocaine exposure is associated with markedly reduced levels of striatal dopamine. The dopamine reduction in

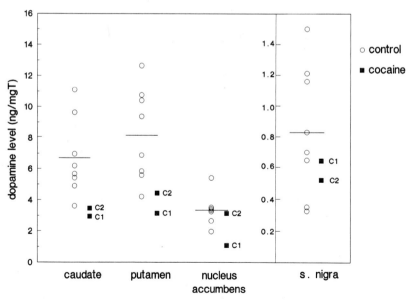

FIGURE 2. Dopamine levels in control ($n = 8$) and cocaine abused ($n = 2$) human basal ganglia (ng/mg tissue).

human striatum could be explained by an acute, reversible decrease in dopamine synthesis or by a permanent neurotoxic effect on dopaminergic nerve terminals.

In order to determine whether long-term cocaine exposure causes actual neurodegeneration we will include in a future study, a representative number of cocaine abusers who have been withdrawn from the drug for an extended period of time prior to death, for measurement of a variety of neurochemical parameters (including uptake binding sites and tyrosine hydroxylase activity) as indices of dopaminergic neuronal integrity.

Repeated Injection of Cocaine Potentiates Methamphetamine-induced Toxicity to Dopamine-containing Neurons in Rat Striatum

MARK S. KLEVEN AND LEWIS S. SEIDEN

Department of Pharmacological and Physiological Sciences
Department of Psychiatry
The University of Chicago
Chicago, Illinois 60637

INTRODUCTION

Adverse effects of cocaine and methamphetamine (MA) abuse may result from compulsive use over the course of several days. This pattern of abuse can result in a behavioral state which is indistinguishable from an acute psychotic episode. While cocaine itself does not appear to be neurotoxic, exposure to high doses of MA has been shown to result in neurotoxicity characterized by depletions of brain dopamine (DA) and/or 5-HT, decreased numbers of presynaptic high-affinity uptake sites, and neuronal degeneration.[1] These effects are consistent with the ablation of DA and/or 5-HT-containing nerve terminals. We now report that repeated injection of cocaine for two weeks enhances neurotoxic effects of MA on DA neurons in the rat.

METHODS

Male Sprague-Dawley rats (Harlan, IN; 200–250 g) were housed individually in stainless steel cages in a room with lights on from 07.00 h–19.00 h and temperature maintained at approximately 24°C. Food (Teklad, Winfield, IA) and water were freely available. Rats (n = 6/group) were treated with single daily injections of cocaine HCL (20 mg/kg/inj.; NIDA) or saline for 15 days and, beginning 24 h after the last injection of cocaine or saline, subjected to a 4-day regimen of MA HCl (Sigma Chemical Co., St. Louis, MO) consisting of twice daily injections at 12-h intervals. Rats were killed by guillotine 2 weeks after the last injection of MA or saline and brain sections were obtained, wrapped individually in aluminum foil, stored in liquid nitrogen, and assayed for monoamines and metabolites using HPLC-EC as previously described.[2]

RESULTS

Repeated administration of cocaine did not have long-lasting effects on DA levels in striatum (13.4 ± 0.41 vs. 11.9 ± 0.72, saline vs. cocaine, respectively) or nucleus

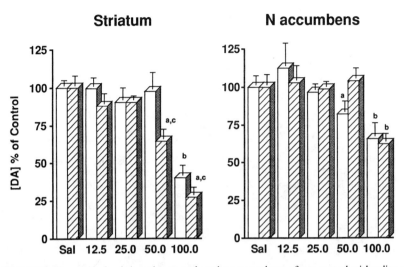

FIGURE 1. Dopamine levels in striatum and nucleus accumbens of rats treated with saline or cocaine (20 mg/kg/inj) once daily for 15 consecutive days followed by methamphetamine (0–100 mg/kg/day × 4 days) and sacrificed two weeks after the last injection. Data were transformed to a percentage of their respective control means (see text). Bars represent the mean ± SEM (n = 5–6/group); *open bars*, repeated saline pretreatment; *hatched bars*, repeated cocaine pretreatment. Data were analyzed for statistical significance using two-way ANOVA followed by individual comparisons using Dunnett's test. [a]$p < 0.05$; [b]$p < 0.01$ vs. saline-treated rats; [c]$p < 0.05$; [d]$p < 0.01$ vs. repeated saline pretreatment.

accumbens (7.9 ± 0.46 vs. 8.0 ± 0.52, saline vs. cocaine). The 4-day regimen of MA caused significant, dose-related depletions of DA in both striatum and nucleus accumbens (FIG. 1) with effects ranging from 25–62% of control. In the striatum, the lowest effective dose of MA to significantly deplete DA in saline-pretreated rats was 100 mg/kg/day. In contrast, a lower daily dose of MA (50 mg/kg/day) produced significant decreases in DA and metabolites in rats pretreated with cocaine (65 ± 6.0 vs. 97 ± 11% of control, cocaine vs. saline pretreatment, respectively). Potentiation of MA-induced depletions of DA was not observed in the nucleus accumbens (FIG. 1).

DISCUSSION

Repeated injection of cocaine enhanced the depletions of striatal DA caused by MA, both decreasing the threshold dose and augmenting depletions following the highest dose. This effect was not observed in the nucleus accumbens. Different effects of repeated cocaine in striatal and mesolimbic regions have already been reported.[3-5] Repeated cocaine has been reported to enhance K[+]-, amphetamine-, and cocaine-stimulated DA release for a period of several weeks[6-9] indicating that cocaine pretreatment should enhance neurochemical effects of amphetamine. The present data are consistent with the idea that neurotoxicity is caused by amphetamine-induced release of DA[1] and suggest that frequent cocaine use may enhance susceptibility to neurotoxic effects of MA.

REFERENCES

1. SEIDEN, L. S. & G. A. RICAURTE. 1987. *In* Psychopharmacology: The Third Generation of Progress. H. Y. Meltzer, Ed.: 359–366. Raven Press. New York.
2. KOTAKE, C., T. HEFFNER, G. VOSMER & L. S. SEIDEN. 1985. Pharmacol. Biochem. Behav. 22: 85–89.
3. KLEVEN, M. S., B. D. PERRY, W. L. WOOLVERTON & L. S. SEIDEN. 1990. Brain Res. 532: 265–270.
4. GOEDERS, N. E. & M. J. KUHAR. 1987. Alcohol Drug Res. 7: 207–216.
5. IZENWASSER, S. & B. M. COX. 1990. Brain Res. 531: 338–341.
6. PERIS, J., S. J. BOYSON, W. A. CASS, P. CURELLA, L. P. DWOSKIN, G. LARSON, L. LIN, R. P. YASUDA & N. R. ZAHNISER. 1990. J. Pharmacol. Exp. Ther. 253: 38–44.
7. KALIVAS, P. W., P. DUFFY, L. A. DUMARS & C. SKINNER. 1988. J. Pharmacol. Exp. Ther. 245: 485–492.
8. YI, S. J. & K. M. JOHNSON. 1990. Neuropharmacology 29: 475–486.
9. AKIMOTO, K., T. HAMAMURA & S. OTSUKI. 1989. Brain Res. 490: 339–344.

Effect of Acute and Chronic Ethanol on Nonadrenergic, Noncholinergic Neurotransmission[a]

EDWARD T. KNYCH

Department of Pharmacology
University of Minnesota–Duluth
Duluth, Minnesota 55812

The anococcygeus muscle (ANO) is innervated by inhibitory nonadrenergic, noncholinergic neurons (NANC). Recent studies suggest that the neurotransmitter which mediates relaxation induced in the ANO by NANC stimulation is nitric oxide (NO) or by a substance which releases NO.[1,2] Ethanol inhibits the action of endothelium-dependent vasodilators whose action is mediated by the release of NO.[3] This study was therefore designed to investigate the effect of acute and chronic ethanol administration on NANC-induced relaxation of the rat ANO.

Male Sprague-Dawley rats weighing 350–400 g were used in this study. All protocols were approved by the University Animal Care and Use Committee. Chronic ethanol administration consisted of the oral administration of ethanol twice daily for 2 days according to Majchrowicz.[4] This treatment protocol produces tolerance to ethanol-induced changes in plasma corticosterone, body temperature, and ethanol-induced contraction of the rat aorta.[5,6] The ANO was removed from either ethanol-naive control or chronic ethanol-treated tolerant rats after sacrifice with ether. The muscle was mounted between platinum electrodes in a 10 ml muscle bath containing Krebs Ringer bicarbonate buffer, pH 7.4, at 37°C and aerated with 95% O_2:5% CO_2. It was equilibrated at an initial tension of 1 g for 45 min. Guanethidine (20 μM) was added to contract the muscle and to block any further release of norepinephrine. When the contraction stabilized a frequency-response curve was generated by transmurally stimulating the NANC nerves at varying frequencies (0.5–16 Hz) for 20 seconds every 2 min. The frequencies were randomly varied in each experiment.

In those experiments designed to study the effect of ethanol on NANC-induced relaxation of the ANO, the NANC nerves were stimulated at 2 Hz for 20 seconds every 2 min until a stable response was obtained. At this time ethanol was added in cumulatively increasing concentrations. The response to nerve stimulation was allowed to equilibrate before each addition of ethanol. The concentration of ethanol which produced a 50% decrease (EC_{50}) in the relaxation induced by nerve stimulation in the absence of ethanol was determined using linear regression analysis. Mean responses of control and ethanol-tolerant ANO were compared using repeated measure ANOVA or unpaired student t-test, as appropriate. A $p \leq 0.05$ was considered significant.

Initial experiments confirmed previous observations[1,2] that the relaxation induced

[a] This study was supported in part by Grant AA-06272 from the NIAAA.

by stimulation of NANC neurons was inhibited by methylene blue and by N^{ω}-nitro-l-arginine (NOARG). The inhibition by NOARG was reversed by l-arginine but not by d-arginine. These results support the hypothesis that the NANC neurotransmitter is nitric oxide or a substance which liberates nitric oxide.

Increasing the frequency of stimulation of NANC neurons produced an increased relaxation of the ANO. The maximal relaxation observed in control ANO was 42.6 ± 9.4%. Half-maximal relaxation was observed at a frequency of approximately 2 Hz. In contrast, 2 days of ethanol treatment significantly increased the maximal relaxation induced by NANC stimulation to 78.1 ± 7.9%. While the response induced in ethanol treated ANO by NANC stimulation was greater at each frequency, the sensitivity of the response was not significantly different. Half maximal relaxation in ethanol-treated ANO was also observed at approximately 2 Hz. These observations suggest that ethanol treatment induces an increase in either the synthesis or release of NO from NANC nerves.

Ethanol, added acutely to the muscle bath, inhibited the relaxation of the ANO induced by NANC stimulation. The EC_{50} dose for ethanol in control ANO was 165 ± 51 mM. Two days of ethanol treatment produced tolerance to the inhibitory effect of acutely administered ethanol. The EC_{50} dose for ethanol in ethanol-tolerant ANO was 351 ± 43 mM.

This study demonstrates that ethanol inhibits NANC-induced relaxation of the rat ANO and tolerance can be demonstrated to this effect after two days of ethanol administration. This tolerance may be due to an increase in the synthesis or release of the proposed NANC neurotransmitter, nitric oxide.

REFERENCES

1. GILLESPIE, J. S., X. LIU & W. MARTIN. 1989. Br. J. Pharmacol. **98:** 1080–1082.
2. LI, C. G. & M. J. RAND. 1989. Clin. Exp. Pharmacol. Physiol. **16:** 933–938.
3. KNYCH, E. T. 1986. Pharmacologist **28:** 143.
4. MAJCHROWICZ, E. 1975. Psychopharmacologia **43:** 245–254.
5. KNYCH, E. T. & J. R. PROHASKA. 1981. Life Sci. **28:** 1987–1994.
6. KNYCH, E. T., C. M. S. GUIMARAES & S. BOIVIN. 1984. Life Sci. **35:** 611–617.

Opioid Modulation of Alcohol Intake in Monkeys by Low Doses of Naltrexone and Morphine

M. KORNET AND C. GOOSEN

Institute of Applied Radiobiology and Immunology-TNO
Lange Kleiweg 151
2280 HV Rijswijk, the Netherlands

J. M. VAN REE

Department of Pharmacology
Rudolf Magnus Institute
University of Utrecht
Vondellaan 6
3521 GD, Utrecht, the Netherlands

INTRODUCTION

Opioid modulation can influence alcohol consumption in experimental animals, but the underlying mechanisms are still unclear.[1,2] Here we report on the effects of low doses of the opioid antagonist naltrexone and the opioid agonist morphine, on alcohol consumption in experienced (over two years), free-choice alcohol drinking rhesus monkeys (*Macaca mulatta*). After periods of imposed abstinence (up to seven days), rhesus monkeys resumed alcohol drinking with elevated alcohol intake immediately at renewal of the alcohol supply.[3] Therefore, the effect of opioid modulation on elevated alcohol drinking after a period of imposed abstinence, was studied also.

MATERIALS AND METHODS

The subjects were eight adult male rhesus monkeys (between 8 and 15.4 kg of body-weight) which had *ad libitum* access to two ethanol/water solutions and tap water. Individual net ethanol intakes were on average 2–6 ml·kg^{-1} per day. Doses of naltrexone and morphine were administered once as a single intramuscular injection at 15.30 h, a) during continuous daily supply of alcohol and water and b) after alcohol supply had been interrupted for two days. Interruption started at 16.00 h and was terminated 48 h later at 16.00 h. Doses of naltrexone administered were 0.02, 0.06, 0.17, 0.5, 1.0 and 1.5 mg·kg^{-1}; doses of morphine were 0.03, 0.06, 0.17, 0.5 and 1.5 mg·kg^{-1}. Each injection was placebo-controlled.

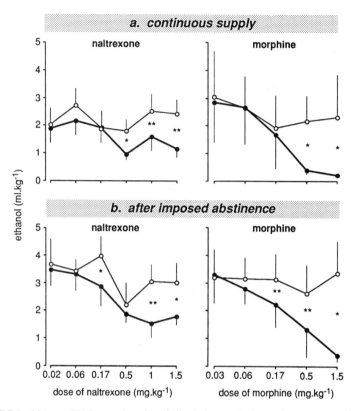

FIGURE 1. Mean (+SEM) net ethanol intake by 8 rhesus monkeys, after naltrexone (*left, black circles*), morphine (*right, black circles*) and matched placebo injections (*open circles*), **a** during continuous supply of water and alcohol and **b** after 2 days of imposed abstinence of alcohol. Wilcoxon matched pairs test $*p < 0.05$ $**p < 0.01$.

RESULTS

Figure 1 shows the mean net ethanol intake measured from 16.00 h to 09.00 h the next day, after administration of naltrexone (*left*) and morphine (*right*) and the matched placebo injections (*open circles*) as a function of the doses, a) during continuous supply (*top*) and b) after imposed abstinence (*bottom*). During continuous supply, naltrexone reduced net ethanol intake, compared to placebo, after doses 0.5, 1.0 and 1.5 mg·kg^{-1}. Morphine also reduced net ethanol intake after doses of 0.5 and 1.5 (the dose of 1.0 mg·kg^{-1} was not tested!). After imposed abstinence, a significant reduction by naltrexone was accomplished after doses of 0.17, 1.0 and 1.5 mg·kg^{-1}; by morphine after doses 0.17, 0.5 and 1.5 mg·kg^{-1}. When treated with placebo, implementation of abstinence always led to elevated ethanol intakes, during the first two hours of renewed access. After doses 0.17, 1.0 and 1.5 mg·kg^{-1} of naltrexone and after doses 0.17 and 0.5 mg·kg^{-1} of morphine, post-abstinence intakes were no longer significantly different from pre-abstinence intakes; after 1.50 mg·kg^{-1} of morphine, ethanol intake was even below pre-abstinence level. Effects of opioid modulation never lasted longer than 24 hours.

Under the condition of continuous supply, opioid modulation led to a shortlasting reduction in water drinking (from 16.00 to 18.00 h) at the two highest doses of naltrexone and the highest dose of morphine. After imposed abstinence, water drinking was not significantly affected by naltrexone, nor by morphine. During the interruption of alcohol supply, no overt signs of physical withdrawal could be observed. At all doses of naltrexone and morphine, the monkeys remained active and alert.

DISCUSSION

Opioid modulation in monkeys reduced uninterrupted alcohol drinking as well as alcohol consumption after a period of abstinence. After implementation of abstinence, effects were selective for alcohol. It is well-known that human alcoholics, despite periods of abstinence, frequently relapse into their previous drinking style.[4] The presented results suggest that endogenous opioids play a special role in alcohol intake after abstinence, and therefore perhaps in relapses into addictive drinking.

Both the antagonist naltrexone and the agonist morphine produced similar results in the monkeys. The results suggest that within the used dose range, naltrexone effectuated smaller reductions in alcohol drinking than morphine. The effects of morphine seem in agreement with the "endorphin compensation" hypothesis,[2] saying that alcoholics have some deficiency in opioid activity which can be compensated for by alcohol as well as by morphine. The suppressive function of naltrexone might be attributed to blocking the reinforcing effects of alcohol, leading to extinction of alcohol consumption.[2] The present findings on morphine are opposite to those in rats.[1] This study compels to some reflection on predicted effects of opioid agonists in human alcohol addiction.[1,2]

REFERENCES

1. HUBBELL, C. L. & L. D. REID. 1990. *In* Opioids, Bulimia and Alcohol Abuse & Alcoholism. L. D. Reid, Ed.: 145–174. Springer Verlag. New York.
2. VOLPICELLI, J. R., C. P. O'BRIEN, A. I. ALTERMAN & M. HAYASHIDA. 1990. *In* Opioids, Bulimia and Alcohol Abuse & Alcoholism. L. D. Reid, Ed.: 195–214. Springer Verlag. New York.
3. KORNET, M., C. GOOSEN & J. M. VAN REE. 1990. Alcohol & Alcoholism 4: 407–412.
4. DOLE, V. P. 1986. Alcohol Clin. Exp. Res. 10: 361–363.

Evaluation of Anxiolytic Action of Ondansetron in Rats during Withdrawal from Chronic Chlordiazepoxide

S. MEHDI REZAZADEH, PAUL L. PRATHER,
MICHAEL W. EMMETT-OGLESBY,
AND HARBANS LAL[a]

Department of Pharmacology
Texas College of Osteopathic Medicine
Fort Worth, Texas 76107-2690

An early symptom of withdrawal which commonly occurs following cessation of chronic administration of benzodiazepines is anxiety.[1] Such anxiety in humans may signal the oncoming of more severe signs and symptoms and thus result in a resumption of drug use. Hence, there has been a need for novel anxiolytics that do not have dependence-producing potential. Drugs that reduce 5-hydroxytryptamine (5-HT) neurotransmission through a variety of mechanisms exhibit anxiolytic efficacy.[2] Ondansetron diminishes 5-HT activity through antagonism of 5-HT$_3$ receptors,[3] and its long-term administration in animals does not result in the development of dependence.[4] The aim of the present experiments was to further characterize the anxiolytic effects of ondansetron in rats during withdrawal from chronic chlordiazepoxide (CDP) utilizing the elevated plus-maze (EPM).[5]

Male hooded rats of the Long-Evans strain were used throughout the investigation. Animals were trained to consume a nutritionally complete liquid diet containing CDP (final dose = 100 mg/kg/d) in two equally divided doses for 7 days.[6] A separate group of rats were also administered a control liquid diet (CDP free) in the same manner. Twelve hours after presentation of the last ration of diet, and 15 min after a final dose of CDP (injected i.p.), withdrawal was precipitated by an i.p. injection of flumazenil (20 mg/kg). Animals were then tested on the EPM 15 min later. Following a 5-min habituation period, the test animal was placed gently on the center of the EPM facing an open arm and observed for 5 min. The entries made onto each arm (open or closed), and the total time spent on each type of arm were recorded. The percent of open-arm entries (%OAE), the percent time spent on the open-arms (%OAT), and the total number of arm entries were computed and statistically analyzed.

In naive rats, ondansetron did not produce a significant change in either total arm entries or the %OAE. However, ondansetron did increase the %OAT. In rats withdrawn from chronic CDP and injected with flumazenil, there was a significant reduc-

---

[a] Author to whom correspondence should be sent.

tion in percentage of both the entries onto and the time spent on the open-arms, when compared to rats maintained on a CDP-free diet. This behavior is similar to that produced by classic anxiogenic drugs such as pentylenetetrazol (PTZ). In contrast, ondansetron pretreatment dose-dependently blocked this withdrawal-induced behavior as reflected by an increase in the %OAE and %OAT. In addition, during withdrawal the total number of arm entries was significantly decreased. This reduction was reversed by administration of ondansetron except at the highest dose (*i.e.*, 0.16 mg/kg).

Earlier studies suggest that ondansetron produced effects similar to those exhibited by known anxiolytics in various animal models of anxiety proposed to represent naturalistic behaviors.[4,7] Ondansetron has also been shown to inhibit behavioral consequences of withdrawal from chronic administration of ethanol, nicotine, cocaine or diazepam.[4,8]

We have previously reported that drugs which stimulate the GABA/BZD complex reverse the anxiogenic behaviors observed during precipitated CDP withdrawal utilizing drug discrimination methodology.[6,9] Our present results indicate that although ondansetron shows little efficacy in naive animals, it exhibits significant anxiolytic activity in rats withdrawn from chronic CDP. However, other studies in our laboratory have demonstrated that ondansetron was ineffective in blocking the interoceptive discriminative stimulus or the behavioral alterations in the EPM produced by the anxiogenic drug PTZ (unpublished data). Based on differential anxiolytic efficacy of ondansetron in various animal models, additional studies are needed to reach any conclusions regarding its clinical applications.

REFERENCES

1. WOODS, J. H., J. L. KATZ & G. WINGER. 1987. Pharmacol. Rev. **39**: 251–413.
2. CHOPIN, P. & M. BRILEY. 1987. TIPS **8**: 383–388.
3. BUTLER, A., J. M. HILL, S. J. IRELAND, C. C. JORDAN & M. B. TYERS. 1988. Br. J. Pharmacol. **94**: 397–412.
4. COSTALL, B., A. M. DOMENEY, M. E. KELLY, R. J. NAYLOR & M. B. TYERS. 1987. Br. J. Pharmacol. **91**: 420P.
5. HANDLEY, S. L. & S. MITHANI. 1984. Naunyn-Schmiedeberg's Arch. Pharmacol. **327**: 1–5.
6. IDEMUDIA, S. O. & H. LAL. 1989. Drug Dev. Res. **16**: 23–29.
7. JONES, B. J., B. COSTALL, A. M. DOMENEY, M. E. KELLY, R. J. NAYLOR, N. R. OAKLEY & M. B. TYERS. 1988. Br. J. Pharmacol. **93**: 985–993.
8. COSTALL, B., B. J. JONES, M. E. KELLY, R. J. NAYLOR, E. S. ONAIVI & M. B. TYERS. 1990. Pharmacol. Biochem. Behav. **36**: 339–344.
9. EMMET-OGLESBY, M. W., D. A. MATHIS, R. T. Y. MOON & H. LAL. 1990. Psychopharmacology **101**: 292–309.

Seizure Incidence Enhancement with Increasing Alcohol Intake

RICHARD LECHTENBERG

AND THERESA M. WORNER

The Long Island College Hospital
Brooklyn, New York 11201
and
Berlex Laboratories
300 Fairfield Road
Wayne, New Jersey 07470-7358

Acute ethanol withdrawal precipitates seizures in alcoholic individuals, but increasing evidence suggests that chronic ethanol consumption may also play a role in the high prevalence of seizure activity in alcoholic individuals.[1-5] In part this increased seizure activity independent of acute withdrawal may be attributable to the kindling effect of recurrent withdrawals.[5-7] Although individual episodes need not produce seizures, the effect over time of recurrent ethanol withdrawals would be to lower the individual's seizure threshold and make him or her more susceptible to seizures.

Alternatively, the amount of ethanol an individual consumes may also contribute to the probability of new-onset seizures which are independent of withdrawal.[4] Whether or not this apparent increase in incident seizures is an artifact in a population at high risk for recurrent ethanol withdrawal episodes or is an independent phenomenon increasing seizure prevalence in alcoholic individuals is controversial. We sought to determine whether there was any correlation between the dose of ethanol an individual consumed and the probability that a seizure independent of alcohol withdrawal would occur. A concurrent objective in this study was to determine if any patterns emerging from the data differed for women compared to men.

METHODS

A total of 500 patients admitted to the alcohol detoxification unit were evaluated, 83 of whom were women. All patients analyzed met DSM-III-R criteria for alcoholism. Admission to the detoxification unit was justified if the patient typically had disabling or dangerous withdrawal symptoms, if he or she was at high risk for delirium tremens, seizures, or hallucinations, if he or she had failed in outpatient detoxification efforts, or if he or she had an unstable social situation. Patients were excluded if they exhibited violent behavior, suicidal ideation, or evolving medical problems.

Discriminant function analysis was used to establish correlations between presence or absence of seizure activity and independent variables, which included illicit drug use, daily ethanol consumption, lifetime ethanol consumption, age, duration of alcoholism, and number of detoxification hospitalizations.

474

TABLE 1. Comparison between 417 Men and 83 Women of Age, Number of Detoxification Admissions and Quantity and Duration of Alcohol Consumption[a]

	Total Group (n = 500)	Men (n = 417)	Women (n = 83)
Age (years)	41.0 ± 10.4	41.4 ± 10.1	38.9 ± 11.4
Number of detox. admissions	2.1 ± 2.6	2.2 ± 2.7	1.5 ± 2.1
Age first ETOH	16.4 ± 5.9	16.2 ± 5.7	17.2 ± 6.7
ETOH consumption			
Years	24.6 ± 10.6	25.3 ± 10.4	21.9 ± 11.6
G/day	293 ± 245	303 ± 226	238 ± 327

[a] ($\bar{x}$ ± SD) Probability of difference between sexes—p—not significant.

OBSERVATIONS

Patient characteristics are displayed in TABLE 1. Seizures were reported for 98 patients of whom 55 were alleged to have had ethanol withdrawal seizures. Correlations were not evident between seizure prevalence and drug history, and the probability of seizure activity did not increase with the use of multiple illicit drugs. Correlations were evident for seizure activity and total hospitalizations, detoxification admissions, average daily

TABLE 2. Discriminant Analysis of Variables Evaluated for Correlation with Seizure Histories

Variable	R2-Ad	F Value	F Probability
Men and women (n = 500)			
Total admissions	.054	20.3	<0.0001
Detoxifications	.041	15.1	<0.0001
G/day × years	.034	12.7	0.0004
G/day alcohol	.029	10.8	0.0010
Nondetox. admissions	.019	7.0	0.0081
Years of alcohol	.007	2.6	0.1064
Men (n = 417)			
Total admissions	.051	16.3	0.0001
Detoxifications	.035	11.0	0.0009
G/day × years	.019	6.0	0.0147
G/day alcohol	.011	3.4	0.0669
Nondetox. admissions	.025	7.9	0.0051
Years of alcohol	.009	2.7	0.1033
Women (n = 83)			
Total admissions	.072	4.2	0.0454
Detoxifications	.076	4.4	0.0396
G/day × years	.170	11.0	0.0016
G/day alcohol	.190	12.6	0.0008
Nondetox. admissions	.001	0.1	0.8191
Years of alcohol	.002	0.1	0.7490

ethanol consumption, and estimated lifetime ethanol consumption (TABLE 2). There was no correlation between the age at onset of alcoholism, the years of alcoholism, or the age of the patient and the prevalence of seizures.

CONCLUSIONS

Our data confirm the correlation between seizure history and recurrent ethanol detoxifications and support a correlation between average daily ethanol consumption and the likelihood of seizure activity. High ethanol consumption rates are associated with a positive seizure history. This correlation was independent of other substance exposure. Kindling readily explains the increased seizure activity seen with repeated detoxifications, but another mechanism must be responsible for any lowering of the seizure threshold directly attributable to long-term ethanol consumption. The toxic effect of ethanol on inhibitory circuits may underlie the epileptogenic potential of ethanol exposure.

REFERENCES

1. VICTOR, M. & C. BRAUSCH. 1967. Epilepsia **8:** 1–20.
2. HILLBOM, M. E. & M. HJELM-JAGER. 1984. Acta Scand. Neurol. **69:** 39–42.
3. LECHTENBERG, R. & T. M. WORNER. 1990. Arch. Neurol. **47:** 535–538.
4. NG, S. K. C., W. A. HAUSER, J. C. M. BRUST & M. SUSSER. 1988. N. Engl. J. Med. **319:** 666–673.
5. BROWN, M. E., R. F. ANTON, R. MALCOLM & J. C. BALLENGER. 1988. Biol. Psychiatr. **23:** 507–514.
6. McCOWN, T. J. & G. R. BREESE. 1990. Alcohol Clin. Exp. Res. **14:** 394–399.
7. BALLENGER, J. C. & R. M. POST. 1978. Br. J. Psychiatr. **133:** 1–14.

Effects of Imipramine and Ethanol on the Activity of a Neuronal L-Type Calcium Channel

JOSEPH J. McARDLE,[a] JAY J. CHOI,
AND GUO-JIE HUANG

Departments of Pharmacology & Toxicology and Anesthesiology
New Jersey Medical School—UMDNJ
185 South Orange Avenue
Newark, New Jersey 07103-2757

Tricyclic antidepressants help patients undergoing withdrawal from chronic ethanol ingestion.[1] The basis for this therapeutic action is not clear because of the broad spectrum of effects tricyclic antidepressants have on central nervous system (CNS) function.[2] Furthermore, these CNS functions are certainly altered with chronic ethanol ingestion.[3,4] For example, chronic exposure of experimental preparations to ethanol increases both the number of dihydropyridine binding sites[5-7] and the amplitude of the currents which the related L-type calcium channels mediate (I_{Ca}).[8] Since the prototypic tricyclic antidepressant imipramine is known to suppress I_{Ca} in neuroblastoma cells,[9] such an effect may enable imipramine to substitute for ethanol by suppressing the enhanced I_{Ca} brought about by alcoholism.

In order to test this hypothesis we compared the acute effects of ethanol and imipramine on whole cell and single channel currents through an L-type calcium channel in the membrane of neurons in cultured dorsal root ganglia. Details of the methodology are described elsewhere.[10] Within 1 min after exposure to 200 mg% ethanol, I_{Ca} increased by 11% of the control value. This facilitatory effect was associated with an increase in the probability of single channel opening (FIG. 1). However, facilitation was not sustained since I_{Ca} decreased by 20% of the control amplitude after 10 min of exposure to 200 mg% ethanol. At the same time, the probability of single channel opening was greatly reduced (see FIG. 1C). 25 mg% ethanol did not decrease I_{Ca} but produced a slight increase in the frequency of single channel opening at both the 1 and 10 min time points. The delayed reduction of I_{Ca} by 200 mg% ethanol did not occur if cultures were incubated with 200 ng/ml of pertussis toxin (PTX) for 3 h. In fact, there was now a sustained facilitation of I_{Ca}. Imipramine inhibited I_{Ca} at all concentrations tested. This inhibitory action, like that of ethanol, was dependent upon an intact G protein since pretreatment with PTX or cell dialysis with GDP-βS significantly protected I_{Ca} from the depressant effect of imipramine.

These data demonstrate a dose- and time-dependent biphasic effect of acute exposure to ethanol on the activity of a neuronal L-type calcium channel. The inhibitory

[a] Address all correspondence to Dr. McArdle at the Department of Pharmacology & Toxicology; Tel.: (201) 456-4428; Fax: (201) 456-4554.

A   B   C

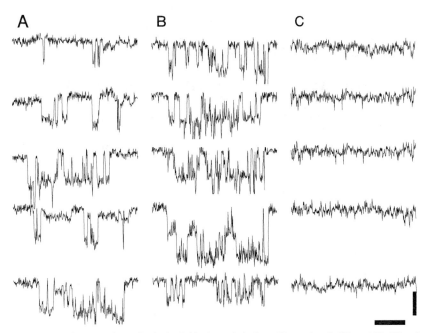

FIGURE 1. Currents through single Ca^{2+} channels before (**A**), and at 1 (**B**) and 10 (**C**) min after exposure to 200 mg% ethanol. Calibration, 1 pA and 20 ms. Cell-attached patch. Holding potential, -40 mV; command potential, 0 mV.

effect of ethanol and that of imipramine depends upon an intact G protein which modulates the activity of the channel. This common site of action of ethanol and imipramine may contribute to the beneficial action of imipramine during withdrawal from ethanol.

REFERENCES

1. SHAPIRO, E. N. 1990. Recent approaches in treatment medications for alcoholics. ADAMHA News **XVI**(6): 9.
2. BALDESSARINI, R. J. 1990. Drugs and the treatment of psychiatric disorders. *In* The Pharmacological Basis of Therapeutics, 8th edit. A. G. Gilman, T. W. Rall, A. S. Nies & P. Taylor, Eds.: 409. Pergamon Press. New York.
3. AIKEN, S. P., J. L. GLEITSMAN & J. J. MCARDLE. 1991. Tolerance to alcohol at the neuromuscular junction of long-sleep and short-sleep mice. Alcohol **8**: 207–209.
4. SHAFIK, E. N., S. P. AIKEN & J. J. MCARDLE. 1991. Regional catecholamine levels in brains of normal and ethanol-tolerant long-sleep and short-sleep mice. Brain Res. **563**: 44–48.
5. HARPER, J. C., C. H. BRENNAN & J. M. LITTLETON. 1989. Genetic up-regulation of calcium channels in a cellular model of ethanol dependence. Neuropharmacology **28**: 1299–1302.
6. BRENNAN, C. H., J. CRABBE & J. M. LITTLETON. 1990. Genetic regulation of dihydropyridine-sensitive calcium channels in brain may determine susceptibility to physical dependence on alcohol. Neuropharmacology **29**: 429–432.
7. LITTLETON, J., H. LITTLE & R. LAVERTY. 1992. Role of neuronal calcium channels in ethanol dependence: From cell cultures to the intact animal. N.Y. Acad. Sci. **654**: 324–334. This volume.

8. AIKEN, S. P., G.-J. HUANG & J. J. McARDLE. 1990. Influence of chronic ethanol treat-
    ment on sleep time and hippocampal calcium currents of long- and short-sleep mice. Soc.
    Neurosci. **16:** (Abstr.) 57.9.
9. OGATA, N., M. YOSHII & T. NARAHASHI. 1989. Psychotropic drugs block voltage-gated
    ion channels in neuroblastoma cells. Brain Res. **476:** 140–144.
10. HUANG, G.-J. & J. J. McARDLE. 1991. Novel suppression of an L-type calcium channel
    in neurones of murine dorsal root ganglia by the chemical phosphatase 2,3-butanedione
    monoxime. J. Physiol. (London) **447:** 257–274.

Studies of the Mechanism of Inhibition of the Dopamine Uptake Carrier by Cocaine *in Vitro* Using Rotating Disk Electrode Voltammetry[a]

JAMES S. McELVAIN[b] AND JAMES O. SCHENK[b–e]

[b] Department of Biochemistry and Biophysics
[c] Department of Chemistry
[d] Program in Pharmacology/Toxicology
Washington State University
Pullman, Washington 99164-4630

The mechanism of action of the abused drug, cocaine, is thought to be related to its ability to inhibit neuronal uptake of dopamine (DA) in the CNS.[1] Although studies of the action of cocaine on the DA uptake carrier have been made, its specific molecular mechanism of action is not fully understood.[1,2] In this study we have used rotating disk electrode (RDE) voltammetric methods[3] with 50 msec resolution to study the mechanism of DA uptake and its inhibition by cocaine.

Individual rat striatal suspensions[4] were incubated at 37°C in 500 μL of physiological buffer in the presence or absence of 0.5, 1.0, 2.0, 4.0, or 8.0 μM cocaine. Inorganic ion dependence of DA uptake was studied in physiological buffers where Na^+ and Cl^- were substituted with choline and isethionate, respectively, in the presence or absence of cocaine. Either exogenous (by direct addition) or endogenous (by KCl stimulation) non-radioactively labeled DA was introduced into the striatal suspension and its uptake or reuptake, respectively, was monitored by the RDE (FIG. 1). The initial uptake rate data was analyzed by non-linear regression analyses of the Michaelis-Menten equation[5] and Eadie-Hofstee graphical procedures.[5] Further terreactant analyses were conducted using methods outlined by Fromm.[6]

The velocity of DA uptake was found to be proportional to the extracellular [DA], [Cl^-], and [Na^+] values. Cocaine uncompetitively inhibited the uptake of exogenous DA added to nonstimulated suspensions and non-competitively inhibited the reuptake of endogenous DA released by KCl. The results of non-linear regression curve fitting of the uptake profiles suggested reaction orders of 1, 1, and 2, for DA, Cl^-, and Na^+, respectively, and cocaine competitively inhibited both Na^+ and Cl^- dependent uptake (see TABLE 1 for the kinetic observations and interpretations). Finally, the results of terreactant studies suggested that DA uptake occurs in a partially random se-

[a] Research reported in this paper was supported by the Washington Alcohol and Drug Abuse Program (Legislative Initiative 171).

[e] Address correspondence to James O. Schenk, Ph.D. at the Department of Chemistry; Tel.: (509) 335-7517 (-4300); Fax: (509) 335-8867.

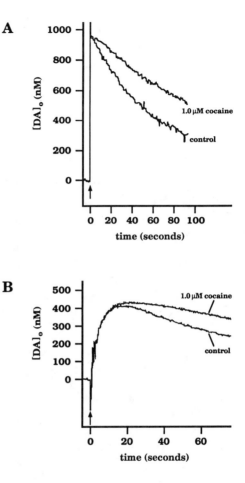

FIGURE 1. The time courses of uptake of exogenously or endogenously added DA monitored by the RDE and the influence of 1.0 μM cocaine. **A** shows that cocaine inhibits the uptake of 1.0 μM DA exogenously added to the striatal suspension (*arrow*). **B** demonstrates that 1.0 μM cocaine also inhibits reuptake of endogenous DA, released by stimulating the striatal suspension with 30 mM KCl (*arrow*). Initial rate data was taken from the apparent zero order kinetic region of the profile which was obtained over the initial 25-sec time period following the maximally observed extracellular DA concentration, $[DA]_o$.

TABLE 1. Summary of the Results of Mechanistic Studies of Cocaine Inhibition of Dopamine Uptake

Conditions of Study	Substrate Studied	Reaction Order	Mechanism of Inhibition[a] (constant parameter)	Interpretation of Result (Coc = cocaine)
Resting	Dopamine	1	Uncompetitive (V_{max}/K_m)	Coc binds to DA-carrier complex
Resting	Sodium[b]	2	Competitive (V_{max})	Coc binds at sodium site
Resting	Chloride[c]	1	Competitive (V_{max})	Coc binds at chloride site
Stimulated	Dopamine	1	Noncompetitive (K_m)	Coc binds at non-DA binding site

[a] Determined by Eadie-Hofstee analysis of initial rate data at cocaine concentrations ranging from 0.5–8.0 μM. The mechanism of inhibition is indicated by the experimental observation of a constant kinetic parameter of V_{max}, K_m, or V_{max}/K_m in parenthesis.

[b] Isosmotically replaced with choline.

[c] Isosmotically replaced with isethionate.

quential, as opposed to a ping-pong, mechanism where DA and Na^+ first bind in random order to the DA transporter and C^- binds last. These data suggest that cocaine cannot inhibit the DA uptake process until DA is bound to the transporter and that it acts by competing at the Na^+-binding site. The finding that cocaine was also competitive at the Cl^- site may result from the possibility that Cl^- binding follows Na^+ binding.[7]

REFERENCES

1. PITTS, D. K. & J. MARWAH. 1987. Neurobiology of drug abuse. Monogr. Neural Sci. **13:** 34–54.
2. HORN, A. S. 1990. Prog. Neurobiol. **34:** 387–400.
3. SCHENK, J. O., T. A. PATTERSON & J. S. McELVAIN. 1990. Trends Anal. Chem. **9:** 325–330.
4. McELVAIN, J. S. & J. O. SCHENK. 1991. Neuropharmacology. In press.
5. FERSHT, A. 1985. Enzyme Structure and Mechanism, 2nd edit. W. H. Freeman and Co. New York.
6. FROMM, H. J. 1975. Initial Rate Enzyme Kinetics. Springer Verlag. New York.
7. MONOD, J., J.-P. CHANGEUX & F. JACOB. 1963. J. Mol. Biol. **6:** 306–329.

Evidence for a Possible Role of the 5-HT$_2$ Antagonist Ritanserin in Drug Abuse

T. MEERT AND G. CLINCKE

Janssen Research Foundation
Department of Neuropsychopharmacology
B-2340 Beerse, Belgium

Ritanserin is a potent central 5-HT$_2$ antagonist. In animals, low doses increase slow wave sleep and markedly disinhibit behavior induced by natural aversive stimuli. Up to high doses, normal behavior is not affected. In humans, ritanserin also markedly increases slow wave sleep and improves mood and drive in dysthymic and depressed patients. Occasional observations over the past 5 years indicated that ritanserin may be of value in subjects withdrawing from drugs of abuse.[1] Such patients may experience similar problems in coping with daily life as dysthymic/depressed patients. Different studies were conducted in order to test a possible role of ritanserin in drug abuse.

In an oral drinking procedure in rats, ritanserin was demonstrated to reduce drug intake and drug preference in animals given the choice between the drug of abuse and water after a period of forced drug exposure. Activity started at doses ⩾0.04 mg/kg ritanserin once daily. Adaptations of the test procedure by prolonging the drug exposure time, by building in a withdrawal phase and by changing the treatment schedules, did not essentially change the activity of ritanserin. Ritanserin was found active against three different agents of abuse: alcohol, cocaine, and fentanyl (see FIG. 1). The concentrations of the tested drugs, obtained in pilot trials testing for an optimal preference rate, were 3% alcohol, 0.1 mg/ml cocaine and 0.02 mg/ml fentanyl. As opposed to the effects on the drugs of abuse, ritanserin could not attenuate the preference for a non-addictive substance sucrose, excluding a non-specific effect of ritanserin on preference. At no time did ritanserin interfere with total fluid intake or any consummatory physiological processes. Additional drinking experiments indicated that ritanserin did not create aversion for the various substances tested. Also a direct interaction between ritanserin and the various drugs of abuse could be ruled out on the basis of various other interaction studies.

Ritanserin did not affect 1) duration of the loss of the righting reflex induced by intraperitoneal injections of high doses of alcohol; 2) cocaine-induced agitation and locomotor stimulation; and 3) opioid-induced analgesia. In a drug discrimination test procedure in rats, ritanserin did not affect the stimulus properties of alcohol, cocaine, and fentanyl. Also with regard to other drugs of abuse, ritanserin did not produce any stimulus generalization to or an antagonism of the stimulus properties of various drugs except for LSD and DOM, two 5-HT$_2$-mediated cues, where an antagonism of the discriminative stimulus properties was observed after ritanserin treatment. Ritanserin

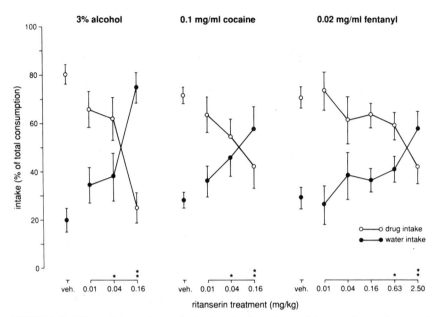

FIGURE 1. Effects of ritanserin on the intake of various drugs of abuse and water in an oral choice drinking paradigm in rats. Presented are the average (±SEM) intake of either alcohol, cocaine and fentanyl or water over the entire period of choice (5 days) after a period of forced drug exposure (10 days). The data on intake are expressed as a percentage of total intake. Ritanserin was given once daily in the morning. Differences with the vehicle conditions were evaluated using the Mann-Whitney U-test (two-tailed; * $p < 0.05$; ** $p < 0.01$).

itself was demonstrated to be devoid of internal stimulus properties. Because ritanserin is also not self-administered and there is no development of conditioned place preference, the drug appears to lack abuse potential.

In the conditioned place preference paradigm, ritanserin attenuated the conditioned place preference induced by d-amphetamine, diazepam, morphine,[2] and fentanyl without having any intrinsic activity.

Also with regard to withdrawal from drugs of abuse, there is evidence indicating a role for ritanserin in drug abuse. For opioids, ritanserin reduced naloxone-induced withdrawal tics in chronically morphine treated mice.[3] In rats barpressing for food, ritanserin blocked the effects on responding of a quasi-morphine[4] and a fentanyl withdrawal. For cocaine, 0.63 mg/kg ritanserin attenuated the sleep–wakefulness alterations in rats during withdrawal from cocaine administration. Acute effects of cocaine on sleep could not be antagonized. Doses ranging from 0.04 to 10.0 mg/kg ritanserin overcame an inhibition of exploratory behavior observed during withdrawal from chronic cocaine treatment in the open field test. The activity was present in terms of a reduction in the latency to enter the open field and in terms of an increase in the duration of time spent in the open field as well as in the number of entries into the open area (see Fig. 2). In control rats, receiving a chronic treatment with vehicle instead of cocaine, ritanserin had no intrinsic effects on exploratory behavior.

Because ritanserin 1) reduces the preference for different substances of abuse in an

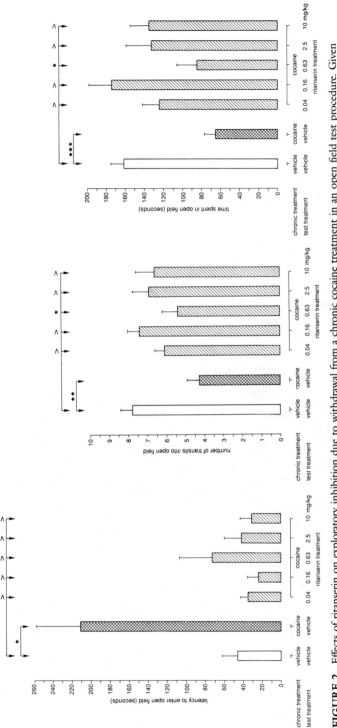

FIGURE 2. Effects of ritanserin on exploratory inhibition due to withdrawal from a chronic cocaine treatment in an open field test procedure. Given are average (±SEM) groups data in terms of latency to enter the open field, number of transits into the open field, and time spent in the open field. Ritanserin or vehicle were given 23 h after a 10 days chronic cocaine treatment and 1 h before testing. Differences with the control condition (vehicle-vehicle group) were evaluated using the Mann-Whitney U-test (two-tailed; > p > 0.05; * p < 0.05).

oral drinking procedure and attenuates conditioned place preference; 2) appears to overcome some of the withdrawal reactions after cessation of chronic treatment with various drugs of abuse; and 3) apparently lacks any direct interaction with substances of abuse, ritanserin might be a good candidate for treatment of problems related to drugs of abuse.

REFERENCES

1. MONTI, J. M. & P. ALTERWEIN. 1991. The Lancet **337:** 60.
2. NOMIKO, G. G. & C. SPYRAKI. 1988. Pharmacol. Biochem. Behav. **30**(4): 853–858.
3. HANDLEY, S. L., A. SINGH & L. SINGH. 1986. Br. J. Pharmacol. **89:** 647P.
4. NEAL, B. S. & S. B. SPARBER. 1990. Psychopharmacology **100:** 258–266.

Prenatal Neurochemistry of Cocaine

JERROLD S. MEYER

Department of Psychology
Neuroscience and Behavior Program
Tobin Hall
University of Massachusetts
Amherst, Massachusetts 01003

A number of physiological and behavioral abnormalities have been reported following prenatal cocaine exposure.[1] Although cocaine is known to bind to recognition sites on monoaminergic nerve terminals and to inhibit neurotransmitter reuptake in adult brain,[2] its mechanism of action during early development is still unknown. In an effort to understand the prenatal neurochemistry and pharmacology of cocaine, we investigated 1) the kinetic characteristics and prenatal ontogeny of cocaine binding sites in rat brain, and 2) synaptosomal uptake of dopamine (DA) and the potency of cocaine in inhibiting such uptake during development.

METHODS

Whole fetal brains were obtained from timed-pregnant Sprague-Dawley rats. Membranes were prepared from P2 (crude synaptosomal) fractions and [^{3}H]cocaine binding was determined using standard filtration methods. On gestational (GD) 20, saturation analyses were performed using a range of ligand concentrations from 0.3 nM to either 300 nM or 1 μM. Nonspecific binding was defined by means of 1 mM unlabeled cocaine. A fixed concentration of 10 nM [^{3}H]cocaine was used to study the ontogeny of cocaine-binding sites. Temperature-dependent synaptosomal DA uptake was investigated by incubating P2 fractions with [^{3}H]DA at either 37°C or 0°C. To determine the kinetics of uptake at GD20, incubations were performed with DA concentrations ranging from 0.05 to 0.50 μM and the results were analyzed by a double-reciprocal plot. In the cocaine inhibition study, synaptosomes were incubated with 0.05 μM [^{3}H]DA in the absence or presence of cocaine at concentrations ranging from 10^{-8} to 10^{-4} M. Resulting inhibition curves were subjected to log-probit analysis.

RESULTS AND CONCLUSIONS

Saturable cocaine binding was found in GD20 fetal rat brain. Kinetic parameters determined by EDBA/LIGAND were as follows: K_D = 176 ± 88 nM, B_{Max} = 612 ± 150 fmol/mg protein (1-site model); K_{DS} = 20 ± 7 nM and 2.1 ± 1.1 μM, B_{MaxS} = 98 ± 47 fmol/mg protein and 2.1 ± 0.6 pmol/mg protein for the high- and low-affinity sites, respectively (2-site model). Scatchard plots were consistently curvilinear, although the 1-site model was not statistically rejected in most experiments. Cocaine

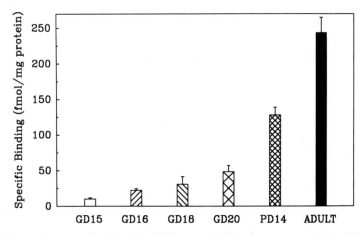

FIGURE 1. Ontogeny of whole-brain [^{3}H]cocaine binding from gestational day (GD) 15 to adulthood. Membrane preparations were incubated with 10 nM [^{3}H]cocaine with or without 1 mM unlabeled cocaine to define nonspecific binding. Values shown represent the mean ± SEM for 3–4 litters at each prenatal time point and 6 individual male brains at postnatal day (PD) 14 and adulthood.

TABLE 1. Synaptosomal Dopamine (DA) Uptake and Cocaine Inhibition at Gestational Day 20

DA Uptake Kinetics	
K_m: 0.154 ± 0.019 μM	V_{Max}: 1.73 ± 0.14 pmol/min/mg protein

Cocaine Inhibition of DA Uptake
IC_{50} (at 0.05 μM DA): 0.591 ± 0.069 μM

binding measured using a 10 nM concentration of ligand was detected as early as GD15 and gradually increased across pre- and postnatal development (FIG. 1).

Synaptosomal DA uptake was present at GD20, and this uptake could be inhibited by cocaine with a potency comparable to that found in adult brain (TABLE 1). In contrast, when several cocaine concentrations were tested at GD15, the dose-response curve was shifted to the right, indicating a lower potency at this earlier stage of development (data not shown).

The present studies demonstrate the presence of cocaine binding and cocaine inhibition of DA uptake in fetal brain. These processes may contribute to the abnormal development found in humans and animals exposed to cocaine *in utero*.

REFERENCES

1. NEUSPIEL, D. R. & S. C. HAMEL. 1991. Cocaine and infant behavior. Dev. Behav. Pediatr. **12**: 55–64.
2. GAWIN, F. H. 1991. Cocaine addiction: Psychology and neurophysiology. Science **251**: 1580–1586.

Ingested Ethanol as a Factor in Double Vision[a]

R. J. MILLER

Department of Psychology
209 Johnson Tower
Washington State University
Pullman, Washington 99164-4820

A frequent symptom of ethanol intoxication is double vision (*diplopia*), a deterioration of the ability to combine the two eyes' images into one percept (*i.e.*, to achieve fusion). One aspect of fusion ability is fusion latency, the time required to achieve fusion once a target is binocularly visible. A major contributor to successful fusion is the ability to converge or diverge the eyes to an angle appropriate for the distance of the target. Several studies[1] have shown that intoxicated observers can neither diverge nor converge to the extremes possible when they are sober, although vergence for intermediate distances remains unaffected. Thus, it might be expected that alcohol would increase fusion latency for far and near, but not for intermediate, targets.

Subjects were 8 male volunteers, age 21–24 years. All had excellent vision and were moderate drinkers. Each subject participated, in counterbalanced order, in two sessions. Preceding each session, he was given 20 min to consume a drink. For the placebo (PL) session, the drink was pure diluent. For the alcohol (AL) session, the drink was 1.4 ml/kg of 190 proof (95%) ethanol, plus diluent.

Fusion latency was assessed with an amblyoscope (FIG. 1), with viewing tubes set at vergence angles corresponding to viewing distances of 10.0, 11.1, 12.5, 14.3, 16.7, 20.0, 25.0, 33.3, 50.0, and 100.0 cm, and infinity. Each trial began with the opening of the shutter for the dominant eye's target. The subject viewed the target for 5 sec; then the second shutter opened. The subject pressed a button as soon as he achieved fusion. The elapsed time between the opening of the second shutter and the subject's response defined fusion latency for that trial. Such a trial was conducted for each of the 11 stimulus vergence distances. This set of trials was repeated every 15 min, for 6 h, with an Intoximeter assessment of blood alcohol level (BAL) preceding each set.

As BAL increased, fusion latencies increased for near and far, but not for intermediate, targets (FIG. 2). A 4 × 11 (BAR × target distance) ANOVA showed both independent variables and the interaction to be statistically significant ($p < .01$). Newman-Keuls analyses showed that at 10 cm, BAR1 differed from BAR3 and BAR4, $p < .05$. At 11.1 cm, BAR1 differed from BAR3 ($p < .05$), and from BAR4 ($p < .01$), and BAR2 differed from BAR4 ($p < .05$). At infinity, all BAR values differed from one another ($p < .01$). The far point of fusion (the maximum distance at which fusion could be attained) decreased significantly as BAL increased.

[a] This investigation was supported in part by funds provided for medical and biological research by the State of Washington (Legislative Initiative 171).

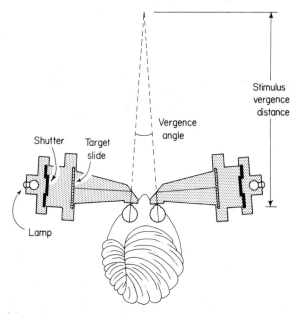

FIGURE 1. Schematic representation of amblyoscope, viewed from above.

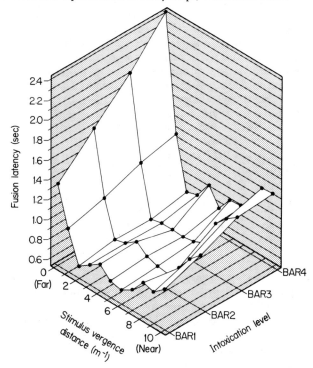

FIGURE 2. Fusion latencies as functions of stimulus vergence distance and intoxication level. *Note:* BAR1: BAL = 0–0.04%; BAR2: BAL = 0.05–0.06%; BAR3: BAL = 0.07–0.08%; BAR4: BAL = 0.09% and above.

Several conclusions are supported by these results:

1. Measurable increases in fusion latency occur even with relatively low levels of intoxication. Tasks requiring rapid detection and recognition (*e.g.*, unexpected objects on the highway) could be affected because, even when such targets can be fused, doing so requires more time as BAL increases.

2. These effects increase progressively with BAL.

3. Alcohol induces changes in fusion latency for far and near targets, but not (at least at the dosage used in this experiment) for intermediate distances.

REFERENCE

1. MILLER, R. J., R. G. PIGION & M. TAKAHAMA. 1986. Percept. Psychophys. **39:** 25–31.

Effect of Haloperidol on Craving and Impaired Control following Alcohol Consumption in Alcoholic Subjects[a]

JACK G. MODELL[b] AND JAMES M. MOUNTZ[c]

Departments of [b] Psychiatry and [c] Nuclear Medicine
University of Alabama School of Medicine
Birmingham, Alabama 35294-0018

We recently proposed that craving and impaired control following alcohol ingestion in alcohol-dependent and alcohol-abusing individuals (herein referred to as "alcoholic[s]") are produced or exacerbated by the alcohol-induced increase in nigrotegmental dopaminergic-inhibitory input to the striatoaccumbens.[1] This study tests the hypothesis that antagonism of the dopaminergic effects of intoxication should, therefore, specifically diminish craving and impaired control in alcoholic individuals following alcohol ingestion.

METHODS

Eight subjects (5 male, 3 female; ages 27–60) with a diagnosis of alcohol-dependence or alcohol-abuse (DSM-IIIR) have thus far participated in a double-blind, placebo-controlled, crossover study in which the effects of the D_2 antagonist haloperidol on alcohol preference following an oral alcohol challenge were assessed. Subjects were otherwise healthy and taking no medications. All subjects were actively engaged in our alcoholism treatment program and were between 2 and 14 weeks abstinent prior to study participation. Subjects were pre-selected to include only those individuals who reported that: 1) the usual amount of craving for an alcoholic beverage two days after their last drink was at least five on a zero to ten scale (0 = none; 10 = extreme) and 2) the amount of difficulty that would be encountered in attempting to cease drinking after consumption of two standard drinks was also at least five on this scale. The study was approved by the University of Alabama Investigational Review Board and informed consent was obtained from all subjects prior to participation.

Subjects were admitted to our research unit for two overnight stays, 48 h apart.

[a] Supported by the National Institute of Health, Department of Research Resources Clinical Research Center Grant Numbers MO1-RR00032 (University of Alabama) and MO1-RR00042 (University of Michigan).
[b] Address correspondence to Jack G. Modell, M. D., Department of Psychiatry, Smolian 403, UAB Station, Birmingham, AL 35294-0018; (204) 934-4301.

Upon presentation for study participation on both days, each subject received a urine drug screen, blood alcohol concentration (BAC) by breath testing (Alco-Sensor III®), and the questionnaire shown in FIGURE 1. All subjects proved drug and alcohol free at the start of the experiments. Each subject then received 0.015–0.020 mg/kg haloperidol or 2 ml normal saline intravenously (balanced crossover), followed by a repeat of the assessment battery after 15 min to assess the effects of the injection. At this time only, passive motor tone in the arm was assessed using a scale of zero to four (0 = no passive resistance; 4 = rigid) and subjects were asked whether they believed the in-

---

For each of the items below, please mark an **X** on the line at the place that best describes how you are feeling at this moment.

1. My mood right now is:

    Extremely   Extremely
    Depressed   Happy
        0-----1-----2-----3-----4-----5-----6-----7-----8-----9-----10

2. My level of desire (craving) right now for an alcoholic beverage is:

    None   Extreme
        0-----1-----2-----3-----4-----5-----6-----7-----8-----9-----10

3. If offered an alcoholic beverage right now, resisting drinking it would be:

    Extremely   Extremely
    Easy   Difficult
        0-----1-----2-----3-----4-----5-----6-----7-----8-----9-----10

4. Right now, I feel:

    Not at all   Extremely
    Intoxicated   Intoxicated
        0-----1-----2-----3-----4-----5-----6-----7-----8-----9-----10

5. If $100 were handed to me to keep (no strings attached) right now, I would be:

    Not at all   Extremely
    Pleased   Pleased
        0-----1-----2-----3-----4-----5-----6-----7-----8-----9-----10

6. Right now, I feel:

    Not at all   Extremely
    Thirsty   Thirsty
        0-----1-----2-----3-----4-----5-----6-----7-----8-----9-----10

7. Right now, I feel:

    Not at all   Extremely
    Sleepy   Sleepy
        0-----1-----2-----3-----4-----5-----6-----7-----8-----9-----10

FIGURE 1. Assessment battery for subjectively rated mood, craving for an alcoholic beverage, degree of difficulty resisting consumption of an alcoholic beverage if offered, intoxication, hedonic capacity, thirst, and sleepiness, administered at: 1) pre-injection (baseline); 2) 15 min following the injection; 3) 15 min following 0.4 g/kg orally administered ethanol; 4) 15 min following optional consumption of an additional 0–0.2 g/kg orally administered ethanol. These items have been previously validated by the authors (unpublished data).

jection contained the active drug or placebo. Each subject then received 0.4 g/kg ethanol orally as 12 ounces of his/her favorite beverage, to be consumed within 5 min. The subject then rested for another 15 min, at which time the questionnaire was re-administered and the BAC was measured. Each subject was then offered the option of drinking a second alcoholic beverage containing 0.2 g/kg ethanol and was instructed to drink any amount of this beverage desired over 5 min. After 15 min, the questionnaire and BAC testing were repeated.

RESULTS

Numeric results of the variables for which significant differences were found following haloperidol administration relative to the saline control are presented in TABLE 1. Compared with the experimental control, pre-treatment with haloperidol resulted in a significant decrease in optional alcohol consumption (t_{14} = -2.0, p = 0.03); and, over the course of the experiment, significant suppression of subjectively rated desire for additional alcohol ($F_{3,14}$ = 4.50, p = 0.01) and a trend towards a decrease in subjectively rated effort required to resist drinking an additional alcoholic beverage ($F_{3,14}$ = 2.4, p = 0.08). There was a significant increase over the course of the experiment in subjectively rated sleepiness following haloperidol administration relative to that reported following administration of saline ($F_{3,14}$ = 4.5, p = 0.01), but there were no significant relative differences in reported levels of intoxication, hedonic capacity, or thirst. There was no correlation between reported sleepiness and alcohol consumption. Additionally, there were no measurable differences between groups in BACs attained following alcohol consumption, and no perceptible changes in muscle tone following haloperidol administration (mean = 0.4 saline; 0.3 haloperidol: ns). Of note, the subjects could not reliably distinguish injected haloperidol from normal saline

TABLE 1. Significant Results[a]

Item/Group	Pre-Injection	Post-Injection	Post-Required Drink	Post-Optional Drink
Craving (q. 2): NS	4.6 (0.7)	4.2 (0.8)	6.6 (0.7)	6.1 (0.6)
Craving: Hal	5.1 (0.9)	4.1 (1.0)	4.5 (0.9)	3.3 (0.9)
Difficulty Refusing More Alcohol (q. 3): NS	4.1 (1.2)	4.8 (0.9)	6.1 (1.1)	6.6 (0.9)
Difficulty Refusing More Alcohol: Hal	4.5 (1.0)	3.9 (1.2)	5.0 (0.8)	3.4 (0.9)
Sleepiness (q. 7): NS	2.2 (0.8)	2.4 (0.8)	2.1 (0.8)	2.5 (0.8)
Sleepiness: Hal	1.9 (0.9)	3.2 (1.2)	4.4 (1.1)	4.0 (1.0)
Optional alcohol consumption (g/kg): NS	0.20 (0.00)			
Optional alcohol consumption (g/kg): Hal	0.13 (0.03)			

[a] Mean and (SEM) at each of the four assessment periods of the questionnaire items (q.) for which differences were found (*top*) and of optional alcohol consumption (*bottom*) following haloperidol (Hal) administration relative to the normal saline (NS) control.

(χ^2_1 = 1.5, p = 0.3). Finally, no subject returned to uncontrolled drinking as a result of participation in this study.

DISCUSSION

The data suggest that the D_2 antagonist haloperidol can specifically reduce craving and impaired control following alcohol consumption in alcoholic individuals. These preliminary findings support the hypothesis that these phenomena are mediated by the dopaminergic effects of alcohol ingestion, and are consistent with the proposed etiologic role in alcoholism for nigrotegmental dopaminergic-inhibitory input to the striatoaccumbens.

REFERENCE

1. MODELL, J. G., J. M. MOUNTZ & T. P. BERESFORD. 1990. J. Neuropsychiatry Clin. Neurosci. 2: 123–144.

Effects of Cocaine on Evoked Field Potentials in the Rat Striatum

KWAKU D. NANTWI AND EUGENE P. SCHOENER

Wayne State University School of Medicine
Department of Pharmacology
Detroit, Michigan 48201

The nigro-striatal pathway has important dopaminergic components.[1] Evoked field potentials represent a useful tool for the study of ensemble neuronal masses[2] and can disclose interaction phenomena that may be elusive at the single unit level. The present studies aimed to characterize cocaine/dopamine (DA) interactions at the cellular level.

Male Sprague-Dawley rats (250–275 g) were used in all experiments. Animals were anesthesized with urethane (1 g/kg), and a femoral vein and artery cannulated to administer fluids and measure arterial blood pressure. The arterial cannula was physically connected to a pressure transducer that was electrically connected to an amplifier on a Grass Physiograph. Animals were tracheotomized to allow for ventilatory assist if necessary and mounted in a stereotaxic apparatus. A limited fronto-temporal craniotomy performed, and the brain surface was kept moist with warm 0.9% saline. Body temperature was maintained at $37 \pm 1°C$ in all cases.

Glass-coated, platinum-iridium electrodes for extracellular recording were manufactured in the laboratory after Wohlbarsht *et al.*[3] Each electrode was inserted via hydraulic microdrive manipulator into the striatum. A small, coaxial, bipolar stimulating electrode was inserted through a separate burr hole into the substantia nigra. Brief trains of stimuli were applied to evoke field potentials in the neostriatum. The putative role of dopamine receptors in cocaine's actions was examined in a test/retest paradigm with specific pharmacologic antagonists for DA receptors.

RESULTS

Multiphasic field potentials were evoked and recorded as shown in FIGURE 1. At low doses, cocaine facilitated or depressed the neuronal activity while at a dose of 1.0 mg/kg, depression was predominant (TABLE 1). Field potentials that were depressed following cocaine, regularly showed a P1 resistance to change while other waves were reduced.

In 6 out of 8 experiments, cocaine-induced changes were completely blocked by the selective dopamine-2 receptor antagonist, eticlopride. For example, in two experiments enhancement of P1 (mean of $62 \pm 17.0\%$) and P2 (mean of $63 \pm 12.60\%$) waves was blocked following the intervention. Similarly, in 4 experiments where depression resulted, the magnitude of depression in P1 and P2 waves was blocked. In this series, N waves were not altered by either drug treatment.

In 4 of 6 experiments with the selective dopamine-1 receptor antagonist,

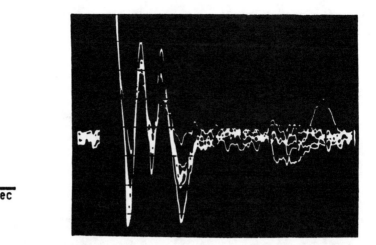

FIGURE 1. A multiphasic evoked field potential characteristic of the type encountered in the striatum. A prominent stimulus artifact preceded the positively and negatively deflected waves. The latency to onset of evoked activity was 2.5 msec.

TABLE 1. Effects of Cocaine on Evoked Field Potentials

Cocaine Dose (mg/kg)	n	Percent Excited	Percent Depressed	Percent Biphasic	% No Change
0.25	10	40	50	10	0
0.50	8	62.5	37.5	0	0
1.00	7	28.5	72.5	0	0

SCH23390, cocaine-induced depressions in N1 and P1 waves were attenuated—however, this effect was not statistically significant. In the other two experiments, neither cocaine nor SCH23390 provoked any change in activity.

The short, constant latency of the field potentials was consistent with previous reports[4,5] and suggested an antidromic nature.[6,7] It may be concluded that effects of cocaine on neostriatal evoked field potentials are mediated by postsynaptic dopamine-2 receptors.

REFERENCES

1. ANDEN, N. E., A. CARLSSON, A. DAHLSTROM, K. L. FUXE, N. A. HILLARP & K. LARSSON. 1964. Demonstration and mapping out of neostriatal dopamine neurons. Life Sci. **3**: 523–530.
2. MITZDORF, U. 1985. Current source-density method and application in cat cerebral cortex: Investigation of evoked potentials and EEG phenomena. Physiol. Rev. **65**(1): 37–100.
3. WOHLBARSHT, M. L., E. F. MACNICHOL, JR. & H. G. WAGNER. 1960. Glass-coated platinum microelectrode. Science **132**: 1309–1310.

4. FREGYESI, T. L. & D. P. PURPURA. 1967. Electrophysiological analysis of reciprocal caudate-nigral relations. Brain Res. **6:** 440–456.
5. FELTZ, P. & D. ALBE-FESSARD. 1972. A study of an ascending nigro-caudate pathway. Electroen. Neurophysiol. **33:** 179–193.
6. HUBBARD, J. I., R. LLINAS & D. M. J. QUASTEL. 1969. Extracellular field potentials in the central nervous system. *In* Electrophysiological Analysis of Synaptic Transmission. H. Davson, A. D. M. Greenfield, R. Whittam & G. S. Brindley, Eds. Williams and Williams. Baltimore.
7. GRACE, A. A. & B. S. BUNNEY. 1983. Intracellular and extracellular electrophysiology of nigral dopaminergic neurons. 1. Identification and characterization. Neuroscience **10:** 301–315.

Locomotor Responses of FAST and SLOW Mice to Several Alcohols and Drugs of Abuse[a]

TAMARA J. PHILLIPS,[b-d] SUE BURKHART-KASCH,[c,d]
COURTNEY C. GWIAZDON,[c,d] AND JOHN C. CRABBE[c-e]

c Research Service (151-W)
Department of Veterans Affairs Medical Center
3710 S.W. U.S. Veterans Hospital Road
Portland, Oregon 97201

Departments of d Medical Psychology and e Pharmacology
3181 S.W. Sam Jackson Park Road
Oregon Health Sciences University
Portland, Oregon 97201-3098

Selectively bred animal lines provide a powerful means for detecting genetic correlations among traits.[1] We used mice selectively bred for differential sensitivity to the locomotor stimulant effects of ethanol to explore the notion that common genes, and thus, a common biological substrate, mediate the stimulant effects of several alcohols and abused drugs. Mice of the two replicate FAST lines are more sensitive to ethanol's locomotor stimulant actions than are mice of the two replicate SLOW lines.[2] Simplistically, if some or all of the genes determining sensitivity to these stimulant effects also determine sensitivity to other drugs with stimulant actions, then the greater sensitivity of FAST relative to SLOW mice should generalize to other drugs.

METHODS

The locomotor responses of FAST and SLOW mice to several drugs (see TABLE 1) were examined using Omnitech automated activity monitors. Horizontal locomotor activity was recorded by computer as photocell beam interruptions.[2] Generally, mice were injected i.p. with vehicle or one dose of a drug, placed immediately into the center of the monitor, and activity counts were accumulated for 15 min. Dose-response curves were obtained in separate experiments for each drug, and each study included a vehicle-treated control group. Each mouse was tested only once, gender varied among experiments as dictated by availability, and mice ranged in age from 53

a Supported by a grant from the Department of Veterans Affairs, by PHS-NIAAA Grants AA06498, AA08621, and AA07468 and by NIDA Contract No. 271-90-7405.
b Address all correspondence to Tamara J. Phillips, Ph.D., at the Department of Veterans Affairs Medical Center.

TABLE 1. Locomoter Responses of FAST and SLOW Mice to Several Alcohols and Drugs of Abuse[a]

Drug	Dose	General Response		Line × Dose Interaction
		FAST	SLOW	
Methanol	1.5–3.0 g/kg	Stim	None	$F[4,178] = 7.3, p < .001$
t-Butanol	0.2–0.6 g/kg	Stim	None	$F[3,112] = 6.1, p < .001$
n-Propanol	0.2–1.2 g/kg	Stim	Depr	$F[5,207] = 21.7, p < .001$
Pentobarbital	10–40 mg/kg	Stim	Stim (F > S)	$F[4,140] = 3.6, p < .01$
Nicotine	0.5–2.0 mg/kg	Depr	Depr (F = S)	NS
d-Amphetamine	2.5–10 mg/kg	Stim	Stim (F = S)	NS
Diazepam	1.0–8.0 mg/kg	None	Depr	$F[4,140] = 7.9, p < .001$
Caffeine	2.5–20 mg/kg	Stim	Stim (F = S)	NS

[a] When general drug responses of the two lines are in the same direction, relative line comparisons are shown in parentheses. Group size per line, replicate and dose was 8–11 mice. Doses listed do not include the vehicle control group for each drug. Stim = stimulant response, Depr = depressant response, None = no significant response. NS = not significant.

to 132 days. Data were statistically evaluated with ANOVA, simple main effect analyses, and Newman Keuls mean comparisons, when appropriate.

RESULTS

TABLE 1 provides a list of the results across all drugs. When *Stim* or *Depr* is listed under *General Response*, the locomotor activity of the line was stimulated or depressed at several doses of the drug. When *None* is listed, the line was generally unresponsive to the drug, although some response may have been elicited by one dose. Differences were seen in the shape of the dose-response curves across drugs; some patterns of response were biphasic, while others were linear. In general, SLOW mice were unsusceptible to alcohol-induced stimulation, whereas FAST mice were highly susceptible. Only two other drugs differentiated the selected lines. FAST mice exhibited greater relative sensitivity to pentobarbital-induced stimulation, and SLOW mice exhibited greater sensitivity to diazepam-induced locomotor depression.

DISCUSSION

The results presented here suggest that sensitivity to the locomotor-stimulant effects of several alcohols and ethanol are determined by some common genes. Thus, these drugs may produce locomotor stimulation via similar biological mechanisms. Pentobarbital may also share this mode of action. FAST and SLOW mice did not differ in stimulant response to *d*-amphetamine or caffeine, suggesting that genes other than those differentiated during their selection may determine sensitivity to these drugs. The absence of stimulant responses to some drugs may also be due to differences in mode of action between these drugs and ethanol. Alternatively, the dose ranges may have been inappropriate for detecting stimulant effects.

In general, our results indicate that drugs with stimulant actions do not share a completely common mechanism of action. Genetic selection for ethanol sensitivity may have altered biochemical systems that have indirect roles in determining general magnitude of stimulant response, in which case only those drugs which share this initial route of action differentiate FAST and SLOW lines.

REFERENCES

1. CRABBE, J. C., T. J. PHILLIPS, A. KOSOBUD & J. K. BELKNAP. 1990. Estimation of genetic correlation: Interpretation of experiments using selectively bred and inbred animals. Alcoholism: Clin. Exp. Res. **14:** 141–151.
2. PHILLIPS, T. J., S. BURKHART-KASCH, E. S. TERDAL & J. C. CRABBE. 1991. Response to selection for ethanol-induced locomotor activation: Genetic analyses and selection response characterization. Psychopharmacology **103:** 557–566.

GABA and Nucleus Accumbens Glutamate Neurotransmission Modulate Ethanol Self-Administration in Rats[a]

STEFANIE RASSNICK,[b,e] ELIZABETH D'AMICO,[c]
EDWARD RILEY,[c] LUIGI PULVIRENTI,[b]
WALTER ZIEGLGÄNSBERGER,[d]
AND GEORGE F. KOOB[b]

[b] Department of Neuropharmacology
The Scripps Research Institute
10666 North Torrey Pines Road
La Jolla, California 92037

[c] San Diego State University
San Diego, California 92120

[d] Max-Planck-Institute for Psychiatry
800 München 40 Germany

Previous research suggests that ethanol (EtOH) facilitates the activity of the γ-aminobutyric acid (GABA)/benzodiazepine (BZ) receptor complex[1] and inhibits the activity of the N-methyl-D-aspartate (NMDA) subtype of the glutamate receptor.[2] The nucleus accumbens (N.Acc.) is a mesolimbic-forebrain region that receives glutamatergic afferent projections from the amygdala and hippocampus[3] and is an important neuroanatomical substrate for the reinforcing effects of psychostimulant drugs.[4] The present study examined the effects of isopropylbicyclophosphate (IPPO), a picrotoxin ligand[5] and RO 15-4513, a BZ inverse agonist, in rats trained to orally self-administer EtOH in a free-choice operant task. To examine the role of glutamate receptors in mediating EtOH reinforcement, the effects of systemic administration of acamprosate, a non-selective glutamate receptor antagonist[6] and microinjection of 2-amino-5-phosphopentanoic acid (AP-5), a competitive NMDA receptor antagonist, into the nucleus accumbens were tested.

Male rats were trained to orally self-administer EtOH in a free-choice operant task using a variant of Samson's sucrose fading technique,[7] with saccharin used to overcome EtOH's taste aversive properties. Behavioral testing was conducted in operant

[a] Research was supported by grants provided by the National Institute on Alcohol Abuse and Alcoholism: AA05297 and AA06420, and The Alcoholic Beverage Medical Research Foundation.
[e] Author to whom correspondence should be addressed.

TABLE 1. Effects of IPPO and RO 15-4513 on EtOH Self-Administration[a]

Treatment	(n)	EtOH Responses % of Baseline Mean (±SEM)	Water Responses % of Baseline Mean (±SEM)
Alcohol preferring rats	(8)		
IPPO 0 µg/kg		101.0 (10.7)	122.6 (21.35)
5 µg/kg		74.5 (11.6)	75.3 (22.7)
10 µg/kg		63.9 (10.9)*	120.4 (61.3)
20 µg/kg		26.9 (21.0)*	20.7 (12.4)
Wistar rats	(10)		
RO 15-4513 0 mg/kg		88.2 (15.4)	94.0 (13.2)
.375 mg/kg		41.2 (11.1)*	53.2 (19.4)
.75 mg/kg		43.9 (9.8)*	63.5 (12.9)
1.5 mg/kg		43.3 (10.0)*	101.3 (20.8)
3.0 mg/kg		43.4 (19.1)*	47.6 (15.2)
6.0 mg/kg		28.8 (14.6)*	37.8 (18.0)*

[a] A two-lever free choice task was used where responses on a fixed ratio schedule-1 (FR-1) resulted in the delivery of response-contingent EtOH (10% w/v) or water reinforcements. Each experiment was conducted using a within-subjects latin-square design of drug administration with a minimum of 2 non-drug days elapsing between drug treatments. RO 15-4513 was prepared as a suspension (.05% emulpher, 0.05% of 10% EtOH and 0.95% saline) and administered 20 min i.p. prior to testing. IPPO was dissolved in saline and administered 10 min i.p. prior to testing. Mean (± standard error of the mean) baseline responses for EtOH and water for the IPPO experiment were 51.8 (5.3) and 24.1 (2.5); and for the RO 15-4513 experiment 52.8 (5.4), and 14.5 (1.5). * $p < 0.05$, as compared to responding following vehicle injection, Newman-Keul's tests for comparison of individual means.

chambers equipped with 2 levers and 2 adjacent stainless steel drinking cups. Responses on a fixed ratio schedule –1 (FR-1) at one lever delivered EtOH (10% w/v: 0.1 ml/response), while responses at the other lever delivered the same quantity of water (30 min daily sessions), with the EtOH side alternated daily. All free-choice responding was conducted in the absence of water and food deprivation, without sweeteners in the EtOH drinking solution, so the results of drug administration on this operant behavior allow for an interpretation of drug effects on the pharmacological properties of EtOH reinforcement.

The results demonstrate that IPPO (5 µg/kg i.p.), and RO 15-4513 (.375, .75, and 1.5 mg/kg i.p.), selectively reduced responses for EtOH, while higher doses of these drugs (IPPO 20 µg/kg; RO 15-4513 at 3.0 & 6.0 mg/kg) suppressed both EtOH and water responses (TABLE 1). Since saccharin self-administration in a free-choice task with access to saccharin (0.05%) and water was unaffected by RO 15-4513 (data not shown, Rassnick and Koob, unpublished observations), the effects of RO 15-4513 on EtOH responding are selective for EtOH and do not necessarily generalize to other reinforcers. Acamprosate (100 mg/kg i.p.), and intra-N.Acc. infusion of AP-5 (3.0, 6.0 µg), selectively reduced EtOH-reinforced responding (TABLE 2). Mean blood EtOH levels ranged from 28 (±6) to 39 (±4) mg%.

These results indicate that GABA and glutamate may be important neurochemical mediators of the acute reinforcing properties of EtOH and that the N.Acc. is an anatomical substrate comprising part of the neural circuitry that modulates the mildly

TABLE 2. Effects of CAOTA and Intra-Nucleus Accumbens Injection of AP-5 on EtOH Self-Administration[a]

Treatment		(n)	EtOH Responses % of Baseline Mean (±SEM)	Water Responses % of Baseline Mean (±SEM)
Wistar Rats		(12)		
Acamprosate	0 mg/kg		102.7 (9.0)	113.0 (19.1)
	0 mg/kg		77.7 (8.2)	76.2 (17.9)
	25 mg/kg		83.4 (12.5)	77.5 (23.0)
	50 mg/kg		71.3 (2.4)	95.2 (22.6)
	100 mg/kg		40.0 (10.0)*	114.9 (23.5)
Wistar rats		(8)		
AP-5	0 μg		103.0 (9.2)	101.1 (37.6)
	3.0 μg		72.3 (9.8)*	93.2 (27.4)
	6.0 μg		68.4 (12.1)*	90.7 (23.6)

[a] A two-lever free choice task was used where responses on a fixed ratio schedule-1 (FR-1) resulted in the delivery of response-contingent EtOH (10% w/v) or water reinforcements. Each experiment was conducted using a within-subjects latin-square design of drug administration with a minimum of 2 non-drug days elapsing between drug treatments. Acamprosate was dissolved in saline and administered 30 min i.p. prior to testing. AP-5 was dissolved in saline and 1 μl was infused bilaterally at a rate of 0.95 μl/min into cannulae aimed at the N.Acc. immediately before the test session (stereotaxic coordinates[9] were: AP: +3.2 mm, lat: 1.7 ± mm to bregma at the skull surface and V: 4.8 mm). Mean (± standard error of the mean) baseline responses for EtOH and water for the acamprosate experiment were 45.4 (2.9), 13.5 (1.1); and for the AP-5 experiment 28.7 (4.2) and 22.3 (2.6). * $p < 0.05$, as compared to responding following vehicle injection, Newman-Keul's tests for comparison of individual means.

intoxicating/reinforcing properties of EtOH associated with EtOH-seeking behavior. Previous studies have suggested that the neural circuitry underlying the activating and reinforcing properties of other drugs of abuse includes an allocortical-limbic-accumbens-palhdal pathway.[8] The present results suggest that N.Acc. glutamatergic afferents originating in allocortical areas and GABA neurotransmission may mediate, in part, the reinforcing properties of EtOH. However other factors such as anticipation of access or motivation related to obtaining EtOH, and other neurotransmitter systems may contribute to the maintenance of ethanol-reinforced responding.

ACKNOWLEDGMENTS

Alcohol-preferring rats were kindly provided by Drs. L. Lumeng and T.-K. Li of Indiana University School of Medicine, Indianapolis, Indiana. The authors thank Dr. R. F. Squires of the Nathan S. Kline Institute for Psychiatric Research, Orangeburg, NY for providing IPPO.

REFERENCES

1. SUZDAK, P. D., R. D. SCHWARTZ, P. SKOLNICK & S. PAUL. 1986. Proc. Natl. Acad. Sci. USA 83: 4071–4075.

2. HOFFMAN, P. L., C. S. RABE, F. MOSES & B. TABAKOFF. 1989. J. Neurochem. **52:** 1937–1940.
3. WALAAS, I. 1981. Neuroscience **6:** 399–405.
4. KOOB, G. F. & F. E. BLOOM. 1988. Science **242:** 715–723.
5. SQUIRES, R. F., J. E. CASIDA, M. RICHARSON & E. SAEDERUP. 1983. Mol. Pharmacol. **23:** 326–336.
6. ZEISE, M. L., S. KASPAROW, M. CAPOGNA & W. ZIEGLGÄNSBERGER. 1990. *In* Taurine Functional Neurochemistry, Physiology and Cardiology. H. Pasantes-Morales, W. Shain, D. L. Martin & R. Martin del Río, Eds.: 237–242. Wiley-Liss, Inc. New York.
7. SAMSON, H. H. 1986. Alcohol. Clin. Exp. Res. **10:** 436–442.
8. SWERDLOW, N. R. & G. F. KOOB. 1987. Behav. Brain Sci. **10**(2): 197–245.
9. PELLEGRINO, L. J., A. S. PELLEGRINO & A. CUSHMAN. 1979. A stereotaxic atlas of the rat brain. Plenum Press. New York.

Ethanol Produces Rapid Biphasic Hedonic Effects[a]

FRED O. RISINGER[b]

AND CHRISTOPHER L. CUNNINGHAM

Department of Medical Psychology (L470)
The Oregon Health Sciences University
3181 S.W. Sam Jackson Park Road
Portland, Oregon 97201-3098

Paradoxically, DBA/2J mice are especially sensitive to the rewarding effects of ethanol in the place-conditioning paradigm and particularly sensitive to the aversive effects of ethanol using the taste-conditioning paradigm.[1,2] One reason for these apparently disparate outcomes may be related to differences in the dynamics of ethanol's rewarding and aversive effects in each of these conditioning situations. It has been hypothesized that ethanol possesses positive reinforcing qualities early after exposure during the rising limb of the BEL time curve, and aversive effects during the falling limb of the BEL time curve.[3] Thus, establishment of ethanol-induced place preference may depend, in part, on whether the early positive effects can be isolated sufficiently in time to overlap with environmental conditioned stimuli. Ethanol-induced aversion or a failure to see preference could be due to delayed negative hedonic effects overlapping with and offsetting the influence of initial positive effects. The present experiment tested this possibility by varying the interval between exposure to ethanol and environmental stimuli in a place conditioning paradigm.

METHOD AND RESULTS

The place conditioning apparatus consisted of 12 identical chambers (30 × 15 × 15 cm) enclosed in ventilated, light and sound attenuating boxes. Occlusion of infrared light beams was used both as a measure of general activity and to determine the animal's position in the chamber. The floor of each box consisted of interchangeable halves with one of two distinctive textures: "hole" floors were made from perforated stainless steel; "grid" floors were composed of stainless-steel rods.

Male DBA/2J mice received four 30-min pairings of one floor stimulus after ethanol injections (CS+ Trials) and the alternate floor stimulus after saline injections (CS− Trials). The experiment concluded with a 60-min preference test offering a choice between the grid floor and hole floor. Each mouse was weighed and injected (i.p.) with

[a] Research presented in this paper was supported by NIAAA Grants AA07702, AA07468, and AA08621.
[b] Author to whom correspondence should be addressed.

either saline or ethanol (3 g/kg). The No-delay group was immediately placed in the apparatus. The Delay-30 group was returned to the home cage for a 30-min waiting period subsequent to being placed in the apparatus. The Delay-60 group was returned to the home cage for a 60-min waiting period before placement in the apparatus. For preference testing, all subjects received saline injections before placement in the apparatus with half grid floor and half hole floor (left/right position counterbalanced).

FIGURE 1 (A) depicts mean activity counts per minute (+SEM) on the first ethanol trial and first saline trial for each group. Ethanol increased overall activity for each group with the Delay-30 group showing the highest level of activation under ethanol. Analysis of variance indicated significant effects of delay, drug treatment, and delay × drug treatment [all Fs(1,138) > 7.9].

Preliminary analysis of preference test performance revealed greater group differences during the last half of the session. FIGURE 1 (B) depicts mean seconds per minute (+SEM) on the grid floor for all groups during the last 30 min of testing. The No-delay groups showed conditioned place preference. The Delay-30 groups showed conditioned place aversion. The Delay-60 groups showed no evidence of place conditioning. Three-way analysis of variance produced a significant effect of delay × conditioning group × time [F(58,1856) = 1.5].

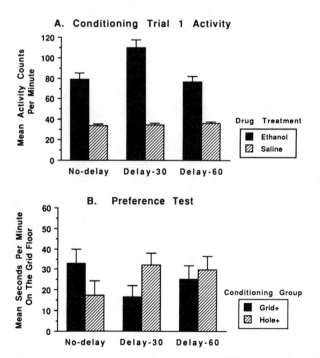

FIGURE 1. A depicts mean activity counts per minute (+SEM) on the first ethanol conditioning trial (*solid bars*) and first saline conditioning trial (*hatched bars*). Ethanol and saline trials were given in an alternating counterbalanced order. **B** depicts mean seconds per minute (+SEM) spent on the grid floor for each group. *Solid bars* depict the Grid+ conditioning groups while *hatched bars* depict Hole+ conditioning groups. Place conditioning is indexed by comparing the difference between adjacent bars (Grid+ vs. Hole+ conditioning groups).

DISCUSSION

These results suggest that ethanol's initial rewarding effects (0 to 30 min after injection) are replaced by aversive effects (30 to 60 min after injection). Presumably, blood and brain ethanol levels were high in all groups, as evidenced by the effect of ethanol on locomotor activity. Ethanol-induced activation did not predict performance during the preference test.

REFERENCES

1. CUNNINGHAM, C. L., D. H. MALOTT & L. K. PRATHER. 1990. Alcohol. Clin. Exp. Res. 14: 280.
2. RISINGER, F. O., S. I. LAWLEY & C. L. CUNNINGHAM. 1990. Soc. Neurosci. Abstr. 16: 754.
3. REID, L. D., G. A. HUNTER, C. M. BEAMAN & C. L. HUBBELL. 1985. Pharmacol. Biochem. Behav. 22: 483–487.

Role of Dopamine Receptors in the Nucleus Accumbens in the Rewarding Properties of Cocaine

PATRICIA ROBLEDO,
RAFAEL MALDONADO-LOPEZ,
AND GEORGE F. KOOB

Department of Neuropharmacology
The Scripps Research Institute
10666 North Torrey Pines Road
La Jolla, California 92037

INTRODUCTION

Studies with intravenous self-administration strongly point to dopaminergic mechanisms in the reinforcing properties of psychomotor stimulants. Dopamine agonists function as positive reinforcers in the monkey[1,2] and the rat,[3] and lesion studies suggest that, at least in part, the dopaminergic system in the nucleus accumbens plays a role as a neuroanatomical substrate for cocaine reinforcement in the rat.[4,5] Further, it is well known that low doses of both D_1 and D_2 dopaminergic antagonists will increase the response rates for intravenous injections of cocaine.[6-9] This increase in self-administration behavior is thought to be a compensatory mechanism for decreases in the magnitude of the reinforcer, similar to the rate increase observed when the dose of the self-administered stimulant is reduced.[4] The purpose of the following study was to explore the hypothesis that dopamine D_1 and/or D_2 receptor subtypes in the nucleus accumbens are responsible for the rewarding properties of cocaine. Hence, the present study evaluated the effects of D_1 and D_2 dopamine receptor antagonists directly infused into the nucleus accumbens on cocaine self-administration behavior in the rat.

METHOD

Thirty male albino Wistar rats weighing 260–300 g (Charles River, Kingston) were used in this study. Animals were housed in groups of three and maintained in a temperature- and light-controlled environment. The rats had free access to food and water except during testing sessions. They were maintained on a 12-h light-dark cycle, and tested during the light phase. Rats were anesthetized with halothane and a polyethylene catheter was implanted in the jugular vein as previously described.[10] Animals were then trained in operant chambers with extendible levers on a fixed ratio 5 (FR5) schedule of reinforcement. Completion of the FR5 resulted in an intravenous injection of 0.1 ml cocaine (Sigma Chemical Co., St. Louis, MO) dissolved in saline

509

(0.25 mg/injection) in a dose of approximately 0.75 mg/kg/injection administered over a period of 4 sec. The duration of the session was 3 h during training and testing. Following completion of training, rats were stereotaxically implanted with bilateral chronic indwelling stainless steel guide cannulae (23 gauge) aimed at the nucleus accumbens (AP +3.2, ML ± 1.7, DV −4.8). A recovery period of at least 3 days was given prior to testing. Microinjections were administered through 30 gauge internal cannula which were inserted such that the tip extended 3 mm below the guide cannulae. The injection volume for all drugs was 0.5 µl per side and was completed in 1 min and 10 sec. The injection cannulae were left in place for an additional minute to allow for diffusion away from the cannulae tip. Statistical analyses were carried out using the Wilcoxon Rank non-parametric test. SCH 23390 maleate (SCH; Schering) was dissolved in distilled water at concentrations of 0.5, 1.0, and 2.0 µg/µl. Haloperidol (HAL; Sigma) was diluted with vehicle solution (1.8 mg methylparaben, 0.2 mg propylparaben in 1 ml dilute lactic acid). The final concentrations of HAL were 0.5, 1.0 and 2.0 µg/µl.

RESULTS

TABLE 1 shows the effect of the selective D_1 dopaminergic antagonist SCH 23390 on self-administration of cocaine. Results are expressed as percent variation from baseline rate of responding. When injected into the nucleus accumbens, SCH 23390 increased responding rates for cocaine at all doses. The maximum effect was observed with the dose of 2 µg, and a significant augmentation was found with the dose of 1 µg ($p < 0.01$). The effect of the preferential D_2 dopaminergic antagonist haloperidol on the self-administration rate of cocaine is also shown on TABLE 1. Haloperidol increased the self-administration of cocaine when injected into the nucleus accumbens at all the doses tested, and the maximum effect was found with the dose of 1 µg which was significantly ($p < 0.05$) different from vehicle. FIGURE 1 displays a representative response record for animals self-administering cocaine on a FR5 schedule. Each mark

TABLE 1. Effects of SCH 23390 and Haloperidol Injected into the Nucleus Accumbens on Cocaine Self-Administration, Percent Variation from Baseline Rate of Responding

	Vehicle	0.5 µg/µl	1 µg/µl	2 µg/µl
Haloperidol				
Median (n = 8)	102.7	106.4	126.1*	109.5
25th Percentile–	96.9–	99.3–	103.4–	68.5–
75th Percentile	108.1	122.0	146.2	157.6
SCH 23390				
Median (n = 8)	110.9	123.5	129.2**	153.5
25th Percentile–	107.9–	113.0–	114.8–	78.2–
75th Percentile	116.2	139.0	143.5	163.3

* $p < 0.05$, ** $p < 0.01$; Wilcoxon Rank test.

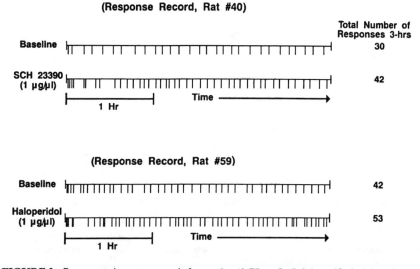

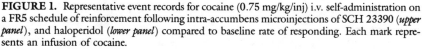

FIGURE 1. Representative event records for cocaine (0.75 mg/kg/inj) i.v. self-administration on a FR5 schedule of reinforcement following intra-accumbens microinjections of SCH 23390 (*upper panel*), and haloperidol (*lower panel*) compared to baseline rate of responding. Each mark represents an infusion of cocaine.

represents an infusion of the drug. In the top panel note the higher rate of responding following an intra-accumbens infusion of SCH 23390 compared to baseline rate. The lower panel illustrates the increase in responding for cocaine produced by an infusion of haloperidol into the nucleus accumbens.

DISCUSSION

It is well known that dopaminergic antagonists (D_1 as well as D_2), injected systemically, produce increases in cocaine self-administration behavior.[6-9] Our results show that both the selective D_1 dopamine receptor antagonist SCH 23390 and the preferential D_2 dopamine receptor antagonist haloperidol directly injected into the nucleus accumbens can also increase the rate of cocaine self-administration in rats. Increases in stimulant self-administration behavior have been interpreted as revealing a decrease in the reward value of the stimulant.[4] Our data are consistent with previous findings suggesting a role of the dopaminergic system in the nucleus accumbens in cocaine reward.[5] Most importantly however, our data extend previous work suggesting that both dopamine receptor subtypes in the nucleus accumbens are involved in the rewarding properties of self-administered cocaine in rats. Finally, these findings show that the increase in responding for cocaine previously observed with systemic administration of D_1 and D_2 antagonists may involve receptors in the region of the nucleus accumbens. These data add further evidence for a competitive interaction with dopamine and the reinforcing actions of cocaine.

REFERENCES

1. GILL, C. A., W. C. HOLTZ, C. L. ZIRKLE & H. HILL. 1978. Pharmacological modification of cocaine and apomorphine self-administration in the squirrel monkey. *In* Proceedings of the Tenth Congress of the Collegium International Neuro-Psychopharmacologicum. P. Deniker, C. Radouco-Thomas & A. Villeneuve, Eds.: 1477–1484. Pergamon Press. New York.
2. IORO, L. C., A. BARNETT, F. H. LEITZ, V. P. HOUSER & C. A. KORDUBA. 1983. SCH 23390, a potential benzazepine antipsychotic with unique interactions on dopaminergic systems. J. Pharmacol. Exp. Ther. **226**: 462–468.
3. YOKEL, R. A. & R. A. WISE. 1978. Amphetamine-type reinforcement by dopamine agonists in the rat. Psychopharmacology (Berlin) **58**: 289–296.
4. KOOB, G. F. 1988. Separate neurochemical substrates for cocaine and heroin reinforcement. *In* Quantitative Analyses of Behavior: Biological Determinants of Behavior. Vol. 7. R. M. Church, M. L. Commons, J. Stellar & A. R. Wagner, Eds.: 55–66. Lawrence Erlbaum Assoc., Inc. Hillsdale, NJ.
5. ROBERTS, D. C. S., G. F. KOOB, P. KLONOFF & H. C. FIBIGER. 1980. Extinction and recovery of cocaine self-administration following 6-hydroxydopamine lesions of the nucleus accumbens. Pharmacol. Biochem. Behav. **12**: 781–787.
6. DEWIT, H. & R. A. WISE. 1977. Blockade of cocaine reinforcement in rats with dopamine blocker pimozide but not with the noradrenergic blockers phentolamine or phenoxybenzamine. Can. J. Psychol. **31**: 195–203.
7. ETTEMBERG, A., H. O. PETIT, F. BLOOM & G. F. KOOB. 1982. Heroin and cocaine self-administration in rats: Mediation by separate neural systems. Psychopharmacology **78**: 204–209.
8. ROBERTS, D. C. S. & G. VICKERS. 1984. Atypical neuroleptics increase self-administration of cocaine: An evaluation of a behavioral screen for anti-psychotic activity. Psychopharmacology **82**: 135–139.
9. KOOB, G. F., H. T. LE & I. CREESE. 1987. The D1 receptor antagonist SCH 23390 increases cocaine self-administration in the rat. Neurosci. Lett. **79**: 315–320.
10. ROBERTS, D. C. S. & G. F. KOOB. 1982. Disruption of cocaine self-administration following 6-hydroxydopamine lesions of the ventral tegmental area in rats. Pharmacol. Biochem. Behav. **17**: 901–904.

Dramatic Depletion of Mesolimbic Extracellular Dopamine after Withdrawal from Morphine, Alcohol or Cocaine: A Common Neurochemical Substrate for Drug Dependence

ZVANI L. ROSSETTI, FRANCO MELIS,
SUSANNA CARBONI, AND GIAN L. GESSA

"B.B. Brodie" Department of Neurosciences
University of Cagliari
09124 Cagliari, Italy

Withdrawal from drugs of abuse is associated with major neurological and vegetative signs of abstinence and with subjective aversive symptoms, such as anxiety, dysphoria, anhedonia, and craving for the drug.[1] The objective neurological and vegetative signs of abstinence, which constitute the so-called physical dependence, differ in each drug dependence or are even absent, as after withdrawal from cocaine.[2] In contrast, the subjective aversive symptoms of abstinence are common to withdrawal of all drugs of abuse. These symptoms are considered to constitute the most compelling motivation for continuing drug intake; that is, they constitute the so-called psychological dependence.

The neurochemical mechanism(s) underlying the aversive subjective symptoms of alcohol, morphine and cocaine withdrawal is not known. However, withdrawal syndromes can be considered the result of adaptive changes to the initial effects of the drugs. Since the mesolimbic dopamine (DA) system is considered to play a crucial role in mediating the rewarding effects elicited by different drugs abused by man,[3-7] we studied the changes in extracellular dopamine after withdrawal of chronic morphine, ethanol, and cocaine in the rat ventral striatum, an area innervated by the mesolimbic DA system.

Ethanol

In ethanol-dependent rats (5 g/kg p.o. every 6 h for 6 days),[8] 8–10 h after suspension of the treatment a marked withdrawal symptomatology was observed. Extracellular DA levels progressively decreased and reached about 25% of controls. DA output remained to such low levels for about 12 h. The inhibition of extraneuronal DA was temporally correlated to the onset of behavioral signs of withdrawal (FIG. 1A).

513

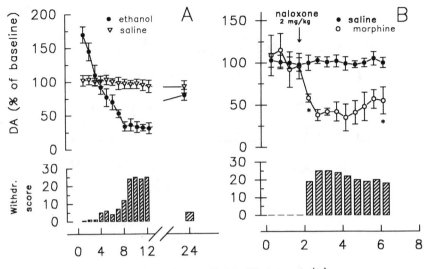

FIGURE 1. A. Course of the time of the changes in extraneuronal DA concentrations after withdrawal of ethanol in dependent rats. Chronic ethanol was administered intragastrically (5 g/kg every 6 h) for 6 days. **B.** Effect of naloxone (2 mg/kg i.p.) on extraneuronal DA concentration in morphine-dependent rats. Chronic morphine was administered by implanting under light ether anesthesia one morphine pellet (75 mg morphine base) every day for 5 days. Pellets were removed immediately before the experiment, on day 6. Abstinence symptomatology was evaluated on 8–10 behavioral items scored according to an arbitrary scale. Values represent mean ± SEM from 6 animals per group. * $p < 0.01$ with respect to controls, two-way ANOVA followed by Newman-Keuls test.

Morphine

In morphine-dependent rats (s.c. morphine pellets, 70 mg of free base for 5 days), after pellet removal, the administration of naloxone induced a marked withdrawal symptomatology and a dramatic reduction in extraneuronal DA concentrations to about 25% of controls. The fall in DA release was temporally correlated to the onset of withdrawal symptomatology (FIG. 1B).

Cocaine

In chronic cocaine-treated rats (15 mg/kg twice per day for 18 days) one day after the last cocaine injection, DA output was not significantly different from control group. However, after 3 days DA release was about 45% lower than in controls, and such reduced levels were maintained for at least 5 days after the last treatment. At this time, animals showed behavioral signs resembling reserpine-like sedation.

Microdialysis was performed as already described 24 h after probe implantation transversely through the ventral striatum.[9]

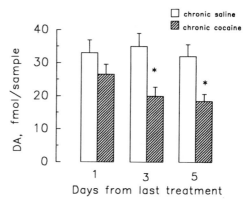

FIGURE 2. Course of the time of the extraneuronal DA concentrations after withdrawal of cocaine in chronically treated rats. Chronic cocaine was administered intraperitoneally 15 mg/kg twice a day for 18 days. Values represent means ± SEM from 5–7 animals per group. * $p < 0.01$ with respect to saline-treated animals. Student's *t*-test.

Consistent with recent results,[10-12] the present investigation demonstrates that withdrawal from chronic morphine, ethanol, and cocaine results in a progressive, marked reduction in extraneuronal DA in the ventral striatum. The mechanism underlying the fall in the extraneuronal concentration of DA during withdrawal is not known. However, our results are consistent with the hypothesis that dopaminergic activity in the limbic areas is suppressed during withdrawal from different drugs of abuse and this inhibition may constitute a relevant common neurochemical correlate of different withdrawal syndromes. This possibility is supported by the close parallelism in the time-course of the fall in DA output and withdrawal signs as well as by the fact that a bolus administration of the withdrawn drug reverted both phenomena (results not shown).

As to the functional relevance of changes in DA output, if one considers that activation of the mesolimbic dopaminergic system may play an important role in the mediation of the reward by different drugs of abuse,[3-7] it is reasonable to conclude that inhibition of DA neurotransmission during abstinence might be responsible for the psychological aversive symptoms, such as dysphoria and anhedonia, during withdrawal.

REFERENCES

1. JAFFE, J. H. 1990. *In* Goodman and Gilman's The Pharmacological Basis of Therapeutics, 8th edit. A. G. Gilman, T. W. Rall, A. S. Nies & P. Taylor, Eds.: 522–573. Pergamon Press. New York.
2. GAWIN, F. H. 1989. Cocaine dependence. Ann. Rev. Med. **40:** 149–161.
3. WISE, R. A. & M. A. BOZARTH. 1987. A psychomotor stimulant theory of addiction. Psychol. Rev. **94:** 469–492.
4. KOOB, G. F. & F. E. BLOOM. 1988. Cellular and molecular mechanisms of drug dependence. Science **242:** 715–723.
5. DI CHIARA, G. & A. IMPERATO. 1988. Drugs abused by humans preferentially increase synaptic dopamine concentrations in the mesolimbic system of freely-moving rats. Proc. Natl. Acad. Sci. USA **85:** 5274–5278.
6. WISE, R. A. & P.-P. ROMPRE. 1989. Brain dopamine and reward. Ann. Rev. Psychol. **40:** 191–225.
7. LIEBMAN, J. M. & S. J. COOPER. 1989. The neuropharmacological basis of reward. Oxford University Press. New York.
8. MAJCHROWITZ, E. 1975. Induction of physical dependence upon ethanol and associated

behavioral changes in rats. Psychopharmacologia **43:** 245–251.

9. PANI, L., A. KUZMIN, M. DIANA, G. DE MONTIS, G. L. GESSA & Z. L. ROSSETTI. 1990. Calcium receptor antagonists modify cocaine effects in the central nervous system differently. Eur. J. Pharmacol. **190:** 217–221.

10. ROSSETTI, Z. L., F. MELIS, S. CARBONI & G. L. GESSA. 1990. Dopamine release during tolerance and withdrawal from chronic morphine or alcohol. Neurosci. Lett. **39**(Suppl.): S184.

11. ROBERTSON, M. W., C. A. LESLIE & J. P. BENNET, JR. 1991. Apparent synaptic dopamine deficiency induced by withdrawal from chronic cocaine treatment. Brain Res. **538:** 337–339.

12. ROSSETTI, Z. L., F. MELIS, S. CARBONI & G. L. GESSA. 1991. Marked decrease of extraneuronal dopamine after alcohol withdrawal in rats: Reversal by MK-801. Eur. J. Pharmacol. **200:** 371–372.

System of Aldehyde Metabolism in Brain of Rats during Development of Tolerance to the Hypnotic Effect of Ethanol

V. I. SATANOVSKAYA

Institute of Biochemistry
Academy of Sciences of BSSR
BLK 50, Grodno, 230009, Belarus

The diminished response of animals to ethanol after repeated exposure may be not only a result of adaptive changes in the metabolism of ethanol; in addition to the direct effects of alcohol, many indirect toxic effects are ascribed to the first oxidative metabolite, acetaldehyde.[1] Acetaldehyde is also known to have its own pharmacologic effects, some of which are antagonistic to the effect of ethanol. Therefore, the overall pharmacologic effects of alcohol in an individual might depend on the equilibrium between direct ethanol and antagonistic acetaldehyde effects.[2,3]

In the brain, acetaldehyde is metabolized by aldehyde dehydrogenase (ALDH, EC 1.2.1.3). An important function of ALDH is to oxidize aldehydes formed during the catabolism of biogenic amines.[4] The competitive inhibition of oxidation of these aldehydes by acetaldehyde is a possible mechanism involved in the pharmacologic effects of ethanol.[5] In the presence of acetaldehyde, the biogenic aldehydes accumulate, and this might lead to an increased reduction of aldehydes to the corresponding alcohol catalyzed by aldehyde reductase (AR, EC 1.1.1.2).

Heterogeneous stock male albino rats were used to study ALDH and AR in some brain structures during development of tolerance to ethanol. Ethanol (i.p., 3.5 g/kg body weight) was administered singly every day in the morning, and the duration of ethanol-induced sleep was recorded. After 24 hours the activities of ALDH and AR were measured with acetaldehyde and *p*-nitrobenzaldehyde as substrates.[6,7] Four groups of animals were studied following 1, 4, 7, and 10 ethanol injections.

As tolerance developed, the sleep time shortened (125 ± 12, 35 ± 7, 14 ± 4, and 15 ± 4 min, respectively). In addition, the number of awake animals increased.

In the large hemispheres, we observed an activation of AR and a decrease of ALDH activity; *i.e.*, the aldehyde metabolism was switched over from the dehydrogenase pathway to the reductase one (TABLE 1). The cerebellum showed an increased capacity to utilize acetaldehyde, the AR activity remaining stable. Variations in the enzyme activities and the soluble protein content were noted in the brain stem.

Following one and four ethanol injections a negative correlation was found between the ethanol-induced sleep time and the ALDH activity in the brain stem ($r =$

TABLE 1. ALDH and AR Activities (μM NAD(P)H/hour/g of protein) in Rat Brain during Development of Tolerance to Ethanol (n = 10)

	Group 1	Group 2	Group 3	Group 4
Large Hemisphere				
ALDH	75.2 ± 4.3	92.3 ± 5.8[a]	146.7 ± 8.3[a,b]	95.8 ± 6.5[a,c]
AR	240 ± 9	240 ± 14	250 ± 16	290 ± 15[a,b]
Cerebellum				
ALDH	95.2 ± 5.1	99.4 ± 5.0	119.8 ± 3.9[a,b]	124.0 ± 6.1[a,b]
AR	340 ± 22	340 ± 9	330 ± 22	380 ± 22
Brain Stem				
ALDH	156.6 ± 11.2	195.8 ± 6.7[a]	128.7 ± 12.0[b]	136.2 ± 9.7[b]

Means ± SD.
[a] p: 0.01–0.001, compared to group 1.
[b] p: 0.01–0.001, compared to group 2.
[c] p: 0.01–0.001, compared to group 3.

-0.72, $p < 0.001$) and the cerebellum ($r = -0.68$, $p < 0.001$). It should be noted that the correlations of the ALDH activities among the studied brain regions were enhanced in rats injected with 4 doses of ethanol.

In conclusion, the data obtained illustrate not only the metabolic heterogeneity of brain regions but also a qualitative nonuniformity of the processes adaptive to ethanol which are involved in the system of aldehyde metabolism.

REFERENCES

1. ERIKSSON, C. J. P. & R. A. DEITRICH. 1983. Metabolic mechanisms in tolerance and physical dependence on alcohol. *In* The Biology of Alcoholism. B. Kissin & H. Begleiter, Eds. Vol. 7: 253–283. Plenum Press. New York.
2. VON WARTBURG, J. P. 1990. On the importance of the psychotropic effects of alcohol. Drug Alcohol Depend. 25(2): 135–139.
3. LI, T. K. 1990. Genetic and neurobiological substrates of alcohol-seeking behavior and alcoholism. Pharmacol. Toxicol. Suppl. 67(1): 12–18.
4. WEINER, H. & B. ARDELT. 1984. Distribution and properties of aldehyde dehydrogenase in regions of rat brain. J. Neurochem. 42(1): 109–115.
5. LAHTI, R. A. & E. MAJCHROWICZ. 1974. Ethanol and acetaldehyde effects on metabolism and binding of biogenic amines. Q. J. Stud. Alcohol A35(1): 1–14.
6. ERWIN, V. G. & R. A. DEITRICH. 1966. Brain aldehyde dehydrogenase. Localisation, purification and properties. J. Biol. Chem. 241(15): 3533–3539.
7. TABAKOFF, B. & V. G. ERWIN. 1970. Purification and characterization of a reduced nicotinamide adenine dinucleotide phosphate-linked aldehyde reductase from brain. J. Biol. Chem. 245(12): 3263–3268.

Morphine Withdrawal in
the Hamster

P. SCHNUR

Department of Psychology
University of Southern Colorado
Pueblo, Colorado 81001

Previous research has demonstrated that environmental cues can function as Pavlovian conditioned stimuli to elicit conditioned withdrawal in opiate-dependent animals and humans.[1,2] The present work investigated Pavlovian conditioning of naloxone-precipitated withdrawal in morphine-pelleted hamsters and tested the effects of MK-801, clonidine, verapamil, and nifedipine on conditioned and naloxone-precipitated withdrawal.

Animals were implanted with morphine (75 mg) or placebo pellets. On five post-implant days, they were observed in a plastic cage for 40 min; 10 min before and 30 min after a naloxone (1 mg/kg) injection. On several post-explant days, animals were observed in the plastic cage 10 min before and 30 min after a saline injection. Behavior was sampled continuously for signs of withdrawal: paw tremors, wet dog shakes, abdominal writhing, yawning, and teeth chattering. Conditioned withdrawal responses were those withdrawal signs occurring during the 10 min pre-naloxone periods on the 5 post-implant days as well as those withdrawal signs occurring before or after the saline

FIGURE 1. Mean withdrawal signs as a function of post-implant days during the 10 min pre-naloxone period. Morphine-pelleted animals withdrawn in the test environment (Group SAL) developed conditioned withdrawal in that environment compared with a placebo control group (PLC) and with a group withdrawn in the home cage environment (UNP). In addition, a 0.1 mg/kg dose of MK-801 facilitated the development of conditioned responding, whereas a 0.3 mg/kg dose inhibited the development of conditioned responding.

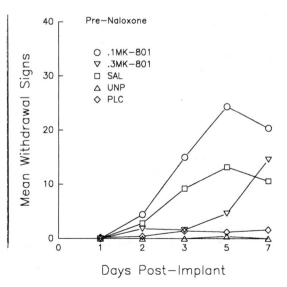

519

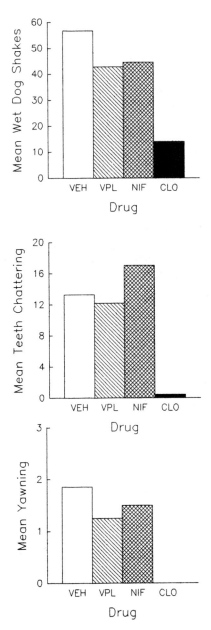

FIGURE 2. Mean withdrawal signs as a function of drug administered prior to naloxone-precipitated withdrawal in morphine-pelleted animals. Drugs injected i.p. were either verapamil (20 mg/kg), nifedipine (20 mg/kg), clonidine (0.4 mg/kg), or vehicle. The top, middle, and bottom panels show wet-dog shakes, teeth chattering and yawning, respectively, on the five post-implant days. Only clonidine suppressed these withdrawal signs.

injection on post-explant days. To investigate pharmacological antagonism of withdrawal, drugs were injected prior to placing animals in the plastic cage.

In Experiment 1, naloxone-precipitated withdrawal was shown to be a direct function of the number of implanted morphine pellets (1, 2, or 4). In addition, conditioned withdrawal to the plastic cage developed in animals implanted with 2 or 4 morphine pellets, but did not develop in placebo pellet controls nor in morphine-implanted controls withdrawn in the home cage instead of in the plastic cage. Conditioned withdrawal was evident for up to 30 days post explant and conditioned withdrawal extinguished following repeated exposures to the plastic cage in the absence of precipitated withdrawal.

In Experiment 2, the effects of the noncompetitive NMDA antagonist MK-801 (0.1, 0.3 mg/kg) on opiate withdrawal were investigated. At the lower dose, MK-801 enhanced both naloxone-precipitated withdrawal and conditioned withdrawal. At the higher dose, MK-801 retarded the development of conditioned withdrawal (FIG. 1), but it did not affect naloxone-precipitated withdrawal, a result consistent with the hypothesis that MK-801 interferes with associative mechanisms subserving the development of dependence.[3]

In Experiment 3, the effects of the α-2 adrenergic agonist, clonidine (0.4 mg/kg), and of the calcium channel antagonists, verapamil (20 mg/kg) and nifedipine (20 mg/kg), on opiate withdrawal were investigated. Neither of the calcium channel antagonists affected withdrawal. Clonidine, however, significantly reduced wet-dog shakes, teeth chattering and yawning (FIG. 2), but not paw tremors or writhing. Compared with vehicle controls none of the drugs tested had a significant effect on conditioned withdrawal or on general locomotor activity.

It is concluded that precipitated withdrawal in the morphine-pelleted hamster provides a convenient and useful animal model for investigating environmental and pharmacological influences on opiate withdrawal.

REFERENCES

1. O'BRIEN, C. P., T. TESTA, T. J. O'BRIEN, J. P. BRADY & B. WELLS. 1977. Science 195: 1000–1002.
2. WIKLER, A. & F. T. PESCOR. 1967. Psychopharmacolgia 10: 255–284.
3. TRUJILLO, K. A. & H. AKIL. 1991. Science 251: 85–87.

Assessment of Dopamine Release by *in Vivo* Microdialysis in the Nucleus Accumbens of Rats following Acute and Chronic Administration of Desipramine[a]

RONALD E. SEE, LEAH ADAMS-CURTIS,
AND MARY ANN CHAPMAN

Department of Psychology
Washington State University
Pullman, Washington 99164-4820

One approach for facilitating abstinence during cocaine withdrawal has utilized the tricyclic antidepressant, desipramine (DMI). In a recent study,[1] DMI-treated cocaine users showed significantly greater abstinence and reduced craving when compared to both placebo-treated and lithium-treated cocaine users. Although DMI preferentially blocks reuptake of norepinephrine, it has also been shown to significantly inhibit dopamine (DA) uptake.[2] The effects of DMI on DA function may be related to its reported success in clinical treatment of cocaine withdrawal. The present study focused on changes in DA release and metabolism in the nucleus accumbens of rats following acute or chronic administration of DMI.

Male rats were implanted with bilateral guide cannulae at the following coordinates from bregma: A/P +1.6 mm, D/V −5.4 mm, M/L +1.5 mm. The animals were allowed to recover for 1 week prior to first insertion of a dialysis probe. For the first day of dialysate collection, rats were administered DMI (10 mg/kg, IP) or distilled water vehicle. For the next 12 days, rats were injected once daily with either DMI or vehicle. The animals were then reprobed on the contralateral side and dialysis collection initiated on day 14 of DMI administration. Dialysis probes were inserted and left in place overnight prior to beginning infusion. The next day, perfusion began 1 h prior to collecting baseline samples. Probes were perfused (2 μl/min) with dialysate buffer and samples collected in vials containing 20 μl of mobile phase. Three consecutive samples collected at 20 min intervals for 1 h provided a baseline prior to injection, after which samples were collected at 20 min intervals for 5 h. Each sample was directly injected into the HPLC system and electrochemical detection was used to detect DA, DOPAC, HVA, and 5HIAA.

[a] This investigation was supported in part by funds provided for medical and biological research by the State of Washington (Legislative Initiative Measure No. 171).

No significant differences in basal concentrations were seen between groups on either day 1 or day 14 of drug administration. FIGURE 1 shows changes in levels of DA, DOPAC, HVA, and 5HIAA over time following acute injection of DMI (day 1). Values are expressed as percentage of the mean of 3 baseline samples taken prior to injection of DMI or vehicle. There were no significant changes from baseline in the DMI or control group. However, on day 14 of treatment, injection of DMI, but not vehicle, produced an increase in DA, DOPAC, HVA, and 5HIAA (FIG. 2). This increase was significant for DOPAC at 80 and 120 min after injection and at the last time point tested (5 h) for DA, HVA, and 5HIAA.

Several lines of evidence suggest that chronic DMI potently affects DA function, particularly in mesolimbic pathways. These include increases in intracranial self-stimulation of ventral tegmental DA regions[3] and facilitation of locomotor responses to DA agonists.[4] Utilizing *in vivo* microdialysis, the present study did not find any differences in basal concentrations of DA or DA metabolites after either acute or chronic DMI, a finding in accord with a recent study[5] that also found no differences in basal extracellular concentrations of DA after chronic DMI. However, extracellular levels of DA, DOPAC, HVA, and 5HIAA were elevated shortly after the last injection of DMI. The prolonged period of increased levels may be due in part to the pharmacokinetics of DMI, which can have a delayed plasma peak 12 h after administration, a half-life of approximately 20–22 h, and show nonlinear rises in plasma concentration after chronic dosing.[6] Since there were no differences in basal levels just prior to the final injection, the increases seen may have been transient. The present results support previous findings of altered mesolimbic DA function following repeated DMI ad-

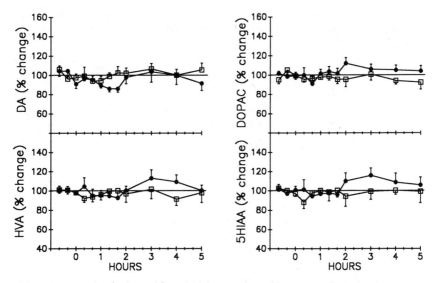

FIGURE 1. Levels of DA (*top left*), DOPAC (*top right*), HVA (*bottom left*), and 5HIAA (*bottom right*) in the nucleus accumbens of rats following initial (day 1) injection of DMI (●—●) or vehicle control (□—□). Data (means ± SEM) are expressed as % of the mean of 3 baseline values obtained prior to injection (time 0).

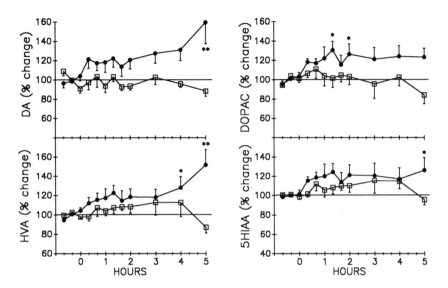

FIGURE 2. Levels of DA (*top left*), DOPAC (*top right*), HVA (*bottom left*), and 5HIAA (*bottom right*) in the nucleus accumbens of rats following final (day 14) injection of DMI (●—●) or vehicle control (□—□). Data (means ± SEM) are expressed as % of the mean of 3 baseline values obtained prior to injection (time 0). (* $p < 0.05$, ** $p < 0.01$, Newman-Keuls test).

ministration. Such effects may be due to the direct actions of DMI on DA function or through more indirect effects such as a primary action of DMI on norepinephrine reuptake.

REFERENCES

1. GAWIN, F. H., H. D. KLEBER, R. BYCK, B. J. ROUNSAVILLE, T. R. KOSTEN, P. I. JATLOW & C. MORGAN. 1989. Desipramine facilitation of initial cocaine abstinence. Arch. Gen. Psychiatry **46:** 117–121.
2. RANDRUP, A. & C. BRAESTRUP. 1977. Uptake inhibition of biogenic amines by newer antidepressant drugs: Relevance to the dopamine hypothesis of depression. Psychopharmacology **53:** 309–314.
3. FIBIGER, H. C. & A. G. PHILLIPS. 1981. Increased intracranial self-administration in rats after long-term administration of desipramine. Science **214:** 683–685.
4. SPYRAKI, C. & H. C. FIBIGER. 1981. Behavioral evidence for supersensitivity of postsynaptic dopamine receptors in the mesolimbic system after chronic administration of desipramine. Eur. J. Pharmacol. **74:** 195–206.
5. NOMIKOS, G. G., G. DAMSMA, D. WENKSTERN & H. C. FIBIGER. 1991. Chronic desipramine enhances amphetamine-induced increases in interstitial concentrations of dopamine in the nucleus accumbens. Eur. J. Pharmacol. **195:** 63–73.
6. SALLEE, F. R. & B. G. POLLOCK. 1990. Clinical pharmacokinetics of imipramine and desipramine. Clin. Pharmacokinet. **18**(5): 346–364.

Weak Base Model of Amphetamine Action

DAVID SULZER,[a] EMMANUEL POTHOS,[b]
HELEN MINJUNG SUNG,[b] NIGEL T. MAIDMENT,[c]
BARTLEY G. HOEBEL,[b] AND STEPHEN RAYPORT[a]

[a] Department of Psychiatry
Columbia University
New York, New York 10032
and
New York State Psychiatric Institute
722 West 168th Street
New York, New York 10032

[b] Department of Psychology
Princeton University
Princeton, New Jersey 08544

[c] Department of Psychiatry
University of California, Los Angeles
Los Angeles, California 90024

Like other rewarding psychostimulants, amphetamine (AMPH) increases extracellular dopamine (DA) levels in the nucleus accumbens.[1] Unlike cocaine, which appears to act by blocking the plasma membrane DA uptake transporter,[2] AMPH's mechanism of action has not been well understood. The apparent high-affinity uptake of AMPH[3,4] suggests that its site of action may be intracellular. Indeed, AMPH (as well as cocaine) can release catecholamines from isolated transmitter storage vesicles.[5,6]

We have suggested a model for the action of AMPH and some other psychostimulants[7] stemming from the observations that most psychostimulants are amphiphilic weak bases and that monoamine accumulation by synaptic vesicles depends on an interior-acidic pH gradient.[8] These psychostimulants in pharmacologically relevant concentrations, as well as protonophores and *classic* weak bases such as ammonium (added as NH_4Cl) or chloroquine, reduce intracellular pH gradients of synaptic vesicles and other acidic organelles, increasing release and reducing uptake of monoamines from storage vesicles.[7] A crucial prediction of this model has now been borne out: weak bases that are not abused act like AMPH when applied directly to the nucleus accumbens or cultured DA neurons. In the cultures we have further determined that the increase in extracellular DA due to weak bases is attenuated by uptake blockers, suggesting that AMPH is taken up by the DA transporter and that elevated cytosolic DA is released by reverse transport.

In the nucleus accumbens of freely moving rats, reverse microdialysis of NH_4Cl caused a large increase in DA release (FIG. 1). Other weak bases including chloroquine and benzylamine, as well as AMPH, caused similar increases in extracellular DA levels.

525

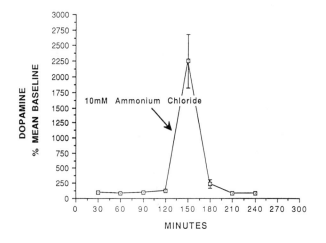

FIGURE 1. Local infusion of weak bases in the nucleus accumbens increases extracellular DA. Ammonium applied as NH_4Cl or $(NH_4)_2SO_4$ (*not shown*) were infused by reverse microdialysis and DA was measured by HPLC as reported previously.[1] DA increases were also seen after local infusion of AMPH and other weak bases that are not normally abused, including chloroquine and benzylamine.

In postnatal ventral midbrain cultures AMPH or NH_4Cl caused significant increases in extracellular DA (FIG. 2, *open bars*). A similar increase was seen after incubation with the cationic ionophore monensin, which reduces intracellular pH gradients by a different mechanism. In the cultures, the DA uptake blocker benztropine completely blocked the proportion of DA increase due to AMPH. This could be due to blockade of AMPH uptake and/or blockade of reverse DA transport. However, since benztropine also significantly attenuated the DA release induced by NH_4Cl (FIG. 2, *striped bars*) and monensin (data not shown) and these compounds are not known substrates for the DA uptake transporter, benztropine must act in part to block *efflux* of DA from the cytosol.[9] Normally such compounds do not cause large-scale DA release after oral or i.v. self-administration because they are excluded by the blood-brain barrier, undergo rapid first-pass clearance by the liver or kidneys, do not undergo sufficient neuronal uptake, or never reach psychostimulant dose levels due to toxicity.

These observations suggest the following model: 1) AMPH enters cells by lipophilic diffusion and is further concentrated in monoamine cells by uptake transporters.[3,4] A component of AMPH action may be due to competition with DA for transporter sites. 2) Weak bases such as AMPH partition into acidic intracellular compartments according to the proton gradient such that $[base]_{in}/[base]_{out} = [H^+]_{in}/[H^+]_{out}$ (ref. 8); in the case of AMPH this appears to be reserpine-insensitive.[7] For some amines $\Delta\psi$ may also play a role in vesicular uptake. 3) After the vesicle's buffering capacity is exceeded, the reduced proton gradient reduces the driving force for transmitter uptake, which is due to the electrochemical gradient such that $\log([DA]_{in}/[DA]_{out}) = \Delta\psi/Z + 2\Delta pH$ (ref. 8). Owing to this relationship, an alkalinization of as little as 0.3 pH units, as seen with 100 μM AMPH,[7] would decrease vesicular DA accumulation by 75%. AMPH also competes with DA for protons so that the resulting uncharged DA will tend to diffuse from the vesicle following its concentration gradient. Although the

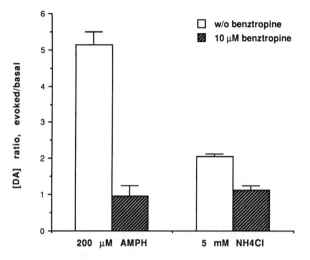

FIGURE 2. AMPH and classic weak bases release DA from ventral midbrain cultures. Both AMPH and NH₄Cl caused significant increases in extracellular DA (*open bars*); 10 μM benztropine inhibited the DA release elicited by NH₄Cl and AMPH (*striped bars*), as well as other weak bases and protonophores (*not shown*). Cultures from rat ventral midbrain containing approximately 10% dopaminergic neurons were grown for 2 weeks.[7] After two washes, the increase in basal extracellular [DA] without and with 10 μM benztropine was determined by HPLC. Benztropine alone increased basal extracellular DA levels from 0.24 to 0.92 pmoles DA/30 min because of blockade of DA reuptake. Cultures were then exposed to drugs without or with benztropine for 30 min. The data are presented as a ratio of basal release without or with benztropine as appropriate: therefore, the effect of benztropine on AMPH- and NH₄Cl-evoked release should reflect *drug uptake* and/or *reverse transport* of DA. Drug effects were concentration-dependent so that higher doses of NH₄Cl, for example, caused greater release than AMPH.

relative importance of the vesicular pool is controversial,[10] so far all compounds including AMPH that abolish the vesicular pH gradient reduce uptake and increase release of monoamines from isolated vesicles.[5-8] 4) Elevated cytosolic DA is released from the cell, at least in part, by reverse action of the uptake transporter. This model differs from earlier ideas where the uptake transporter acts as a mobile carrier that flips between the intracellular and extracellular faces of the plasma membrane; reverse transport, on the other hand, can occur even if the transporter is a channel for neurotransmitter. Cocaine, which also potently inhibits the vesicular pH gradient,[7] may block efflux of cytosolic DA released from vesicles by also blocking the transporter.

Although our evidence does not contradict earlier models, the weak base actions of AMPH on synaptic vesicles, in concert with reverse action of the plasma membrane transporter, appear to quantitatively account for most of the effects of AMPH on DA uptake and release.

REFERENCES

1. HERNANDEZ, L., F. LEE & B. G. HOEBEL. 1987. Brain Res. Bull. **19:** 623–628.
2. RITZ, M. C., R. J. LAMB, S. R. GOLDBERG & M. J. KUHAR. 1987. Science **237:** 1219–1223.

3. BONISCH, H. 1984. Naunyn-Schmiedeberg's Arch. Pharmacol. **327**: 267–272.
4. ZACZEK, R., S. CULP & E. B. DE SOUZA. 1991. J. Pharmacol. Exp. Ther. **257**: 830–835.
5. SCHUMANN, H. J. & A. PHILIPPU. 1962. Nature. **193**: 890–891.
6. KNEPPER, S. M., G. L. GRUNEWALD & C. O. RUTLEDGE. 1988. J. Pharmacol. Exp. Ther. **247**: 487–494.
7. SULZER, D. & S. RAYPORT. 1990. Neuron. **5**: 797–808.
8. JOHNSON, R. G. 1988. Physiol. Rev. **68**: 232–307.
9. RAITERI, M., F. CERRITO, A. M. CERVONI & G. LEVI. 1979. J. Pharmacol. Exp. Ther. **208**: 195–202.
10. PARKER, E. M. & L. X. CUBEDDU. 1986. J. Pharmacol. Exp. Ther. **237**: 179–203.

Morphine-induced Downregulation of μ-Opioid Receptors and Peptide Synthesis in Neonatal Rat Brain[a]

ANN TEMPEL AND KATHRYN ESPINOZA

Department of Psychiatry
Hillside Hospital/LIJMC
P.O. Box 38
Glen Oaks, New York 11004

Chronic administration of opioid agonists during pre- and/or postnatal development may alter opioid receptor ontogeny and, concomitantly, sensitivity to opioid drugs. In order to address this issue, we examined changes in brain opioid receptors and peptides of neonates chronically exposed to morphine either *in utero* or beginning on postnatal day one.

METHODS

Drug Treatment

1) Pregnant Sprague-Dawley rats were implanted subcutaneously with either a single morphine pellet (75 mg) or placebo pellets on gestation day 16. 2) Newborn Sprague-Dawley rats, reared in litters of 10 pups per mother, were each given one daily subcutaneous injection of morphine sulfate (5 mg/kg) or saline beginning on postnatal day 1. Rat pups were sacrificed by decapitation on postnatal day 0, 4, 8, 16, 21, or 28.

Opiate Receptor Autoradiography

Coronal brain sections (20 μM thick) were processed for *in vitro* autoradiography as previously described.[1] Autoradiograms were analyzed by the MCID Image Analysis System.

Northern Blot Analysis and Quantification

Cellular RNA was isolated by the chloroform-phenol method as previously described.[2] Northern blots were hybridized to the proenkephalin (PPE) probe and then

[a] This work was supported by NIDA Grant DA-05440.

to the neutral probe, 1B15 and were analyzed by densitometry. Normalization of PPE mRNA levels for the amount of RNA loaded was accomplished by taking the ratio of PPE mRNA to 1B15 mRNA for each sample. Ratio values from each brain region from drug treated and control animals were compared to calculate changes in mRNA levels.

RESULTS

Four days of postnatal (PN) morphine treatment induced a total loss of μ-opiate receptors in the patches of the striatum with a small significant loss in the matrix area as revealed by autoradiography. This loss of μ receptors was no longer observed with increased duration (8 days) of morphine treatment. Four days of PN morphine treatment produced a 24% increase in striatal PPE mRNA levels relative to saline-treated animals. No significant changes in the level of 1B15 mRNA were apparent following agonist treatment. Longer durations of morphine treatment (PN 1–14) induced a 39% decrease in PPE mRNA levels. This decrease is similar to what is seen in adult striatum following chronic morphine treatment.[3]

DISCUSSION

The results of this study demonstrate that morphine treatment leads to a loss of μ striatal opiate receptors while PPE synthesis in the striatum of neonatal rat brain is initially increased. Our data suggest that there are different mechanisms underlying opiate addiction in the developing central nervous system. We suggest that these differences may be due to interactions with the G-protein/cAMP system.

REFERENCES

1. TEMPEL, A. & R. S. ZUKIN. 1987. Proc. Natl. Acad. Sci. USA **84:** 4308–4312.
2. TEMPEL, A., J. A. KESSLER & R. S. ZUKIN. 1990. J. Neurosci. **10**(3): 741–747.
3. UHL, G. R., J. P. RYAN & J. P. SCHWARTZ. 1988. Brain Res. **459:** 391–397.

Methylxanthines (Caffeine and Theophylline) Blocked Methamphetamine-induced Conditioned Place Preference in Mice but Enhanced That Induced by Cocaine

DANILO Bv. TUAZON,[a,b,c] TSUTOMU SUZUKI,[b]
MIWA MISAWA,[b] AND SHIGERU WATANABE[a]

[a] Department of Psychology
Keio University
Mita-2-Chome, Minato-Ku
Tokyo 108, Japan

[b] Department of Applied Pharmacology
Hoshi University
Ebana-2-Chome, Shinagawa-Ku
Tokyo 142, Japan

Caffeine (CAF) can be considered to be the most widely used behaviorally active drug in the world. Its frequency and pattern of use in foodstuffs and beverages increases the likelihood of its joint usage and possible interaction with other drugs.[3] Given the high prevalence and persistence of CAF use, it has been identified as a drug of abuse. However, despite of its abundant use, few studies have examined its rewarding properties. CAF and theophylline (TPL) are methylated xanthines (MXT). They share in common several pharmacological action of therapeutic interest. The purpose of this study is to show the effects of the interaction of MXT (CAF and TPL) with metamphetamine (MAP) and cocaine (COCA).

The biased CPP procedure was used to examine the effects of MXT on the MAP- and COCA-induced CPP in ddY mice. MAP (0.5, 1.0, 2.0 and 4.0 mg/kg), COCA (1.25, 2.5, 5.0 and 10.0 mg/kg), CAF and TPL (both 1.0, 3.0, 6.0, 9.0, 13.5, 27.0 and 36.0 mg/kg) and with 9.0 mg/kg CAF or TPL were intraperitoneally (i.p.) administered. Conditioning was conducted using a rectangular box with 2 compartments (15 × 30 × 15 cm). The first chamber has black walls and a smooth floor while the other has white walls and a rough floor. A middle barrier restricted the animals to one area during training. Conditioning was one hour a day for 6 days, alternating the injection of saline and drugs. On test day, neither drug nor saline was injected.

[c] Present address: Concordia College, Portland, Oregon/Christ College, Irvine, California–Japan Office Room 103, 1-2-32, Fujimi, Chiyoda-ku, Tokyo 102, Japan.

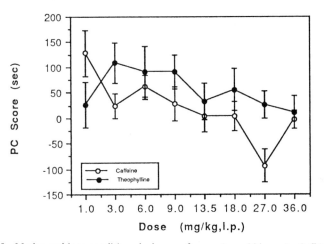

FIGURE 1. Methyxanthines conditioned place preference (n = 10/group). Caffeine showed CPP at low dose (1.0 mg/kg) and CPA at high dose (27.0 mg/kg). Theophylline showed CPP at low dose (3.0 mg/kg). (PC score: Drug minus baseline score.)

The barrier was removed and the time spent by each animal in the 2 compartments was measured for 15 min. Alone data showed that for all doses of MAP tested and for 2.5, 5.0, and 10.0 mg/kg COCA produced significant CPP. CAF produced a biphasic effect; a lower dose (1.0 mg/kg) was rewarding, whereas a higher dose (27.0 mg/kg) produced aversion. TPL showed CPP at 3.0 mg/kg. However, when 9.0 mg/kg CAF or TPL was combined, all the MAP-induced CPP was reduced significantly while the COCA-induced CPP was unaffected.

The CPP for caffeine agrees with the findings of Brockwell et al.[1] Lower CAF

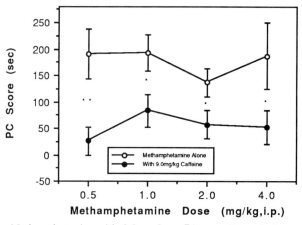

FIGURE 2. Methamphetamine with 9.0 mg/kg caffeine conditioned place preference (n = 10/group). MAP showed CPP at all doses tested but the effect was reduced significantly by CAF. (PC score: Drug minus baseline score.)

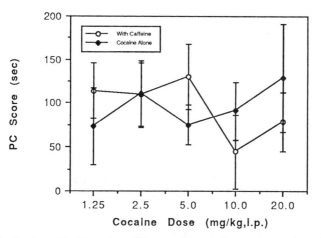

FIGURE 3. Cocaine with 9.0 mg/kg caffeine conditioned place preference (n = 10/group). COCA showed CPP at 2.5, 5.0, and 10.0 mg/kg and was unaffected by CAF. (PC score: Drug minus baseline score.)

doses may be associated with enhanced central dopamine (DA) release by indirectly stimulating the pre- and post-synaptic DA receptors.[5] The CPP-blocking effect of CAF or TPL-MAP combinations can be due to the overstimulation of DA systems resulting in depolarization-induced inactivation of DA neurons.[2] The difference in the case of COCA can be attributed to mechanisms of the influence on DA. MAP causes the release of endogenous DA while COCA blocks the reuptake of DA.[4] The level of the released DA caused by the tested doses of MAP is probably much higher than the reuptake DA caused by COCA.

REFERENCES

1. BROCKWELL, N. T., R. EIKELBOOM & R. J. BENINGER. 1991. Pharmacol. Biochem. Behav. **38:** 513–517.
2. GRACE, A. A. & B. S. BUNNEY. 1986. J. Pharmacol. Exp. Ther. **238:** 1092–1100.
3. HARLAND, R. D., D. V. GAUVIN, R. C. MICHALIS, J. M. CARNEY, T. W. SEALE & F. A. HOLLOWAY. 1988. Pharmacol. Biochem. Behav. **32:** 1017–1023.
4. MCMILLEN, B. A. 1983. Trends Pharmacol. Sci. **4:** 429–432.
5. WATANABE, H. & H. URAMOTO. 1986. Neuropharmacology **25**(6): 577–581.

Comparison of Evoked Potentials in Men and Women Admitted for Alcohol Detoxification

THERESA M. WORNER[a]

AND RICHARD LECHTENBERG

The Long Island College Hospital
Brooklyn, New York 11201

Berlex Laboratories, Inc.
300 Fairfield Road
Wayne, New Jersey 07470-7358

Electrophysiologic studies of brain dysfunction have revealed abnormalities in men undergoing alcohol detoxification and drug withdrawal. CNS hyperexcitability routinely occurs during the acute withdrawal of these substances. Improvement in the patient's clinical status and electrophysiologic parameters occur with abstinence.[1] Visual evoked potentials (VEPs) have augmented wave amplitudes and increased symmetry of potentials after alcohol withdrawal.[2] Encephalopathy associated with liver disease may increase the latencies of brainstem auditory evoked potentials (BAERs).[3] At least in men, BAER amplitudes decrease during alcohol withdrawal. Evoked potential (EP) studies focusing on female alcoholics to assess whether or not there are any gender-specific effects of alcoholism have not been done. By reviewing VEPs and BAERs of alcoholics undergoing detoxification, we tried to determine whether or not there are differences in the VEPs and BAERs of men compared to women and whether there is any correlation between markers of alcohol consumption and EP characteristics.

METHODS

Of 203 subjects evaluated, 70 were female. All patients met DSM-III-R criteria for alcoholism. Subjects were admitted if they manifested withdrawal signs or symptoms, had failed in out-patient treatment, or were in an unstable social situation. Subjects were excluded from admission if they were suicidal, homicidal, or exhibited serious medical problems.

OBSERVATIONS

Correlations were not evident in either sex between evoked potential patterns and daily alcohol consumption, breath ethanol level at the time of admission, serum B12

[a] Address for correspondence: Dr. T. M. Worner, 322 E. 50th St., New York, NY 10022.

TABLE 1. Characteristics of Men and Women Admitted for Detoxification ($\bar{x} \pm$ SD)

	Women (n = 70)	Men (n = 133)	p
Age (years)	36.0 ± 11.1	41.6 ± 10.1	0.0006
ETOH consumption			
Years	20.8 ± 11.1	26.0 ± 9.6	0.0029
Grams/day	227.4 ± 152.6	280.7 ± 220.4	NS
Laboratory tests			
Breath alcohol (mg%)	32.3 ± 65.8	47.1 ± 70.5	NS
Serum B12 (pg/ml)	556.3 ± 336.0	571.6 ± 300.7	NS
Serum folate (ng/ml)	7.7 ± 4.6	7.2 ± 3.9	NS
GGTP (IU)	155.5 ± 379.7	151.6 ± 195.4	NS
Hematocrit (%)	39.3 ± 5.4	44.0 ± 4.1	<0.00005
MCV (fl)	92.0 ± 7.4	93.1 ± 6.7	NS

content, serum folate level, GGTP, or MCV. Unfortunately, our populations of men and women exhibited some significant differences, such as median age and years of alcoholism, which could have influenced evoked potential patterns (TABLE 1). Despite this, VEP measurements were remarkably similar for men and women (TABLE 2). Specific components of the auditory evoked potentials did, however, have some con-

TABLE 2. Comparison of Visual and Brainstem Auditory Evoked Potential Latencies (msec) in Men and Women Admitted for Alcohol Detoxification ($\bar{x} \pm$ SD)

	Women	Men	p
Right visual	99.2 ± 7.4	101.6 ± 8.0	NS
Left visual	98.5 ± 6.5	100.6 ± 7.1	NS
Left auditory			
I	1.56 ± 0.20	1.6 ± 0.16	NS
II	2.78 ± 0.14	2.80 ± 0.22	NS
III	3.72 ± 0.15	3.86 ± 0.26	<0.00005
IV	4.90 ± 0.33	5.04 ± 0.24	0.0093
V	5.60 ± 0.20	5.77 ± 0.28	<0.00005
I–III	2.11 ± 0.18	2.26 ± 0.24	<0.00005
III–V	1.91 ± 0.37	1.90 ± 0.22	NS
I–V	3.95 ± 0.32	4.16 ± 0.26	0.0001
Right auditory			
I	1.65 ± 0.56	1.62 ± 0.21	NS
II	2.84 ± 0.44	2.83 ± 0.22	NS
III	3.68 ± 0.25	3.83 ± 0.21	0.0003
IV	4.85 ± 0.46	4.98 ± 0.26	NS
V	5.56 ± 0.26	5.69 ± 0.32	0.0001
I–III	2.09 ± 0.16	2.17 ± 0.30	0.0273
III–V	1.92 ± 0.33	1.90 ± 0.21	NS
I–V	3.95 ± 0.21	4.06 ± 0.49	NS

sistently significant differences in latencies for men compared to women. These were limited to components III and V of the BAERs. Interpeak latencies for waves I-III were significantly longer for men compared to women. Despite the differences between the groups, the latencies recorded for both groups were within the normal limits for the laboratory doing the testing. Men also exhibited a more asymmetric pattern of BAERs with latency recorded for the left side generally being longer than those recorded for the right side. Despite this apparent asymmetry, evoked response latencies were within normal limits on both sides of the head in both sexes. When groups were matched for age, all significant correlations persisted. When the groups were matched for years of alcohol consumption, the left VEP in men was significantly longer than that observed in women ($p = 0.024$). Likewise, except for BAER wave IV on the left, results reported in TABLE 2 remained significantly different in men compared to women when the groups were matched for alcohol consumption.

DISCUSSION

Interpeak latencies for alcoholic men and women were significantly different on BAER testing at least for peaks I-III, but the interpeak latencies for both groups of alcoholic individuals were within normal limits. Delays involving the interpeak latencies of components I-III and III-V on the BAER suggest diffuse brainstem disease.[4] The intersex difference in brainstem latencies is consistent with observations in normal subjects, with women exhibiting shorter latencies than men.[5] In both sexes the degree of CNS disease in the brainstem must have been relatively slight in view of the integrity of the evoked potential responses.[6]

REFERENCES

1. EMMERSON, R. Y., R. E. DUSTMAN, D. E. SHEARER & H. M. CHAMBERLIN. 1987. Alcohol 4: 241–248.
2. LEVY, L. J. & M. S. LOSOWSKY. 1987. Alcohol and Alcoholism 22: 355–357.
3. CHU, N. S. & S. S. YANG. 1987. Alcohol 4: 225–230.
4. EPSTEIN, C. M. 1988. Neurol. Clin. 6: 771–790.
5. BEAGLEY, H. A. & J. B. SHELDRAKE. 1978. Br. J. Audiol. 12: 69–77.
6. ROWE, M. J. 1978. Electroencephal. Clin. Neurophysiol. 44: 459–470.

Cocaine Administration: D₁ Dopamine Receptor Function and Dopamine Clearance/Diffusion in Rat Striatum and Nucleus Accumbens[a]

NANCY R. ZAHNISER,[b,c,e] R. DAYNE MAYFIELD,[b]
WAYNE A. CASS,[b] AND GREG A. GERHARDT[b,c,d]

[b] Department of Pharmacology, C-236
[c] Neuroscience Program
[d] Department of Psychiatry
University of Colorado Health Sciences Center
4200 East Ninth Avenue
Denver, Colorado 80262

Repeated cocaine administration results in persistent sensitization of locomotor and stereotyped behaviors. These behaviors are produced by activation of dopamine (DA) pathways projecting to nucleus accumbens (NAc) and striatum, respectively. Alterations in these two areas that may contribute to behavioral sensitization include changes in postsynaptic DA receptors and presynaptic DA nerve terminals.

Based on the observation that repeated cocaine administration produces a persistent and selective enhancement of the electrophysiological sensitivity of D₁ DA receptors in NAc,[1] we investigated whether repeated cocaine administration also induces long-lasting increases in D₁ DA receptor density, affinity and/or stimulated adenylyl cyclase activity. Male Sprague-Dawley rats were injected once-daily for 6 days with either saline or cocaine-HCl (15 mg/kg; i.p.) and then withdrawn for 1 week. Cocaine-induced head bobbing, rated on days 1 and 6 of drug treatment, showed that the cocaine-treated rats were behaviorally sensitized. Quantitative autoradiography (QAR) showed that D₁ receptor densities and affinities were similar between brain areas and between treatment groups. Furthermore, the maximal activity and affinity of DA-stimulated adenylyl cyclase were not different in NAc or striatum. While not ruling out changes in other D₁ DA receptor-mediated events, these results indicate that repeated cocaine administration does not produce persistent changes in D₁ DA receptor density, affinity for either the antagonist ³H-SCH 23390 or the agonist DA, or stimulated adenylyl cyclase activity in NAc or striatum.

Cocaine administration preferentially increases extracellular DA concentrations mea-

[a] This work was supported by USPHS Grants DA04216, AA07464, AG 06434 and NS09199.
[e] Address correspondence to Dr. Zahniser at the Department of Pharmacology; Tel.: (303) 270-5288; Fax: (303) 270-7097.

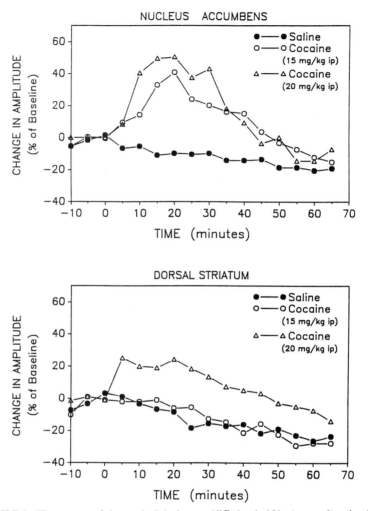

FIGURE 1. Time course of changes in DA clearance/diffusion in NAc (*top panel*) and striatum (*bottom panel*) of urethane-anesthetized rats following a single injection at time 0 of saline or cocaine (15 or 20 mg/kg, i.p.). Extracellular DA concentrations were measured with an *in vivo* electrochemical recording electrode in response to DA, pressured-ejected at 5-min intervals throughout the experiment. The amplitudes of the signal at 5 min prior to injection of saline or cocaine and immediately after injection were averaged to obtain a baseline value. The values at each time point were calculated as percent change from baseline. Representative data are shown from six rats, each of which received a single injection of either saline or cocaine.

sured with *in vivo* microdialysis in NAc, as compared with striatum.[2] This could be due to the ability of cocaine to increase DA release and/or decrease DA uptake to a greater extent in NAc. Prior to studying presynaptic changes induced by repeated cocaine administration, we measured DA clearance/diffusion with *in vivo* electrochemistry in NAc and striatum in response to a single, systemic dose of cocaine in order

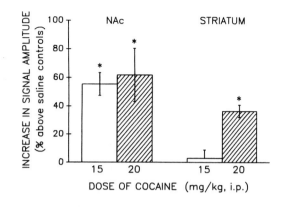

FIGURE 2. Comparison of DA clearance/diffusion in NAc and striatum 20 minutes after injection of cocaine (15 or 20 mg/kg, i.p.). The procedure was the same as described in FIGURE 1. Mean values ± SEM are shown for *n* = 4 rats for each group. * p < 0.05, compared to saline controls (analysis of variance followed by Newman-Keuls comparisons).

to investigate whether a differential effect of cocaine on DA uptake could explain this observation. Nafion-coated carbon fiber electrodes were positioned in NAc or dorsal striatum of urethane-anesthetized rats. When a finite amount of DA (25–100 nl, 200 μM barrel concentration) was pressure-ejected at 5-min intervals from a micropipette positioned 300 ± 30 μm from the electrode, transient (t$^{1/2}$ = 9–59 seconds) and reproducible increases in DA (0.35–3.16 μM) were detected. Changes in this signal constitute an *in vivo* measure of DA clearance/diffusion. In response to 15 mg/kg cocaine-HCl (i.p.), the signal from pressure-ejected DA concentrations increased in NAc indicating significant inhibition of the DA transporter (FIGS. 1 and 2). The time course of the DA increase paralleled that of the behavioral changes in nonanesthetized rats receiving the same dose of cocaine. In contrast, no change in the DA response amplitude was detected in dorsal striatum; however, when the dose of cocaine was increased to 20 mg/kg, enhancement of the DA signal occurred in both brain areas (FIGS. 1 and 2). QAR analysis of ^{3}H-mazindol binding was used to directly investigate the DA transporter. Competition curves revealed that the affinity of the DA transporter for cocaine did not differ between NAc and striatum. However, in agreement with others,[3] the density of binding sites in NAc was only 40% of that in dorsal striatum. Our results suggest that the greater apparent sensitivity of NAc to cocaine, as compared with dorsal striatum, is due to fewer DA transporter molecules for cocaine to inhibit, rather than to a higher affinity of the transporter for cocaine.

ACKNOWLEDGMENTS

The authors thank Mr. Gaynor Larson and Ms. Pam Curella for technical assistance.

REFERENCES

1. HENRY, D. J. & F. J. WHITE. 1991. J. Pharmacol. Exp. Ther. In press.
2. CARBONI, E., A. IMPERATO, L. PEREZZANI & G. DI CHIARA. 1989. Neuroscience **28:** 653–661.
3. MARSHALL, J. F., S. J. O'DELL, R. NAVARRETE & A. J. ROSENSTEIN. 1990. Neuroscience **37:** 11–21.

Vasopressin System Is Impaired in Rat Offspring Prenatally Exposed to Chronic Nicotine[a]

VLASTA K. ZBUZEK[b] AND VRATISLAV ZBUZEK

Department of Anesthesiology
University of Medicine and Dentistry
New Jersey Medical School
185 South Orange Avenue, MSB E-594
Newark, New Jersey 07103-2714

Contrary to the known stimulatory effect of acute nicotine on the vasopressin (VP) release from the hypothalamo-neurohypophyseal (HT-NH) system, nicotine (NIC) administered chronically to adult rat markedly suppresses the activity of VP-ergic system.[1] Since VP may play a significant role during maturation of the central nervous system[2] and the prenatal exposure to NIC has adverse effects on the developing rat brain,[3] we investigated the effect of chronic NIC administered to pregnant rats on the VP-ergic system of the offspring.

Timed pregnant Sprague-Dawley rats were infused subcutaneously via Alzet osmotic pumps with a daily dose of 6 mg NIC free base per kg body weight, throughout the whole gestation period. After the parturition the NIC-treated dams were replaced by intact nursing dams to secure a complete NIC withdrawal in the offspring. VP was measured by the RIA[4] within 1 day after the birth and 1,2,3,4 and 6 weeks of age in serum (pooled from both sexes), neurointermediate lobe (NIL), and hypothalamus (HT). In addition, the NILs of pups at 3,4, and 6 weeks of age were individually superfused, employing the technique described elsewhere,[4] to assess the rate of VP release. The data were analyzed by two-way ANOVA and are presented as % change in the pups prenatally treated with NIC, compared to the intact pups (TABLE 1).

The administration of chronic NIC did not affect litter size nor the sex distribution in it and caused only transient reduction in the body weight of newborn pups. A significant decline in the VP release occurred in NIC-treated pups of both sexes at the age of 3 weeks, followed by decline in serum VP concentration and VP content in the NIL at the age of 4 weeks, and a decrease in the VP content in the HT at week 6 (TABLE 2).

In summary, the activity of HT-NH VP-system is markedly suppressed during the development and maturation of the offspring prenatally exposed to NIC. The NIC-induced changes in the studied markers of VP-system were not revealed until the third week of postnatal life (*i.e.*, the period when VP-system becomes fully developed[5]) even though nicotinic binding sites in different areas of the brain are already detectable at the late embryonic stages.[3]

[a] Supported by Smokeless Tobacco Research Council Grant 0140.
[b] Author to whom correspondence should be addressed.

TABLE 1. The Percent Changes in Indices of VP Activity of Offspring Prenatally Exposed to Nicotine, Related to the Values of Control Pups, Set equal to 100%

	Age of Offspring (Weeks)					
	0	1	2	3	4	6
Females						
VP content in NIL	↑8.3[a]	↑8.3	↓7.1	↓4.6	↓46.0*	↓20.8*
Total VP release	–	–	–	↓30.8*	↓22.4[b]	↓21.1[b]
VP content in HT	↓8.0	↓10.0	↓5.0	↓7.0	↓8.0	↓44.5*
Males						
VP content in NIL	↓5.0	↓0.2	↓3.4	↓11.4	↓28.3*	↓25.1*
Total VP release	–	–	–	↓36.1*	↓23.4[b]	↓38.3*
VP content in HT	↓5.0	↓10.2	↓10.2	↓14.2	↓18.6	↓32.7*
Serum VP concentration						
(pooled from both sexes)	↓6.5	↑9.0	↑11.0	↓19.0	↓22.6*	↓36.4*

[a] ↑↓ Direction of change; * $p < 0.05$; [b] not significant owing to a large scatter.

TABLE 2. Differences in Actual Values of VP Release, Serum VP Concentration, VP Content in the NIL and HT between the Control and Prenatally Treated Pups, as They Consecutively Occurred during the Period of Maturation

		Control	Nicotine[a]
3 Weeks			
Total VP release	females:	62.6 ± 3.0	43.3 ± 3.2
(ng/NIL/170 min)	males:	63.5 ± 3.6	40.6 ± 2.9
4 Weeks			
Serum VP concentration (pg/ml)			
pooled from both sexes		3.99 ± 0.42	3.09 ± 0.40
VP content in the NIL	females:	790.73 ± 37.86	427.40 ± 48.68
(ng/gland)	males:	795.78 ± 74.33	570.30 ± 15.98
6 Weeks			
VP content in the HT (ng/HT)	females:	39.87 ± 1.25	22.10 ± 0.81
	males:	39.40 ± 1.34	26.50 ± 1.70

[a] All values (mean ± SE) shown for nicotine-treated pups are significantly lower than those of the controls at $p < 0.05$.

REFERENCES

1. ZBUZEK, V. K. & V. ZBUZEK. 1991. J. Neuroendocrinol. **3:** 107–112.
2. TRIBOLLET, E., M. GOUMAZ, M. RAGGENBASS, M. DUBOIS-DAUPHIN & J. J. DREIFUSS. 1991. Dev. Brain Res. **58:** 13–24.
3. LICHTENSTEIGER, W., U. RIBARY, M. SCHLUMPF, B. ODERMATT & H. R. WIDMER. 1988. Prog. Brain Res. **73:** 137–157.
4. ZBUZEK, V., V. K. ZBUZEK & W. WU. 1984. Neuroendocrinology **39:** 538–548.
5. BOER, G. J. 1987. *In* Vasopressin, Principles and Properties. D. M. Gash & G. J. Boer, Eds.: 117–174. Plenum Press. New York.

Index of Contributors